PRACTITIONER'S GUIDE TO EMPIRICALLY BASED MEASURES OF ANXIETY

D1613486

AABT CLINICAL ASSESSMENT SERIES

Series Editor

Sharon L. Foster
California School of Professional Psychology, San Diego, California

---

PRACTITIONER'S GUIDE TO EMPIRICALLY BASED MEASURES OF ANXIETY
Edited by Martin M. Antony, Susan M. Orsillo, and Lizabeth Roemer

PRACTITIONER'S GUIDE TO EMPIRICALLY BASED MEASURES OF DEPRESSION
Edited by Arthur M. Nezu, George F. Ronan, Elizabeth A. Meadows, and Kelly S. McClure

---

A Continuation Order Plan is available for this series. A continuation order will bring delivery of each new volume immediately upon publication. Volumes are billed only upon actual shipment. For further information please contact the publisher.

PRACTITIONER'S GUIDE TO EMPIRICALLY BASED MEASURES OF ANXIETY

Edited by

Martin M. Antony

St. Joseph's Healthcare, Hamilton, and McMaster University
Hamilton, Ontario, Canada

Susan M. Orsillo

VA Boston Healthcare System and Boston University School of Medicine
Boston, Massachusetts

and

Lizabeth Roemer

University of Massachusetts at Boston
Boston, Massachusetts

Published under the auspices of the Association for Advancement of Behavior Therapy

Kluwer Academic / Plenum Publishers
New York   Boston   Dordrecht   London   Moscow

Library of Congress Cataloging-in-Publication Data

Practitioner's guide to empirically based measures of anxiety/edited by Martin M.
Antony, Susan M. Orsillo, and Lizabeth Roemer.
    p.   ; cm. — (AABT clinical assessment series)
    Includes bibliographical references and index.
    ISBN 0-306-46582-5
       I. Anxiety—Diagnosis. I. Antony, Martin, M., 1964–   II. Orsillo, Susan M., 1964–   III. Roemer
Lizabeth, 1967–   IV. Series.
       [DNLM: 1. Anxiety Disorders—diagnosis—Handbooks. 2. Anxiety
Disorders—therapy—Handbooks. 3. Psychiatric Status Rating Scales—Handbooks.   WM
34 P8947 2001]
    RC531 .P73 2001
    616.85′223—dc21

                                                                                          2001023683

ISBN 0-306-46582-5

©2001 Kluwer Academic / Plenum Publishers
233 Spring Street, New York, N.Y. 10013

http://www.wkap.nl/

10 9 8 7 6 5 4 3 2 1

A C.I.P. record for this book is available from the Library of Congress.

Printed in the United States of America

Contributors

Martin M. Antony • Anxiety Treatment and Research Centre, St. Joseph's Healthcare, Hamilton, and Department of Psychiatry and Behavioural Neurosciences, McMaster University, Hamilton, Ontario L8N 4A6, Canada

Sonja V. Batten • National Center for PTSD–Women's Health Sciences Division, Boston VA Healthcare System, and Boston University School of Medicine, Boston, Massachusetts 02130

J. Gayle Beck • Department of Psychology, State University of New York at Buffalo, Buffalo, New York 14260

Bruce F. Chorpita • Department of Psychology, University of Hawaii at Manoa, Honolulu, Hawaii 96822

John P. Forsyth • Department of Psychology, University at Albany, State University of New York, Albany, New York 12222

Steven Friedman • Department of Psychiatry, State University of New York, Health Science Center at Brooklyn, Brooklyn, New York 11203

Charity Hammond • National Center for PTSD–Women's Health Sciences Division, Boston VA Healthcare System, and Boston University School of Medicine, Boston, Massachusetts 02130

Larry W. Hawk, Jr. • Department of Psychology, State University of New York at Buffalo, Buffalo, New York 14260-4110

Maria Karekla • Department of Psychology, University at Albany, State University of New York, Albany, New York 12222

Randi E. McCabe • Anxiety Treatment and Research Centre, St. Joseph's Hospital, and Department of Psychiatry and Behavioural Neurosciences, McMaster University, Hamilton, Ontario L8N 4A6, Canada

Eden Medaglia • Department of Psychology, University of Massachusetts at Boston, Boston, Massachusetts 02125

Jennifer S. Mills • Department of Psychology, York University, Toronto, Ontario M3J 1P3, Canada

Susan M. Orsillo • National Center for PTSD–Women's Health Sciences Division, Boston VA Healthcare System, and Boston University School of Medicine, Boston, Massachusetts 02130

Lizabeth Roemer • Department of Psychology, University of Massachusetts at Boston, Boston, Massachusetts 02125

Melinda A. Stanley • Department of Psychiatry and Behavioral Sciences, University of Texas Health Sciences Center at Houston, Houston, Texas 77025

Laura J. Summerfeldt • Department of Psychology, Trent University, Peterborough, Ontario K9J 7B8, Canada

Alissa A. Taylor • Department of Psychology, University of Hawaii at Manoa, Honolulu, Hawaii 96822

Andrew R. Yartz • Department of Psychology, State University of New York at Buffalo, Buffalo, New York 14260-4110

Series Preface

"Where can I find a copy of ...?"

"I have a client coming in who's anxious—do you have any good measures?"

Several times a year I look up from my desk to answer questions like these from graduate students and colleagues. My answers invariably disappoint them: I recite a litany of not very fruitful alternatives for finding the measures they seek. "Well, you can check the original article, but that probably won't have a copy. Or you can call the originator of the instrument. If you can't find the person or if he or she doesn't return your call, you can try getting a copy from someone who's used the instrument. But be sure to ask if it's copyrighted. Then make sure you look up the literature on its reliability and validity...."

Difficulties in locating assessment devices and finding evaluative information on their psychometric properties vex researchers and clinicians alike. Such difficulties likely contribute to failure to use assessment tools that could greatly enhance a clinician's practice and may fuel continuing complaints about the schism between research and practice. Indeed, although many mental health professionals receive training in the scientific foundations of clinical practice, numerous surveys question their application of this training in practice settings after graduate school ends (e.g., Morrow-Bradley & Elliott, 1986; Swan & MacDonald, 1978).

The need for scientifically sound but practical clinical tools is relevant for clinical assessment, intervention, and research. Increasing demands from third-party payers for accountability information have produced increased needs for practical assessment tools that yield useful information about changes in clients' functioning over time. Yet many graduate training courses provide little instruction in assessment other than traditional personality and intellectual assessment approaches (Aiken, West, Sechrest, & Reno, 1990), leaving many mental health professionals with limited information about alternatives to these approaches. As mentioned, obtaining copies of assessment devices for particular problem areas is a challenge because many are not readily available. Finally, although occasional reviews of assessment devices appear in the literature, few sources exist that enable clinicians and researchers to appraise reliability and validity evidence for particular assessment tools and to compare different instruments. This kind of information is essential in deciding whether the psychometric properties of measurement instruments are sufficiently strong to warrant their use.

The AABT Clinical Assessment Series, developed by the Association for Advancement of Behavior Therapy, addresses these issues. Each volume examines a different clinical problem area and provides critical overviews of key assessment issues and available assessment tools for use in the area. Convenient summary tables compare and contrast different instruments in terms of their time requirements and suitability for different assessment purposes. Finally, and most importantly, each volume provides a summary of reliability and validity information about each instrument along with sample copies of the instruments, or, for commercially available instruments, samples of the instrument content and information about how to purchase the assessment device. These compendia of information provide valuable resources for practicing clinicians and for researchers who wish to develop state-of-the-science assessment strategies for clinical problems and to make informed choices about which devices best suit their purposes. This volume, the second in the series, addresses anxiety disorders in adult populations. It follows the first volume in the series on depression (Nezu, Ronan, Meadows, & McClure, 2000). The third volume will focus on child behavior problems in school settings.

The AABT Clinical Assessment Series was the brainchild of a number of individuals at the Association for Advancement of Behavior Therapy with the imagination and initiative to bring this project into being. Lizette Peterson and Linda Sobell deserve special recognition for their vision and persistence in launching this project. David Teisler provided invaluable support and liaison work between the editors and the organization. Mariclaire Cloutier at Kluwer Academic/Plenum Publishers greatly assisted with the production of the volume and in supporting the efforts required to bring this project to fruition. And of course, the editors of this volume-Marty Antony, Sue Orsillo, and Liz Roemer—collected massive amounts of information and carefully selected the topics and instruments they would cover to offer state-of-the-science approaches that are also relevant to the concerns of practicing clinicians.

WHO SHOULD USE THIS BOOK?

This book is written for practitioners who assess and treat anxious clients and who wish to make their assessment practices more systematic, want to have assessment devices readily available, and want to expand their assessment practices with the most up-to-date approaches. Although the volume is produced in conjunction with the Association for Advancement of Behavior Therapy, the volume is not for behaviorists only—any empirically minded clinician should find this compendium valuable. In addition, the volume should prove useful for researchers who wish to compare and contrast various measurement tools for assessing depression and related constructs. Finally, the volume will prove invaluable for professors like myself in helping students and colleagues find easy answers to questions like those posed at the beginning of this preface.

REFERENCES

Aiken, L. S., West, S. G., Sechrest, L., & Reno, R. R. (1990). Graduate training in statistics, methodology, and measurement in psychology: A survey of Ph.D. programs in North America. *American Psychologist, 45,* 721–734.

Morrow-Bradley, C., & Elliott, R. (1986). Utilization of psychotherapy research by practicing psychotherapists. *American Psychologist, 41,* 188–197.

Nezu, A. M., Ronan, G. F., Meadows, E. A., & McClure, K. S. (Eds.) (2000). *Practitioner's guide to empirically based measures of depression.* New York: Kluwer Academic/Plenum Publishers.

Swan, G. E., & MacDonald, M. L. (1978). Behavior therapy in practice: A national survey of behavior therapists. *Behavior Therapy, 8,* 799–807.

Sharon L. Foster
San Diego, CA

Preface

According to recent estimates, one in four people will experience an anxiety disorder at some time in his or her life. Anxiety disorders can negatively affect all aspects of an individual's quality of life, including the ability to establish and maintain satisfying relationships and to succeed in the workplace. In rare cases, sufferers can become housebound. Furthermore, a number of studies have found that anxiety disorders pose a substantial economic burden, both on those who suffer from anxiety and on society as a whole. To further complicate matters, anxiety disorders frequently co-occur with one another, and with other psychological disorders, including depression, substance use disorders, somatoform disorders, and eating disorders, which can result in a complicated and unwieldy presentation.

Despite the high prevalence and severe impairment that is often associated with anxiety disorders, people who suffer from anxiety are often undiagnosed or misdiagnosed, and as a result may fail to find appropriate treatment. In addition, many clinicians are unfamiliar with the range of instruments and scales that are available to assess individuals suffering from anxiety. The purpose of this book is to provide a resource that contains information on almost all of the measures that have been demonstrated to be useful for measuring the presence and severity of anxiety and related problems. This is the second volume in the AABT Clinical Assessment Series, following the initial volume on assessment instruments for depression.

This book includes reviews of more than 200 instruments for measuring anxiety-related constructs in adults, including self-report instruments and clinician-administered scales. It includes chapters on instruments for particular anxiety disorders (e.g., panic disorder, specific and social phobias, generalized anxiety disorder, obsessive compulsive disorder, posttraumatic and acute stress disorders) as well as anxiety measures that do not emphasize the features of a particular disorder. This volume also includes brief review chapters on related topics such as behavioral and psychophysiological assessment, and assessment of anxiety in special populations (e.g., across cultures, in older adults). Finally, there are a number of appendixes that almost all clinicians and researchers who work with anxious individuals will find invaluable. Appendix A includes a series of quick-view guides summarizing the main features of the measures reviewed in this book. Appendix B contains reprinted versions of more than 75 of the most popular instruments for assessing anxiety. Finally, a Glossary is included to provide the reader with definitions of terms that are used throughout this book.

We would like to thank a number of people for helping us bring this volume to completion. First, we thank our students and colleagues who assisted us with the seemingly endless process of organizing the materials for Part 2 and the appendixes, and for ensuring that all of the details are as accurate as possible. In particular, we thank the authors of the measures we included, who provided us with essential information and feedback throughout this process. A heartfelt thank-you also goes to Uppala Chandrasekera, Charity Hammond, Eden Medaglia, Robin Smith, and Lisa Young for their invaluable help. We also wish to thank Sharon Foster, Debra Hope, Art Nezu, Linda Sobell, and David Teisler for helping to get this project off the ground and for inviting us to participate in this important series. Thanks also to the staff at Kluwer Academic/Plenum Publishers, especially Mariclaire Cloutier, Teresa Krauss, and Andrea Macaluso, for their support, assistance, and patience during the preparation of this manuscript. Finally, we wish to thank those in our lives who saw significantly less of us than we all would have liked while we worked on this book. Thanks to our friends, family, colleagues, and students for being so understanding.

Martin M. Antony
Toronto, ON

Susan M. Orsillo
Boston, MA

Lizabeth Roemer
Boston, MA

Contents

Part II.   Assessment Strategies for Anxiety Disorders

Chapter 8
PANIC DISORDER AND AGORAPHOBIA: A BRIEF OVERVIEW AND
Randi E. McCabe

Introduction

Martin M. Antony

BACKGROUND

Anxiety disorders are among the most prevalent of psychological disorders, affecting up to 25% of individuals in the general population at some time in their lives (Kessler et al., 1994). Despite their high prevalence, however, anxiety disorders often go undiagnosed and untreated, especially in primary care settings (e.g., Weiller, Bisserbe, Maier, & Lecrubier, 1998). In addition, there is evidence that those individuals who do receive treatment for an anxiety disorder are often treated with an intervention that is not empirically supported (e.g., Rowa, Antony, Brar, Summerfeldt, & Swinson, 2000).

Recently, there has been increased attention to the identification and dissemination of empirically supported treatments for psychological problems (e.g., Chambless & Hollon, 1998; Kendall, 1998; Nathan & Gorman, 1998). With interest in empirically supported treatments on the rise, the need for evidence-based assessment strategies is greater than ever before. It is this need for readily available assessment strategies that has led to the development of the AABT Clinical Assessment Series. This is the second volume in the series, following the initial volume on assessment instruments for depression (Nezu, Ronan, Meadows, & McClure, 2000).

The purpose of this book is to provide clinicians and researchers with a single comprehensive resource on assessment measures for anxiety disorders in adults, including detailed descriptions of relevant measures and, where possible, reprinted copies of the scales. Although other resources on assessment instruments exist (e.g., American Psychiatric Association, 2000; Corcoran & Fischer, 2000; Schutte & Malouff, 1995), they have typically been much broader in scope, covering instruments for many different types of psychological problems, reviewing only a small number of anxiety-related scales. In addition, there exists one volume devoted entirely to measures for stress, trauma, and adaptation (Stamm, 1996). However, ours is the first book to focus exclusively on assessment scales for anxiety disorders, while covering a full range of anxiety-related problems.

Martin M. Antony • Anxiety Treatment and Research Centre, St. Joseph's Healthcare, Hamilton, and Department of Psychiatry and Behavioral Neurosciences, McMaster University, Hamilton, Ontario L8N 4A6, Canada.

STRUCTURE OF THE BOOK

This book is organized into two main parts. Part 1 includes six brief chapters on general topics related to the assessment of anxiety disorders, including an overview of assessment strategies for anxiety, behavioral assessment methods, psychophysiological assessment, biological challenges in the assessment of anxiety, cultural issues in assessing anxiety, and the assessment of anxiety in older adults. Part 2 includes chapters describing the assessment of each of the main anxiety disorders, including panic disorder with and without agoraphobia, specific phobia, social phobia, generalized anxiety disorder, obsessive compulsive disorder, and posttraumatic stress disorder. In addition, we have included a chapter describing anxiety-related measures that are not tied to any particular anxiety disorder. For each of the anxiety disorders covered in Part 2, we have included a brief chapter providing an overview of assessment for the disorder, followed by a thorough review of available instruments for the disorder.

A series of appendixes follow Part 2 of the book. Appendix A includes seven quick-view guides, summarizing the key features of the instruments reviewed earlier in the book. These tables provide easily accessed information regarding the format of each measure, the purpose of the instrument, the time to administer the scale, any costs involved, and whether the instrument is available in alternate forms (e.g., brief versions, computerized versions, languages other than English). Appendix B includes reprinted versions of more than 75 of the instruments that are reviewed in Part 2 of the book. Finally, Appendix C is a glossary that defines many of the terms that are used throughout this book.

Format of Instrument Descriptions

Chapters 7, 9, 11, 13, 15, 17, and 19 include descriptions of instruments for anxiety-related problems. Each of these chapters begins with a series of extended descriptions of instruments. In the second part of each chapter are brief descriptions of additional measures. Decisions regarding whether to include an instrument as either an extended entry or a brief entry were based on a number of factors. Instruments were more likely to be described in brief entries if (1) they were relatively new and if only preliminary psychometric data on the instrument were available, (2) they were older measures that are now rarely used, or (3) they assessed a construct that was only somewhat related to anxiety disorders (e.g., the chapter on obsessive compulsive disorder scales includes only brief descriptions of related OCD spectrum disorders such as body dysmorphic disorder, tic disorders, and trichotillomania).

For instruments that are described in the *brief format*, we provide information regarding the title, format, and purpose of the scale, relevant citations, and contact information for the author, when available. These measures are not reprinted in Appendix B, whereas we reprinted all measures from the extended format section for which we were able to obtain permission.

For instruments described in the *extended format*, more detailed information is provided according to the following standard outline:

Title. The title of the scale is provided, along with the most commonly used acronym.

Original citation. This section includes the original reference(s) for the scale (e.g., the journal article in which the scale is published, the manual for the instrument). To save space, these original citations are not reprinted again in the reference section at the end of each chapter.

Purpose. This section describes the purpose of the particular instrument.

Description. This section provides a description of the instrument, including the format (e.g., self-report versus clinician-administered), the number of items, the scale on which items are rated (e.g., 0–100), and a description of any subscales.

Administration and scoring. This section includes information about administration (e.g., the time taken to complete the instrument) and instructions on how to score the instrument. In cases where scoring is complicated or time-consuming (e.g., more than a few minutes), we also include an estimate of the time needed to score the instrument. Scoring instructions generally include information regarding the items that make up each subscale and information about which items are reverse-scored. In cases where we were unable to obtain permission to reprint a scale, scoring instructions may be limited. In these cases, readers should contact the author or publisher of the measure for complete scoring instructions.

A *reverse-scored item* is one that is scored by transposing the ratings made by the respondent for the reverse-scored item with the "opposite" rating. For example, if the possible ratings on an item range from 1 to 5, before adding up the ratings for the items in the scale, reverse scored items would be rerated as follows: a score of 1 would be replaced with a score of 5; a score of 2 would be replaced with a score of 4; a score of 4 would be replaced with a score of 2; a score of 5 would be replaced with a score of 1. A score of 3 would remain unchanged.

Psychometric properties. This section provides information regarding sample scores and norms (e.g., means and standard deviations for various groups), as well as research on the reliability and validity of the instrument.

Alternative forms. This section provides information on the availability of the instrument in formats other than the standard English version for adults, including translations, child versions, abbreviated versions, versions for special populations, and computerized versions of the scale. This section was not included for those measures for which there are no alternative forms.

Source. In this section, we provide information on where to obtain the scale as well as up-to-date contact information on the author of the instrument. Information about the instrument's cost, if any, is included in this section. Because contact information frequently changes, we cannot guarantee that the information provided will remain accurate in the period after this book is published.

SELECTION OF MEASURES FOR INCLUSION

A concerted attempt was made to review almost all measures for anxiety and anxiety disorders in this book. As was the case for the first volume in this series, methods used to find instruments included multiple advertisements in relevant journals, comprehensive literature reviews, multiple computer searches, and letters to numerous anxiety disorder experts asking them to suggest instruments that we should review and inquiring about new instruments that were in development. Despite these efforts, we expect that some instruments were missed and we apologize for any omissions.

The criteria used to select measures for inclusion were similar to those used in the depression volume by Nezu et al. (2000): (1) all instruments were required to be available in English, (2) all instruments were required to assess some aspect of anxiety or an anxiety disorder (e.g., severity of anxiety symptoms, hypothesized mediators of anxiety, causal factors in anxiety), (3) priority was given to instruments with clinical utility, particularly those that are likely to be useful for clinicians who use cognitive and behavioral techniques in their practices, and (4) the measure had to have established psychometric properties (preferably published in a peer-reviewed journal).

SOME ADDITIONAL POINTS TO KEEP IN MIND

Definitions and Acronyms

The Glossary (Appendix C) contains definitions of most of the technical terms used in this book. A number of acronyms that we used throughout the book are: PD (panic disorder), PDA (panic disorder with agoraphobia), GAD (generalized anxiety disorder), OCD (obsessive compulsive disorder), PTSD (posttraumatic stress disorder), and *SD* (standard deviation).

Space Restrictions

One of the biggest challenges in preparing this book was the limited amount of space we had to review such a large number of instruments. Whereas the first volume in this series reviewed about 90 instruments for depression, this volume contains more than 200 reviews, as well as many more reprinted instruments compared to the depression volume. For this reason, we were unable to provide extended reviews of all instruments. In addition, we were unable to review all psychometric studies for each measure.

Reprinted Measures in Appendix B

We did not edit the content of the instruments that are reprinted in Appendix B. Therefore, any items that are worded poorly and any grammatical irregularities are in most cases present in the original version. In a few cases, we did alter the formatting of instruments to reduce the amount of space needed to reprint the scale. Also, although many of the scales in Appendix B are administered with an alternate title or with no title at all, we chose to reprint the title of the instrument and the most commonly used acronym at the top of each scale. In several cases, we note the typical way the measure is identified in the description of the measure.

REFERENCES

American Psychiatric Association (2000). *Handbook of psychiatric measures*. Washington, DC: Author.

Chambless, D. L., & Hollon, S. D. (1998). Defining empirically supported therapies. *Journal of Consulting and Clinical Psychology, 66*, 7–18.

Corcoran, K., & Fischer, J. (2000). *Measures for clinical practice: A sourcebook. Volume 2: Adults* (3rd ed.). New York: Free Press.

Kendall, P. C. (1998). Empirically supported psychological therapies. *Journal of Consulting and Clinical Psychology, 66*, 3–6.

Kessler, R. C., McGonagle, K. A., Zhao, S., Nelson, C. B., Hughes, M., Eshleman, S., Wittchen, H.-U., & Kendler, K. (1994). Lifetime and 12-month prevalence of DSM-III-R psychiatric disorders in the United States: Results from the National Comorbidity Survey. *Archives of General Psychiatry, 51*, 8–19.

Nathan, P. E., & Gorman, J. M. (Eds.) (1998). *A guide to treatments that work*. London: Oxford University Press.

Nezu, A. M., Ronan, G. F., Meadows, E. A., & McClure, K. S. (Eds.) (2000). *Practitioner's guide to empirically based measures of depression*. New York: Kluwer Academic/Plenum Publishers.

Rowa, K., Antony, M. M., Brar, S., Summerfeldt, L. J., & Swinson, R. P. (2000). Treatment histories of patients with three anxiety disorders. *Depression and Anxiety, 12*, 92–98.

Schutte, N. S., & Malouff, J. M. (1995). *Sourcebook of adult assessment strategies*. New York: Plenum Press.

Stamm, B. H. (1996). *Measurement of stress, trauma, and adaptation*. Lutherville, MD: The Sidran Press.

Weiller, E., Bisserbe, J.-C., Maier, W., & Lecrubier, Y. (1998). Prevalence and recognition of anxiety syndromes in five European primary care settings: A report from the WHO study on psychological problems in general health care. *British Journal of Psychiatry, 173*(Suppl. 34), 18–23.

PART I
General Issues in the Assessment of Anxiety Disorders

Chapter 1
Assessment of Anxiety and the Anxiety Disorders: An Overview

Martin M. Antony

This chapter provides an overview of issues related to the assessment of anxiety and anxiety disorders. It begins with a discussion of the nature of fear and anxiety, the features that comprise these emotions, and a listing of the anxiety disorders as defined in the Diagnostic and Statistical Manual of Mental Disorders (DSM-IV; American Psychiatric Association, 2000). Next, the chapter discusses the functions of assessment for anxiety as well as key areas that should be covered during an evaluation. The most important methods of assessment are reviewed, as are a number of additional issues that should be taken into account when planning and carrying out an evaluation. Any instruments mentioned in this chapter that do not include citations are described in the chapters from Part 2 of this book, along with full references.

OVERVIEW OF ANXIETY AND THE ANXIETY DISORDERS

DSM-IV defines *anxiety* as an "apprehensive anticipation of future danger or misfortune accompanied by a feeling of dysphoria or somatic symptoms of tension" (American Psychiatric Association, 2000, p. 820). Related to anxiety is the basic emotion of *fear*. Although some

Martin M. Antony • Anxiety Treatment and Research Centre, St. Joseph's Healthcare, Hamilton, and Department of Psychiatry and Behavioural Neurosciences, McMaster University, Hamilton, Ontario L8N 4A6, Canada.

theorists do not differentiate between the states of fear and anxiety, others (e.g., Antony & Barlow, 1996) have argued that these states are distinct from one another. Anxiety is a future-oriented emotional state characterized by high negative affect, a sense that upcoming events are uncontrollable and unpredictable, difficulty concentrating, and a tendency to worry. For example, an individual who is anxious about performance situations might experience anxiety when anticipating an upcoming presentation. Or, an individual who is anxious about dogs might feel anxious while anticipating visiting a friend who lives with a large dog.

In contrast to anxiety, fear is a focused, all-or-nothing, alarm reaction in which there is an intense motivation to escape from a potential danger, and in which the organism is mobilized (both physically and cognitively) for action (Antony & Barlow, 1996). For example, an individual might experience the emotion of fear while giving a stressful presentation or while exposed to a large, unfamiliar, growling dog. David H. Barlow has argued that the experience of panic (e.g., panic attacks, as defined in DSM-IV) is essentially indistinguishable from the emotion of fear (e.g., Antony & Barlow, 1996).

Many theorists and researchers have discussed anxiety and fear in terms of their component parts. For example, in their tripartite theory of anxiety and depression, Clark and Watson (1991) argued that anxiety consists of two separate factors: elevated *negative affect* (e.g., psychological tension, agitation, distress, worry), which is also associated with depressed mood, and *physiological hyperarousal* (e.g., racing heart, sweating, shaking), which appears to be more pronounced in anxiety than in depression.

Other investigators, such as Peter Lang (1971), emphasized the value of conceptualizing fear and anxiety as a constellation of three different response channels: cognitive, behavioral, and physiological. Examples of the *cognitive* response channel include the anxious predictions, assumptions, beliefs, and information processing biases that are often held by anxious individuals. The *behavioral* response channel includes avoidance behaviors, compulsions, distraction, and various overprotective behaviors that are used to reduce discomfort or to prevent an anticipated danger. Finally, the *physiological* response channel includes the physical sensations that an individual experiences when feeling anxious or frightened. These may include palpitations, dizziness, sweating, and a number of other symptoms that are associated with physical arousal. Because these three response channels are often not highly intercorrelated (e.g., Rachman, 1990; Rachman & Hodgson, 1974), some investigators have argued that it is important to assess these response components separately (e.g., Lehrer & Woolfolk, 1982). Many of the instruments reviewed in this book focus on particular aspects of anxiety and fear, consistent with Lang's response channels.

DSM-IV describes 12 different anxiety disorders, which are listed in Table 1 along with brief descriptions of their key features. Note that anxiety and fear are associated with a wide range of psychological problems that are not all technically defined as anxiety disorders. For example, hypochondriasis (a somatoform disorder) is associated with intense anxiety and fear over the possibility of having a serious medical illness. Similarly, eating disorders are typically associated with intense anxiety over gaining weight or eating certain foods. Measures of anxiety and related constructs (especially those described in Chapter 7) may be helpful for the assessment of anxiety that occurs in the context of other problems.

FUNCTIONS OF ASSESSMENT

Assessment of anxiety disorders has several different functions, including differential diagnosis, clinical description, case formulation, treatment planning, and evaluating outcome.

Table 1. Anxiety Disorders Defined in DSM-IV-TR

Anxiety disorders	Key features
Panic Disorder without Agoraphobia	Recurrent, unexpected panic attacks, associated with persistent concern about the attacks
Panic Disorder with Agoraphobia	Panic disorder associated with agoraphobia (i.e., fear and avoidance of situations in which escape might be difficult or embarrassing, or in which help might not be available in the event of a panic attack or paniclike sensations)
Agoraphobia without History of Panic Disorder	The presence of agoraphobia in an individual who has never met full criteria for panic disorder
Specific Phobia	Clinically significant anxiety, fear, and avoidance related to a specific object or situation (e.g., heights, animals, blood, injections, flying, enclosed places)
Social Phobia	Clinically significant anxiety, fear, and avoidance related to social and performance situations, associated with a fear of embarrassment or humiliation
Obsessive Compulsive Disorder	The presence of obsessions (thoughts, urges, or images that are distressing and intrusive) and compulsions (repetitive behaviors meant to reduce anxiety or prevent perceived danger)
Posttraumatic Stress Disorder and Acute Stress Disorder	Reexperiencing a traumatic event, accompanied by symptoms of increased arousal and avoidance of situations and thoughts that remind the individual of the event
Generalized Anxiety Disorder	Persistent, excessive, and uncontrollable worry for at least 6 months, associated with a number of additional symptoms such as irritability, muscle tension, and difficulties sleeping or concentrating
Anxiety Disorder Due to a General Medical Condition	Anxiety symptoms that are the direct consequence of a general medical condition (e.g., panic attacks caused by hyperthyroidism)
Substance-Induced Anxiety Disorder	Anxiety symptoms that are the direct consequence of a substance (e.g., cocaine)
Anxiety Disorder Not Otherwise Specified	Disorder with prominent anxiety or phobic avoidance not meeting criteria for a specific anxiety disorder or for which there is inadequate or contradictory information

Differential Diagnosis

One important function of assessment is to determine an appropriate diagnosis. Differential diagnosis is particularly important in cases where different diagnoses are likely to lead to different treatments. For example, although both pharmacotherapy and cognitive-behavioral treatments are appropriate for panic disorder with agoraphobia, there is no evidence that medications are useful for specific phobias. For cases of specific phobia, exposure-based interventions are the only empirically supported treatments (for a review, see Antony & Swinson, 2000). Therefore, to select an appropriate treatment, it may be important to adequately distinguish a specific phobia of flying from panic disorder with agoraphobia associated with a fear of flying.

Clinical Description

The assessment process allows the clinician to obtain important descriptive information about an individual's anxiety problem, including the development and course of the problem, the associated cognitive features, patterns of avoidance, and associated symptoms.

Case Formulation

A thorough assessment is necessary for the development of a thoughtful case formulation. For example, the assessment may provide important information regarding the functional relationship between an individual's alcohol abuse and his or her social anxiety (i.e., determining whether one problem is causing or maintaining the other), which would help in developing appropriate treatments focusing either on one problem or the other, or perhaps on both problems concurrently.

Planning Treatment

The information gathered during the assessment can be used to develop a detailed treatment plan. For example, identifying the specific situations that an individual fears and avoids, as well as the variables that influence his or her fear in a particular situation, can help with the development of an appropriate plan for exposure-based treatment.

In addition, knowing what types of treatments an individual has tried in the past can help to identify treatments that may be effective currently. One empirically supported measure that can be used to assess previous treatments for anxiety disorders is the Psychosocial Treatments Interview for Anxiety Disorders (PTI). The PTI has a standard 42-item version and an abridged 22-item version. This interview asks about the extent to which an individual has received treatments from a variety of modalities including pharmacotherapy, relaxation training, behavior therapy, cognitive therapy, supportive therapy, and psychodynamic psychotherapy. An initial study on the reliability of the PTI found that the scale had adequate levels of interrater reliability and internal consistency (Steketee et al., 1997). Interestingly, studies based on the PTI (e.g., Goisman et al., 1993; Goisman, Warshaw, & Keller, 1999) suggest that most people with anxiety disorders fail to obtain evidence-based psychotherapies for their conditions.

Assessment of Treatment Outcome

Assessment should not end when treatment begins. Rather, the clinician should continue the process of assessment throughout treatment and periodically after treatment has terminated. Repeated assessments provide empirical data regarding whether a patient's symptoms have improved or worsened and whether improvements have been maintained after a particular intervention has ended.

AREAS TO FOCUS ON DURING THE ASSESSMENT

A thorough assessment should cover a broad range of areas, including diagnostic information, the primary symptoms of the problem, and factors related to the etiology, maintenance, and treatment of the condition. Table 2 is a list of variables that should be assessed before beginning treatment with an individual suffering from an anxiety disorder.

Table 2. Areas to Focus on During the Assessment

Assessment topic	Examples
Diagnostic features	Establish DSM-IV diagnosis; assess for presence of comorbid conditions
Symptom severity	Intensity of symptoms; frequency of panic attacks or other symptoms; associated distress; functional impairment
Key features of the problem	Physical symptoms associated with anxiety and fear; content of anxious thoughts, worries, obsessions, and so on; patterns of avoidance, subtle avoidance and overprotective behaviors, presence of compulsions, anxiety over physical arousal symptoms or other aspects of fear response; variables that affect the individual's fear in the situation
Skills deficits	Poor communication skills contributing to social phobia; poor driving skills contributing to specific phobia of driving
Development and course of the problem	Traumatic events contributing to the onset; chronic course versus waxing and waning course
Treatment history, treatment preferences	Which treatments have been tried in the past? What has worked? What hasn't worked? Does the individual have any preferences for one treatment modality over another?
Family factors	Accommodation by family members (e.g., helping the individual to avoid feared situations), potential for family members to help with treatment, family history of anxiety disorders
Medical and health issues	Medical conditions that may account for symptoms; medical conditions that may impact on treatment

TYPES OF ASSESSMENT STRATEGIES

Screening Questions and Instruments

Assessment of anxiety disorders typically begins with screening questions, administered either during a clinical interview or using standard questionnaires designed to screen for psychopathology. Positive responses to initial screening questions may indicate possible difficulties with anxiety and should be followed up by more detailed assessment of the anxiety-related problems. The overview chapters for each disorder reviewed in Part 2 of this book provide examples of brief screening questions that may be used by the clinician to assess for the key features of each anxiety disorder.

In addition, there are a number of self-report scales and semistructured interviews that screen for anxiety symptoms, anxiety disorders, and other forms of psychopathology. Examples of popular screening instruments and interviews with sections that assess anxiety and related disorders are provided in Table 3. A more detailed review of these and other instruments may be found elsewhere (e.g., Bufka, Crawford, & Levitt, in press; Summerfeldt & Antony, in press).

Clinical Interviews

Clinical interviews are perhaps the most commonly used method of collecting information during a psychological assessment. Table 2 lists the areas that should be asked about during an assessment. Many of these topics tend to be covered during the clinical interview.

In many clinical settings, interviews are not standardized or structured. However, as mentioned previously, there are a number of semistructured interviews that provide informa-

Table 3. Examples of Instruments that Screen for Anxiety

Instrument	Anxiety-related features
Anxiety Disorders Interview Schedule for DSM-IV (ADIS-IV; Brown, Di Nardo, & Barlow, 1994)	A semistructured interview that assesses all of the diagnostic criteria of each anxiety disorder, as well as a range of other DSM-IV disorders, and provides severity ratings of all present disorders
Minnesota Multiphasic Personality Inventory (MMPI-2) (Butcher, Dahlstrom, Graham, Tellegen, & Kraemmer, 1989)	A 567-item self-report instrument that includes 10 clinical scales, of which several measure anxiety-related symptoms. Psychasthenia scale measures anxiety-related symptoms; social introversion scale measures symptoms of social anxiety; a PTSD scale may be derived from the MMPI-2 (see Chapter 19)
Psychiatric Diagnostic Screening Questionnaire (PDSQ) (Zimmerman & Mattia, 1999)	A 90-item self-report scale that includes questions about 13 different DSM-IV categories, including several anxiety disorders (e.g., PTSD, phobias, GAD)
Symptom Checklist-90-R (SCL-90-R) (Derogatis, 1994)	A 90-item self-report scale that includes nine primary symptom scales, several of which measure anxiety-related symptoms (e.g., anxiety, interpersonal sensitivity, obsessive compulsive, phobic anxiety). A briefer, 53-item version (the Brief Symptom Inventory, Derogatis & Melisaratos, 1983) is also available
Structured Clinical Interview for DSM-IV (SCID-IV) (First, Spitzer, Gibbon, & Williams, 1996)	A semistructured interview that assesses all of the diagnostic criteria of each anxiety disorder, as well as a range of other DSM-IV disorders

tion on the diagnostic features of individuals suffering from anxiety disorders (see Table 3 for examples). Semistructured interviews have the advantage of being empirically supported, with demonstrated reliability and validity. These interviews ensure that questions about particular symptoms are asked in a systematic way so that important questions are not missed. Ideally, the diagnostic features of a problem should be assessed using a semistructured interview, while adding further questions about other important features of the problem, as suggested in Table 2.

Self-Report Scales

Self-report scales are a powerful way of providing information about an individual's problem from the patient's perspective, uninfluenced by the clinician's biases and expectations. Several guiding principles should be used when choosing among these instruments. First, the clinician should consider the goals of the assessment. For example, some instruments are best used to assess the diagnostic criteria for a particular disorder, whereas others are most useful as a measure of severity for a particular problem and therefore are well-suited to measuring outcome following treatment. If the goal of the assessment is just to identify the presence of a particular problem (e.g., to provide an appropriate referral), a less detailed assessment may be necessary than in cases where the goal is to develop a detailed treatment plan and measure outcome.

Second, the clinician should try to select multiple measures that target different domains of a particular problem. For example, when assessing people with panic disorder, an appropriate assessment battery should include measures of agoraphobic avoidance (e.g., Mobility

Inventory), panic frequency (e.g., a panic attack diary), cognitive features (e.g., Agoraphobic Cognitions Scale), and anxiety over physical sensations (e.g., Anxiety Sensitivity Index). In addition, it is often helpful to include measures of associated features, such as depression.

Third, the clinician should select measures that are likely to help with treatment planning, if he or she is likely to end up treating the individual. For example, measures of phobic cognitions are useful for planning a cognitively based intervention. Similarly, detailed assessment of the situations that are avoided by the individual, as well as any safety behaviors that the person relies on, are important for developing a hierarchy for exposure-based treatments.

Fourth, the measures should be selected to test out particular hypotheses that arise during the clinical interview. For example, if the patient seems depressed or sad during the clinical interview, even though he or she denies any symptoms of depression, a detailed self-report measure of depression may provide insight into whether the individual is experiencing symptoms of depression that were not reported during the interview.

Finally, the assessment should begin very generally and become more focused as additional information is obtained. For example, before the initial appointment, a patient might be asked to complete general measures of anxiety and depression (e.g., the Depression Anxiety Stress Scales), a psychopathology screening measure (e.g., Psychiatric Diagnostic Screening Questionnaire), and measures of functional impairment, medical history, and family background. After the clinician has a better idea of the types of problems that an individual is having, a more focused assessment, including measures of particular symptoms (e.g., agoraphobic avoidance, social anxiety, obsessions, and compulsions) may be warranted.

Behavioral Assessment

Behavioral assessment is frequently used when assessing individuals with anxiety disorders. Commonly used behavioral assessment techniques include the behavioral approach test (e.g., asking an individual to enter a feared situation and measuring his or her reactions) and self-monitoring diaries (e.g., completing panic attack diaries each time a panic attack occurs). Behavioral assessment techniques are reviewed in Chapter 2.

Psychophysiological Assessment

As discussed earlier, the three channels (physiological, cognitive, behavioral) through which anxiety and fear may be measured are often independent of one another. Measuring heart rate or other indices of physiological responding can provide additional information over and above interviews, self-report scales, and behavioral assessments. Chapter 3 provides a detailed review of how heart rate assessment can be included as part of a comprehensive assessment for individuals with anxiety disorders.

OTHER ASSESSMENT ISSUES TO CONSIDER

Age, Cultural Background, and Sex of the Individual

When choosing assessment scales, it is important to consider demographic variables such as age, culture, and sex. Many of the instruments reviewed in this book have only been examined in certain populations and, in some cases, they may not be appropriate for individuals from particular cultures or age groups (e.g., children, older adults). Although several of the scales reviewed in this book have been adapted for use with children, this volume reviews only the adult versions. More detailed discussions of issues related to assessment of anxiety across cultures and in older adults are provided in Chapters 5 and 6, respectively.

Intellectual Limitations

Many of the instruments included in this book are based on the assumption that the individual completing the scale does not have any significant intellectual limitations. When interpreting findings from standard assessment scales, it is important to take into account any intellectual or cognitive deficits, language difficulties, impaired concentration, or other problems that may impact on an individual's ability to complete the scales accurately. The descriptions of measures provided in Part 2 of this book include information about available translations for many instruments.

Available Resources

When choosing among measures, clinicians in some settings may need to attend to practical issues such as the cost of a particular instrument and the amount of time needed to complete a scale. Information related to these issues is provided in the descriptions of instruments in Part 2 of this book as well as in Appendix A.

Reactivity to Assessment Instruments

Reactivity refers to the tendency for an individual's symptoms to change as a result of the assessment process. Clinicians should be sensitive to the possibility that their assessment procedures may affect an individual's functioning in unexpected ways. For example, having a person confront a feared situation during a behavioral approach test may have the effect of reducing the individual's fear through the process of exposure. In addition, having an individual record his or her anxious thoughts and behaviors in diaries may lead to changes in these symptoms. Reactivity is often unavoidable. Nevertheless, it is an issue that should be attended to during the assessment process and data that are collected during the assessment should be interpreted in light of the possible effects of reactivity.

SUMMARY AND CONCLUSIONS

The purpose of this chapter was to provide an introduction to some of the key issues that arise when assessing individuals with anxiety disorders. Many of these issues are discussed in more detail elsewhere in this book. The chapter begins with an overview of anxiety, fear, and the anxiety disorders, followed by a discussion of the functions of assessment and the areas that should be focused on during the evaluation. The chapter closes with a discussion of the types of strategies that are used for assessing people with anxiety disorders and some additional issues that should be kept in mind during the assessment process.

REFERENCES

American Psychiatric Association. (2000). *Diagnostic and statistical manual of mental disorders* (4th ed., Text revision). Washington, DC: Author.

Antony, M. M., & Barlow, D. H. (1996). Emotion theory as a framework for explaining panic attacks and panic disorder. In R. M. Rapee (Ed.), *Current controversies in the anxiety disorders* (pp. 55–76). New York: Guilford.

Antony, M. M., & Swinson, R. P. (2000). *Phobic disorders and panic in adults: A guide to assessment and treatment.* Washington, DC: American Psychological Association.

Brown, T. A., Di Nardo, P., & Barlow, D. H. (1994). *Anxiety Disorders Interview Schedule for DSM-IV.* San Antonio, TX: The Psychological Corporation.

Bufka, L. F., Crawford, J. I., & Levitt, J. T. (in press). Brief screening assessments for managed care and primary care. In M.M. Antony & D.H. Barlow (Eds.), *Handbook of assessment, treatment planning, and outcome evaluation: Empirically supported strategies for psychological disorders.* New York: Guilford.

Butcher, J. N., Dahlstrom, W. G., Graham, J. R., Tellegen, A., & Kraemmer, B. (1989). *Minnesota Multiphasic Personality Inventory—2 (MMPI-2): Manual for administration and scoring.* Minneapolis: University of Minnesota Press.

Clark, L. A., & Watson, D. (1991). Tripartite model of anxiety and depression: Psychometric evidence and taxonomic implications. *Journal of Abnormal Psychology, 100,* 316–336.

Derogatis, L. R. (1994). *Symptom Checklist-90-R administration, scoring, and procedures manual* (3rd ed.). Minneapolis, MN: National Computer Systems.

Derogatis, L. R., & Melisaratos, N. (1983). The Brief Symptom Inventory: An introductory report. *Psychological Medicine, 13,* 596–605.

First, M. B., Spitzer, R. L., Gibbon, M., & Williams, J. B. W. (1996). *Structured Clinical Interview for DSM-IV Axis I Disorders–Patient Edition (SCID-I/P, Version 2.0).* New York: Biometrics Research Department, New York State Psychiatric Institute.

Goisman, R. M., Rogers, M. P., Steketee, G. S., Warshaw, M. G., Cuneo, P., & Keller, M. B. (1993). Utilization of behavioral methods in a multicenter anxiety disorders study. *Journal of Clinical Psychiatry, 54,* 213–218.

Goisman, R. M., Warshaw, M. G., & Keller, M. B. (1999). Psychosocial treatment prescriptions for generalized anxiety disorder, panic disorder, and social phobia, 1991–1996. *American Journal of Psychiatry, 156,* 1819–1821.

Lang, P. J. (1971). The application of psychophysiological methods to the study of psychotherapy and behavior modification. In A. E. Bergin & S. L. Garfield (Eds.), *Handbook of psychotherapy and behavior change* (pp. 75–125). New York: Wiley.

Lehrer, P. M., & Woolfolk, R. L. (1982). Self-report assessment of anxiety: Somatic, cognitive, and behavioral modalities. *Behavioral Assessment, 4,* 167–177.

Rachman, S. (1990). *Fear and courage* (2nd ed.). San Francisco: Freeman.

Rachman, S., & Hodgson, R. I. (1974). Synchrony and desynchrony in fear and avoidance. *Behaviour Research and Therapy, 12,* 311–318.

Steketee, G., Perry, J. C., Goisman, R. M., Warshaw, M. G., Massion, A. O., Peterson, L. G., Langford, L., Weinshenker, N., Farreras, I. G., & Keller, M. B. (1997). The Psychosocial Treatments Interview for Anxiety Disorders: A method for assessing psychotherapeutic procedures in anxiety disorders. *Journal of Psychotherapy Practice and Research, 6,* 194–210.

Summerfeldt, L. J., & Antony, M. M. (in press). Structured and semi-structured interviews. In M. M. Antony & D. H. Barlow (Eds.), *Handbook of assessment, treatment planning, and outcome evaluation: Empirically supported strategies for psychological disorders.* New York: Guilford.

Zimmerman, M., & Mattia, J. I. (1999). The reliability and validity of a screening questionnaire for 13 DSM-IV Axis I disorders (the Psychiatric Diagnostic Screening Questionnaire) in psychiatric outpatients. *Journal of Clinical Psychiatry, 60,* 677–683.

Chapter 2
Behavioral Assessment of Anxiety Disorders

Bruce F. Chorpita and Alissa A. Taylor

For the past 40 years, behavioral assessment has played an important role in the identification, case formulation, and treatment of anxiety and continues to be the cornerstone of empirically based clinical practice with anxiety disorders (Barlow, Chorpita, & Turovsky, 1996). For example, many of the recently advanced multimodal treatment protocols for anxiety disorders are built on the foundations of self-monitoring, behavioral observation, repeated measurement, and individualized review of eliciting events and specific anxiety responses.

Behavioral assessment is often best understood in terms of its uniqueness relative to other approaches such as diagnostic assessment and *traditional* assessment (the term *traditional* assessment, widely employed in the past to refer to personality, group-referenced, or nomothetic techniques, can now be somewhat misleading, in that behavioral assessment has actually become a dominant "tradition" in its own right). Diagnostic assessment involves the classification of patterns of symptoms in terms of discrete classes or disorders, and although the modern system of classification is explicitly atheoretical in nature, diagnostic classification implicitly suggests an underlying constellation of learning history, neurological, physiological, and biological events associated with each disorder. Relative to diagnosis, traditional assessment more explicitly emphasizes that behavior is the result of internal mental processes, with a frequent emphasis on understanding how an individual differs from group norms on particular trait dimensions. In contrast, behavioral assessment neither classifies individuals nor measures them against others, but rather is aimed at identifying the relations between one's environment and behavioral events. Some have therefore highlighted the theoretical incompatibility of diagnosis and traditional assessment with behavioral assessment, suggesting that diagnostic and traditional assessment are not necessary parts of behavioral case formulation

Bruce F. Chorpita and Alissa A. Taylor • Department of Psychology, University of Hawaii at Manoa, Honolulu, Hawaii 96822.

(Nelson & Hayes, 1979). On the other hand, modern behavioral assessment now advocates a more complementary perspective, according to which behavior is perceived to be the result of the individual's current environment and other unique variables (past learning history, neurological, physiological, and biological states; e.g., McGlynn & Rose, 1998). Some aims of behavioral assessment for anxiety are as follows:

1. Identification of *target behaviors* (i.e., behavioral excesses or deficits) as the focus of treatment. These are the behaviors that if changed would produce the greatest difference in the client's life and would be most socially meaningful.
2. Identification of alternative behaviors (those that can replace the maladaptive behavior), and functional classes of behaviors (different behaviors controlled by the same contingencies).
3. Selection, design, and continual evaluation of the interventions and their effects.
4. Identification of controlling variables that trigger the target behavior.
5. Identification of individual strengths, reinforcers, and goals.
6. Emphasis on current problems and difficulties, as opposed to historical events.

TECHNIQUES OF BEHAVIORAL ASSESSMENT FOR ANXIETY DISORDERS

Within the area of anxiety disorders, there are numerous available techniques involving behavioral assessment (Nietzel, Bernstein, & Russell, 1988; McGlynn & Rose, 1998). Indeed, the most critical aspects of behavioral assessment involve proper selection of techniques and their systematic application to arrive at individualized case formulation (i.e., understanding of causal relations between anxiety responses and environmental or interoceptive events) and to measure approximations of the therapeutic goals. For a more comprehensive review of the theoretical underpinnings of behavioral assessment, one should consider Barrios (1988), Haynes (1990, 1998), Haynes and O'Brien (2000), and Nelson and Hayes (1979).

Behavioral assessment of anxiety can be organized into three broad domains: (1) verbal reports, (2) behavioral acts, and (3) physiological events (e.g., cardiac activity, electrodermal activity). This organization draws from the conceptualization of Lang (1968), who highlighted that individuals' thoughts, behaviors, and feelings represented unique and often desynchronous response domains with respect to the emotions of fear and anxiety that can supply different information about the anxiety an individual is experiencing (McGlynn & Rose, 1998). This discussion will focus only on the assessment of verbal reporting and behavioral acts; psychophysiological assessment is discussed in a separate chapter.

Verbal Reporting

Situational Ratings. Situational ratings involve the subjective report of the intensity of fear that is being experienced. A common method of measuring client discomfort is the Subjective Unit of Discomfort Scale (SUDS; Wolpe & Lazarus, 1966), a simple but effective means of assessing anxiety that has been applied to a wide variety of disorders and behaviors (Kaplan, Smith, & Coons, 1995). When using the SUDS, 100 represents the worst anxiety ever felt or that could be imagined and 0 represents feeling completely calm and relaxed. The individual thus provides a rating in response to an anxiety-provoking situation. This technique has a wide variety of applications but has been most studied in the context of systematic desensitization and exposure. Research has shown a positive relation between frequency, length, and intensity of exposure and decreases in SUDS ratings (Kazdin & Wilcoxin, 1976).

In addition to the SUDS, there are other useful methods of obtaining subjective anxiety ratings. Examples include fear thermometers (FT; Walk, 1956) and visual analogues (e.g., McGlynn, Rose, & Lazarte, 1994). When using the FT, the client is told that the thermometer is to measure how much anxiety he or she is experiencing, usually on a 1 (completely calm) to 10 (absolute terror) point scale. When using a visual analogue scale, the individual places a mark along a line that has two anchors such as "calm" on one end and "terror" on the other.

There has been some research examining the validity of SUDS ratings. Thayer, Papsdorf, Davis, and Vallecorsa (1984) investigated the relation of SUDS to other measures of anxiety (i.e., heart rate and peripheral vasoconstriction, digit temperature) and found significant positive correlations between SUDS and these criterion measures. In another investigation, participants reported higher SUDS ratings and that it took them longer to relax when they were imagining phobic stimuli compared with neutral scenes (Milby, Mizes, & Giles, 1986). Kaplan et al. (1995) also found moderate positive correlations between SUDS and state anxiety, providing additional support for the concurrent validity of the SUDS.

Self-Monitoring. Haynes (1978) defined self-monitoring as a form of behavioral assessment that requires an individual to self-observe and systematically record the occurrence of behaviors and their parameters (e.g., intensity, duration, frequency, antecedents, consequences). As alluded to above, self-monitoring is not only a valuable assessment tool, but also a critical component of any empirically supported psychosocial treatment for anxiety disorders. Self monitoring provides a picture of what behaviors will be most useful targets and allows the tracking of how those targets change as a function of treatment (Nelson, Hay, Devany, & Koslow-Green, 1980).

Watson and Tharp (1985) suggested that for self-monitoring to be effective, materials should be available when the target behavior occurs, easy to use, and inexpensive. Examples of self-monitoring materials include fear hierarchies (FH), thought records, and journals or diaries to record aspects of specific behaviors, events, or exposure exercises (Mavissakalian & Michelson, 1983). FHs provide an invaluable tool for treatment and the continual assessment of treatment effects. An FH is typically designed in a collaborative process between the therapist and the client, whereby they identify stimuli, situations, cues, and sensations that produce anxiety and fear. The client is then asked to give a subjective rating of anxiety (e.g., SUDS or FT score) in response to each item. A diversity of items (e.g., 10 to 12) should be agreed on representing different cues, stimuli, and gradations of fear. A sample item may read "Being 20 feet away from a caged snake." The items are then used to guide treatment, and daily subjective ratings of hierarchy items can be used to monitor treatment progress (Wolpe, 1973).

Similarly, daily thought records, journals, or diaries, in which the client records anxiety-provoking or unwanted thoughts, can provide information on the client's cognitions and possible treatment targets and on the circumstances, time of day, or events that lead to a certain behavior. They can vary in complexity and form in accordance with the client's ability and also provide information on how an individual's mood or anxiety may change throughout the day (Beidel, Neal, & Lederer, 1991). Again, the goal is to provide prospective evidence on the temporal sequence and possible causal linkages among events and responses related to anxiety. New technology is also aiding and facilitating the practice of self-monitoring. For example, Taylor, Fried, and Kenardy (1990) found that hand-held computers were a feasible means of monitoring for some individuals.

A primary difficulty with self-monitoring is compliance. Clients may fail to complete monitoring in a timely fashion leading to retrospective recall of events, fail to complete the monitoring altogether, or complete the monitoring in a cursory fashion (Taylor et al., 1990, Thorpe & Olson, 1990). There are also issues of client reactivity (i.e., behavior change as a result of the measurement itself; e.g., Ciminero & Drabman, 1977), inaccuracy of reporting, especially if the behavior is socially undesirable (Thorpe & Olson, 1990), as well as other idiosyncratic sources of error (Haynes, 1978).

Behavioral Acts

Behavioral acts are usually measured by means of a performance test, often called a behavioral avoidance test or a behavioral approach test (BAT). The BAT is designed to determine actual parameters of behavior through controlled measurement and observation. This test can serve not only as components of initial assessment, but also as a means by which to monitor treatment progress or to validate the accuracy of subjective reporting (de Beurs, Lange, Van Dyck, Blonk, & Koele, 1991).

Agras, Leitenberg, and Barlow (1968) gave individuals with agoraphobia instructions to walk a course from the clinic to a shopping mall while fear was measured three ways, namely, heart rate, SUDS, and distance traveled. Beidel, Turner, and Jacob (1989) found that an impromptu speech was a valid way to measure behavior, cognition, and physiology in social phobics, and others have found that imaginal speech tasks can also be an expedient alternative to their *in vivo* counterpart (Monfette, Boisvert, & Ivers, 1998). For other anxiety conditions, a feared stimulus (e.g., spider, dog) can be brought into the clinic setting. Perhaps most interestingly, behavior tests can involve the presentation of internal or *interoceptive* stimuli as well. For example, a common challenge procedure for individuals with panic disorder requires the performance of activities (e.g., hyperventilation, running in place, or spinning in a chair, or more complex procedures such as inhalation of carbon dioxide-enriched air) designed to induce particular feared physiological sensations (e.g., dizziness, shortness of breath).

Although the centerpiece of BATs is the observation of actual behavior in the presence of a feared object or event, BATs are frequently and successfully used in combination with the other techniques reviewed earlier. BATs can be used with SUDS or FT ratings to provide the therapist with information about the intensity of fear through the exercise. This can be an effective illustration for the client as well, in that the level of anxiety should decrease noticeably with prolonged exposure to an anxiety-provoking stimulus. Psychophysiological measures can also be used in conjunction with BATs to highlight the patterns of physiological habituation over the course of exposure or treatment (e.g., Holden & Barlow, 1986).

Despite their demonstrated utility, behavior tests are not without some limitations. For example, McGlynn and Rose (1998) correctly noted that some *contrived* BATs can lack internal validity due to their contextual demands and should be used as a precursor to BATs in a natural setting, because behavior in the contrived situation may not predict or represent behavior in a naturalistic setting. Another drawback to BATs is that they are narrow in scope and thus may not be a useful assessment tool for individuals with a heterogeneity of feared stimuli or with diffuse apprehensions as with generalized anxiety disorder. Along different lines, Mavissakalian and Hamann (1986) concluded that BATs are time consuming and often do not provide information above that provided by other measures of anxiety. Finally, research has shown that the results of BATs are particularly sensitive to therapist instruction, and thus special care must be taken in the directions that are given (e.g., Trudel, 1979).

CONCLUSIONS

Behavioral assessment for anxiety disorders encompasses a variety of sophisticated techniques. However, such assessment involves far more than the application of its constituent procedures (Haynes, 1990). It is important to consider that behavioral assessment has as its primary goal the understanding and identification of causal factors associated with an individual's anxiety response. Thus, careful application of behavioral assessment procedures involves individualized selection of those techniques that will most efficiently serve to reveal the factors that elicit or maintain the target behavior. Once selected, the repeated application of such measurement techniques is clearly one of the most important aspects of understanding what contributes to positive therapeutic change. Thus, the contributions of behavioral assessment not only to case formulation but also to efficacious treatment of anxiety are substantial and abundant. Clearly, as research continues, these contributions will increase.

REFERENCES

Agras, S., Leitenberg, H., & Barlow, D. H. (1968). Social reinforcement in the modification of agoraphobia. *Archives of General Psychiatry, 19*, 423–427.

Barlow, D. H., Chorpita, B. F., & Turovsky, J. (1996). Fear, panic, anxiety, and the disorders of emotion. In D. A. Hope (Ed.), *Perspectives on anxiety, panic, and fear* (Vol. 43, pp. 251–328). Lincoln: University of Nebraska Press.

Barrios, B. A. (1988). On the changing nature of behavioral assessment. In A. S. Bellack & M. Hersen (Eds.), *Behavioral assessment: A practical handbook.* (3rd ed., pp. 3–41). New York: Pergamon Press.

Beidel, D. C., Neal, A. M., & Lederer, A. S. (1991). The feasibility and validity of a daily diary for the assessment of anxiety in children. *Behavior Therapy, 22*, 505–517.

Beidel, D. C., Turner, S. M., & Jacob, R. G. (1989). Assessment of social phobia: Reliability of an impromptu speech task. *Journal of Anxiety Disorders, 3*, 149–158.

Ciminero, A. R., & Drabman, R. S. (1977). Current advances in the behavioral assessment of children. In B. B. Lahey & A. E. Kazdin (Eds.), *Advances in child clinical psychology* (Vol. 1, pp. 47–82). New York: Plenum Press.

de Beurs, E., Lange, A., van Dyck, R., Blonk, R., & Koele, P. (1991). Behavioral assessment of avoidance in agoraphobia. *Journal of Psychopathology and Behavioral Assessment, 13*, 285–300.

Haynes, S. N. (1978). *Principles of behavioral assessment.* New York: Gardener.

Haynes, S. N. (1990). Behavioral assessment of adults. In G. Goldstein & M. Hersen (Eds.), *Handbook of psychological assessment* (2nd ed., pp. 423–463). New York: Pergamon Press.

Haynes, S. N. (1998). The changing nature of behavioral assessment. In A. Bellack & M. Hersen (Eds.), *Behavioral assessment: A practical handbook* (4th ed., pp. 1–21). Boston: Allyn & Bacon.

Haynes, S. N., & O'Brien. W. O. (2000). *Principles and practice of behavioral assessment.* New York: Kluwer Academic/Plenum Publishers.

Holden, A. R., & Barlow, D. H. (1986). Heart rate and heart rate variability recorded in vivo in agoraphobics and nonphobics. Behavior Therapy, 17, 26–42.

Kaplan, D. M., Smith, T., & Coons, J. (1995). A validity of the subjective unit of discomfort (SUD) score. *Measurement and Evaluation in Counseling and Development, 27*, 195–199.

Kazdin, A. E., & Wilcoxin, L. A. (1976). Systematic desensitization and nonspecific treatment effects: A methodological evaluation. *Psychological Bulletin, 83*, 729–758.

Lang, P. J. (1968). Fear reduction and fear behavior: Problems in treating a construct. In J. M. Schlein (Ed.), *Research in psychotherapy* (Vol. 3, pp. 90–103). Washington, DC: American Psychological Association.

Mavissakalian, M., & Hamann, M. S. (1986). Assessment and significance of behavioral avoidance in agoraphobia. *Journal of Behavioral Avoidance in Agoraphobia, 8*, 317–327.

Mavissakalian, M. & Michelson, L. (1983). Self-directed in vivo exposure practice in behavioral and pharmacological treatments of agoraphobia. Behavior Therapy, 14, 506–519.

McGlynn, F. D., & Rose, M. P. (1998). Assessment of anxiety and fear. In A. Bellack & M. Hersen (Eds.), *Behavioral assessment: A practical handbook* (4th ed., pp. 179–209). Boston: Allyn & Bacon.

McGlynn, F. D., Rose, M. P., & Lazarte, A. (1994). Control and attention during exposure influence arousal and fear among insect phobics. *Behavior Modification, 18,* 371–388.

Milby, J. B., Mizes, J. S., & Giles, T. R. (1986). Assessing the process of desensitization therapy: Five practical measures. *Journal of Psychotherapy and Behavioral Assessment, 8,* 241–252.

Monfette, M. E., Boisvert, J. M., & Ivers, H. (1998, November). *Comparisons of in vivo and imaginal presentations of a behavioral approach test for social anxiety: The impromptu speech task.* Paper presented at the meeting of the Association for Advancement of Behavior Therapy, Washington, DC.

Nelson, R. O., Hay, L. R., Devany, J., & Koslow-Green, L. (1980). The reactivity and accuracy of children's self-monitoring: Three experiments. *Child Behavior Therapy, 2,* 1–24.

Nelson, R. O., & Hayes, S. C. (1979). Some current dimensions of behavioral assessment. *Behavioral Assessment, 1,* 1–16.

Nietzel, M. T., Bernstein, D. A., & Russell, R. L. (1988). Assessment of anxiety and fear. In A. S. Bellack & M. Hersen (Eds.), *Behavioral assessment: A practical handbook* (3rd ed., pp. 280–312). New York: Pergamon Press.

Taylor, C. B., Fried, L., & Kenardy, J. (1990). The use of real-time computer diary for data acquisition and processing. *Behaviour Research and Therapy, 28,* 93–97.

Thayer, B. A., Papsdorf, J. D., Davis, R., & Vallecorsa, S. (1984). Automatic correlates of the subjective anxiety scale. *Journal of Behavior Therapy and Experimental Psychiatry, 15,* 3–7.

Thorpe, G. L., & Olson, S. L. (1990). *Behavior therapy: Concepts, procedures, and applications.* Boston: Allyn & Bacon.

Trudel, G. (1979). The effects of instructions, level of fear, duration of exposure and repeated measures on the behavioral avoidance test. *Behaviour Research and Therapy, 17,* 113–118.

Walk, R. D. (1956). Self-ratings of fear in fear-invoking situation. *Journal of Abnormal and Social Psychology, 52,* 171–178.

Watson, D. L., & Tharp, R. G. (1985). *Self-directed behavior: Self-modification for personal adjustment* (4th ed.). Monterey, CA: Brooks/Cole.

Wolpe, J. (1973). *The practice of behavior therapy.* New York: Pergamon Press.

Wolpe, J., & Lazarus, A. A. (1966). *Behavior therapy techniques.* New York: Pergamon Press.

Chapter 3
Psychophysiological Assessment of Anxiety: Tales from the Heart

Andrew R. Yartz and Larry W. Hawk, Jr.

Psychophysiological assessment of anxiety has traditionally been restricted to academic settings. However, decreases in the cost of equipment and training, coupled with growing evidence supporting the utility of several physiological measures, have made such assessment more feasible for clinicians. The purpose of this chapter is to briefly review some of the pros and cons of physiological measures, and to focus on the clinical relevance and application of one particularly useful and accessible measure: heart rate (see Table 1).

Anxiety, like other emotions, is often conceptualized in terms of three response domains: subjective/verbal, behavioral, and physiological. The subjective/verbal domain is virtually always assessed, and for good reason. Self-report typically offers the most rapid and least expensive information about a client's situation and symptomatology. However, it is clear that self-report offers a limited perspective, which is often incomplete or even contrasts with information from other domains. Such *desynchrony* (see Lang, Cuthbert, & Bradley, 1998; Turpin, 1991) is a primary reason for including behavioral and physiological indices. While behavioral measures, such as behavioral approach tasks (BATs; see Chorpita & Taylor, this volume), are now widely employed in clinical practice, several impediments to the inclusion of physiological techniques in standard anxiety care remain.

In addition to cost and training restrictions, psychophysiology has generally been under-utilized due to misunderstandings about the logical utility and application of these measures. It is important to recognize that physiological processes play a number of important roles, the

Andrew R. Yartz and Larry W. Hawk, Jr. • Department of Psychology, State University of New York at Buffalo, Buffalo, New York 14260-4110.

Table 1. Applications of HR
Reactivity Measures
to the Assessment of Anxiety

Diagnosis
  Distinguish clinical from subclinical anxiety
  Assist in differential diagnosis
Prognosis
  Predict response to treatment
  Predict natural course of disorder
Treatment process
  Maximize engagement during exposure
  Assist in hypothesis testing

most vital of which is the maintenance of various bodily functions within specific homeostatic limits (e.g., delivery of oxygen to cells, body temperature). Consequently, no psychophysiological measure has a one-to-one correspondence with the experience of fear or anxiety (see Cacioppo & Tassinary, 1990), and for the majority of these measures, clinical cutoff scores do not exist. Regarding their applicability to anxiety assessment, psychophysiological data are often misrepresented as an *alternative* to self-report, as they are commonly perceived or proposed as more objective measures that are less susceptible to bias. While it is true that many physiological processes are not susceptible to the *same* biases that affect self-report (e.g., volitional deceit, social desirability), other factors do influence psychophysiological indices (e.g., movement artifact, equipment settings, diet). The important point is that each response domain has its relative strengths and weaknesses, and the inclusion of information from multiple domains may increase the validity of the assessment. In the following pages, we will provide several examples to support this position.

FOCUS ON THE HEART

There are numerous psychophysiological measures that are relevant to the assessment of anxiety. Peripheral measures reflecting sweat gland, respiratory, and muscle activity, as well as central techniques like the electroencephalogram and functional magnetic resonance imaging, have all contributed to our understanding of normal and abnormal fear and anxiety (Cacioppo, Tassinary, & Berntson, 2000; Lang, Bradley, & Cuthbert, 1998). However, the remainder of this review will be primarily focused on heart rate (HR), which offers arguably the best combination of clinical utility research and practical functionality for daily clinical practice.

Before discussing the logistics of utilizing HR assessment in clinical practice, it is important to be aware of the basic biological processes underlying this measure. HR is influenced by both the sympathetic (SNS) and parasympathetic (PNS) branches of the autonomic nervous system, which receives input regarding homeostasis from the brainstem and information concerning emotional and cognitive processes from higher-order brain regions. The SNS and PNS function like the gas and brake pedals of a car, respectively, allowing for rapid and fine-tuned modifications of the rate at which the heart pumps oxygen-rich blood to tissues throughout the body. Consistent with "fight-or-flight" notions, HR typically increases during times of perceived threat or challenge as a means of preparation for action.

While many readers have likely measured HR from the neck or wrist pulse, this method can be intrusive or unreliable in many circumstances (e.g., imagine a client attempting to monitor her pulse during a panic attack). Fortunately, the heart is a large muscle, and the electrical activity associated with its contractions can be easily and inexpensively recorded using sensors placed on the skin. From this electrocardiogram (ECG or EKG), HR is readily calculated manually or electronically.

Resting HR varies widely. For example, men typically have lower resting HRs than women, and higher levels of aerobic fitness are generally associated with lower resting HRs. Therefore, it is not surprising that resting HR alone is rather uninformative regarding anxiety diagnosis or response to treatment. Instead, it is more useful to measure the *change* in HR from rest (baseline) to the *in vivo* or imaginal presentation of feared stimuli, including animals or blood (specific phobias), contaminants (as in OCD), worries (as in GAD), interoceptive stimuli (as in panic), or traumatic recollections (as in PTSD).

This seems straightforward enough. However, there are a number of potential factors that can decrease the validity of HR change assessments. For example, "resting" HR measured during a typical session may actually be elevated in anticipation of exposure to feared stimuli. Thus, repeated baseline measurements of HR, including sessions in which the client anticipates no aversive stimuli, are recommended. Furthermore, HR will normally increase during postural movements and/or speech production, making it important that the client be seated in a comfortable position and given instructions to remain as still and quiet as possible during the presentation of the phobic stimulus.

Given these interpretational problems, why not just measure subjective fear and anxiety ratings? As it turns out, HR responses can assist clinicians in diagnosis, prognosis, and the evaluation and facilitation of the therapy process. Examples of each of these applications are provided next.

Diagnosis

HR responses to trauma-relevant stimuli (but not other stressors) are generally greater among combat veterans and victims of motor vehicle accidents, with PTSD versus those without PTSD (e.g., Blanchard, Hickling, Taylor, Loos, & Gerardi, 1994; Keane et al., 1998; Orr, 1994). In fact, using the criterion of a HR increase of at least 2 beats per minute in response to trauma-relevant cues, persons with PTSD were identified with a sensitivity of .69 and a specificity of .78 (Blanchard et al., 1996). HR responses to trauma-related stimuli may therefore be useful in making PTSD diagnoses, perhaps especially in cases where the influence of secondary gain on self-report is of concern (e.g., clients seeking financial compensation related to the trauma).

There is also evidence that HR during affective imagery may distinguish anxiety diagnoses. For example, HR responses during personalized phobic imagery are greatest for persons with a specific phobia, least for panic disorder with agoraphobia patients, and intermediate among social phobics (Cook, Melamed, Cuthbert, McNeil, & Lang, 1988). These findings were interpreted as reflecting the relative coherence of the fear networks in each disorder, with greater HR responding during phobic imagery reflecting more focal, coherent associative networks (Cook et al., 1988). Notably, not all anxiety is associated with increased HR. Worry, the core aspect of GAD, may lead to *decreased* HR responses to perceived threat. Interestingly, the reduction in HR and related autonomic indices may actually reinforce, and thereby maintain, dysfunctional worry (see Borkovec, Ray, & Stober, 1998). In addition, blood/injection phobia is associated with a HR decrease to phobic stimuli, which often precipitates fainting (e.g., Ost, Sterner, & Lindahl, 1984; Page, 1994).

Prognosis

HR responses to feared stimuli can also predict treatment outcome. In studies of persons with OCD, panic disorder, social and specific phobias, the pattern is generally the same. Larger initial HR increases to imagery of highly feared situations, followed by decreases in HR responses within and across exposure sessions, are associated with better treatment response (see reviews by Foa & Kozak, 1998; Lang et al., 1998). It has been proposed that these HR changes predict treatment outcome because they reflect more thorough activation, and consequently greater reprocessing, of fear neural networks. Through this activation and reprocessing, it is thought that a change in the meaning (i.e., threat value) of fear stimuli occurs, resulting in clinical improvement (see Foa & Kozak, 1998).

In the absence of intervention, HR reactivity may also predict the natural course of anxiety. For example, smaller initial HR responses to trauma-relevant videotapes were associated with the remission of PTSD symptoms 1 year later, with a sensitivity of .65 and specificity of .84 (Blanchard et al., 1996). Similarly, lower HR on presentation to the emergency room following a variety of traumatic events, had unique predictive power for the development of PTSD over the next 4 months, even after accounting for demographics, trauma history, and trauma severity (Shalev et al., 1998). Thus, HR may be used to help determine who would benefit most from treatment following traumatic experiences.

Treatment Process

Although not yet tested, a logical extension of the work examining HR's prognostic value would be to use HR responses as a form of feedback to amend treatment. For example, the absence of HR increases to highly feared situations might lead the clinician to consider whether elements should be added to increase the strength of the exposure sessions (e.g., use a different contagion or additional imagery descriptors). It is also important to consider the possibility that the client is subtly avoiding exposure (and appropriate reprocessing) via well-established distraction techniques. In this way, HR responses may help to ensure maximally effective exposure sessions by acting as a manipulation check of anxiety induction.

HR data also provide a quantitative, objective measure that can be useful for hypothesis testing, an important part of cognitive–behavioral therapy. In a recent case report (Hofmann & Barlow, 1996), one day of ambulatory HR monitoring was used to effectively challenge a client's beliefs that her cardiac symptoms were catastrophic and that her symptoms and panic were unpredictable. The authors note that such "medical tests" may have more weight than "the psychologist's word" (p. 60), or the client's own questioning of the evidence. Although firm conclusions certainly await further research, this case study suggests that the monitoring of feared physiological symptoms may be especially valuable in the treatment of panic.

In sum, HR is clinically useful for the assessment of anxiety. There is evidence that HR reactivity to feared stimuli aids in diagnosis and can predict response to treatment, as well as the natural course of recovery from traumatic events. HR reactivity can also be useful as a treatment outcome measure and may even facilitate the treatment process. Of course, not all of these findings hold true across all anxiety disorders, but there certainly are many circumstances in which clients with anxiety can benefit from the addition of HR assessment.

Acquiring HR Monitors

Ambulatory HR monitors are readily available for very reasonable prices from a variety of sources. The most common types include a separate transmitter belt and output device. The transmitter belt is discretely worn around the chest under the clothing, and consists of a plastic band (within which are embedded sensors that pick up the cardiac signals) that is connected to an elastic strap. The output device, which displays HR in real time, typically resembles a wristwatch. Some output devices will store HR data (sampling every 15 or 60 seconds) for up to several days, allowing for the collection of ambulatory HR data (as in the Hofmann–Barlow study mentioned above). The data can later be reviewed through the output device, or even uploaded to a personal computer.

Prices vary depending on the desired features, but basic HR monitors that can be used for real-time HR assessment are readily available for $50–100 (Polar, a leading brand, can be contacted at www.polarusa.com; see www.bodytrends.com/heartrate.htm for information on several monitors). Additional features such as programmable alarms for HR zones, recovery time (i.e., return to baseline following HR increases), HR average over a given period of time, data storage capabilities, and PC interfacing are available for $100–200 more.

THE FUTURE

Many questions remain concerning the most effective use of HR assessment in clinical settings. Application of this measure by front-line clinicians may yield the most informed opinions and ideas about what issues to pursue next.

Beyond HR, theoretical and technological advances in the application of several additional measures of anxiety are occurring rapidly, and more are expected. The startle eyeblink reflex (measured electromyographically with a pair of sensors beneath the eye) is noteworthy in this regard. Over the past 15 years, studies of the potentiation of startle during negative emotional states, including fear, have suggested that this measure may have unique assessment capabilities. Because startle is reflexive, but is not part of the autonomic nervous system, it offers many of the advantages of HR without some of the disadvantages (see Foa & Kozak, 1998; Lang et al., 1998; for more comprehensive reviews, see Dawson, Schell, & Bohmelt, 1999). More generally, as advances in the application of HR, startle, and other techniques to anxiety assessment continue, it is hoped that psychophysiological measurement will become increasingly useful to, and informed by, standard clinical practice.

REFERENCES

Blanchard, E. B., Hickling, E. J., Taylor, A. E., Loos, W. R., Forneris, C. A., & Jaccard, J. (1996). Who develops PTSD from motor vehicle accidents? *Behaviour Research and Therapy, 3,* 1–10.

Blanchard, E. B., Hickling, E. J., Taylor, A. E., Loos, W. R., & Gerardi, R. J. (1994). The psychophysiology of motor vehicle accident related posttraumatic stress disorder. *Behavior Therapy, 25,* 453–467.

Borkovec, T. D., Ray, W. J., & Stober, J. (1998). Worry: A cognitive phenomenon intimately linked to affective, physiological, and interpersonal behavioral processes. *Cognitive Therapy and Research, 22*(6), 561–576.

Cacioppo, J. T., & Tassinary, L. G. (1990). Inferring psychological significance from physiological signals. *American Psychologist, 45,* 16–28.

Cacioppo, J. T., Tassinary, L. G., & Berntson, G. G. (Eds.). (2000). *Handbook of psychophysiology.* London: Cambridge University Press.

Cook, E. W., III, Melamed, B. G., Cuthbert, B. N., McNeil, D. W., & Lang, P. J. (1988). Emotional imagery and the differential diagnosis of anxiety. *Journal of Consulting and Clinical Psychology, 56,* 734–740.

Dawson, M. E., Schell, A. M., & Bohmelt. A. H. (1999). *Startle modification.* London: Cambridge University Press.

Foa, E. B., & Kozak, M. J. (1998). Clinical applications of bioinformational theory: Understanding anxiety and its treatment. *Behavior Therapy, 29,* 675–690.

Hofmann, S. G., & Barlow, D. H. (1996). Ambulatory psychophysiological monitoring: A potentially useful tool when treating panic relapse. *Cognitive and Behavioral Practice, 3,* 53–61.

Keane, T. M., Kolb, L. C., Kaloupek, D. G., Orr, S. P., Blanchard, E. B., Thomas, R. G., Hsieh, F. Y., & Lavori, P. W. (1998). Utility of psychophysiology measurement in the diagnosis of posttraumatic stress disorder: Results from a Department of Veteran's Affairs cooperative study. *Journal of Consulting and Clinical Psychology, 66,* 914–923.

Lang, P. J., Bradley, M. M., & Cuthbert, B. N. (1998). Emotion, motivation, and anxiety: Brain mechanisms and psychophysiology. *Biological Psychiatry, 44,* 1248–1263.

Lang, P. J., Cuthbert, B. N., & Bradley, M. M. (1998). Measuring emotion in therapy: Imagery, activation, and feeling. *Behavior Therapy, 29,* 655–674.

Orr, S. P. (1994). An overview of psychophysiological studies of PTSD. *PTSD Research Quarterly, 5,* 1–7.

Öst, L., Sterner, U., & Lindahl, I. (1984). Physiological responses in blood phobics. *Behaviour Research and Therapy, 22.* 109–117.

Page, A. C. (1994). Blood injury phobia. *Clinical Psychology Review, 14,* 443–461.

Shalev, A. Y., Sahar, T., Freedman, S., Peri, T., Glick, N., Brandes, D., Orr, S. P., & Pitman, R. K. (1998). A prospective study of heart rate response following trauma and the subsequent development of posttraumatic stress disorder. *Archives of General Psychiatry, 55,* 553–559.

Turpin. G. (1991). The psychophysiological assessment of anxiety disorders: Three-systems measurement and beyond. *Psychological Assessment, 3,* 366–375.

Chapter 4
Biological Challenge in the Assessment of Anxiety Disorders

John P. Forsyth and Maria Karekla

OVERVIEW

Procedures known collectively as biological challenges have a long and somewhat checkered history in the assessment of anxiety-related disorders. Biological challenge procedures include, but are not limited to, ingestion of caffeine, infusions of yohimbine and isoproterenol, high- and low-dose carbon dioxide inhalation, sodium lactate infusion, epinephrine infusion, and voluntary room-air hyperventilation (Gorman, 1987; see also Rapee, 1995; Uhde & Tancer, 1989, for reviews of such procedures). Such procedures are unique in that they often reliably induce a topography of physiological and self-reported symptoms that closely approximate panic attacks or fearful responding. The noun form of the word *challenge*, therefore, denotes the notion that exposure to the effects of such procedures is inherently aversive or provocative (i.e., challenging) in susceptible individuals, whereas the term *biological* refers to the fact that each of these procedures has been studied extensively and almost exclusively in the context of identifying putative biological mechanisms involved in the etiology and maintenance of panic disorder (Rapee, 1995; van den Hout, 1988). Though this literature is indeed impressive, and much has been learned about the biological functions of different panicogens (Gorman, 1987), it has not yielded the kind of knowledge that might be of use by those interested in applying such procedures in assessment of anxiety disorders. Here, we take the view that assessment technology and procedures, of which biological challenge agents are one part, can yield knowledge that (1) contributes to scientific understanding (i.e., knowledge for knowledge's sake) and (2) leads to more effective action (i.e., knowledge for what it can accomplish to achieve practical ends). Practitioners are largely concerned with what knowl-

John P. Forsyth and Maria Karekla • Department of Psychology, University at Albany, State University of New York, Albany, New York 12222.

edge can accomplish, whereas researchers are concerned primarily with knowledge for the sake of understanding. The typical application of biological challenge procedures in the assessment of anxiety disorders has succeeded as to count (1), but has failed as to count (2).

Space restrictions obviously limit a detailed explication of such issues. Thus, we will provide a brief overview of some of the more robust findings from the biological challenge literature that, in our view, have some practical utility in the assessment of anxiety-related disorders. Here we will use a pragmatic definition of utility, where knowledge from assessment yields information that leads to more effective action on the part of the therapist in alleviating human suffering. As most biological challenge procedures are invasive (e.g., yohimbine infusion, lactate infusion) and produce comparable effects (Rapee, 1995), we will restrict our coverage to noninvasive procedures (e.g., carbon dioxide inhalation, hyperventilation provocation, minimally invasive interoceptive exposure exercises) since they have the greatest likelihood of making their way into routine assessment.

WHAT ARE BIOLOGICAL CHALLENGES AND WHY ARE THEY PANICOGENIC?

Biological challenges describe a class of agents that, in most cases, reliably induce panicogenic symptoms in patients and, to a lesser extent, in nonpatient populations (but see Forsyth, Eifert, & Canna, 2000). Efforts to identify the relation between response to biological change and psychological factors is a more recent development. This emerging body of work suggests that panicogenic challenges are aversive precisely because they evoke a direct or indirectly acquired tendency to catastrophically respond to autonomic symptoms (Salkovskis & Clark, 1990) accompanied by a direct or indirectly acquired powerful (and often rigidly applied) action tendency to avoid and/or escape the private experience. Most so-called biological challenges evoke such psychological tendencies to respond fearfully to one's own responses, particularly in individuals with long histories of doing so (McNally & Eke, 1996). The potential practical value of such procedures in terms of assessment, therefore, rests in their use to evoke relevant aspects of a client's repertoire of responding to their own responses, and particularly how such tendencies restrict, and interfere with, other aspects of the client's life.

HOW ARE BIOLOGICAL CHALLENGES HELPFUL IN THE ASSESSMENT OF ANXIETY DISORDERS?

As indicated, invasive and noninvasive panicogenic challenges produce comparable autonomic symptoms that are similar in many respects to the experience of panic (e.g., dizziness, tachycardia, dyspnea, chest tightness). Indeed, one of the assets of such procedures is that one can reliably induce such symptoms in a controlled setting, and thereby assess how clients respond to the effects of such procedures so as to identify possible targets for intervention.

In terms of assessment, some of the more robust individual difference factors that seem to predict psychological responding to panicogenic challenge agents include high anxiety sensitivity, suffocation fear, and perceived uncontrollability (McNally & Eke, 1996; Zvolensky, Eifert, Lejuez, & McNeil, 1999). Further, it is generally well established that such challenge procedures are reliably panicogenic in persons suffering from panic disorder, and clients with other anxiety-related disorders where panic attacks are a prominent feature (Rapee, Brown, Antony, & Barlow, 1992; Schmidt, Telch, & Jaimez, 1996). Finally, and perhaps most importantly, the literature suggests that panicogenic challenges most reliably induce panic when there is a close match between the effects produced by the challenge and those that are often problematic for the patient (Sanderson, Rapee, & Barlow, 1989). Such a match or mismatch may provide important information about a client's problematic responses, pointing the way to more effective and efficient behavioral targeting in treatment. For example, high- and low-dose carbon dioxide inhalation and voluntary hyperventilation are capable of producing a wide range of panicogenic symptoms via stimulation of the cardiorespiratory system. One would expect, therefore, that such minimally invasive provocation agents will likely evoke panic that is similar, but not necessarily identical, to naturally occurring panic in patients with predominant cardiorespiratory complaints (e.g., suffocation, smothering, dyspnea, tachycardia, dizziness, chest pain; Barlow, 1988). Such information, in turn, could prove valuable in selecting targets for treatment as one could evoke the problematic behavior in session in a manner analogous to how it occurs in the client's natural environment. At present, we are unaware of any studies that have used aversive psychological challenge procedures for the purposes of selecting optimal treatment (but see Forsyth et al., 2000; Schmidt, Forsyth, Santiago, & Trakowski, 2000, for a possible means to do so). However, several studies have shown that challenge procedures can be used effectively in interoceptive exposure, and that patient response to such challenges (i.e., repeated 35% vital capacity CO_2 inhalation) can be attenuated following cognitive–behavioral treatment for panic (Schmidt, Trakowski, & Staab, 1997).

Briefly then, one may be able to use challenge agents, such as CO_2 inhalations and room air hyperventilation, to (1) identify problematic responses for a client and predispositions to respond fearfully to unwanted symptoms of arousal, (2) as a means of interoceptive exposure in treatment, and/or (3) to assess and monitor treatment outcome (see Rapee et al., 1992, for a comparison of both procedures in assessment of anxiety-related disorders).

WHAT ARE THE PRACTICAL CONSIDERATIONS IN USING PANICOGENIC CHALLENGE METHODS?

Traditional panicogenic challenge procedures are often impractical for practitioners to use routinely in therapy (Hoffman, Bufka, & Barlow, 1999). As a result, most practitioners will likely see minimally invasive provocations, such as hyperventilation, exercise, breath holding, breathing through a straw, and the like, as more cost effective and easier to implement. Yet, use of such minimally invasive procedures may also come at a cost in that they are typically weak by comparison with other challenges, and involve a significant degree of client control; just the opposite of what typically occurs in the case of panic attacks in the natural environment. Arguably, use of high- and low-dose CO_2 challenge routinely in assessment may appear prohibitive; however, it is our experience that the cost of equipment is minimal, and it does not require medical consultation to implement safely.

For instance, the basic equipment required for manual administration of CO_2 costs about $500 and includes a Y- or three-way valve, balloon reservoir, and respiratory C-Pap mask, and a premixed canister of CO_2-enriched air (see Lejuez, Forsyth, & Eifert, 1998, for detailed descriptions of CO_2 delivery methods). Though doses typically range from as low as 4% over several minutes to 35% in a single vital capacity inhalation procedure (e.g., Bourin, Baker, & Bradwejn, 1998), we have found inhalations of approximately 20% CO_2 for 20 to 25 seconds to be quite effective in producing reliable panic-like symptoms in panic patients, and to a lesser extent in nonclinical healthy controls. Yet, we should add that little is known about CO_2 dose–response effects, and there is also considerable intra- and interindividual variability that influences the effectiveness of CO_2 inhalation in inducing panic. Finally, though high-dose 35% CO_2 challenge does not appear to pose any long term-risk for development of panic attacks or panic disorder (Harrington, Schmidt, & Telch, 1996), inhalations of CO_2 should *not* be used with every client, particularly those presenting with any of the following conditions: asthma, heart disease and related cardiorespiratory conditions, hypertension, renal disease, stroke, any seizure disorders and head injury, and the possibility of pregnancy.

Another advantage of CO_2 challenge is that its effects are largely involuntary and relatively short-lived (minutes to recovery). Thus, one may quickly and reliably assess a client's sensitivity to panicogenic sensations in a controlled fashion. Such information, when combined with interview, direct observation, paper-and-pencil self-report, self-monitoring, and perhaps some form of ambulatory or clinic-based physiological assessment, may be valuable in assisting case formulation and functional analysis, selection of treatment targets, and ultimately increased accountability and better outcomes. Further, one could also test hypotheses about the role of other psychological and experiential processes that may potentiate or depotentiate a client's panic and/or avoidance. For instance, a therapist may modify inhalations of CO_2-enriched air to make them controllable (real or imagined), predictable or unpredictable, to change the client's attribution as to expected outcomes, to examine how responding changes over multiple repeated inhalations and time, and to examine the role of other stressors and safety cues in moderating severity of panicogenic responding to bodily symptoms. Clients could be taught skills to manage the onset of naturally occurring panicogenic symptoms and practice using such strategies in response to symptoms induced by CO_2-enriched air within the safe confines of the therapy setting.

Lastly, it is our view that the correspondence between subjective distress and panic on the one hand, coupled with extent of physiological arousal on the other, might prove useful in delineating a client's particular subtype of panic attack (Barlow, Brown, & Craske, 1994), and hence assist in treatment matching efforts. For example, our work with nonclinical populations suggests that a two-dimensional scheme (*self-report distress*: high versus low; *extent of physiological arousal*: high versus low; cf. Forsyth et al., 2000; Schmidt et al., 2000) is a reliable way to discriminate between three main classifications of panic attacks (e.g., *prototypic panic*: high distress plus high physiological arousal; *cognitive panic*: high distress plus low physiological arousal; and *nonfearful panic*: low distress plus high arousal). Though we have not explored the implications of this classification for treatment outcome, it is conceivable that patients showing a cognitive presentation of panic would likely benefit most from cognitive interventions, whereas those showing prototypic panic attacks would likely require both cognitive and direct interoceptive exposure exercises.

Before concluding, we would be remiss if we did not mention hyperventilation, as it seems to be a comparatively easier and less expensive panicogenic procedure compared with CO_2 challenge. Room air hyperventilation requires the therapist to simply instruct the client to "take deep, hard breaths, as if you are blowing up a balloon," for a period varying between 90 seconds and 2 minutes (Antony, Brown, & Barlow, 1997). This method of anxiety induction is advantageous for clinicians for a number of reasons, including (1) low cost, (2) ease of implementation, and (3) reliability in inducing some of the more physiological symptoms of panic such as dizziness, lightheadedness, confusion, derealization, breathlessness, increase in heartbeat, numbness and tingling sensations. The main disadvantages of hyperventilation provocation versus CO_2 inhalation are that it typically produces (1) fewer psychological symptoms of panic, (2) requires a significant degree of client control to implement (i.e., voluntary paced breathing), and (3) is less effective in inducing panic symptoms that closely resemble naturally occurring panic attacks (e.g., Antony et al., 1997; Rapee et al., 1992).

SUMMARY AND CONCLUSIONS

The widespread use of so-called "biological" challenges in the anxiety disorders has produced an impressive literature that has helped elucidate the nature and phenomenology of panic attacks. Yet, researchers have barely scratched the surface in terms of demonstrating the practical relevance and utility of such procedures in the routine assessment and treatment of anxiety-related disorders. What seems needed are studies showing that the use of such procedures contributes to better, more efficient, and accurate treatment targeting and outcome. That is, it will require demonstrating practical utility. The challenge for those using panicogenic procedures is to show their practical relevance in clinical settings.

REFERENCES

Antony, M. M., Brown, T. A., & Barlow, D. H. (1997). Response to hyperventilation and 5.5% CO_2 inhalation of subjects with types of specific phobia, panic disorder, or no mental disorder. *American Journal of Psychiatry*, *154*, 1089–1095.

Barlow, D. H. (1988). *Anxiety and its disorders: The nature and treatment of anxiety and panic*. New York: Guilford.

Barlow, D. H., Brown, T. A., & Craske, M. G. (1994). Definitions of panic attacks and panic disorder in the DSM-IV: Implications for research. *Journal of Abnormal Psychology*, *103*, 553–564.

Bourin, M., Baker, G. B., & Bradwejn, J. (1998). Neurobiology of panic disorder. *Journal of Psychosomatic Research*, *44*, 163–180.

Forsyth, J. P., Eifert, G. H., & Canna, M. (2000). Evoking analogue subtypes of panic attacks in a nonclinical population using carbon dioxide-enriched air. *Behaviour Research and Therapy*, *38*, 559–572.

Gorman, J. M. (1987). Panic disorders. *Modern Problems of Pharmacopsychology*, *22*, 36–90.

Harrington, P. J., Schmidt, N. B., & Telch, M. J. (1996). Prospective evaluation of panic potentiation following 35% CO_2 challenge in nonclinical subjects. *American Journal of Psychiatry*, *153*, 823–825.

Hoffman, S. G., Bufka, L. F., & Barlow, D. H. (1999). Panic provocation procedures in the treatment of panic disorder: Early perspectives and case studies. *Behavior Therapy*, *20*, 305–317.

Lejuez, C. W., Forsyth, J. P., & Eifert, G. H. (1998). Devices and methods for administering carbon dioxide-enriched air in experimental and clinical settings. *Journal of Behavior Therapy and Experimental Psychiatry*, *29*, 239–248.

McNally, R. J., & Eke, M. (1996). Anxiety sensitivity, suffocation fear, and breath-holding duration as predictors of response to carbon dioxide challenge. *Journal of Abnormal Psychology*, *105*, 146–149.

Rapee, R. M. (1995). Psychological factors influencing the affective response to biological challenge procedures in panic disorder. *Journal of Anxiety Disorders*, *9*, 59–74.

Rapee, R. M., Brown, T. A., Antony, M. M., & Barlow, D. H. (1992). Response to hyperventilation and inhalations of 5.5% carbon dioxide-enriched air across the DSM-III-R Anxiety Disorders. *Journal of Abnormal Psychology*, *101*, 538–552.

Salkovskis, P. M., & Clark, D. M. (1990). Affective responses to hyperventilation: A test of the cognitive model of panic. *Behaviour Research and Therapy*, *28*, 51–61.

Sanderson, W. C., Rapee, R. M., & Barlow, D. H. (1989). The influence of illusion of control on panic attacks induced by 5.5% carbon dioxide enriched air. *Archives of General Psychiatry*, *46*, 157–162.

Schmidt, N. B., Forsyth, J. P., Santiago, H. T., & Trakowski, J. H. (2000). Panic attack typology in panic disorder: Using concordance/discordance of subjective and physiological arousal. Manuscript under review.

Schmidt, N. B., Telch, M. J., & Jaimez, T. L. (1996). Biological challenge manipulation of PCO_2 levels: A test of Klein's (1993) suffocation alarm theory of panic. *Journal of Abnormal Psychology*, *105*, 446–454.

Schmidt, N. B., Trakowski, J. H., & Staab, J. P. (1997). Extinction of panicogenic effects of a 35% CO_2 challenge in patients with panic disorder. *Journal of Abnormal Psychology, 106,* 630–638.

Uhde, T. W., & Tancer, M. E. (1989). Chemical models of panic: A review and critique. In P. Tyrer (Ed.), *Psychopharmacology of anxiety. British Association for Psychopharmacology monograph, No. 11* (pp. 109–131). New York: Oxford University Press.

van den Hout, M. A. (1988). The explanation of experimental panic. In S. Rachman & J. D. Maser (Eds.), *Panic: Psychological perspectives* (pp. 237–257). Hillsdale, NJ: Erlbaum.

Zvolensky, M. J., Eifert, G. H., Lejuez, C. W., & McNeil, D. W. (1999). The effects of offset control over 20% carbon-dioxide-enriched air on anxious responding. *Journal of Abnormal Psychology, 108,* 624–632.

Chapter 5
Cultural Issues in the Assessment of Anxiety Disorders

Steven Friedman

As minority groups continue to grow in number in the United States, demographers predict that by the mid-twenty-first century Caucasians will make up less than 50% of the population (Ponterotto & Casas, 1991). Mental health professionals, particularly in urban settings, are increasingly called on to provide culturally relevant services to diverse groups. In the twenty-first century, ethnic and cultural groups will continue to travel and intermingle in an unprecedented manner, complicating the task of assessment and treatment for mental health clinicians. Much of the research on developing assessment instruments for anxiety has been performed by North American researchers. Even with empirically validated assessment tools, such as in this edited volume, the assumption has been that anxiety is experienced and communicated to others in similar ways across the world. However, as Kirmayer (1997) and other cross-cultural researchers have noted, recent developments in emotion theory highlight the place of culture in the emotional and expressive experience of anxiety. Whereas cross-cultural epidemiological surveys (Horwath & Weissman, 1997; Weissman et al., 1997) have found very similar rates of anxiety disorders across cultures, there appear to be variations in how anxiety symptoms are described and experienced across the world. In this chapter I will briefly review some of the issues that culture and ethnicity pose in the assessment of anxiety, and the implications of these issues for clinical practice in ethnically diverse societies.

Steven Friedman • Department of Psychiatry, State University of New York, Health Science Center at Brooklyn, Brooklyn, New York 11203.

CULTURE AND ANXIETY

Culture is a complex construct that is often difficult to define and measure objectively. Sociodemographic variables such as gender, age, race, education, language, religion, country of origin, and immigration status are all variables that may be measured to capture components of this concept. However, more subtle aspects such as an individual's sense of origin, values, and belief systems are not easily captured by standardized assessment tools. Although it would be desirable to have a standardized assessment tool to measure the construct of culture, it is highly unlikely that any measure would be complex enough to capture the phenomenon and simple enough to be useful to the clinician.

Anxiety is also a complex construct and its expression appears to differ across cultures. In its simplest sense, anxiety is a descriptive label for how one feels. In the cross-cultural medical and psychiatric literature, complaints regarding "anxiety" and other negative emotions are seen as an "idiom of distress" (Kleinman & Good, 1985), a term used by anthropologists to describe how people communicate in meaningful forms their distress to others. Therefore, what constitutes "anxiety" or an anxiety disorder is affected by multiple variables such as antecedent events, one's appraisals of these events, physiological reactivity, response by oneself and others to these events, and labeling of one's responses by oneself and others. Cross-cultural approaches emphasize that the way people label their reactions is dependent on their social reality and is different in significant ways across cultures. Therefore, what constitutes "anxiety" has multiple components, and the disposition to act on this anxiety is informed by the client's cultural perspective.

Well-constructed and validated assessment instruments are developed by thoughtfully operationalizing and standardizing questions and obtaining data on reliability as well as validity. However, there are a number of important issues and steps that may be missed when utilizing instruments in different cultural settings than for whom they were originally developed. For example, in using translations of well-known instruments such as the Beck Anxiety Inventory (Beck & Steer, 1990) an appropriate cross-cultural step is to translate the test from English into the native version and back to English to see if the translations hold up. Even when done this way, final versions of the instrument may show variations from the original English one, since often there may not be identical translations of a word from one culture to another. In addition, the translated version may still fail to capture all of the relevant phenomenological experience. The reason for this is that if one does not assess for the presence of a particular symptom that is typical of a cultural group, it will not appear as an item on the final version.

ISSUES IN ASSESSING ANXIETY ACROSS CULTURES

There are a number of important issues to consider when assessing anxiety across cultures. These include view of the self, the use of language, how symptoms are experienced, and the clinician's knowledge of the possible variations in the expression of anxiety symptoms across cultures. First among these issues is the recognition that different cultural groups differ in their view of "self" (Kitayamu & Markus, 1994). On a continuum, the role of self can range from being seen as "egocentric"(as in many westernized countries) versus "sociocentric views" (in traditional societies). This variation in a view of the role of self will clearly affect how language is used to express an emotion. For example, in Western cultures, clients may easily label or endorse items such as "I am anxious or depressed," whereas in some other ethnic groups such language may not exist or may be seen as insulting or degrading their family or group, and therefore likely to be ignored or suppressed. In addition, whether a client from a particular culture even makes distinctions between mood, physical symptoms, or behavior is not always apparent. For example, cross-cultural research (Kleinman & Good, 1985) has documented that in much of the world people do not necessarily make clear distinctions between thoughts, feelings, and bodily experiences. When assessing for anxiety in clients from different cultural groups, these clients may experience symptoms as part of their disorder that are more commonly viewed in Western practice as depression or somatization disorder. If not aware of this, the clinician will either miss or mislabel important symptoms.

Evidence for the above points is present in the repeated demonstration that factor structures and analysis for symptoms of depression and anxiety may differ across gender and cultural groups (Good & Kleinman, 1985). For the clinician, the important message is that culture influences whether symptoms that are experienced are even discussed or presented as targets for treatment. As noted above, it is also possible that reported symptoms may not meet the clinician's expectations of how symptoms should present or cluster together. For example, Zinbarg et al. (1994) found that in the field trials for DSM-IV, 15–20% of the Hispanic clients who met criteria for "anxiety disorder, not otherwise specified" actually seemed to experience symptoms that were similar to the category of mixed depression/anxiety.

Even well-designed instruments for the assessment of anxiety may miss or mislabel symptoms. For example, it has been shown that African patients from Nigeria (Awaritefe, 1988) may complain of "worms or parasites in the head." This is viewed as a nondelusional form of anxiety. The description of symptoms such as "heat in the head" is also common in some African clients. Similarly, in some South Asian cultures, the concern of "loss of semen through urine" may be a nonspecific form of anxiety. However, as far as I am aware, no current instruments that measure anxiety, including those in this volume, consider such symptoms.

Culture-bound syndromes (Mezzich, Kleinman, Fabrega, & Parron, 1996) are a concept recognized by many Western clinicians. For example, Western clinicians may be familiar with a prevalent anxiety-related syndrome in Japan called Taijin Kyofusho. This syndrome is sometimes viewed as a form of social phobia, in which the key phenomenological feature is the fear that the client will make the *other* person uncomfortable. This contrasts with typical Western clients' social phobia, in which the fear is that one will embarrass *oneself*. In our own experience in working with African-Caribbean clients, we find that our clients consistently use words such as *paranoid* when they actually mean they are socially fearful. Similarly, the stigma of mental illness appears so intense in many African-Caribbeans that they are reluctant to admit to any feelings of anxiety, panic, or obsessions because they fear being labeled "crazy" or "psychotic."

In Hispanic patients, "ataques de nervious" (Guarnaccia & Rogler, 1998) involves many symptoms and may fulfill criteria for a variety of disorders such as depression, panic, somatoform, and adjustment disorder. Ataques de nervious includes as its primary symptoms "screaming uncontrollably, as well as attacks of anger." These symptoms are unlikely, if present in a Western client, to be viewed by the clinician as anxiety or panic. The above examples highlight that the assessment of anxiety by any empirically validated instruments, even if "cross-validated" for use with other cultural groups, is limited by the types of symptoms that are included in the original version, and the willingness of the client to endorse items on the test.

In summary, as Good and Kleinman (1985) state, cross-cultural research makes it clear that the phenomenology of disorders, or the "meaningful forms in which distress is articulated and constitute a social reality, varies in quite significant ways across cultures" (p. 298). The take home message for the clinician should be that standardized assessment tools are to be used cautiously across cultures other than those for which they were developed.

SUGGESTIONS FOR CLINICIANS IN CROSS-CULTURAL SETTINGS

Clinicians need to be flexible and assess for a wide range of possible symptoms. In addition to an assessment of "anxiety" symptoms, a culturally sensitive approach to the patient should include: an assessment of religious and spiritual affiliations, understanding of the client's reference group, and a broad ranging assessment of the person's culture and "idioms of distress." In addition, clinicians need to be aware that in treatment settings, comorbidity (i.e., having more than one disorder) is the rule rather than the exception (Maser & Dinges, 1993). Furthermore, comorbidity may be even more common among clients who are from minority backgrounds or who are recent immigrants (de Girolamo & McFarlane, 1996). Rates of traumatic events, with their subsequent sequelae, appear to be extremely high in these populations and may complicate the assessment and treatment of anxiety. Table 1 outlines some issues for the clinician to consider when assessing for anxiety across cultures.

Each cultural or ethnic group also has its own unique expression of symptoms, stressors, and strengths, which need to be understood to develop a thorough plan for assessment and treatment. For example, regarding the assessment of clients with panic disorder or other anxiety disorders, there are reports suggesting that isolated sleep paralysis (i.e., an altered state of consciousness experienced while falling asleep or on awakening in which the individual reports a short episode of paralysis with paniclike symptoms such as rapid heartbeat and fear) occurs more frequently in African-Americans than in European-Americans (Paradis, Friedman, & Hatch, 1997). Similarly, the role of religion and extended family support network has important implications for treatment with African-American clients. Standardized structured interviews, such as the Anxiety Disorders Interview Schedule for DSM-IV (Brown, Di Nardo, & Barlow, 1994), need to be modified accordingly (Neal-Barnett & Smith, 1997).

Overall, the task for clinicians working across cultures is to become educated regarding the above-noted "idioms of distress" and the impact they have on their clients. To obtain a comprehensive assessment, therapists need to broaden their knowledge and insight into cultural groups other than their own. Obviously, when working across cultures one should not assume that all members of a particular cultural group will experience and communicate their distress in exactly similar ways. There is great variability within cultures and clinicians should not be blinded by cultural stereotypes of how particular cultural groups respond to assessment batteries. Clinicians do need to be aware of, and respond therapeutically, to the multicultural nature of contemporary urban societies. Respecting and educating themselves regarding the cultural complications of anxiety, the unique strengths and problems of different ethnic and cultural groups, is a task all clinicians will increasingly face. Some efforts have been made to address these issues in specially edited volumes on cross-cultural approaches to assessment

Table 1. Issues in the Assessment of Anxiety Across Cultures

What are acceptable/common expressions of emotional distress for this particular ethnic group?
How does this particular group view "anxiety" or any emotional distress?
What are the group's expectations and beliefs regarding people who experience and express symptoms of "anxiety"?
What are the expected treatments for this emotional disorder?
What is the role of the client, family, and community regarding this disorder and its treatment?
What is this group's expectations regarding the health professional's role in assessment and treatment?
What are the unique stressors this group may experience?
What are some of the strengths of this client and group?

and treatment issues (Aponte, Rivers, & Wohl, 1995; Mezzich, Kleinman, Fabrega & Parron, 1996; Ponterotto & Casas, 1991) but current efforts are woefully inadequate for this important and long neglected task. The development of casebooks on assessing and treating anxiety across cultures (Friedman, 1997) would be useful in sensitizing the clinician to the complex interplay between culture and anxiety.

REFERENCES

Aponte, J. F., Rivers, R. Y., & Wohl, J. (Eds.). (1995). Psychological interventions and cultural diversity. Boston: Allyn & Bacon.

Awaritefe, A. (1988). Clinical anxiety in Nigeria. *Acta Psychiatrica Scandinavica, 77,* 729–735.

Beck, A. T., & Steer, R. A. (1990). *Beck Anxiety Inventory manual.* San Antonio, TX: The Psychological Corporation.

Brown, T. A., Di Nardo, P., & Barlow, D. H. (1994). *Anxiety Disorders Interview Schedule for DSM-IV.* San Antonio, TX: The Psychological Corporation.

de Girolamo, G., & McFarlane, A. C. (1996). The epidemiology of PTSD: A comprehensive review of the international literature. In A. J. Marsella, M. J. Friedman, E. T. Gerrity, & R. M. Scurfield (Eds.), *Ethnocultural aspects of posttraumatic stress disorders: Issues, research, and clinical applications* (pp. 33–86). Washington, DC: American Psychological Association.

Good, B. J., & Kleinman, A. M. (1985). Culture and anxiety: Cross cultural evidence for the patterning of anxiety disorders. In A. H. Tuma, & J. D. Maser (Eds.), *Anxiety and the anxiety disorders* (pp. 297–323). Hillsdale, NJ: Erlbaum.

Friedman, S. (Ed.). (1997). *Cultural Issues in the Treatment of Anxiety.* New York: Guilford.

Guarnaccia, P. J., & Rogler, L. H. (1999). Research on culture bound syndromes. *American Journal of Psychiatry, 156,* 1322–1327.

Horwath, E., & Weissman, M. M. (1997). Epidemiology of anxiety disorders across cultural groups. In S. Friedman (Ed.), *Cultural issues in the treatment of anxiety* (pp. 21–39). New York: Guilford.

Kirmayer, L. J. (1997). Culture and anxiety: A clinical and research agenda. In S. Friedman (Ed.), *Cultural issues in the treatment of anxiety* (pp. 225–251). New York: Guilford.

Kitayamu, S., & Markus, H. R. (Eds.). (1994). *Emotion and culture: Empirical studies of mutual influence.* Washington, DC: American Psychological Association.

Kleinman, A., & Good, B. (Eds.). (1985). *Culture and depression: Studies in the anthropology and cross-cultural psychiatry of affect and disorder.* University of California Press.

Maser, J. D., & Dinges, N. (1993). Comorbidity: Meaning and uses in cross-cultural clinical research. *Culture, Medicine and Psychiatry, 16,* 409–425.

Mezzich, J. E., Kleinman, A., Fabrega, H., & Parron, D. L. (1996). *Culture and psychiatric diagnosis: A DSM-IV perspective.* Washington, DC: American Psychiatric Press.

Neal-Barnett, A. M., & Smith, J. (1997). African Americans. In S. Friedman (Ed.), *Cultural issues in the treatment of anxiety* (pp. 154–174). New York: Guilford.

Paradis, C. M., Friedman, S., & Hatch, M. (1997). Isolated sleep paralysis in African Americans with panic disorder. *Cultural Diversity and Mental Health, 3,* 69–76.

Ponterotto, J. G., & Casas, J. M. (1991). *Handbook of racial/ethnic minority counseling research.* Springfield, IL: Thomas.

Thakker, J., Ward, T., & Strongman, K. T. (1999). Mental disorder and cross-cultural psychology: A constructivist perspective. *Clinical Psychology Review, 19,* 843–874.

Weissman, M. M., Bland, R. C., Canino, G. J., Faravelli, C., Greenwald, S., Hwu, H. G., Joyce, P. R., Karam, E. G., Lee, C. K., Lellouch, J., Lepine, J. P., Newman, S. C., Oakley-Browne, M. A., Rubio-Stipee, M., Wells, J. E., Wickramaratne, P. J., Wittchen, H. V., & Yeh, E. K. (1997). The cross-national epidemiology of panic disorder. *Archives of General Psychiatry, 54,* 305–309.

Zinbarg, R. E., Barlow, D. H., Liebowitz, M. R., Street, L. L., Broadhead, E., Katon, W., Roy-Byrne, P., Lepine, J., Teherani, M., Richards, J., Brantley, P., & Kraemer, H. (1994). The DSM-IV field trial for mixed anxiety-depression. *American Journal of Psychiatry, 151,* 1153–1162.

Chapter 6
Assessment of Anxiety Disorders in Older Adults: Current Concerns, Future Prospects

J. Gayle Beck and Melinda A. Stanley

Perhaps as a result of significant and notable advances in the assessment of anxiety in general, recent efforts have begun to address the evaluation of anxiety in the elderly. These efforts are particularly timely, given that the population of older adults is steadily growing, due to improved medical knowledge, better health status, and a higher level of resources relative to the situation 50–100 years ago (Arean, 1993). Although anxiety disorders represent a salient mental health concern in older adults (Regier et al., 1988), considerably greater attention has been devoted to mood disorders in the elderly (Reynolds, Lebowitz, & Schneider, 1993). This chapter will present an overview of the current state of measurement strategies designed to address anxiety-based disorders in older adults, with particular attention to three salient issues: (1) examination of whether we can use well-established instruments to evaluate anxiety in older adults, (2) consideration of special concerns associated with the assessment of anxiety in the elderly, and (3) determination of clinical applicability and utility. Although specific measurement instruments will be discussed elsewhere in this book, this overview will help to orient the reader to issues that are distinct and idiosyncratic to the assessment of older adults.

J. Gayle Beck • Department of Psychology, State University of New York at Buffalo, Buffalo, New York 14260.   Melinda A. Stanley • Department of Psychiatry and Behavioral Sciences, University of Texas Health Sciences Center at Houston, Houston, Texas 77030.

CAN WE USE WELL-ESTABLISHED INSTRUMENTS TO EVALUATE ANXIETY IN THE ELDERLY?

A central issue in the assessment of anxiety in the elderly is whether instruments that have been developed and established with young and middle-aged adults are valid and useful for older adults. Underlying this issue are questions concerning the nature of anxiety across the life span. One could envision that older adults might experience anxiety-based problems differently, based on aging-related physical and cognitive changes, generational differences in the identification and labeling of affective states, and the shifting nature of "current concerns" that occurs across the life span. Alternatively, one might argue that the signs and symptoms of anxiety disorders (as defined by DSM-IV; American Psychiatric Association, 1994) should be relatively invariant across age cohorts. Although a detailed discussion of this issue is beyond the scope of this brief chapter (see Averill & Beck, 2000; Hersen & Van Hasselt, 1992; Stanley & Beck, 1998), it is important to note that insufficient data are available to answer this question at present. Some studies report differences in anxiety between young, middle-aged, and older adults (e.g., Shapiro, Roberts, & Beck, 1999) while others do not (e.g., Stanley, Beck, & Zebb, 1996). Nevertheless, the field has evolved two general approaches to address the assessment of anxiety problems in the elderly (see Table 1 for a summary of assessment instruments that are appropriate for older adults).

Approach 1: Develop measures specific to older adults. A small handful of instruments have appeared that are targeted specifically for the elderly. For example, the Worry Scale for Older Adults (Wisocki, Handen, & Morse, 1986) is a 35-item self-report measure designed expressly to evaluate the nature and severity of older adults' worry. This instrument was developed to systematically assess worry about finances, health, and social functioning, with the assumption that these issues are particularly salient for older adults. The psychometric properties (e.g., internal consistency, test–retest reliability, convergent validity) of the Worry Scale for Older Adults appear to be acceptable overall (Stanley et al., 1996; Stanley, Novy, Bourland, Beck, & Averill, 2001) suggesting that future work with this scale would be beneficial, particularly studies that examine the utility of the Worry Scale for Older Adults to differentiate older anxious adults from elders with other psychiatric conditions.

Similarly, preliminary efforts are under way to develop a behavioral coding system for observational analysis of anxiety in the elderly (Novy et al., 1997). This type of effort could potentially prove useful in situations where an older adult is not able to report anxiety symptoms (e.g., following a stroke). Future work in this domain could benefit geriatric assessment to a considerable extent.

Table 1. Summary of Instruments Appropriate for Assessment of Anxiety in Older Adults

Clinician-administered	Self-report
Anxiety Disorders Interview Schedule	Worry Scale for Older Adults
Structured Clinical Interview for DSM-IV	Penn State Worry Questionnaire
Hamilton Anxiety Rating Scale	State–Trait Anxiety Inventory
	Zung Self-Rating Anxiety Scale
	Beck Anxiety Inventory
	Padua Inventory
	Fear Questionnaire
	Hopkins Symptom Checklist

Approach 2: Evaluate established measures to determine their validity and utility for the elderly. There has been considerably more work reported using this approach (e.g., Stanley et al., 1996) most likely owing to economy of research effort. In particular, both clinician-administered and self-report instruments have been examined in this regard. For example, DSM-III-R versions of both the Anxiety Disorders Interview Schedule (Di Nardo & Barlow, 1988; updated for DSM-IV by Brown, Di Nardo, & Barlow, 1994) and the Structured Clinical Interview for DSM-III-R (Spitzer, Williams, & Gibbon, 1987; updated for DSM-IV by First, Spitzer, Gibbon, & Williams, 1996) have been examined for their utility with older adults, with promising results (e.g., Beck, Stanley, & Zebb, 1995; Segal, Hersen, Van Hasselt, Kabacoff, & Roth, 1993). Additionally, the Hamilton Anxiety Rating Scale (Hamilton, 1959) has been shown to be useful in assessing anxiety in older adults with and without diagnosable psychiatric complaints (Beck, Stanley, & Zebb, 1999). Continued support for these instruments will further strengthen their psychometric status and permit greater comparison of data derived from older versus younger samples.

Similar efforts have been undertaken with respect to self-report instruments. In particular, data have addressed the appropriateness of the State-Trait Anxiety Inventory (Spielberger, 1983; Spielberger, Gorsuch, Lushene, Vagg, & Jacobs, 1983), the Hopkins Symptom Checklist (Derogatis, Lipman, Rickels, Uhlenhuth, & Covi, 1973), the Zung Self-Rating Anxiety Scale (Zung, 1971), the Penn State Worry Questionnaire (Meyer, Miller, Metzger, & Borkovec, 1990), the Beck Anxiety Inventory (Beck & Steer, 1990), the Padua Inventory (Sanavio, 1988), and the Fear Questionnaire (Marks & Mathews, 1979), for their use with older adults (for summary see Stanley & Beck, 1998). These efforts generally indicate that most well-established self-report instruments perform adequately in the evaluation of older adults.

HOW DO WE ACCOMMODATE SPECIAL CONCERNS IN THE EVALUATION OF ANXIETY IN THE ELDERLY?

Although there is preliminary support for the use of well-established assessment instruments with anxious older adults, this conclusion belies the fact that aging-related issues need to be considered when addressing the elderly. In particular, we have scant data available to help to differentiate between the symptoms of anxiety and depression (Alexopoulos, 1991; Flint, 1994; for an exception, see Wetherell & Arean, 1997). Although mood and anxiety disorders share considerable overlap in younger adults, comorbidity rates in older adults have been reported to exceed those observed in younger samples (e.g., Lindesay, Briggs, & Murphy, 1989), suggesting that clear differentiation of anxiety and depression may be especially difficult in the elderly. Thus, one issue of continuing concern in this arena is the development of instruments that can clearly differentiate between anxious and depressed mood symptoms in older persons.

Another special concern that arises in the evaluation of older adults involves the higher rates of medical conditions. Aging is often associated with an increased prevalence of disease and disability, some of which can produce anxiety-like symptoms (e.g., cardiovascular disease, hypothyroidism, visual and auditory impairments; Cohen, 1991). It is important to recognize that one must differentiate between the physical sequelae of a specific disease that may mimic an anxiety problem (e.g., palpitations resulting from cardiovascular disease) and the psychological consequences of being diagnosed with a chronic, potentially fatal disease (e.g., a normal increase in anxiety and worry). To date, research on this topic is scant and thus, there are few guidelines (other than clinical judgment) for differential diagnosis of this sort.

As well, issues of cognitive impairment are germane in the evaluation of older adults. Although the overlap between dementia and depression has received considerable discussion (e.g., Meyers, 1998), there has been little parallel work with respect to anxiety. Initial efforts at the examination of assessment-related issues in older adults with anxiety problems typically have targeted the "young old" (e.g., individuals aged 65–74; Beck et al., 1999). These individuals are considerably less likely to suffer from cognitive impairment, relative to older individuals. As such, greater consideration of how anxiety-related problems interrelate with cognitive functioning in the "old old" would be particularly important in this regard.

A number of practical issues arise when evaluating an older adult. These concerns are not specific to the assessment of anxiety but rather reflect general clinical considerations that one must take into account when working with geriatric populations. Examples of these concerns are outlined in Table 2.

HOW DO WE DETERMINE WHICH MEASURES ARE MAXIMALLY USEFUL FOR DELIVERING CLINICAL SERVICES OF ANXIOUS OLDER ADULTS?

A neglected aspect of the available literature on the assessment of anxiety in older adults is clinical applicability. Included under this heading are issues such as the demand that a given assessment instrument places on the client, the cost of administering a specific instrument, and how well an instrument can be streamlined into a managed care system (e.g., Hayes, Barlow, & Nelson-Gray, 1999). Because most older adults in the United States receive their primary health coverage from Medicare, these issues are salient in the selection of assessment instruments. To date, there is no published literature evaluating clinical applicability of various assessment devices. Common sense, however, suggests that semistructured interviews are more costly than self-report questionnaires, indicating that research examining the sensitivity and specificity of various self-report instruments in the detection of DSM-IV (American Psychiatric Association, 1994) anxiety disorders in the elderly would be a welcome addition to the literature. In this vein, consideration of how to integrate psychological assessment instruments into primary medical care settings would be important, given that most older adults either do not seek help for mental health problems or consult their internist (Lasoski, 1986;

Table 2. Special Issues Involved in the Assessment of Older Adults

---

Medical concerns: Has the patient received a thorough medical evaluation in the previous year? Is the patient receiving multiple medications that may have a synergistic effect on mood and memory? How many physicians are prescribing medication for the patient? For which conditions?

Scheduling: Is the patient easily fatigued? If so, consider scheduling the evaluation to span several short appointments, instead of one long appointment. Is the patient reluctant to drive at night or during times when traffic is heavy? Is the patient concerned about logistical issues (not finding the office, difficulty parking)?

Sensory decline: Is the print size of the questionnaires adequate for an older adult? Is there sufficient lighting in the evaluation room? Is the environment free of distracting noise? (particularly important for patients with hearing aids)

Accuracy of reporting: Would it be useful to interview another informant (e.g., spouse, adult child, close neighbor) about the patient? Will the use of less "psychologically oriented" terms be more acceptable to the patient (e.g., *wound-up* as opposed to *muscle tension*)?

Memory aids: If you would like the patient to bring additional information to the next appointment, will it help to provide a written list of the desired information?

Wong & Pan, 1994). It would be useful to develop instruments that could be used by general medical practitioners as rapid screening devices for anxiety-based disorders in the elderly. Perhaps this effort could begin with examination of existing instruments, given the growing literature on psychometric qualities of these measures when used with the elderly.

SUMMARY

The assessment of anxiety in the elderly is an area that has just begun to receive attention from researchers and clinicians. As such, there are many questions that are unanswered at present. This overview is intended to facilitate continued work in this area, as well as to highlight issues where clinical science could benefit from more systematic information.

REFERENCES

Alexopoulos, G. (1991). Anxiety and depression in the elderly. In C. Salzman & B. Lebowitz (Eds.). *Anxiety in the elderly* (pp. 63–77). New York: Springer.

American Psychiatric Association. (1994). *Diagnostic and statistical manual of mental disorders* (4th ed.). Washington, DC: Author.

Arean, P. A. (1993). Cognitive behavioral therapy with older adults. *the Behavior Therapist, 16*, 236–239.

Averill, P., & Beck, J. G. (2000). Posttraumatic stress disorder in older adults: A conceptual review. *Journal of Anxiety Disorders, 14*, 133–156.

Beck, J. G., Stanley, M. A., & Zebb, B. J. (1995). Psychometric properties of the Penn State Worry Questionnaire in older adults. *Journal of Clinical Geropsychology, 1*, 33–42.

Beck, J. G., Stanley, M., & Zebb, B. (1999). Effectiveness of the Hamilton Anxiety Rating Scale with older generalized anxiety disorder patients. *Journal of Clinical Geropsychology, 5*, 281–292.

Beck, A. T., & Steer, R. A. (1990). *Beck Anxiety Inventory manual.* San Antonio, TX: The Psychological Corporation.

Brown, T. A., Di Nardo, P., & Barlow, D. H. (1994). *Anxiety Disorders Interview Schedule for DSM-IV.* San Antonio, TX: The Psychological Corporation.

Cohen, G. (1991). Anxiety and general medical disorders. In C. Salzman & B. Lebowitz (Eds.). *Anxiety in the elderly* (pp. 47–62). New York: Springer.

Derogatis, L., Lipman, R., Rickels, K., Uhlenhuth, E., & Covi, L. (1973). The Hopkins Symptom Checklist (HSCL): A self-report inventory. *Behavioral Science, 19*, 1–15.

Di Nardo, P., & Barlow, D. H. (1988). *Anxiety Disorders Interview Schedule-Revised.* San Antonio, TX: The Psychological Corporation.

First, M. B., Spitzer, R. L., Gibbon, M., & Williams, J. B. W. (1996). *Structured Clinical Interview for DSM-IV Axis I Disorders-Patient Edition (SCID-I/P, Version 2.0).* New York: Biometrics Research Department, New York State Psychiatric Institute.

Flint, A. (1994). Epidemiology and comorbidity of anxiety disorders in the elderly. *American Journal of Psychiatry, 151*, 640–649.

Hamilton, M. (1959). The assessment of anxiety states. *British Journal of Medical Psychology, 32*, 50–55.

Hayes, S., Barlow, D. H., & Nelson-Gray, R. (1999). *The scientist practitioner: research and accountability in the age of managed care* (2nd ed.). Boston: Allyn & Bacon.

Hersen, M., & Van Hasselt, V. (1992). Behavioral assessment and treatment of anxiety in the elderly. *Clinical Psychology Review, 12*, 619–640.

Lasoski, M. (1986). Reasons for low utilization of mental health services by the elderly. In T. Brink (Ed). *Clinical gerontology* (pp. 1–18). New York: The Haworth Press.

Lindesay, J., Briggs, K., & Murphy, E. (1989). The Guy's/Age Concern Survey: Prevalence rates of cognitive impairment, depression, and anxiety in an urban elderly community. *British Journal of Psychiatry, 155*, 317–329.

Marks, I. M., & Mathews, A. M. (1979). Brief standard self-rating for phobic patients. *Behaviour Research and Therapy, 17*, 263–267.

Meyer, T. J., Miller, M. L., Metzger, R. L., & Borkovec, T. D. (1990). Development and validation of the Penn State Worry Questionnaire. *Behaviour Research and Therapy, 28*, 487–495.

Meyers, B. S. (1998). Depression and dementia: Comorbidities, identification, and treatment. *Journal of Geriatric Psychiatry and Neurology, 11,* 201–205.

Novy, D., Stanley, M., Swann, A., Averill, P., Breckenridge, J., Akkerman, R., & Beck, J. G. (1997, November). *An observational approach to assess anxiety behaviors in elders.* Paper presented at the meeting of the Association for Advancement of Behavior Therapy, Miami Beach, FL.

Regier, D., Boyd, J., Burke, J., Rae, D., Myers, J., Kramer, M., Robins, L., George, L., Karno, M., & Locke, B. (1988). One-month prevalence of mental disorders in the United States: Based on five epidemiological catchment area sites. *Archives of General Psychiatry, 45,* 977–986.

Reynolds, C., Lebowitz, B., & Schneider, L. (1993). Diagnosis and treatment of depression in late life. *Psychopharmacology Bulletin, 29,* 83–85.

Sanavio, E. (1988). Obsessions and compulsions: The Padua Inventory. *Behaviour Research and Therapy, 26,* 169–177.

Segal, D., Hersen, M., Van Hasselt, V., Kabacoff, R., & Roth, L. (1993). Reliability of diagnosis in older psychiatric patients using the Structured Clinical Interview for DSM-III-R. *Journal of Psychopathology and Behavioral Assessment, 15,* 347–356.

Shapiro, A., Roberts, J., & Beck, J. G. (1999). Differentiating symptoms of anxiety and depression in older adults: Distinct cognitive and affective profiles? *Cognitive Therapy and Research, 23,* 53–74.

Spielberger, C. D. (1983). *Manual for the State–Trait Anxiety Inventory STAI (Form Y).* Palo Alto, CA: Mind Garden, Inc.

Spielberger, C. D., Gorsuch, R. L., Lushene, R., Vagg, P. R., & Jacobs, G. A. (1983). *Manual for the State–Trait Anxiety Inventory (Form Y).* Palo Alto, CA: Mind Garden.

Spitzer, R. L., Williams, J. B. W., & Gibbon, M. (1987). *SCID: Structured Clinical Interview for DSM-III-R.* New York: New York State Psychiatric Institute.

Stanley, M., & Beck, J. G. (1998). Anxiety disorders. In M. Hersen & V. B. Van Hasselt (Eds.). *Handbook of clinical geropsychology* (pp. 217–238), New York: Plenum Press.

Stanley, M., Beck, J. G., & Zebb, B. (1996). Psychometric properties of four anxiety measures in older adults. *Behaviour Research and Therapy, 34,* 827–838.

Stanley, M., Novy, D., Bourland, S., Beck, J. G., & Averill, P. (2001). Assessing older adults with generalized anxiety: A replication and extension. *Behaviour Research and Therapy, 39,* 221–235.

Wetherell, J., & Arean, P. (1997). Psychometric evaluation of the Beck Anxiety Inventory with older medical patients. *Psychological Assessment, 9,* 136–144.

Wisocki, P., Handen, B., & Morse, C. (1986). The Worry Scale as a measure of anxiety among homebound and community active elderly. *the Behavior Therapist, 9,* 91–95.

Wong, M., & Pan, P. (1994). Patterns of psychogeriatric referral and attendance at three different settings in Hong Kong. *International Psychogeriatrics, 6,* 199–208.

Zung, W. (1971). A rating instrument for anxiety disorders. *Psychosomatics, 12,* 371–379.

Chapter 7
Measures for Anxiety and Related Constructs

Lizabeth Roemer

ANXIETY CONTROL QUESTIONNAIRE (ACQ)

Original Citation

Rapee, R. M., Craske, M. G., Brown, T. A., & Barlow, D. H. (1996). Measurement of perceived control over anxiety-related events. *Behavior Therapy*, 27, 279–293.

Purpose

To assess perceived control over emotional reactions and external threats.

Description

The ACQ is a relatively new 30-item, factor-analytically derived self-report measure developed specifically to assess perceptions of control over potentially threatening internal and external events and situations. Factor analysis was conducted using a clinical sample of treatment-seeking individuals diagnosed with anxiety disorders. There are two subscales: *events*, which consists of 16 items, and *reactions*, which consists of 14 items. Participants are asked to indicate on a six-point Likert scale the degree to which they agree or disagree with

Lizabeth Roemer • Department of Psychology, University of Massachusetts at Boston, Boston, Massachusetts 02125.

each statement. Scores reflect the degree of control a person perceives; higher scores indicate higher levels of perceived control.

Administration and Scoring

The ACQ can be administered in 5 to 10 minutes. Items 2, 3, 5–9, 14–16, 18, 20, 23–26, 28, and 30 are reverse-scored. A total score is then calculated by summing all items. The *reactions* subscale consists of items 3, 4, 6, 9–11, 13, 17, 18, 21, 22, 26–28; the remaining items comprise the *events* subscale.

Psychometric Properties

Sample Means and Norms.   The original article reports a mean total score of 73.8 (SD = 21.2) for a clinical anxious sample and 96.1 (SD = 18.9) for an undergraduate sample.

Reliability.   Good internal consistency has been shown for both the overall scale and the subscales in a clinically anxious sample (αs range from .80 to .87) and an undergraduate sample (αs range from .82 to .89; Rapee et al., 1996). Good test–retest reliability at 1 week (r = .88) and 1 month (r = .82) has also been shown (Rapee et al., 1996).

Validity.   Although the original article demonstrated the two-factor structure in both a clinical and a nonclinical sample, another study failed to replicate the structure in an undergraduate sample (Zebb & Moore, 1999). The latter study instead revealed a three-factor structure: internal sense of control, lack of helplessness over internal events, and lack of helplessness over external events. The primary difference was that reverse-scored items loaded on distinct factors in the second study. These findings suggest that more work needs to be done on the factor structure of the scale. However, the convergent validity of the overall scale is supported by findings of significant correlations between the ACQ and measures of anxiety and stress (rs range from −.46 to −.51), which were significantly stronger than those between the latter and the Rotter Locus of Control Scale (a more general measure of perceived control). Further, a clinically anxious sample demonstrated significantly lower scores on the ACQ than either nonanxious controls or a group of men with erectile disorder, suggesting that the scale is specific to anxiety-disordered individuals. Finally, treatment sensitivity was demonstrated by the finding that scores increased significantly from pre- to posttreatment and this increase correlated with changes on the Hamilton Anxiety Rating Scale (Rapee et al., 1996).

Source

The ACQ is reprinted in the original article and in Appendix B. Although the full title is written in the version printed here, typically the questionnaire is titled "ACQ." For more information, contact Ronald M. Rapee, Ph.D., Department of Psychology, Macquarie University, Sydney, NSW 2109, Australia; (tel) +61 2 9850 8032; (fax) +61 2 9850 8062; (e-mail) ron.rapee@mq.edu.au.

BECK ANXIETY INVENTORY (BAI)

Original Citation

Beck, A. T., Epstein, N., Brown, G., & Steer R. A. (1988). An inventory for measuring clinical anxiety: Psychometric properties. *Journal of Consulting and Clinical Psychology, 56,* 893–897.

Purpose

To measure symptoms of anxiety that are minimally shared with those of depression.

Description

The BAI is one of the most widely used, well-researched measures of anxiety. It is a 21-item self-report measure designed to assess severity of anxious symptoms within an adult psychiatric population. Respondents report how much they have been bothered by a list of symptoms during the past week on a four-point Likert-type scale from "not at all" to "severely: I could barely stand it." Sample items include: "Shaky" and "Terrified."* Because the BAI was designed specifically to discriminate anxiety from depression, some authors have noted that it is heavily loaded with somatic, paniclike symptoms of anxiety rather than more general, stress-related, anxiety symptoms (e.g., Cox, Cohen, Direnfeld, & Swinson, 1996).

Administration and Scoring

The BAI can be administered in 5 to 10 minutes. The manual (Beck & Steer, 1993) provides guidelines for oral administration, which requires approximately 10 minutes. The measure is scored by summing all items. Possible scores range from 0 to 63. The manual provides the following guidelines for interpretation: scores of 0–7 reflect a minimal level of anxiety, scores of 8–15 reflect mild anxiety, scores of 16–25 indicate moderate anxiety, and scores of 26–63 indicate severe anxiety. Although the manual notes age and gender differences in BAI scores among individuals with anxiety disorders (women and younger patients report higher scores), no age- or gender-adjusted norms have been provided to date.

Psychometric Properties

Sample Means and Norms. The manual reports the following means for individuals with anxiety disorders diagnosed by semistructured interview: PD with agoraphobia, 27.27 (*SD* = 13.11); PD without agoraphobia, 28.81 (*SD* = 13.46); social phobia, 17.77 (*SD* = 11.64); OCD, 21.96 (*SD* = 12.42); and GAD, 18.83 (*SD* = 9.08). In a normative community sample matched to the U.S. national census, a score of 3 fell at the 50th percentile and a score of 10 fell at the 80th percentile (Gillis, Haaga, & Ford, 1995).

Reliability. The BAI shows excellent internal consistency in mixed psychiatric samples (α = .92; Beck et al., 1988) and anxiety disorder samples (αs range from .85 to .93; Beck & Steer, 1993). The original study revealed adequate 1-week test–retest reliability (r = .75), and a subsequent study revealed good 5-week test–retest reliability (r = .83) among individuals diagnosed with PD and agoraphobia (de Beurs, Wilson, Chambless, Goldstein, & Feske, 1997).

Validity. The BAI correlated significantly more strongly with a measure of anxiety (r = .48) than with a measure of depression (r = .25) in a psychiatric sample (Beck et al., 1988). Within a normative student sample, the BAI correlated significantly with measures of anxiety (rs .51 to .69) and with measures of depression (rs .48 to .56; Osman, Kopper, Barrios, Osman, & Wade, 1997). Although the BAI shows moderate correlations with measures of depression, it has been found to discriminate between self-report and diary ratings of anxiety and depression better than the State–Trait Anxiety Inventory–Trait Version (Creamer, Foran, & Bell, 1995; Fydrich, Dowdall, & Chambless, 1992).

Several factor solutions have been derived for the BAI. The original article reports a factor analysis yielding a subjective/panic scale and a somatic scale, whereas the manual reports four clusters emerging from a cluster analysis: neurophysiological, subjective, panic, and autonomic symptoms of anxiety. Support has been found for both a two-factor (Hewitt & Norton, 1993) and four-factor (Osman et al., 1997) solution; differences may be due to the use of different factor analytic techniques (Hewitt & Norton, 1993). Finally, the BAI is treatment sensitive, with comparable effect sizes following intervention for PD with agoraphobia to other anxiety measures (de Beurs et al., 1997).

Alternative Forms

A computerized version of the BAI has been developed and is available from The Psychological Corporation. A Spanish version is also available. French and Turkish translations are reported in the literature.

Source

A complete kit for the BAI (manual and 25 forms) costs $61.00 US and is available from The Psychological Corporation, 555 Academic Court, San Antonio, TX 78204-2498, USA; (tel) 800-211-8378 (USA) or 800-387-7278 (Canada); (webpage) www.psychcorp.com. Spanish record forms are also available.

DEPRESSION ANXIETY STRESS SCALES (DASS)

Original Citations

Lovibond, P. F., & Lovibond, S. H. (1995). The structure of negative emotional states: Comparison of the Depression Anxiety Stress Scales (DASS) with the Beck Depression and Anxiety Inventories. *Behaviour Research and Therapy, 33,* 335–343.

Lovibond, S. H., & Lovibond, P. F. (1995). *Manual for the Depression Anxiety Stress Scales.* Sydney: The Psychology Foundation of Australia.

Purpose

To measure core symptoms of depression, anxiety, and tension/stress with maximum discrimination.

Description

The DASS is a 42-item self-report measure that assesses depression, anxiety, and stress over the previous week. This distinction between anxiety and tension/stress is supported by the DSM-IV (American Psychiatric Association, 1994) distinction between PD and GAD, and Barlow's (in press) distinction between panic and anxious apprehension. According to the authors, nonspecific symptoms of general distress are not represented in the DASS. Each scale consists of 14 items, which are grouped into smaller subscales. For the *depression* scale, subscales are dysphoria, hopelessness, devaluation of life, self-deprecation, lack of interest/ involvement, anhedonia, and inertia; for the *anxiety* scale, subscales are autonomic arousal, skeletal musculature effects, situational anxiety, and subjective experience of anxious affect; and for the *stress* scale, subscales are difficulty relaxing, nervous arousal, easily upset/agitated, irritable/overreactive, and impatient. Respondents indicate how much each statement applied to them over the past week on a four-point Likert-type scale. A 21-item, short form of the scale is also available (DASS21) with seven items per scale.

Administration and Scoring

The DASS can be administered in 5 to 10 minutes. Three scores (one for each scale) are derived by summing items in each scale; for the DASS21, total and subscale sums are multiplied by 2. The manual provides tables for converting scores to z scores. The *depression* (D) scale consists of items 3, 5, 10, 13, 16, 17, 21, 24, 26, 31, 34, 37, 38, and 42; the *anxiety* (A) scale consists of items 2, 4, 7, 9, 15, 19, 20, 23, 25, 28, 30, 36, 40, and 41; the *stress* (S) scale consists of items 1, 6, 8, 11, 12, 14, 18, 22, 27, 29, 32, 33, 35, and 39. The DASS21 consists of the following items in the order they are listed here: 22, 2, 3, 4, 42, 6, 41, 12, 40, 10, 39, 8, 26, 35, 28, 31, 17, 18, 25, 20, and 38 (loading on the same three subscales as in the DASS).

The following guidelines are provided for interpretation: scores of 0–9 (D), 0–7 (A), and 0–14 (S) are considered normal; scores of 10–13 (D), 8–9 (A), and 15–18 (S) are considered mild; scores of 14–20 (D), 10–14 (A), and 19–25 (S) are considered moderate; scores of 21–27 (D), 15–19 (A), and 26–33 (S) are considered severe; and scores of 28+ (D), 20+ (A), and 34+ (S) are considered extremely severe.

Psychometric Properties

Sample Means and Norms. The manual reports the following norms for individuals in a nonclinical sample: *depression*, 6.34 (*SD* = 6.97); *anxiety*, 4.70 (*SD* = 4.91); and *stress*, 10.11 (*SD* = 7.91). Gender- and age-specific norms are also reported in the manual. In addition, means for anxiety disorder groups and individuals with major depressive disorder (MDD) are reported by Antony, Bieling, Cox, Enns, and Swinson (1998) and Brown, Chorpita, Korotitsch, and Barber (1997). In the latter study, a mean of 25.31 (*SD* = 10.24) on the *depression* scale was reported for the MDD group, a mean of 15.48 (*SD* = 8.81) on the *anxiety* scale was reported for the PDA group, and a mean of 22.36 (*SD* = 9.90) on the *stress* scale was reported for the GAD group.

Reliability. Internal consistency has been demonstrated in a student population (αs from .81 to .91; S. H. Lovibond & P. F. Lovibond, 1995), a clinical sample (αs range from .88 to .96, Brown et al., 1997), and using the DASS21 in a clinical sample (αs range from .87 to .94; Antony, Bieling, et al., 1998). Adequate 2-week temporal stability was also demonstrated in a clinical sample (*rs* .71 to .81; Brown et al., 1997).

Validity. The factor structure of the DASS was initially established in an undergraduate sample (Lovibond & Lovibond, 1995). This factor structure has been supported in a clinical sample of individuals with anxiety and mood disorders (Brown et al., 1997). In addition, the factor structure of the DASS21 was supported in a similar clinical and community sample (Antony, Bieling, et al., 1998). Construct validity of the three scales has been demonstrated by findings of significant correlations between the Anxiety scale and measures of anxiety (*rs* = .81 to .84 in the three samples described above) and between the Depression scale and measures of depression (*rs* .74 to .79 in the same samples). In addition, within a clinical population, the Stress scale was more strongly correlated with measures of worry and negative affect than the other two scales, the Depression scale was more strongly correlated with measures of depression and positive affect than the other two scales, and the Anxiety scale was more strongly correlated with measures of anxiety than the other two scales, all supporting the discriminant validity of the three scales (Brown et al., 1997). Also, in the same study, predicted differences between clinical groups were found: Individuals with GAD and MDD reported significantly higher Stress scores, individuals with PDA reported significantly higher Anxiety scores, and individuals with MDD reported significantly higher Depression scores. Finally, scales show specific temporal stability across a period of 3 to 8 years (Lovibond, 1998).

Alternative Forms

As noted above, a 21-item version of the scale that demonstrates good psychometric properties has been developed. Chinese, Spanish, and Persian translations are currently in development. In addition, trait, child, and momentary ("how you feel right now") versions are being developed.

Source

The DASS is reprinted in Appendix B and the DASS21 can be derived from this using the description in the Scoring section above. The questionnaires and scoring template can also be downloaded directly from http://www.psy.unsw.edu.au/dass/. A manual is available for $40 US or $50 Australian from DASS Orders, School of Psychology, University of New South Wales, NSW 2052, Australia; (tel) 61-2-93853047; (fax) 61-2-93853641; (e-mail) P.Lovibond@unsw.edu.au.

FEAR QUESTIONNAIRE (FQ)

Original Citation

Marks, I. M., & Mathews, A. M. (1979). Brief standard self-rating for phobic patients. *Behaviour Research and Therapy, 17*, 263–267.

Purpose

To assess the severity of and monitor change in common phobias as well as associated anxiety and depression.

Description

The FQ is a widely used, well-validated, 24-item self-report measure that was designed specifically to monitor change in patients with phobias. The main scale (also called the Total Phobia Scale) consists of 15 items (items 2–16) and contains three 5-item subscales: *agoraphobia*, *blood/injury*, and *social*. In addition, the FQ includes a *global phobic distress* index, a 5-item *anxiety/depression* scale, and a *main target phobia* scale, along with two items that inquire about other avoided situations and other distressing feelings. Respondents rate severity of avoidance of 15 specific situations, their main phobia, and any other situations on a nine-point Likert-type scale. In addition, respondents indicate how troublesome symptoms are on nine-point Likert-type scales for the *anxiety/depression* scale. Finally, on the *global phobic distress* index, respondents indicate how disturbing/disabling their phobias are on a nine-point Likert-type scale.

Administration and Scoring

It takes less than 10 minutes to administer the FQ. A *total phobia* (FQ-TOT) score is derived by summing responses on items 2 through 16; possible scores range from 0 to 120. Subscale scores are derived by summing appropriate items: *agoraphobia* (FQ-AG), 5, 6, 8, 12, 15; *blood/injury* (FQ-BI), 2, 4, 10, 13, 16; *social* (FQ-SP), 3, 7, 9, 11, 14. An *anxiety/depression* score is derived by summing the five items that comprise that scale and the *global phobic distress* index consists of the response to that single item.

Psychometric Properties

Sample Means and Norms. Means for the initial sample of 20 patients with phobias were 47 (*SD* = 19.3) for the total phobia score, 17 (*SD* = 10.0) for agoraphobia, 15 (*SD* = 10.7) for blood/injury, 15 (*SD* = 8.5) for social, 22 (*SD* = 9.1) for anxiety/depression, and 5.5 (*SD* = 2.7) for global phobic rating. A clinical sample of individuals diagnosed with PDA by structured interview reported a mean of 15.0 (*SD* = 9.4) on the agoraphobia subscale, whereas a sample of individuals diagnosed with social phobia reported a mean score of 22.5 (*SD* = 8.8) on the social subscale (Cox, Swinson, & Shaw, 1991). In a normative community sample matched to the U.S. national census, an FQ-TOT score of 25, an FQ-AG score of 4, an FQ-SP score of 9, and an FQ-BI score of 10 fell at the 50th percentile, whereas scores of 42, 10, 16, and 17, respectively, fell at the 80th percentile (Gillis et al., 1995).

Reliability. The FQ has demonstrated adequate to good internal consistency in a clinical sample, with (rs ranging from .71 to .83 for the three phobia subscales, total phobia score, and anxiety/depression score (Oei, Moylan, & Evans, 1991). Internal consistency for the three phobia subscales was weaker in one nonclinical sample (αs range from .44 to .73; Trull & Hillerbrand, 1990) and acceptable in another (αs range from .71 to .86; Osman, Barrios, Osman, & Markway, 1993). Good 1-week test–retest reliability was demonstrated in the initial study (rs .82 to .96 for phobia subscales, total phobia score, and anxiety/depression score) and good longer term (3–16-week) test–retest reliability was reported for the phobia subscales and the total phobia score (rs .84 to .90; Michelson & Mavissakalian, 1983).

Validity. The three-factor structure for the 15-item total phobia scale has been replicated in a mixed anxiety disorder sample (Oei et al., 1991), in a panic disorder sample (Cox, Swinson, Parker, Kuch, & Reichman, 1993), and in one nonclinical sample (Osman et al., 1993) but not in another (Trull & Hillerbrand, 1990). Correlations between the FQ social phobia scale and other measures of social anxiety tend to be high, ranging from .59 to .83 (Davidson et al., 1991; Osman, Gutierrez, Barrios, Kopper, & Chiros, 1998; Turner, Beidel, & Dancu, 1996). Correlations between the FQ agoraphobia scale and other measures of agoraphobic avoidance are also high, ranging from .44 to .71 (Chambless, Caputo, Jasin, Gracely, & Williams, 1985; Cox, Swinson, Kuch, & Reichman, 1993). Studies have found that individuals with PDA score significantly higher on the agoraphobia subscale than individuals with other anxiety disorders, whereas individuals with social phobia score significantly higher on the social subscale (e.g., Cox et al., 1991; Oei et al., 1991; van Zuuren, 1988). Thus, these two subscales effectively discriminate individuals with PDA and social phobia. Finally, the original article and numerous subsequent studies have shown that the FQ is sensitive to change following treatment.

Alternative Forms

The FQ has been translated into Catalan, Chinese, Dutch, French, German, Italian, and Spanish.

Source

The FQ is reprinted in the original article and in Appendix B. For more information, contact Isaac Marks, M.D., Department of Psychiatry, Charing Cross Hospital, Fulham Palace Road, London W48RF, United Kingdom; (tel) 44-208 846 7390; (e-mail) i.marks@iop.kcl.ac.uk.

FROST MULTIDIMENSIONAL PERFECTIONISM SCALE (FMPS)

Original Citation

Frost, R. O., Marten, P., Lahart, C., & Rosenblate, R. (1990). The dimensions of perfectionism. *Cognitive Therapy and Research, 14*, 449–468.

Purpose

To measure various dimensions of perfectionism.

Description

The FMPS is a 35-item self-report measure that was designed to assess multiple dimensions of perfectionism, a construct that has been associated with general anxiety level and with several anxiety disorders. Items were generated to fit into five theoretically derived scales: personal standards, concern over mistakes, parental expectations, doubting of actions, and organization. Items were factor analyzed in two undergraduate samples and a six-factor solution emerged in which parental expectations was divided into parental expectations and parental criticism. Respondents indicate how much they agree with each statement on a five-point Likert-type scale.

Administration and Scoring

The FMPS can be administered in 10 minutes. Subscales are derived by summing the items in each scale: the *concern over mistakes* (CM) subscale consists of items 9, 10, 13, 14, 18, 21, 23, 25, and 34; the *personal standards* (PS) subscale consists of items 4, 6, 12, 16, 19, 24, and 30; the *parental expectations* (PE) subscale consists of items 1, 11, 15, 20, and 26; the *parental criticism* (PC) scale consists of items 3, 5, 22, and 35; the *doubting of actions* (DA) subscale consists of items 17, 28, 32, and 33; and the *organization* (O) subscale consists of items 2, 7, 8, 27, 29, and 31. A total perfectionism score is derived by summing all subscales except for organization, which assesses a separate but related dimension of perfectionism.

Psychometric Properties

Sample Means and Norms. Antony, Purdon, Huta, and Swinson (1998) reported means for each subscale for nonclinical volunteers and groups of individuals with anxiety disorders. Listed here are nonclinical means for all scales as well as means for specific anxiety disorder groups for those scales that differed significantly from the nonclinical sample's means. Nonclinical volunteers reported the following means on the subscales: CM, 17.43 (SD = 5.25); DA, 7.74 (SD = 3.15); PS, 22.74 (SD = 6.07); PE, 13.63 (SD = 4.31); PC, 8.69 (SD = 3.65); O, 22.57 (SD = 4.38). Significantly elevated clinical group means on *concern over mistakes* were: PD, 24.14 (SD = 8.21); OCD, 21.53 (SD = 7.87); and SP, 27.48 (SD = 8.35). For *doubt over actions*, individuals with OCD reported a mean of 14.44 (SD = 4.34) and individuals with social phobia reported a mean of 13.03 (SD = 4.03). Finally, individuals with social phobia reported a mean of 11.33 (SD = 4.54) on the *parental criticism* subscale.

Reliability. The original article revealed adequate to excellent internal consistency for all subscales and the total score (αs ranging from .77 to .93). No test–retest reliability has been reported.

Validity. There is some evidence that the factor structure of the FMPS may not be stable. One study using a nonclinical sample yielded a different solution (Rhèaume, Freeston, Dugas, Letarte, & Ladouceur, 1995) and another suggested that a four-factor solution may be more appropriate (combining CM and D and combining PE and PC; Stöber, 1998). In a clinical sample of individuals with anxiety disorders, although six comparable factors could be extracted, a three-factor solution was statistically preferable (Purdon, Antony, & Swinson, 1999). Interestingly, again CM and D were combined, as were PE and PC. Convergent validity for the measure is demonstrated by significant correlations between the overall score and other measures of perfectionism and by correlations between the CM and DA scales and various measures of psychiatric symptoms (Frost et al., 1990). In addition, individuals with social phobia reported elevated levels of CM, DA, and PC relative to nonclinical controls, individuals with OCD reported elevations in CM and DA, and individuals with PD reported elevations in CM (Antony, Purdon, et al., 1998). Also, individuals with high levels of CM displayed more negative reactions to a task with high frequency of mistakes (Frost et al., 1995) and also to naturally occurring mistakes (despite comparable frequencies of mistakes; Frost et al., 1997) than individuals with lower levels of CM.

Alternative Forms

The FMPS has been translated into Chinese, French, Egyptian, German, Hebrew, Japanese, Portuguese, and Spanish.

Source

The FMPS items are reprinted in the original article and the scale is reprinted in Appendix B. For more information, contact Randy Frost, Ph.D., Department of Psychology, Smith College, Northampton, MA 01063, USA; (tel) 413-585-3911; (fax) 413-585-3786; rfrost@science.smith.edu.

HAMILTON ANXIETY RATING SCALE (HARS) AND CLINICAL ANXIETY SCALE (CAS)

Original Citation

HARS: Hamilton, M. (1959). The assessment of anxiety states by rating. *British Journal of Medical Psychology, 32,* 50–55.

CAS: Snaith, R. P., Baugh, S. J., Clayden, A. D., Husain, A., & Sipple, M. A. (1982). The Clinical Anxiety Scale: An instrument derived from the Hamilton Anxiety Scale. *British Journal of Psychiatry, 141,* 518–523.

Purpose

To assess degree of generalized anxious symptomatology (as opposed to specific phobic avoidance) among clinically anxious individuals.

Description

The HARS is a widely used clinician-administered scale. It includes a list of symptoms that were initially grouped under 13 symptom clusters. Subsequently, the general somatic cluster was divided into muscular and sensory, resulting in 14 items on the most widely used version of the scale (Hamilton, 1969). The interviewer provides a rating of the severity of each overarching symptom cluster on a scale from 0 (not present) to 4 (very severe/incapacitating). Beyond the general Likert scale descriptors, no guidelines are provided for these ratings. The scale was developed specifically to provide a measure of the severity of anxious symptomatology among already-diagnosed individuals. It is often used as an outcome measure in psychosocial and drug treatment trials.

The CAS was developed by taking ratings of each of the specific HARS symptoms (those listed under the 14 clusters) and determining which symptoms were most strongly correlated with an independent composite measure of severity derived from clinician and patient ratings. The revised scale consists of six items (psychic tension, inability to relax, startle response, worrying, apprehension, and restlessness) as well as a seventh item assessing panic attacks that can be added, but is not included in the total score. The CAS includes explicit instructions for scoring items.

Administration and Scoring

The HARS can be administered in 15 to 30 minutes. An overall score is derived by summing all 14 items. In addition, *psychic* and *somatic* subscale scores can be derived. The psychic subscale consists of the summed severity of items 1–6 and 14, whereas the *somatic* subscale consists of the summed severity of items 7–13. The CAS is scored by summing responses to the six items. Snaith, Harrop, Newby, and Teale (1986) identified the following guidelines for interpretation of CAS scores: scores of 0–4 are considered recovered, 5–10 are considered mild, 11–16 moderate, and 17–24 severe.

Psychometric Properties

Sample Means and Norms. The following mean total scores for the HARS have been reported: 2.40 (*SD* = 2.47) for a sample of normal controls, 20.31 (*SD* = 6.03) for a sample of individuals diagnosed with mood disorders, and 18.95 (*SD* = 8.43) for a sample of individuals diagnosed with anxiety disorders (Kobak, Reynolds, & Griest, 1993).

Reliability. Estimates for the internal consistency of the HARS range from adequate to good (αs ranging from .77 to .81) in one study (Moras, Di Nardo, & Barlow, 1992) to excellent (α = .92) in another (Kobak et al., 1993). In the latter study, 1-week test–retest reliability was also excellent (*r* = .96). In the original study, an interrater reliability of .89 was reported, whereas subsequent studies have reported reliabilities ranging from .65 (Moras et al., 1992) to .74 (Maier, Buller, Philipp, & Heuser, 1988). Two structured interview guides have been developed for administering the HARS; both report excellent interrater and test–retest reliability (Bruss Gruenberg, Goldstein, & Barber, 1994, Shear et al., in press).

Validity. HARS scores have been found to correlate significantly with self-report measures of anxiety in clinical samples (Beck & Steer, 1991; Maier et al., 1988). In addition, individual with anxiety disorders scored substantially higher on the HARS than did normal controls (Kobak et al., 1993). As noted above, the CAS has been found to correlate strongly with patient and independent clinician ratings of anxiety severity (Snaith et al., 1986). The two-factor solution of the HARS has been supported in studies of clinical samples (Maier et al., 1988) and in studies using international samples of individuals with PD (Bech et al., 1992). However, the discriminant and discriminative validity of the HARS has been challenged; in particular, high correlations with measures of depression have been found ($r = .78$) and items on the scale failed to discriminate individuals with GAD from those with MDD (Riskind, Beck, Brown, & Steer, 1987). Based on factor analysis of the HARS with the Hamilton Depression Rating Scale, new versions of both scales were derived with reduced symptom overlap and that more effectively discriminated the two clinical groups (Riskind et al., 1987). However, a subsequent study found that the original and revised scales were comparable in discriminating individuals with anxiety and comorbid mood disorders from those with only anxiety disorders (Moras et al., 1992). Finally, the HARS is sensitive to treatment change and correlates significantly with changes in other anxiety measures, although the somatic scale may also respond to anxiolytic medication side effects (Maier et al., 1988). The CAS is also responsive to treatment (e.g., Hoehn-Saric, McLeod, & Hipsley, 1993) and, because it contains only items from the psychic subscale of the HARS, may be less influenced by anxiolytic side effects.

Alternative Forms

Kobak et al. (1993) have developed a computer-administered version of the HARS, which is highly correlated with the clinician-administered version ($r = .92$). As noted above, several structured interview formats have been developed (Bruss et al., 1994; Shear et al., in press), which may be particularly useful when extensive training is not possible.

Source

The 14-item version of the HARS and the CAS are both reprinted in the original articles and in Appendix B (the format of the HARS is altered slightly to facilitate administration). One structured interview guide (HARS-IG) is reprinted in Bruss et al. (1994); another (SIGH-A) is available from M. Katherine Shear, M.D., Anxiety Disorders Prevention Program, Western Psychiatric Institute and Clinic, University of Pittsburgh, 3811 O'Hara Street, Pittsburgh, PA 15213-2593, USA; (tel) 412-624-1340; (fax) 412-624-6644; (e-mail) shearmk@msx.upmc.edu.

HOSPITAL ANXIETY AND DEPRESSION SCALE (HADS)

Original Citations

Zigmond, A., & Snaith, R. P. (1983). The Hospital Anxiety and Depression Scale. *Acta Psychiatrica Scandinavica, 67,* 361–370.

Snaith, R. P., & Zigmond, A. S. (1994). *The Hospital Anxiety and Depression Scale manual*. Berkshire, UK: NFER-Nelson Publishing Co.

Purpose

To detect states of depression and anxiety in medical (nonpsychiatric) patients.

Description

The HADS is a 14-item self-report measure designed to assess depressive and anxious symptomatology in medically ill individuals. Somatic items were intentionally omitted to allow for assessment of mood state independent of physical symptoms. The 7-item anxiety subscale (HADS-A) assesses anxious mood, restlessness, and anxious thoughts, whereas the 7-item depression subscale (HADS-D) assesses predominantly anhedonic symptoms. Respondents indicate how they have been feeling over the past week on four-point Likert-type scales. Items alternate between whether the most severe response choice is listed first or last; numbers to the side of each option indicate the weight of the response choice.

Administration and Scoring

The HADS can be administered in 5 minutes. Separate anxiety and depression scores are derived by summing items on each subscale. The authors recommend against deriving a total score for the measure. The manual indicated that, for both scales, scores of 0–7 are considered normal, 8–10 mild, 11–14 moderate, and 15–21 severe.

Psychometric Properties

Sample Means and Norms.   Mean scores of 7.48 ($SD = 4.2$) for the HADS-A and 4.37 ($SD = 3.7$) for the HADS-D were reported in a sample of French-Canadian outpatients who were HIV positive (Savard, Laberge, Gauthier, Ivers, & Bergeron, 1998) and means of 5.44 ($SD = 4.07$) for the HADS-A and 3.02 ($SD = 2.98$) for the HADS-D were reported in a large sample of patients with cancer (Moorey et al., 1991). Means of 4.55 ($SD = 3.73$) for the HADS-A and 3.98 ($SD = 3.46$) for the HADS-D were reported in a large Swedish normative sample (Lisspers, Nygren, & Soderman, 1997).

Reliability.   Excellent internal consistency for both scales was demonstrated in both samples described above (αs ranging from .89 to .93) and test–retest reliability (over an average period of 1.69 months) was .72 for both subscales in the sample of outpatients who were HIV positive.

Validity.   The initial study demonstrated significant correlations between interview ratings of anxiety and the HADS-A ($r = .54$) and interview ratings of depression and the HADS-D ($r = .79$) with nonsignificant correlations between each subscale and the other interview rating (among patients who exhibited differences in level of anxious and depressive symptoms). The HADS-A and HADS-D were also significantly correlated with self-report measures of anxiety and depression, respectively, in the study of patients who were HIV positive; however, each scale also correlated with the measure of the other construct (i.e., HADS-A correlated with a measure of depression as well). Despite this challenge to discriminant validity of the scales, the two-factor structure has been supported in both samples described above (Moorey et al., 1991; Savard et al., 1998) and in a normative sample (Lisspers et al., 1997). In addition, excellent concurrence has been found between semistructured interview-based designation of presence or absence of mood and anxiety disturbance and classification using the HADS-suggested ranges in a general hospital setting (Aylard, Gooding, McKenna, & Snaith, 1987). In the latter study, the depression and anxiety scales were not significantly correlated.

Alternative Forms

The HADS has been translated into Arabic, Cantonese, Danish, Dutch, French, German, Hebrew, Italian, Norwegian, Swedish, and Spanish.

Source

The HADS is reprinted in the original article and is also available (along with scoring templates and a manual) from NFER-Nelson Publishing Co., Ltd., Darville House, 2 Oxford Road East, Windsor, Berkshire SF4 1DF, United Kingdom; (tel) 011 44 1753 858 961; (website) http://www.nfer-nelson.co.uk/.

META-COGNITIONS QUESTIONNAIRE (MCQ)

Original Citation

Cartwright-Hatton, S., & Wells, A. (1997). Beliefs about worry and intrusions: The Meta-Cognitions Questionnaire and its correlates. *Journal of Anxiety Disorders, 11*, 279–296.

Purpose

To measure beliefs about worry and intrusive thoughts.

Description

The MCQ is a relatively new, 65-item self-report measure designed to assess beliefs about worry and intrusive thoughts. The measure is derived both from Wells's theory of GAD and from his more general self-regulatory model of vulnerability to psychological disorders (Wells & Matthews, 1994). The scale consists of five factor-derived subscales: *positive worry beliefs* (factor 1); *beliefs about controllability and danger* (factor 2); *beliefs about cognitive competence* (factor 3); *general negative beliefs* (factor 4) (including responsibility, superstition, and punishment); and *cognitive self-consciousness* (factor 5). Items were derived both from interviews with undergraduates and from examination of cognitive therapy transcripts with anxiety outpatients. Respondents are asked to indicate how much they agree with each statement on a four-point Likert-type scale.

Administration and Scoring

The MCQ takes 15–20 minutes to administer. Separate factor scores are calculated by reverse-scoring certain items (indicated by * here) and then summing the appropriate items. The *positive worry beliefs* scale consists of items 1, 9, 12, 22, 26, 27, 30, 32, 35, 38, 44*, 46, 52, 54, 56, 60, 62, 63, and 65. The *beliefs about controllability and danger* scale consists of items 2, 5, 8, 11, 13, 18, 21, 31, 33, 36, 40, 42, 45, 48, 53, and 64. The *beliefs about cognitive competence* consists of items 3, 10, 16, 24, 28, 43, 47, 51, 57, and 58. The *general negative beliefs (including responsibility, superstition, and punishment)* scale consists of items 7, 15, 17, 19, 29, 34, 37, 39, 41*, 49, 50, 55, and 59. The *cognitive self-consciousness* scale consists of items 4, 6, 14, 20*, 23, 25, and 61.

Psychometric Properties

Preliminary psychometric analyses (initially reported in the original article) are summarized below.

Sample Means and Norms. The following means have been reported for samples of individuals diagnosed with GAD, OCD, and nonanxious controls: GAD: Factor 1, 32.9 (SD = 10.0); Factor 2, 47.5 (SD = 7.7); Factor 3, 22.8 (SD = 8.0); Factor 4, 27.7 (SD = 6.2); and Factor 5, 16.5 (SD = 5.4). OCD: Factor 1, 29.4 (SD = 11.1); Factor 2, 51.8 (SD = 8.2); Factor 3, 21.4 (SD = 7.8); Factor 4, 31.1 (SD = 10.5); and Factor 5, 21.9 (SD = 2.6). Nonanxious controls: Factor 1, 29.6 (SD = 8.8); Factor 2, 26.0 (SD = 6.3); Factor 3, 15.5 (SD = 4.2); Factor 4, 19.7 (SD = 6.7); and Factor 5, 14.9 (SD = 4.1).

Reliability. The subscales demonstrate adequate to good internal consistency in an undergraduate and graduate sample (αs ranging from .72 to .89) and adequate to very good test–retest reliabilities over 5 weeks among a university community sample (rs from .76 to .89 with an r of .94 for the total scale).

Validity. The factor structure was replicated by the original authors in a student sample. Although some items showed relatively weak item total correlations, they were retained in the scale to keep the measure comprehensive. All scales correlated significantly with a measure of trait anxiety (rs from .26 to .73), both subscales of the Padua Inventory (rs from .28 to .74), and the Anxious Thoughts Inventory (rs from .36 to .66). The MCQ significantly predicted scores on both scales of the Padua Inventory and the total Anxious Thoughts Inventory even when trait anxiety is controlled for. In these analyses, the subscales of uncontrollability, positive beliefs, and cognitive confidence all contributed to prediction. Finally, the potential clinical utility of the scale was demonstrated in findings of significant differences between clinical groups (individuals with GAD and OCD) and controls on several subscales.

Source

The MCQ is reprinted in Appendix B. For more information, contact Adrian Wells, Ph.D., Department of Clinical Psychology, University of Manchester, Rawnsley Building, Manchester Royal Infirmary, Manchester, United Kingdom; (tel) 44-161-276-5387; (fax) 44-161-273-2135; (e-mail) adrian.wells@man.ac.ak.

POSITIVE AND NEGATIVE AFFECT SCALES (PANAS)

Original Citation

Watson, D., Clark, L. A., & Tellegen, A. (1988). Development and validation of brief measures of positive and negative affect: The PANAS scales. *Journal of Personality and Social Psychology, 54,* 1063–1070.

Purpose

To assess the relatively independent factors of positive and negative affect.

Description

The PANAS is a 20-item self-report measure specifically designed to assess the distinct dimensions of *positive* and *negative* affect (PA and NA, respectively). According to the authors, the dimension of positive affect ranges from a state of enthusiasm and activation to a state of sluggishness and lethargy (i.e., low positive affect), whereas the dimension of negative affect ranges from a state of subjective distress and aversive arousal to a state of calmness and serenity (low negative affect). Items were chosen for inclusion from a larger set of mood descriptors if they loaded on only one of the two factors. Respondents are asked to indicate on a five-point Likert-type scale the extent to which they feel or have felt a list of adjectives over a specified time period. The PANAS has been used with multiple time frames, such as moment, today, past few days, week, past few weeks, year, and general. The use of briefer time intervals makes it a particularly useful measure of state mood changes.

Administration and Scoring

The PANAS can be administered in less than 5 minutes. Separate scores for the PA and NA scales are calculated by summing responses to items within each scale. The *positive affect* scale consists of items 1, 3, 5, 9, 10, 12, 14, 16, 17, and 18, whereas the *negative affect* scale consists of the remaining items.

Psychometric Properties

All psychometric information is from the original article unless otherwise stated.

Norms. Means for scales from a large normative undergraduate population using seven different time frame instructions are reported. For the "at this moment" instructions, the mean for the PA scale was 29.7 (*SD* = 7.9) and for the NA scale 14.8 (*SD* = 5.4). For the "general" instructions, the mean for the PA scale was 35.0 (*SD* = 6.4) and for the NA scale 18.1 (*SD* = 5.9). For an inpatient sample, using the "general" instructions, the mean for the PA scale was 32.5 (*SD* = 7.5) and for the NA scale 26.6 (*SD* = 9.2).

Reliability. Internal consistency estimates for both scales using all time instructions are good to excellent αs ranging from .88 to .90 for the PA scale; αs ranging from .84 to .87 for the NA scale. Test–retest reliabilities increase with longer time frames, ranging from .47 (moment) to .68 (general) for the PA scale and .39 (moment) to .71 (general) for the NA scale. The reliabilities for the PA and NA scales using the "general" instructions suggest adequate temporal stability for trait mood. Good internal consistency also has been demonstrated in small community and psychiatric samples, along with good temporal stability in psychiatric samples.

Validity. The factor structure of the PANAS is supported by findings that items on each scale correlated significantly with the appropriate higher-order factor derived from an expanded mood adjective measure and items did not correlate significantly with the other higher-order factor (i.e., positive affect items did not correlate with the negative affect factor). The factor structure has also been supported by independent investigators (Mackinnon et al., 1999) and within a Spanish-speaking sample (Sandin et al., 1999). The NA scale was significantly correlated with measures of general psychiatric distress ($r = .74$), depression ($r = .58$), and state anxiety ($r = .51$), whereas the PA scale was negatively correlated with measures of depression ($r = -.36$) in a student sample. In addition, the two scales show very modest correlations (*r*s range from $-.12$ to $-.23$) with one another, supporting the discrimination between the two factors.

Further, relatively more depressed individuals reported significantly lower scores on the PA scale than relatively more anxious individuals, whereas the two groups did not differ significantly on the NA scale, suggesting discriminative validity of the scale (Waikar & Craske, 1997). In addition, scores on the NA scale were significantly correlated with anxious and depressive symptoms, whereas scores on the PA scale were significantly negatively correlated with depressive symptoms 6 to 7 years later, supporting the predictive validity of the measure (Watson & Walker, 1996). Finally, although no treatment sensitivity data are available, sensitivity to change has been demonstrated in several findings, for example, increased PA following a social interaction among an undergraduate sample (McIntyre, Watson, Clark, & Cross, 1991).

Alternative Forms

The PANAS has been translated into French, German, Norwegian, Polish, Russian, and Spanish. A child version has also been developed and validated (Laurent et al., 1999). An expanded version of the scale, the PANAS-X, which includes additional scales assessing specific types of affect, is available from the authors.

Source

The PANAS is reprinted in the original article and in Appendix B. For more information and permission to use the scale, contact David B. Watson, Ph.D., Department of Psychology, University of Iowa, 11 Seashore Hall E, Iowa City, IA 52242-1407, USA; (tel) 319-335-3384; (fax) 319-335-0191; (e-mail) david-watson@uiowa.edu. Permission must also be obtained from the copyright holder, the American Psychological Association. There is no cost when the measure is used for noncommercial purposes. A manual for the PANAS is available from the author for a nominal fee.

SELF-RATING ANXIETY SCALE (SAS)

Original Citation

Zung, W. W. K. (1971). A rating instrument for anxiety disorders. *Psychosomatics, 12,* 371–379.

Purpose

To assess symptoms of anxiety as a clinical disorder.

Description

The SAS (which is also referred to as the SRAS and the Zung SAS) is a 20-item self-report measure that was developed to assess symptoms of anxiety disorders, based on diagnostic conceptualizations in DSM-II. It consists primarily of somatic symptoms (15 of the 20 items). The respondent indicates how often he or she has experienced each symptom on a four-point Likert-type scale ranging from "none or a little of the time" to "most or all of the time." In order to counter response bias, several items are reverse-scored.

Administration and Scoring

The SAS can be administered in 5 minutes. Items 5, 9, 13, 17, and 19 are reverse scored and then all items are summed for a raw score. An index is derived by dividing the raw score by the maximal possible score of 80 and then multiplying by 100. A table for conversion of raw scores is provided in the original article.

Psychometric Properties

Norms. The original article reports a mean index score of 58.7 ($SD = 13.8$) for patients with anxiety disorders (as defined by DSM-II) and a mean index score of 33.8 ($SD = 5.9$) for controls.

Reliability. According to the original article, the split-half reliability coefficient revealed adequate internal consistency ($r = .71$). Good internal consistency was found in a sample of Nigerian outpatients ($\alpha = .81$) and adequate internal consistency was revealed in a normal Nigerian sample ($\alpha = .69$; Jegede, 1977). Good test–retest reliability was demonstrated in a sample of individuals meeting DSM-III criteria for agoraphobia over a period ranging from 1 to 16 weeks ($rs = .81$ to $.84$; Michelson & Mavissakalian, 1983).

Validity. The original article revealed a significant correlation between SAS index scores and an interview-based measure of anxiety symptoms ($r = .66$ in a mixed sample, $r = .74$

in an anxiety disorder sample) as well as a moderate correlation between the SAS and another self-report measure of anxiety ($r = .30$). In this study, patients with anxiety disorders scored significantly higher on the SAS than did patients with schizophrenia, depressive disorder, personality disorder, and nonclinical controls. A similar significant difference was revealed between patients and controls in a study using a Nigerian sample (Jegede, 1977). Numerous psychosocial and psychopharmacological studies have demonstrated treatment sensitivity of the SAS.

Alternative Forms

The original article also describes and reprints an interview version of the SAS, the Anxiety Status Inventory, which is less commonly used currently. The SAS has been translated into Chinese, Italian, Portuguese, and Spanish.

Source

The SAS is reprinted in the original article and in Appendix B.

STATE–TRAIT ANXIETY INVENTORY (FORM Y) (STAI)

Original Citation

Spielberger, C. D., Gorsuch, R. L., Lushene, R., Vagg, P. R., & Jacobs, G. A. (1983). *Manual for the State–Trait Anxiety Inventory (Form Y)*. Palo Alto, CA: Mind Garden.

Purpose

To assess state and trait levels of anxiety.

Description

The STAI consists of two 20-item self-report measures that assess state and trait levels of anxiety. Standardized administration involves administering the state version prior to the trait version. Form Y is an altered version of the original Form X; items that seemed more closely related to depression or had weak psychometric properties in younger, less educated, or low-SES groups were replaced. Respondents indicate how much each statement reflects how they feel right *now*, at *this moment* (state version), or how they *generally* feel (trait version) on four-point Likert-type scales. Sample items from the state version include "I feel frightened" and "I feel pleasant." Sample items from the trait version include "I wish I could be as happy as others seem to be," "I am a steady person," and "I have disturbing thoughts."*

*Reproduced by special permission of the distributor, MIND GARDEN, Inc., 1690 Woodside Road #202, Redwood City, CA 94061 (650) 261-3500 from the State–Trait Anxiety Inventory by Charles D. Spielberger. Copyright 1977 by Charles D. Spielberger. All rights reserved. Further reproduction is prohibited without the Distributor's written consent.

Administration and Scoring

Both scales can be administered in 10 minutes. "Anxiety-absent" items on each scale are reverse-scored, and the 20 items of each scale are then summed for total scores. The manual provides percentile ranks for a range of populations, including gender- and age-specific rankings.

Psychometric Properties

Sample Means and Norms. The manual reports the following means for working adults: Men had a mean STAI-S score of 35.72 (SD = 10.40) and mean STAI-T score of 34.89 (SD = 9.19); women had a mean STAI-S score of 35.20 (SD = 10.61) and a mean STAI-T score of 34.79 (SD = 9.22). As noted above, percentile rankings are available in the manual. A review of treatment outcome studies for GAD reports mean pretreatment STAI-T scores for individuals diagnosed with GAD ranging from 47 to 61 (Fisher & Durham, 1999), whereas another study found mean STAI-T scores for individuals diagnosed with PDA ranging from 51 to 54 and for those diagnosed with PD ranging from 44 to 46 (Oei, Evans, & Crook, 1990).

Reliability. The manual reports good to excellent internal consistency for both scales (αs between .86 and .95) in adult, college, high school student, and military recruit samples. Also, adequate 30-day test–retest reliability was found for Form Y with high school students (rs .71 and .75) as well as 20-day test–retest reliability with Form X given to college students (rs .76 and .86).

Validity. Convergent validity for the STAI-T has been demonstrated in significant correlations with other trait measures of anxiety for both Forms X and Y in normal populations (e.g., Creamer et al., 1995; Spielberger et al., 1983). In addition, individuals diagnosed with anxiety disorders scored significantly higher on the STAI-T than did nonclinical volunteer participants (Bieling, Antony, & Swinson, 1998). Support for the validity of the STAI-S stems from findings of elevated scores in an exam situation (Lazarus & Opton, 1966) and decreases from pre- to postsurgery (Auerbach, 1973).

Although the two-factor (state and trait) solution has been supported in a clinical population (Oei et al., 1990), other studies have revealed a four-factor solution (Spielberger et al., 1980) with separate anxiety present and anxiety absent factors for both scales. In addition, a hierarchical model for the STAI-T was supported in a sample of individuals with anxiety disorders, suggesting that in addition to an overall factor, the trait scale contains lower-order factors of anxiety and depression (Bieling et al., 1998).

Several studies have suggested that the STAI does not discriminate well from measures of depression. The Bieling et al. (1998) study described above found the STAI-T was more highly correlated with a measure of depression than it was with a measure of anxiety. Other studies have found comparable correlations between the STAI-T and measures of anxiety and depression (e.g., Creamer et al., 1995), similarly challenging the discriminant validity of the scale.

Finally, the STAI-T is sensitive to change in treatment, as evidenced by a review of GAD treatment studies (Fisher & Durham, 1999). However, reliable change was less evident in this measure than in other measures of anxiety in at least one outcome study (Borkovec & Costello, 1993).

Alternative Forms

A child version of the STAI (STAIC) is available from the publishers. The STAI has been translated into 30 languages including Dutch, French, German, Hindi, Italian, and Spanish. A six-item version of the scale has also been developed (Marteau & Bekker, 1992).

Source

The STAI manual, instrument, and scoring guide are available for a fee of $25 US. The identical items plus permission to reproduce up to 200 copies of the scale may be obtained for $125 US. The STAI and related materials are available from Mind Garden, Inc., 1690 Woodside Rd., Suite 202, Redwood City, CA 94061, USA; (tel) 650-261-3500; (fax) 650-261-3505; (e-mail) info@mindgarden.com; (website) www.mindgarden.com.

THOUGHT CONTROL QUESTIONNAIRE (TCQ)

Original Citation

Wells, A., & Davies, M. (1994). The Thought Control Questionnaire —A measure of individual differences in the control of unwanted thoughts. *Behaviour Research and Therapy*, *32*, 871–878.

Purpose

To assess strategies for controlling unpleasant and unwanted thoughts.

Description

The TCQ is a 30-item self-report measure designed to assess individual differences in the use of different thought control strategies. Because attempts to control unwanted thoughts have been proposed both as maintaining factors in anxiety disorders (e.g., Wegner, 1994) and as treatment strategies (e.g., reappraisal, Beck & Emery, 1985), it is important to better understand the consequences of various strategies used to control thoughts. For this purpose, a large pool of items reflecting various thought control strategies was developed from open-ended interviews with both anxiety disorder patients and nonpatient controls. These items were subjected to two successive factor analyses in large nonclinical samples. Five subscales, of six items each, were derived: *distraction*, *social control*, *worry*, *punishment*, and *re-appraisal*. Respondents are asked to indicate how often they generally use each technique on a four-point Likert-type scale.

Administration and Scoring

The TCQ takes 5 to 10 minutes to complete. Items 5, 8, and 12 are reverse scored. Subscale scores are derived by summing items: *distraction* consists of items 1, 9, 16, 19, 21, and

30; *social control* consists of items 5, 8, 12, 17, 25, and 29; *worry* consists of items 4, 7, 18, 22, 24, and 26; *punishment* consists of items 2, 6, 11, 13, 15, and 28; and *re-appraisal* consists of items 3, 10, 14, 20, 23, and 27. A total score is derived by summing all 30 items (with 5, 8, and 12 reverse-scored).

Psychometric Properties

Sample Means and Norms.   The original article reports means for total score and each subscale, by gender, for a normative sample. Warda and Bryant (1998) report means for two groups of individuals who had experienced a motor vehicle accident: those who were diagnosed with Acute Stress Disorder (ASD) and those who were not. Individuals with ASD reported the following means: *distraction*, 14.60 (*SD* = 3.42); *social control*, 13.30 (*SD* = 4.32); *worry*, 11.85 (*SD* = 3.22); *punishment*, 10.80 (*SD* = 3.92); and *re-appraisal*, 13.60 (*SD* = 3.90). Individuals without ASD reported the following means: *distraction*, 13.95 (*SD* = 4.52); *social control*, 14.10 (*SD* = 3.40); *worry*, 8.45 (*SD* = 2.16); *punishment*, 8.00 (*SD* = 2/05); and *re-appraisal*, 12.00 (*SD* = 3.15).

Reliability.   Internal consistency of the subscales was marginal to adequate in the original normative sample (αs ranging from .64 to .79, punishment and reappraisal were below .70) and similar in a clinical sample of individuals with depression and PTSD (αs ranging from .67 to .78, punishment, reappraisal, and social control were below .70; Reynolds & Wells, 1999). In the original study, 6-week test–retest reliability ranged from .67 to .83 for the subscales and was .83 for the total scale.

Validity.   The original five-factor solution of the TCQ was derived in a normative sample; however, a very similar structure emerged from a clinical sample of individuals with PTSD and depression (Reynolds & Wells, 1999). The distraction factor emerged as two separate factors representing cognitive and behavioral distraction, but because only two items comprised the former factor the authors recommend continued use of the original five factors. The punishment and worry subscales show expected significant associations with measures of anxiety, worry, and neuroticism in the original normative sample. Similar associations were found between these two factors and measures of intrusion, anxiety, and depression in clinical samples (Reynolds & Wells, 1999). In addition, in the latter study, social control was negatively associated with a measure of avoidance, distraction was negatively associated with measures of depression and anxiety, and reappraisal was negatively associated with measures of depression. These findings suggest that whereas punishment and worry may represent maladaptive ways of controlling thoughts, other strategies (such as talking to others) may prove more effective. Consistent with the former conclusion, individuals with OCD, PTSD, ASD, and depression display elevated levels of punishment and worry strategies in comparison with controls (Amir, Cashman, & Foa, 1997; Reynolds & Wells, 1999; Warda & Bryant, 1998). Finally, decreases in punishment and worry and increases in appraisal and distraction are associated with symptom improvement among individuals with PTSD and depression (Reynolds & Wells, 1999), suggesting that increased adaptive and decreased maladaptive thought control strategies correspond to symptom relief.

Source

The items for the TCQ are reproduced in a factor table in the original article and the scale is reprinted in Appendix B. For more information, contact Dr. Adrian Wells, University of

Manchester Department of Clinical Psychology, Rawnsley Building, Manchester Royal Infirmary, Manchester, United Kingdom; (tel) 44-161-276-5387; (fax) 44-161-273-2135; (e-mail) adrian.wells@man.ac.ak.

TRIMODAL ANXIETY QUESTIONNAIRE (TAQ)

Original Citation

Lehrer, P. M., & Woolfolk, R. L. (1982). Self-report assessment of anxiety: Somatic, cognitive, and behavioral modalities. *Behavioral Assessment, 4,* 167–177.

Purpose

To assess somatic, behavioral, and cognitive aspects of anxiety.

Description

The TAQ is a 36-item self-report measure that was developed to separately assess the cognitive, somatic, and behavioral domains of anxiety. The 16 items that make up the somatic scale, the 19 items of the behavioral scale, and the 11 items of the cognitive scale are those items with the highest factor loadings from a larger pool of items used to develop the measure. The individual responds to each statement on a nine-point Likert-type scale indicating how often he or she experiences each item. This scale has also been called the Lehrer–Woolfolk Anxiety Symptom Questionnaire, the Anxiety Symptom Questionnaire, and the Three Systems Anxiety Questionnaire, although the authors' preferred title is the TAQ. The scale is typically administered under the title "Symptom Questionnaire."

Administration and Scoring

The TAQ takes 5 to 10 minutes to administer. Three subscale scores are derived by summing all items on the scale. The *somatic scale* is comprised of items 1, 2, 4, 7, 10, 13, 14, 18, 20, 23, 29–31, and 33–35; the *cognitive scale* is comprised of items 5, 8, 11, 15, 16, 19, 21, 24, 27, 32, and 36; and the *behavioral scale* consists of items 3, 6, 9, 12, 17, 22, 25, 26, and 28.

Psychometric Properties

Sample Means and Norms.   Scholing and Emmelkamp (1992) reported the following means for individuals with social phobia: *somatic,* 31.7 (SD = 12.8), *behavioral,* 28.2 (SD = 8.3), and *cognitive,* 31.3 (SD = 8.2); and for a normal adult sample: *somatic,* 23.5 (SD = 7.1), *behavioral,* 16.1 (SD = 6.0), and *cognitive,* 22.4 (SD = 6.7). Koksal, Power, and Sharp (1991) reported the following means for individuals with phobic disorders: *somatic,* 44.0 (SD = 18.6), *behavioral,* 54.1 (SD = 26.2), and *cognitive,* 52.3 (SD = 18.1); and for individuals with nonphobic anxiety disorders: *somatic,* 37.7 (SD = 17.4), *behavioral,* 37.8 (SD = 19.5), and *cognitive,* 54.2 (SD = 17.6).

Reliability.   Split-half reliabilities for the subscales ranged from .83 to .85 in a college sample and from .91 to .93 in a mixed clinical/community sample (Lehrer & Woolfolk, 1982). Good internal consistency was also demonstrated in a sample of individuals with social phobia (αs range from .83 to .92; Scholing and Emmelkamp, 1992). No data regarding test–retest reliability have been published.

Validity.   The three-factor structure was supported in a sample of individuals with social phobia, a sample of nonclinical adults, and a sample of nonclinical adolescents (Scholing & Emmelkamp, 1992). The validity of the factor structure is further supported by findings of moderate correlations among the three scales (rs between .47 and .66), suggesting the scales measure related but distinct constructs (Lehrer & Woolfolk, 1982). Convergent validity is suggested by significant correlations between all three subscales and a measure of trait anxiety (rs between .60 and .86) as well as a measure of neuroticism (rs between .32 and .67) for both patient and student samples, and significant correlations with a measure of general distress among patients (rs between .60 and .70; Lehrer & Woolfolk, 1982). Differential associations have also been found for subscales in a clinical sample. Whereas only the somatic subscale is significantly correlated with the general anxiety factor of the Hamilton Anxiety Rating Scale ($r = .50$), the behavioral subscale is most strongly correlated with Eysenck's Introversion Scale ($r = .60$; Lehrer & Woolfolk, 1982). Further evidence for the clinical utility of the scale stems from the finding that scores significantly differentiate a sample of socially phobic individuals from a nonclinical adult sample (Scholing & Emmelkamp, 1982), with the behavioral subscale most effectively discriminating the groups. Finally, an analogue intervention study revealed a specific association between intervention and symptom reduction: A cognitive intervention led to significant reduction on the cognitive scale only, whereas a behavioral intervention led to significant reduction on the behavioral scale only (as cited in Lehrer & Woolfolk, 1982).

Alternative Forms

The TAQ has been translated into Dutch.

Source

The TAQ is reprinted in Appendix B. For more information contact Paul Lehrer, Ph.D. Professor of Psychiatry, UMDNJ–RW Johnson Medical School, 671 Hoes Lane, Piscataway, NJ 08854 USA; (tel) 732-235-4413; (fax) 732-235-4430; (e-mail) lehrer@umdnj.edu.

BRIEF DESCRIPTIONS OF ADDITIONAL MEASURES

Acceptance and Action Questionnaire (AAQ)

The AAQ is a very recent nine-item self-report measure that assesses emotional avoidance and emotion-focused inaction (or, conversely, emotional acceptance and action), constructs likely to be related to anxiety and salient in individuals with anxiety disorders. The scale is currently unpublished but its psychometric properties have been established (Hayes et al., 2001). AAQ scores show a significant correlation with measures of anxiety and phobic avoidance in both clinical and nonclinical samples, and individuals diagnosed with agoraphobia score significantly higher on the measure than do nonanxious individuals (Hayes et al., 2000). For more information contact Steven C. Hayes, Ph.D., Department of Psychology/296, University of Nevada, Reno, NV 89557-0062, USA; (tel) 775-784-6829; (fax) 775-784-1126; (e-mail) hayes@scs.unr.edu.

Affective Control Scale (ACS)

This 42-item self-report measure assesses fear of loss of control when experiencing strong affective states. This measure extends the fear of fear construct and includes subscales assessing *fear of anxiety, fear of depression, fear of anger*, and *fear of strong positive affective states*. Items from the scale, along with its psychometric properties in a nonclinical sample, are presented in the original article (Williams, Chambless, & Ahrens, 1997) and a subsequent article reports on validity and reliability in a nonclinical sample (Berg, Shapiro, Chambless, & Ahrens, 1998). For more information about the measure, contact Dianne L. Chambless, Ph.D., Department of Psychology, University of North Carolina at Chapel Hill, Chapel Hill, NC 27599-3270, USA; (tel) 919-962-3989; (fax) 919-962-2537; (e-mail) chambles@email.unc.edu; (website) www.unc.edu/~chambles/questionnaires/index.html.

Anxiety Attitude and Belief Scale (AABS)

The AABS is a newly developed, 36-item self-report measure designed to assess attitudes and beliefs thought to index a psychological vulnerability to anxiety disorder (Brown, Craske, Tata, Rassovsky, & Tsao, 2000). Initial factor analysis in an undergraduate population revealed three factors: *vigilance-avoidance, catastrophizing*, and *imagination*. The scale's items along with its initial psychometric properties (including evidence for predictive validity specific to anxiety versus depression) are presented in the original article. For more information, contact Dr. Gary Brown, Centre for Applied Social and Psychological Development, Salomons Centre, Canterbury Christchurch University College, Turnbridge Wells, TN3 0TG, United Kingdom; (tel) +44 1892 507 704; (fax) +44 1892 507 660; (e-mail) g.brown22@salomons.org.uk.

Anxiety Screening Questionnaire (ASQ-15)

The ASQ-15 is a brief anxiety disorder screening instrument designed for use in a primary care setting (Wittchen & Boyer, 1998). It consists of stem questions for major depressive disorders, panic disorder, social phobia, agoraphobia, PTSD, and GAD, as well as specific questions assessing DSM-IV and ICD-10 criteria for GAD. The scale and a preliminary investigation of its psychometric properties are presented in Wittchen and Boyer (1998).

Anxious Self-Statements Questionnaire (ASSQ)

The ASSQ is a 32-item self-report measure of the frequency of anxiety-related cognitive self-statements. A large pool of theoretically derived items was reduced to those items that significantly discriminated high and low trait-anxious individuals (Kendall & Hollon, 1989). The items, along with psychometric properties of the scale in an undergraduate sample, are presented in the original article. A subsequent study explored the content specificity of the measure along with a measure of depression-related cognitive statements, and found that the scale may be better conceptualized as containing two subscales, one consisting of self-statements about *one's inability to cope* and the other consisting of self-statements reflecting *anxiety/uncertainty about the future* (Safren et al., 2000). The scale has been translated in Spanish. For more information, contact Philip C. Kendall, Ph.D., Department of Psychology, Weiss Hall, Temple University, Philadelphia, PA 19122, USA; (fax) 215-204-5339.

Anxious Thoughts Inventory (AnTI)

The AnTI is a 22-item self-report measure that assesses three dimensions of generalized worry: *social worry*, *health worry*, and *meta-worry*. The scale was derived from factor analysis of a large pool of worry items. The first two scales reflect content areas of worry, whereas the meta-worry scale reflects worrying about the uncontrollability of thoughts, or worrying about worrying. The scale and its psychometric properties are presented in the original article (Wells, 1994). For more information, contact Dr. Adrian Wells, University of Manchester Department of Clinical Psychology, Rawnsley Building, Manchester Royal Infirmary, Manchester, United Kingdom; (tel) 44-161-276-5387; (fax) 44-161-273-2135; (e-mail) adrian.wells@man.ac.ak.

Anxious Thoughts and Tendencies Scale (AT&T)

The AT&T is a self-report measure of a general anxiety-prone cognitive style. The original measure included 19 items and was designed to assess three main anxiety-related cognitive distortions (catastrophizing, selective abstraction, and intrusive thoughts; Ganellen, Matuzas, Uhlenhuth, Glass, & Easton, 1986), although analyses in a clinical sample indicated that the scale was better conceptualized as unidimensional. The AT&T was recently revised so as to clarify and simplify items; analyses in a community sample supported its reliability and validity and suggested that it be reduced to 15 items (Uhlenhuth, McCarty, Paine, & Warner, 1999). For more information about the scale, contact E. H. Uhlenhuth, M.D., University of New Mexico, School of Medicine, Department of Psychiatry, 2400 Tucker, N.E., Albequerque, NM 87131 USA; (tel) 505-272-8876; (fax) 505-272-5572; (e-mail) uhli@unm.edu.

Cardiac Anxiety Questionnaire (CAQ)

The CAQ is an 18-item self-report measure recently developed to assess heart-focused anxiety among individuals with and without heart disease (Eifert et al., 2000). The scale consists of three subscales that assess heart-related *fear*, *avoidance*, and *attention*. The scale, along with its preliminary psychometric properties, is presented in the original article. For more information, contact Georg H. Eifert, Ph.D., 3950 Kalaa Wai, #T-101, Wailea, HI 96753, USA; (e-mail) geifert@aol.com.

Cognition Checklist (CCL)

The CCL is a 26-item self-report measure designed to assess the frequency of depression and anxiety-related automatic thoughts (Beck, Brown, Steer, Eidelson, & Riskind, 1987). It contains a 14-item *depression* and a 12-item *anxiety* subscale (CCL-A). Scales are comprised of items that discriminated between predominantly anxious and predominantly depressed outpatients. The items of the CCL, along with the preliminary psychometric properties of the subscales, are presented in the original article, and an additional psychometric study is reported in Steer, Beck, Clark, and Beck (1994). The latter study found that the CCL-A demonstrated discriminant validity in a clinical, but not in a student, sample. In addition, Taylor, Koch, Woody and McLean (1997) found that both scales had good convergent and discriminant validity. Taylor et al. (1997) also reported that although the CCL-D showed good criterion-related validity, the CCL-A was weaker in this regard. For more information, contact Aaron T. Beck, M.D., Center for Cognitive Therapy, Department of Psychiatry, University of Pennsylvania, Room 754, 3600 Market Street, Philadelphia, PA 19104-2648, USA; (tel) 215-898-4102; (fax) 215-573-3717; (e-mail) becka@landru.cpr.upenn.edu.

Cognitive Somatic Anxiety Questionnaire (CSAQ)

The CSAQ is a 14-item self-report measure designed to assess the *cognitive* and *somatic* components of trait anxiety. The scale is comprised of two separate subscales that assess each dimension. The original article (Schwartz, Davidson, & Goleman, 1978) reprints the scale and presents evidence that each subscale is differentially associated with self-regulation techniques (i.e., physical exercise is associated with less somatic and more cognitive anxiety than meditation). Psychometric data are presented by DeGood and Tait (1987) and Steptoe and Kearsley (1990); means for different anxiety disorder groups are presented by Koksal et al. (1991). The CSAQ has been translated into Spanish. For more information about the scale, contact Gary E. Schwartz, Ph.D., University of Arizona, Department of Psychology, Rm 324, Tucson, AZ 85721, USA; (tel) 520-621-3248; (fax) 520-621-3249; (e-mail) gschwart@u.arizona.edu.

Endler Multidimensional Anxiety Scales (EMAS)

The EMAS is a self-report measure of anxiety with three components: the *state* scale (EMAS-S), the *trait* scale (EMAS-T), and the *perception* scale (EMAS-P). The EMAS-S is a 20-item measure that assesses two components of state anxiety: *autonomic-emotional* and *cognitive* worry. The EMAS-T is a 60-item measure that assesses four general situational dimensions of anxiety: *social evaluation*, *physical danger*, *ambiguous*, and *daily routines*. The EMAS-P consists of 8 items that assess an individual's perception of the type and level of threat during a specific event. Psychometric properties of the scales are presented in the manual (Endler, Edwards, & Vitelli, 1991); support for its factor structure and validity in the differential assessment of anxiety and depression is presented elsewhere (e.g., Endler, Cox, Parker, & Bagby, 1992; Endler, Parker, Bagby, & Cox, 1991). The EMAS is published by Western Psychological Services, 12031 Wilshire Boulevard, Los Angeles, CA 90025, USA; (tel) 213-478-2061; (fax) 213-478-7838; (webpage) www.wpspublish.com.

Fear of Pain Questionnaire III (FPQ-III)

The FPQ-III is a 30-item self-report measure that assesses fears about pain and can be used in chronic pain inpatient, general medical outpatient, and nonpain populations. It assesses fear of specific types of pain and painful situations. The scale and its psychometric properties are presented in McNeil and Rainwater (1998). Additional information can be obtained from Daniel W. McNeil, Ph.D., Department of Psychology, Anxiety and Psychophysiology Research Laboratory and Clinic, West Virginia University, P.O. Box 6040, Morgantown, WV 26506-6040, USA; (tel) 304-293-2001, ext. 622; (fax) 304-293-6606; (e-mail) dmcneil@ wvu.edu.

Four Dimensional Anxiety and Depression Scale (FDADS)

This 24-item self-report measure was developed to assess four dimensions (*emotional, physical, cognitive,* and *behavioral*) of both *anxiety* and *depression*, resulting in eight subscales of three items each (Bystritsky, Waikar, & Vapnik, 1996). The anxiety subscales were derived from a 40-item Four Dimensional Anxiety Scale, by selecting those items that best discriminated between measures of anxiety and depression (Bystritsky, Linn, & Ware, 1990). Items from depression measures that corresponded to each of the four components were added to compose the four depression subscales. The items of the FDADS, along with its psychometric properties, are presented in Bystritsky et al. (1996). For more information, contact Alexander Bystritsky, M.D., Ph.D., Neuropsychiatric Institute and Hospital, Anxiety Disorders Program, 300 UCLA Medical Plaza, Los Angeles, CA 90024-1759, USA; (tel) 310-206-5133; (fax) 310-206-4310; (e-mail) abystritsky@mednet.ucla.edu.

Four Systems Anxiety Questionnaire (FSAQ)

The FSAQ is a 60-item self-report measure designed to assess four components of anxiety: *cognitive, feeling* (affective), *behavioral,* and *somatic.* The authors note that the traditional three-system theory (assessed by the TAQ described earlier) compounds subjective/ feeling states and cognitions into the cognitive system; this scale provides separate scales devoted to each. Koksal and Power (1990) describe the development of the scale and its psychometric properties (including treatment sensitivity); its relationship to other multisystem measures of anxiety (the TAQ and CSAQ, both described in this chapter) across the anxiety disorders is described in Koksal et al. (1991).

Health Anxiety Questionnaire (HAQ)

The HAQ is a 21-item self-report measure developed to assess degree of health-related concern (Lucock & Morley, 1996). Cluster analysis revealed four subscales of the measure: *health worry and preoccupation, fear of illness and death, reassurance-seeking behavior,* and *interference with life.* The original article presents items from the scale along with its psychometric properties. For more information, contact Dr. Stephen Morley, Division of Psychiatry and Behavioral Sciences in Relation to Medicine, School of Medicine, University of Leeds, Leeds, LS2 9LT, United Kingdom.

Looming Maladaptive Style Questionnaire-Revised (LMSQ-R)

The LMSQ-R was developed to assess a general cognitive style, thought to be a unique cognitive vulnerability common to anxiety disorders, which is characterized by the perspective that degree of danger is rapidly intensifying and rising in risk (Riskind, Williams, Gessner, Chrosniak, & Cortina, in press; Riskind & Williams, in press; Riskind, 1997). The measure consists of six brief vignettes of potentially threatening situations followed by eight questions, three of which assess the perception of increasing threat and constitute the *looming maladaptive style* subscale (Riskind et al., 2000). A variety of studies provide support for the validity of the scale, including its ability to predict worry and catastrophic thinking. For the most comprehensive review of the current model of looming vulnerability, research using the scale, and its application to different phenomena and disorders, see Riskind and Williams (in press). For more information, contact John H. Riskind, Ph.D., Department of Psychology, George Mason University, David King Hall MSN 3F5, Fairfax, VA 22030-4444, USA; (tel) 703-993-4094; (fax) 703- 993-1359; (e-mail) jriskind@gmu.edu.

Mood Anxiety Symptom Questionnaire (MASQ)

This 90-item self-report measure was designed specifically to assess Clark and Watson's (1991) tripartite model of anxiety and depression. It consists of five subscales: *general distress: mixed symptoms*, *general distress: depressive symptoms*, *general distress : anxiety symptoms*, *anxious arousal*, and *anhedonic depression*. These scales are proposed to assess the three factors of anxiety and depression, with the first three scales assessing the general distress factor, whereas the latter two scales assess anxiety- and depression-specific symptoms, respectively. Studies have supported the reliability and convergent validity of the subscales, as well as the discriminant validity of the two specific subscales (i.e., anxious arousal and anhedonic depression; Watson, Weber, et al., 1995). The three-factor model of anxiety and depression has been supported in factor analyses of the scale across several samples, although these analyses have suggested the need for refinements in specific items of the five subscales, which are currently under way (Watson, Clark, et al., 1995). A 62-item short form, which omits the *general distress: mixed symptoms* factor, has also been developed (Watson & Walker, 1996). For more information about the MASQ, contact David B. Watson, Ph.D., Department of Psychology, University of Iowa, 11 Seashore Hall E, Iowa City, IA 52242-1407, USA; (tel) 319-335-3384; (fax) 319-335-0191; (e-mail) david-watson@uiowa.edu.

Multidimensional Anxiety Questionnaire (MAQ)

The MAQ is a 40-item self-report measure that assesses a range of anxiety symptoms over the previous month. In addition to providing a total scale score, the MAQ contains four subscales: *physiological-panic*, *social phobia*, *worry-fears*, and *negative affectivity*. The manual (Reynolds, 1999) provides standard scores and clinical cutoffs for the total score and for each subscale score, and also reviews the psychometric properties of the scale. The MAQ and the manual can be obtained from Psychological Assessment Resources, Inc., P.O. Box 998, Odessa, FL 33556, USA; (tel) 800-331-TEST or 813-968-3003; (webpage) www.par-inc.com.

Multidimensional Perfectionism Scale (MPS)

Concurrent with the development of the Frost Multidimensional Perfectionism Scale, Hewitt and Flett (1991) developed a 45-item self-report measure of perfectionism. This scale consists of three subscales: *self-oriented* perfectionism (SO), which reflects a tendency to be perfectionistic with oneself, *other-oriented* perfectionism, which reflects a tendency to expect perfection from other people, and *socially prescribed* perfectionism, which reflects an individual's belief that others expect perfection from him or her. The reliability and validity of the scale have been demonstrated in clinical, community, and student populations. Psychometric properties are presented in the original article (Hewitt & Flett, 1991) and in a subsequent study by the authors (Hewitt, Flett, Turnbull-Donovan, & Mikail, 1991). Antony, Purdon, et al. (1998) present data on perfectionism across the anxiety disorders using both this and Frost's measure. For more information on the MPS, contact Paul L. Hewitt, Ph.D., Department of Psychology, University of British Columbia, 2136 West Mall, Vancouver, BC, V6T 1Z4, Canada; (tel) 604-822-5827; (fax) 604-822-6923; (e-mail) phewitt@cortex.psych.ubc.ca. The scale is published by Multihealth Systems, Inc., 908 Niagara Falls Blvd., North Tonawanda, NY 14120-2060, USA; (tel) 800-456-3003 (USA) or 800-268-6011 (Canada); (fax) 416-492-3343 or 888-540-4484.

Pain Anxiety Symptoms Scale (PASS)

This 40-item self-report measure was designed to measure fear of pain across cognitive, behavioral, and physiological domains. The scale consists of four subscales: *avoidance, cognitive anxiety, fearful thinking,* and *physiological anxiety.* Psychometric properties of the scale are presented in the original article (McCracken, Zayfert, & Gross, 1992) and in later papers (Burns, Mullen, Higdon, Wei, & Lansky, 2000; McCracken & Gross, 1995). For more information, contact Lance McCracken, Ph.D., Pain Management Unit, Royal National Hospital for Rheumatic Diseases, Bath BA1 1RL, United Kingdom; (tel) 44 1225 473403; (fax) 44 1225 473461; (e-mail) lance.mccracken@rnhrd-tr.swest.nhs.uk.

Reactions to Tests (RTT)

The RTT is a 40-item self-report measure that assesses four dimensions of test-related anxiety: *tension, worry, test-irrelevant thinking,* and *bodily symptoms* (Sarason, 1984). Items were derived in part from an earlier test anxiety inventory by the same author, the Test Anxiety Scale (TAS); other items were rationally derived so as to tap the multiple dimensions of test anxiety. The original article describes the development of the scale and initial studies utilizing the measure. For more information about the RTT, contact Irwin G. Sarason, Ph.D., Department of Psychology, Box 351525, University of Washington, Seattle, WA 98195, USA; (tel) 206-543-6542; (fax) 206-685-3157; (e-mail) isarason@u.washington.edu.

Taylor Manifest Anxiety Scale (TMAS)

The TMAS was developed by Taylor in 1953 to assess anxiety. Items from the original MMPI were selected and a 50-item self-report measure with true–false response options was developed. The items of the scale, along with psychometric properties and normative data, are presented in the original article (Taylor, 1953). Although this scale was very popular for many years, it is now used infrequently.

Test Anxiety Inventory (TAI)

The TAI is a 20-item self-report measure that assesses trait levels of test anxiety, with separate scales assessing the *worry* and *emotionality* components of this construct. The TAI has been translated into numerous languages. The scale was developed by Charles Spielberger and can be purchased (along with a manual) from Mind Garden, Inc., 1690 Woodside Rd., Suite 202, Redwood City, CA 94061, USA; (tel) 650-261-3500; (fax) 650-261-3505; (e-mail) info@mindgarden.com; (website) www.mindgarden.com.

White Bear Suppression Inventory (WBSI)

The WBSI is a 15-item self-report measure developed to assess the tendency to suppress thoughts. Thought suppression has been theoretically and empirically associated with many psychiatric symptoms, including obsessive and depressive symptoms (see Wegner, 1994, for a review). The original article (Wegner & Zanakos, 1994) presents the scale items and reviews several studies that support the reliability and validity of the scale. For instance, the WBSI was correlated with anxious affect and obsessional thinking and was associated with failure to physiologically habituate to emotional thoughts. Muris, Merckelbach, and Horselenberg (1996) present further support for the psychometric strength of the measure, and Spinhoven and van der Does (1999) present evidence of its reliability and validity in a clinical sample. For more information about the WBSI, contact Daniel M. Wegner, Ph.D., Department of Psychology, Harvard University, 1470 William James Hall, 33 Kirkland Street, Cambridge, MA 02138, USA; (tel) 617-496-2596; (webpage) http://www.wjh.harvard.edu/~wegner/.

Worry-Emotionality Scale–Revised (WES)

The WES is a 10-item self-report measure of state levels of test anxiety. The scale is based on a two component (*worry* and *emotionality*) conceptualization of test anxiety and evidence that these cognitive and emotional components show differential performance interference and treatment response. The revised version of the scale was derived from factor analysis; each component (i.e., worry-cognitive, emotionality-somatic) is assessed by five items. The scale and its psychometric properties are presented in Morris, Davis, and Hutchings (1981). Further psychometric properties are presented in Steptoe and Kearsley (1990). For more information, contact Dr. Larry W. Morris, Department of Psychology, Middle Tennessee State University, P.O. Box 87, 1301 E. Main St., Murfreesboro, TN 37132, USA; (tel) 615-898-2729; (fax) 615-898-5027; (e-mail) lmorris@frank.mtsu.edu.

REFERENCES

Amir, N., Cashman, L., & Foa, E. B. (1997). Strategies of thought control in obsessive compulsive disorder. *Behaviour Research and Therapy, 35*, 775–777.

Antony, M. M., Bieling, P. J., Cox, B. J., Enns, M. W., & Swinson, R. P. (1998). Psychometric properties of the 42-item and 21-item versions of the Depression Anxiety Stress Scales (DASS) in clinical groups and a community sample. *Psychological Assessment, 10*, 176–181.

Antony, M. M., Purdon, C., Huta, V., & Swinson, R. P. (1998). Dimensions of perfectionism across the anxiety disorders. *Behaviour Research and Therapy, 36*, 1143–1154.

Auerbach, S. M. (1973). Trait–state anxiety and adjustment to surgery. *Journal of Consulting and Clinical Psychology, 40,* 264–271.

Aylard, P. R., Gooding, J. H., McKenna, P. J., & Snaith, R. P. (1987). A validation study of three anxiety and depression self-assessment scales. *Journal of Psychosomatic Research, 31,* 261–268.

Barlow, D. H. (in press). *Anxiety and its disorders: The nature and treatment of anxiety and panic* (2nd ed.). New York: Guilford.

Bech, P., Allerup, P., Maier, W., Albus, M., Lavori, P., & Ayuso, J. L. (1992). The Hamilton Scales and the Hopkins Symptom Checklist (SCL-90): A cross-national validity study in patients with panic disorders. *British Journal of Psychiatry, 160,* 206–211.

Beck, A. T., Brown, G., Steer, R. A., Eidelson, J. I., & Riskind, J. H. (1987). Differentiating anxiety and depression: A test of the cognitive content-specificity hypothesis. *Journal of Abnormal Psychology, 96,* 179–183.

Beck, A. T. B., Emery, G., & Greenberg, R. L. (1985). *Anxiety disorders and phobias: A cognitive perspective.* New York: Basic Books.

Beck, A. T., & Steer, R. A. (1991). Relationship between the Beck Anxiety Inventory and the Hamilton Anxiety Rating Scale with anxious outpatients. *Journal of Anxiety Disorders, 5,* 213–223.

Beck, A. T., & Steer, R. A. (1993). *Beck Anxiety Inventory manual.* San Antonio, TX: Psychological Corporation.

Berg, C. Z., Shapiro, N., Chambless, D. L., & Ahrens, A. H. (1998). Are emotions frightening? II: An analogue study of fear of emotion, interpersonal conflict, and panic onset. *Behaviour Research and Therapy, 36,* 3–15.

Bieling, P. J., Antony, M. M., & Swinson, R. P. (1998). The State–Trait Anxiety Inventory, Trait Version: Structure and content re-examined. *Behaviour Research and Therapy, 36,* 777–788.

Borkovec, T. D., & Costello, E. (1993). Efficacy of applied relaxation and cognitive–behavioral therapy in the treatment of generalized anxiety disorder. *Journal of Consulting and Clinical Psychology, 61,* 611–619.

Brown, G. P., Craske, M. G., Tata, P., Rassovsky, Y., & Tsao, J. C. I. (2000). The anxiety attitude and belief scale: Initial psychometric properties in an undergraduate sample. *Clinical Psychology and Psychotherapy, 7,* 230–239.

Brown, T. A., Chorpita, B. F., Korotitsch, W., & Barlow, D. H. (1997). Psychometric properties of the Depression Anxiety Stress Scales (DASS) in clinical samples. *Behaviour Research and Therapy, 35,* 79–89.

Bruss, G. S., Gruenberg, A. M., Goldstein, R. D., & Barber, J. P. (1994). Hamilton Anxiety Rating Scale interview guide: Joint interview and test–retest methods for inter-rater reliability. *Psychiatry Research, 53,* 191–202.

Burns, J. W., Mullen, J. T., Higdon, L. J., Wei, J. M., & Lansky, D. (2000). Validity of the Pain Anxiety Symptoms Scale (PASS): Prediction of physical capacity variables. *Pain, 84,* 247–252.

Bystritsky, A., Linn, L. S., & Ware, J. E. (1990). Development of a multidimensional scale of anxiety. *Journal of Anxiety Disorders, 4,* 99–115.

Bystritsky, A., Waikar, S. V., & Vapnik, T. (1996). Four-Dimensional Anxiety and Depression Scale: A preliminary psychometric report. *Anxiety, 2,* 47–50.

Chambless, D. L., Caputo, G. C., Jasin, S. E., Gracely, E. J., & Williams, C. (1985). The Mobility Inventory for Agoraphobia. *Behaviour Research and Therapy, 23,* 35–44.

Clark, L. A., & Watson, D. (1991). Tripartite model of anxiety and depression: Psychometric evidence and taxonomic implications. *Journal of Abnormal Psychology, 100,* 316–336.

Cox, B. J., Cohen, E., Direnfeld, D. M., & Swinson, R. P. (1996). Does the Beck Anxiety Inventory measure anything beyond panic attack symptoms? *Behaviour Research and Therapy, 34,* 949–954.

Cox, B. J., Swinson, R. P., Kuch, K., & Reichman, J. T. (1993). Dimensions of agoraphobia assessed by the Mobility Inventory. *Behaviour Research and Therapy, 31,* 427–431.

Cox, B. J., Swinson, R. P., Parker, J. D., Kuch, K., & Reichman, J. T. (1993). Confirmatory factor analysis of the Fear Questionnaire in panic disorder with agoraphobia. *Psychological Assessment, 5,* 235–237.

Cox, B. J., Swinson, R. P., & Shaw, B. F. (1991). Value of the Fear Questionnaire in differentiating agoraphobia and social phobia. *British Journal of Psychiatry, 159,* 842–845.

Creamer, M., Foran, J., & Bell, R. (1995) The Beck Anxiety Inventory in a non-clinical sample. *Behaviour Research and Therapy, 33,* 477–485.

Davidson, J. R. T., Potts, N. L. S., Richichi, E. A., Ford, S. M., Krishnan, R. R., Smith, R. D., & Wilson, W. (1991). The Brief Social Phobia Scale. *Journal of Clinical Psychiatry, 52* (11, Suppl.), 48–51.

de Beurs, E., Wilson, K. A., Chambless, D. L., Goldstein, A. J., & Feske, U. (1997) Convergent and divergent validity of the Beck Anxiety Inventory for patients with panic disorder and agoraphobia. *Depression and Anxiety, 6,* 140–146.

DeGood, D. E., & Tait, R.. (1987). The Cognitive-Somatic Anxiety Questionnaire: Psychometric and validity data. *Journal of Psychopathology and Behavioral Assessment, 9,* 75–87.

Eifert, G. H., Thompson, R. N., Zvolensky, M. J., Edwards, K., Frazer, N. L., Haddad, J. W., & Davig, J. (2000). The Cardiac Anxiety Questionnaire: Development and preliminary validity. *Behaviour Research and Therapy, 38,* 1039–1053.

Endler, N. S., Cox, B. J., Parker, J. D. A., & Bagby, R. M. (1992). Self-reports of depression and state–trait anxiety: Evidence for differential assessment. *Journal of Personality and Social Psychology, 63,* 832–838.

Endler, N. S., Edwards, J. M., & Vitelli, R. (1991). *Endler Multidimensional Anxiety Scales (EMAS) manual.* Los Angeles: Western Psychological Services.

Endler, N. S., Parker, J. D. A., Bagby, R. M., & Cox, B. J. (1991). Multidimensionality of state and trait anxiety: Factor structure of the Endler Multidimensional Anxiety Scales. *Journal of Personality and Social Psychology, 60,* 919–926.

Fisher, P. L., & Durham, R. C. (1999). Recovery rates in generalized anxiety disorder following psychological therapy: An analysis of significant change in the STAI-T across outcome studies since 1990. *Psychological Medicine, 29,* 1425–1434.

Frost, R. O., Trepanier, K. L., Brown, E. J., Heimberg, R. G., Juster, H. R., Makris, G. S., & Leung, A. W. (1997). Self-monitoring of mistakes among subjects high and low in perfectionistic concern over mistakes. *Cognitive Therapy and Research, 21,* 209–222.

Frost, R. O., Turcotte, T. A., Heimberg, R. G., Mattia, J. I., Holt, C. S., & Hope, D. A . (1995). Reactions to mistakes among subjects high and low in perfectionistic concern over mistakes. *Cognitive Therapy and Research, 19,* 195–205.

Fydrich, T., Dowdall, D., & Chambless, D. L. (1992). Reliability and validity of the Beck Anxiety Inventory. *Journal of Anxiety Disorders, 6,* 55–61.

Ganellen, R. J., Matuzas, W., Uhlenhuth, E. H., Glass, R., & Easton, C. R. (1986). Panic disorder, agoraphobia, and anxiety-relevant cognitive style. *Journal of Affective Disorders, 11,* 219–225.

Gillis, M. M., Haaga, D. A. F., & Ford, G. T. (1995). Normative values for the Beck Anxiety Inventory, Fear Questionnaire, Penn State Worry Questionnaire, and Social Phobia and Anxiety Inventory. *Psychological Assessment, 7,* 450–455.

Hamilton, M. (1969). Diagnosis and rating of anxiety. *British Journal of Psychiatry, Special Publication No. 3,* 76–79.

Hayes, S. C., Bissett, R. T., Strosahl, K., Follette, W. C., Polusney, M. A., Pistorello, J., Toarmino, D., Batten, S. V., Dykstra, T. A., Stewart, S. H., Zvolensky, M. J., Eifert, G. H., Bond, F. W., & Bergan, J. (2001). *Psychometric properties of the Acceptance and Action Questionnaire (ACT).* Manuscript in preparation.

Hewitt, P. L., & Flett, G. L. (1991). Perfectionism in the self and social contexts: Conceptualization, assessment, and association with psychopathology. *Journal of Personality and Social Psychology, 60,* 456–470.

Hewitt, P. L., Flett, G. L., Turnbull-Donovan, W., & Mikail, S. F. (1991). The Multidimensional Perfectionism Scale: Reliability, validity, and psychometric properties in psychiatric samples. *Psychological Assessment: A Journal of Consulting and Clinical Psychology, 3,* 464–468.

Hewitt, P. L., & Norton, G. R. (1993). The Beck Anxiety Inventory: A psychometric analysis. *Psychological Assessment, 5,* 408–412.

Hoehn-Saric, R., McLeod, D. R., & Hipsley, P.A. (1993). Effect of fluvoxamine on panic disorder. *Journal of Clinical Psychopharmacology, 13,* 321–326.

Jegede, R. O. (1977). Psychometric attributes of the self-rating anxiety scale. *Psychological Reports, 40,* 303–306.

Kendall, P. C., & Hollon, S. D. (1989). Anxious self-talk: Development of the Anxious Self-Statements Questionnaire (ASSQ). *Cognitive Therapy and Research, 13,* 81–93.

Kobak, K. A., Reynolds, W. M., & Greist, J. H. (1993). Development and validation of a computer-administered version of the Hamilton Anxiety Scale. *Psychological Assessment, 5,* 487–494.

Koksal, F., & Power, K. G. (1990). Four Systems Anxiety Questionnaire (FSAQ): A self-report measure of somatic, cognitive, behavioral, and feeling components. *Journal of Personality Assessment, 54,* 534–544.

Koksal, F., Power, K. G., & Sharp, D. M. (1991). Profiles of DSM-III anxiety disorders on the somatic, cognitive, behavioural, and feeling components of the Four Systems Anxiety Questionnaire. *Personality and Individual Differences, 12,* 643–651.

Laurent, J., Catanzaro, S. J., Joiner, T. E., Rudolph, K. D., Potter, K. I., Lambert, S., Osborne, L., & Gathright, T. (1999). A measure of positive and negative affect for children: Scale development and preliminary validation. *Psychological Assessment, 11,* 326–338.

Lazarus, R. S., & Opton, E. M. (1966). The study of psychological stress: A summary of theoretical formulations and experimental findings. In C.D. Spielberger (Ed.), *Anxiety and behavior* (pp. 225–262). New York: Academic Press.

Lisspers, J., Nygren, A., & Soderman, E. (1997). Hospital Anxiety and Depression Scale (HAD): Some psychometric data for a Swedish sample. *Acta Psychiatrica Scandinavica, 96,* 281–286.

Lovibond, P. F. (1998). Long-term stability of depression, anxiety, and stress syndromes. *Journal of Abnormal Psychology, 107,* 520–526.

Lucock, M. P., & Morley, S. (1996). The Health Anxiety Questionnaire. *British Journal of Health Psychology, 1,* 137–150.

Mackinnon, A., Jorm, A. F., Christensen, H., Korten, A. E., Jacomb, P.A., & Rodgers, B. (1999). A short form of the

Positive and Negative Affect Schedule: Evaluation of factorial validity and invariance across demographic variables in a community sample. *Personality and Individual Differences, 27*, 405–416.

Maier, W., Buller, R., Philipp, M., & Heuser, I. (1988). The Hamilton Anxiety Scale: Reliability, validity and sensitivity to change in anxiety and depressive disorders. *Journal of Affective Disorders, 14*, 61–68.

Marteau, T. M., & Bekker, H. (1992). The development of a six-item short-form of the state scale of the State–Trait Anxiety Inventory (STAI). *British Journal of Clinical Psychology, 31*, 301–306.

McCracken, L. M., & Gross, R. T. (1995). The Pain Anxiety Symptoms Scale (PASS) and the assessment of emotional responses to pain. In L. Vandecreek, S. Knapp, & T. L. Jackson (Eds.), *Innovations in clinical practice: A source book* (Vol. 14, pp. 309–321). Sarasota, FL: Professional Resources Press.

McCracken, L. M., Zayfert, Z., & Gross, R. T. (1992). The Pain Anxiety Symptoms Scale: Development and validation of a scale to measure fear of pain. *Pain, 50*, 67–73.

McIntyre, C. W., Watson, D., Clark, L. A., & Cross, S. A. (1991). The effect of induced social interaction on positive and negative affect. *Bulletin of the Psychonomic Society, 29*, 67–70.

McNeil, D. W., & Rainwater, A. J. (1998). Development of the Fear of Pain Questionnaire -III. *Journal of Behavioural Medicine, 21*, 389–410.

Michelson, L., & Mavissakalian, M. (1983). Temporal stability of self-report measures in agoraphobia research. *Behaviour Research and Therapy, 21*, 695–698.

Moorey, S., Greer, S., Watson, M., Gorman, C., Rowden, L., Tunmore, R., Robertson, B., & Bliss, J. (1991). The factor structure and factor stability of the Hospital Anxiety and Depression Scale in patients with cancer. *British Journal of Psychiatry, 158*, 255–259.

Moras, K., Di Nardo, P. A., & Barlow, D. H. (1992). Distinguishing anxiety and depression: Reexamination of the reconstructed Hamilton Scales. *Psychological Assessment, 4*, 224–227.

Morris, L. W., Davis, M. A., & Hutchings, C. H. (1981). Cognitive and emotional components of anxiety: Literature review and a Revised Worry-Emotionality Scale. *Journal of Educational Psychology, 73*, 541–555.

Muris, P., Merckelbach, H., & Horselenberg, R. (1996). Individual differences in thought suppression. The White Bear Suppression Inventory: Factor structure, reliability, validity and correlates. *Behaviour Research and Therapy, 34*, 501–513.

Oei, T. P. S., Evans, L., & Crook, G. M. (1990). Utility and validity of the STAI with anxiety disorder patients. *British Journal of Clinical Psychology, 29*, 429–432.

Oei, T. P. S., Moylan, A., & Evans, L. (1991). Validity and clinical utility of the Fear Questionnaire for anxiety-disorder patients. *Psychological Assessment, 3*, 391–397.

Osman, A., Barrios, F. X., Osman, J. R., & Markway, K. (1993). Further psychometric evaluation of the Fear Questionnaire: Responses of college students. *Psychological Reports, 73*, 1259–1266.

Osman, A., Gutierrez, P. M., Barrios, F. X., Kopper, B. A., & Chiros, C. E. (1998). The Social Phobia and Social Interaction Anxiety Scales: Evaluation of psychometric properties. *Journal of Psychopathology and Behavioral Assessment, 20*, 249–264.

Osman, A., Kopper, B. A., Barrios, F. X., Osman, J. R., & Wade, T. (1997). The Beck Anxiety Inventory: Reexamination of factor structure and psychometric properties. *Journal of Clinical Psychology, 53*, 7–14.

Purdon, C., Antony, M. M., & Swinson, R. P. (1999). Psychometric properties of the Frost et al. Multidimensional Perfectionism Scale in a clinical anxiety disorders sample. *Journal of Clinical Psychology, 55*, 1271–1286.

Reynolds, M., & Wells, A. (1999). The Thought Control Questionnaire —Psychometric properties in a clinical sample and relationships with PTSD and depression. *Psychological Medicine, 29*, 1089–1099.

Reynolds, W. M. (1999). *Multidimensional Anxiety Questionnaire: Professional manual.* Odessa, FL: Psychological Assessment Resources, Inc.

Rhèaume, J., Freeston, M. H., Dugas, M. J., Letarte, H., & Ladouceur, R. (1995). Perfectionism, responsibility and obsessive-compulsive symptoms. *Behaviour Research and Therapy, 33*, 785–794.

Riskind, J. H. (1997). Looming vulnerability to threat: A cognitive paradigm for anxiety. *Behaviour Research and Therapy, 35*, 685–702.

Riskind, J. H., Beck, A. T., Brown, G., & Steer, R. A. (1987). Taking the measure of anxiety and depression: Validity of the reconstructed Hamilton Scales. *Journal of Nervous and Mental Disease, 175*, 474–479.

Riskind, J. H., & Williams, N. L. (in press). A unique cognitive vulnerability common to all anxiety disorders: The looming maladaptive style. In L. B. Alloy & J. H. Riskind (Eds.), *Cognitive vulnerability to emotional disorders.* Mahwah, NJ: Lawrence Erlbaum.

Riskind, J. H., Williams, N. L., Gessner, T., Chrosniak, L., & Cortina, J. (2000) The looming maladaptive style: Anxiety, danger, and schematic processing. *Journal of Personality and Social Psychology, 79*, 837–852.

Safren, S. A., Heimberg, R. G., Lerner, J., Henin, A., Warman, M., & Kendall, P. C. (2000). Differentiating anxious and depressive self-statements: Combined factor structure of the anxious self-statements questionnaire and the Automatic Thoughts Questionnaire–Revised. *Cognitive Therapy and Research, 24*, 327–344.

Sandin, B., Chorot, P., Lostao, L., Joiner, T. E., Santed, M. A., & Valiente, R. M. (1999). The PANAS Scales of

Positive and Negative Affect: Factor analytic validation and cross-cultural convergence. *Psicothema, 11*, 37–51. (Spanish)

Sarason, I. G. (1984). Stress, anxiety, and cognitive interference: Reactions to tests. *Journal of Personality and Social Psychology, 46*, 929–938.

Savard, J., Laberge, B., Gauthier, J. G., Ivers, H., & Bergeron, M. G. (1998). Evaluating anxiety and depression in HIV-infected patients. *Journal of Personality Assessment, 71*, 349–367.

Scholing, A., & Emmelkamp, P. M. G. (1992). Self report assessment of anxiety: A cross validation of the Lehrer Woolfolk Anxiety Symptom Questionnaire in three populations. *Behaviour Research and Therapy, 30*, 521–531.

Schwartz, G. E., Davidson, R. J., & Goleman, D. J. (1978). Patterning of cognitive and somatic processes in the self-regulation of anxiety: Effects of meditation versus exercise. *Psychosomatic Medicine, 40*, 321–328.

Shear, M. K., Vander Bilt, J., Rucci, P., Endicott, J., Lydiard, B., Otto, M. W., Pollack, M. H., Chandler, L., Williams, J., Ali, A., & Frank, D. M. (in press). Reliability and validity of a structured interview guide for the Hamilton Anxiety Rating Scale (SIGH-A). *Depression and Anxiety.*

Snaith, R. P., Harrop, F. M., Newby, D. A., & Teale, C. (1986). Grade scores of the Montgomery–Asberg Depression and the Clinical Anxiety Scales. *British Journal of Psychiatry, 148*, 599–601.

Spinhoven, P., & van der Does, A. J. W. (1999). Thought suppression, dissociation and psychopathology. *Personality and Individual Differences, 27*, 877–886.

Steer, R. A., Beck, A. T., Clark, D. A., & Beck, J. S. (1994). Psychometric properties of the Cognition Checklist with psychiatric outpatients and university students. *Psychological Assessment, 6*, 67–70.

Steptoe, A., & Kearsley, N. (1990). Cognitive and somatic anxiety. *Behaviour Research and Therapy, 28*, 75–81.

Stöber, J. (1998). The Frost Multidimensional Perfectionism Scale revisited: More perfect with four (instead of six) dimensions. *Personality and Individual Differences, 24*, 481–491.

Taylor, J. (1953). A personality scale of manifest anxiety. *Journal of Abnormal and Social Psychology, 48*, 285–290.

Taylor, S., Koch, W., Woody, S., & McLean, P. (1997). Reliability and validity of the Cognition Checklist with psychiatric outpatients. *Assessment, 4*, 9–16.

Trull, T. J., & Hillerbrand, E. (1990). Psychometric properties and factor structure of the Fear Questionnaire phobia subscale items in two normative samples. *Journal of Psychopathology and Behavioral Assessment, 12*, 285–297.

Turner, S. M., Beidel, D. C., & Dancu, C. V. (1996). *The Social Phobia and Anxiety Inventory manual.* North Tonawanda, NY: Multi-Health Systems Inc.

Uhlenhuth, E. H., McCarty, T., Paine, S., & Warner, T. (1999). The revised Anxious Thoughts and Tendencies (AT&T) scale: A general measure of anxiety-prone cognitive style. *Journal of Affective Disorders, 52*, 51–58.

van Zuuren, F. J. (1988). The Fear Questionnaire: Some data on validity, reliability, and layout. *British Journal of Psychiatry, 153*, 659–662.

Waikar, S. V., & Craske, M. G. (1997). Cognitive correlates of anxious and depressive symptomatology: An examination of the helplessness/hopelessness model. *Journal of Anxiety Disorders, 11*, 1–16.

Warda, G., & Bryant, R. A. (1998). Thought control strategies in acute stress disorder. *Behaviour Research and Therapy, 36*, 1171–1175.

Watson, D., Clark, L. A., Weber, K., Assenheimer, J. S., Strauss, M. E., & McCormick, R. A. (1995). Testing a tripartite model: II. Exploring the symptom structure of anxiety and depression in student, adult, and patient samples. *Journal of Abnormal Psychology, 104*, 15–25.

Watson, D., & Walker, L. M. (1996). The long-term stability and predictive validity of trait measures of affect. *Journal of Personality and Social Psychology, 70*, 567–577.

Watson, D., Weber, K., Assenheimer, J. S., Clark, L. A., Strauss, M. E., & McCormick, R. A. (1995). Testing a tripartite model: I. Evaluating the convergent and discriminant validity of anxiety and depression symptom scales. *Journal of Abnormal Psychology, 104*, 3–14.

Wegner, D. M. (1994). Ironic processes of mental control. *Psychological Review, 101*, 34–52.

Wegner, D. M., & Zanakos, S. (1994). Chronic thought suppression. *Journal of Personality, 62*, 615–640.

Wells, A. (1994). A multi-dimensional measure of worry: Development and preliminary validation of the Anxious Thoughts Inventory. *Anxiety, Stress, and Coping, 6*, 289–299.

Wells, A., & Matthews, G. (1994). *Attention and emotion: A clinical perspective.* Hillsdale, NJ: Erlbaum.

Williams, K. E., Chambless, D. L., & Ahrens, A. (1997). Are emotions frightening? An extension of the fear of fear construct. *Behaviour Research and Therapy, 35*, 239–248.

Wittchen, H. U., & Boyer, P. (1998). Screening for anxiety disorders: Sensitivity and specificity of the Anxiety Screening Questionnaire (ASQ-15). *British Journal of Psychiatry, 34*(Suppl), 10–17.

Zebb, B. J., & Moore, M. C., (1999). Another look at the psychometric properties of the Anxiety Control Questionnaire. *Behaviour Research and Therapy, 37*, 1091–1103.

PART II
Assessment Strategies for Anxiety Disorders

Chapter 8
Panic Disorder and Agoraphobia: A Brief Overview and Guide to Assessment

Randi E. McCabe

INTRODUCTION

Panic disorder (PD) is characterized by recurrent, unexpected panic attacks associated with at least one of the following: (1) fear of having additional panic attacks, (2) worry about the implications or consequences of the panic attack (e.g., losing control or going crazy), or (3) a major change in behavior as a consequence of the attacks (e.g., not going out alone, sitting near bathrooms or exits, avoiding activities or situations). PD is often associated with agoraphobia— fear and avoidance of situations (e.g., being far from home alone, standing in line, shopping malls, public transportation, crowds) where it would be difficult to escape or get help in the event of a panic attack (American Psychiatric Association, 1994).

There are a number of important issues to consider when assessing and treating individuals with PD including: establishing a diagnosis, examining the nature and frequency of the panic attacks, assessing the core features of the disorder (interoceptive anxiety, panic-related cognitions, agoraphobic avoidance), and consideration of associated features (e.g., comorbidity, level of impairment). This chapter will provide a brief overview of these issues (for more detailed review, see Antony & Swinson, 2000; Baker, Patterson, & Barlow, in press; Barlow, in press; Beck & Zebb, 1994).

Randi E. McCabe • Anxiety Treatment and Research Centre, St. Joseph's Hospital, and Department of Psychiatry and Behavioural Neurosciences, McMaster University, Hamilton, Ontario L8N 4A6, Canada.

Table 1. Important Issues in Assessment
of PD with Agoraphobia

Diagnostic specificity and differential diagnosis
  Ruling out medical conditions that may present as panic
  Assessing for substances that may cause panic symptoms
  Distinguishing panic disorder from other anxiety disorders and related conditions
    Identifying uncued panic attacks
    Examining the focus of fear during the panic attack
    Examining the reasons for avoidance of situations
Nature and frequency of panic attacks
Core features of PD
  Interoceptive anxiety
  Panic cognitions
  Agoraphobic avoidance
    Overt avoidance
    Subtle avoidance
Associated features
  Comorbidity
  Impairment
  Course
  Family factors

DIFFERENTIAL DIAGNOSIS

Medical Conditions that May Mimic Panic Symptoms

There are a number of medical conditions that cause symptoms that overlap with those of PD. Thus, it is important for the clinician to ensure that a patient has undergone a complete medical examination to rule out possible medical causes of symptoms (e.g., hyperthyroidism, hypoglycemia) before a diagnosis of PD is considered (for a review, see Dattilio & Salas-Auvert, 2000).

Substances that May Cause Panic Symptoms

Use of or withdrawal from certain substances (e.g., illicit drugs, medications, caffeine, alcohol) may cause panic symptoms and a diagnosis of a substance-induced anxiety disorder may be warranted. However, if the panic symptoms persist in the absence of the substance and after any withdrawal symptoms have subsided, then a diagnosis of PD may be appropriate.

Distinguishing Panic Disorder from Other Anxiety Disorders and Related Conditions

Comprehensive clinical interviews such as the Structured Clinical Interview for DSM-IV (SCID-IV; First, Spitzer, Gibbon, & Williams, 1996) and the Anxiety Disorders Interview Schedule for DSM-IV (ADIS-IV; Brown, Di Nardo, & Barlow, 1994; Di Nardo, Brown, &

Barlow, 1994) are excellent measures for obtaining the information required to make diagnostic decisions and assess comorbidity.

Cued versus Uncued Panic Attacks. Panic attacks, as well as avoidance, often occur in the context of other anxiety disorders (e.g., social phobia, posttraumatic stress disorder) so that careful assessment is required to make a differential diagnosis. A key feature of panic attacks associated with PD is that they are typically uncued and unexpected (i.e., occurring "out of the blue," without any warning or obvious trigger), particularly in the initial stages of the disorder. According to the DSM-IV, a necessary criterion for the diagnosis of PD is a history of recurrent, unexpected, or uncued panic attacks.

In comparison, panic attacks associated with other anxiety disorders are typically cued (i.e., triggered by a particular situation, object, or thought) and may be associated exclusively with a feared stimulus (e.g., an individual with social phobia who has panic attacks exclusively in social situations). Panic attacks that are triggered exclusively by thoughts occurring in the context of other anxiety disorders (e.g., worries about danger in GAD; obsessions about contamination in OCD) should be considered cued (Antony & Swinson, 2000). A good question to ask in this case is "Have you ever had a panic attack when you weren't worrying about _____ or obsessing about _____?"

After an extended period of experiencing panic attacks, patients may start to become aware of internal sensations (e.g., dizziness, palpitations) that cue or trigger their attacks. At this stage in the course of the disorder, some individuals may report that their attacks are no longer uncued. To confirm a history of uncued panic attacks, it is often helpful to focus on the first few panic attacks experienced by the individual, before he or she became aware of internal cues or triggers for the attacks.

Although individuals with hypochondriasis also report anxiety triggered by internal sensations, their panic attacks are typically not associated with agoraphobic avoidance and their anxiety is focused on the development of a serious illness (e.g., cancer) rather than on the possibility of having another panic attack (Antony & Swinson, 2000). In addition, the feared sensations are often not typical panic attack symptoms. For example, people with hypochondriasis might report anxiety about having headaches, feeling lumps, or noticing other symptoms that are typically not associated with panic.

Focus of Apprehension during the Panic Attack. To provide an accurate diagnosis and to select appropriate treatment strategies, it is important to identify the focus of apprehension during the patient's panic attacks. In PD, the focus of the fear is generally on experiencing the panic attack itself (i.e., the physical or psychological symptoms and their consequences) whereas in other anxiety disorders the focus of anxiety and fear is generally on features of the specific situation or triggering stimulus. For example, during a panic attack, an individual with PD is likely to report fears of dying, losing control, going crazy, or having others notice his or her panic attacks. In contrast, individuals with social phobia often are fearful of consequences over and above the effects of others noticing their panic attacks (e.g., saying something stupid, looking incompetent, appearing boring). To identify the patient's focus of apprehension, a good question to ask is "What do you fear will happen during a panic attack?"

Reasons for Avoidance. Individuals with PD may avoid situations that overlap with those avoided by individuals with other anxiety disorders. However, in PD, situations are avoided because of the fear of having a panic attack, whereas in other anxiety disorders, situations are typically avoided because of concerns about other aspects of the situation. For example, an individual with PD may avoid parties for fear of having a panic attack, whereas an individual with social phobia may avoid parties for fear of being embarrassed or having nothing to say to others. Thus, it is important to assess the reasons why an individual avoids a particular situation. Although an individual with PD and an individual with social phobia may both fear similar situations (e.g., being in crowds, riding on public transportation, and shopping in malls), the fears of the individual with social phobia are exclusively focused on the social aspects of the situation (e.g., people staring, being negatively evaluated by others).

In some cases, even the most experienced clinician may have difficulty establishing a differential diagnosis. For example, consider an individual who avoids situations partly for fear of experiencing a panic attack and partly because of a concern that people are staring and thinking negatively about him or her. In this case, a diagnosis of both PD with agoraphobia and social phobia may be warranted if criteria are met for both disorders.

Nature and Frequency of Panic Attacks

In addition to assessing the development and course of the problem and its impact on functioning, it is also important to determine the frequency of panic attacks, the symptoms experienced during a typical panic attack, and the type of panic attacks the person is experiencing (e.g., cued versus uncued or situationally predisposed; nocturnal). These variables may be assessed through clinical interview, self-report measures (e.g., Panic Attack Symptoms Questionnaire; Clum, Broyles, Borden, & Watkins, 1990), and self-monitoring diaries.

Self-monitoring diaries may be constructed by the clinician or a previously published diary may be used (e.g., Barlow & Craske, 2000; de Beurs, Chambless, & Goldstein, 1997; Rapee, Craske, & Barlow, 1990). When instructing a patient to engage in self-monitoring, it is important to clarify the purpose of the self-monitoring (e.g., to provide information on the frequency and severity of panic attacks, common triggers, and emotional or behavioral consequences). It is also helpful to warn the patient that he or she may feel more anxious when monitoring symptoms because of the increased focus on his or her anxiety symptoms. Finally, it is also recommended that patients are taught to differentiate between panic and generalized anxiety, given research showing that patients often mislabel other forms of anxiety as panic (Brown & Cash, 1989). Self-monitoring diaries are extremely useful for recording exposure practices (situational and interoceptive), implementing cognitive techniques (e.g., cognitive restructuring), and measuring progress during treatment.

Assessment of the Core Features of Panic Disorder and Agoraphobia

Interoceptive Anxiety and Panic Cognitions.   According to cognitive–behavioral models of PD, catastrophic misinterpretation of physical sensations (e.g., interpreting a racing heart as a warning sign of a heart attack) and anxiety over experiencing panic-related physical sensations are central characterizing features of PD (Antony & Barlow, 1996; Barlow, in press; Clark, 1986). Measures of sensation-focused anxiety such as the Body Sensations Questionnaire (Chambless, Caputo, Bright, & Gallagher, 1984) and the Anxiety Sensitivity Index (Peterson & Reiss, 1993) are helpful for identifying the specific symptoms feared by a patient, and can be used for choosing interoceptive exposure exercises to be used during treatment. Interoceptive exposure involves exposing the patient to feared bodily sensations repeatedly to enable extinction of the fear response. Before beginning interoceptive exposure, it is important to assess for any medical conditions or physical limitations (e.g., asthma, seizure disorders, heart disease, back and neck injuries) that may interfere with the safe practice of symptom induction exercises.

PD is also associated with characteristic threat-related cognitions including catastrophic thoughts, expectancies of danger, information processing biases, and underlying beliefs about personal control (for review, see Khawaja & Oei, 1998). A variety of self-report measures, such as the Agoraphobic Cognitions Questionnaire (ACQ; Chambless et al., 1984), Panic Attack Cognitions Questionnaire (PACQ; Clum et al., 1990), Body Sensations Interpretation Questionnaire (BSIQ; Clark et al., 1997), and the Catastrophic Cognitions Questionnaire (CCQ; Khawaja, Oei, & Baglioni, 1994), are available to assess panic and agoraphobic cognitions and identify targets for cognitive therapy (e.g., beliefs such as "I will have a heart attack" or "I will be paralyzed by fear"). Of these, the ACQ is the best established, having been used in many studies throughout the world.

Agoraphobic Avoidance.   The clinician can assess overt patterns of avoidance by directly asking about situations that are avoided because of fear of having a panic attack or panic-related sensations. Together with the patient, a detailed list of situations should be developed and the patient should rate his or her fear and avoidance levels for each situation. This list can be used to develop an exposure hierarchy. In addition, self-report measures such as the Mobility Inventory for agoraphobia (Chambless, Caputo, Jasin, Gracely, & Williams, 1985) are useful for assessing common agoraphobic situations.

The behavioral approach test (BAT) is a behavioral measure that involves instructing a patient to enter a feared situation. The BAT is helpful for determining levels of avoidance and fear in specific situations, corroborating information obtained in the clinical interview, and measuring treatment progress and outcome. Variables that can be measured during the BAT include physical symptoms, anxious cognitions, subtle avoidance strategies, escape or refusal to enter a situation, heart rate, and subjective ratings of fear.

An individualized BAT (I-BAT; e.g., Mathews, Gelder, & Johnston, 1981) is specifically tailored to assess an individual's unique fears. However, the I-BAT does not provide an absolute level of functioning and an individual's score is determined by the initial selection of situations, which are subject to bias from the clinician. Thus, it is hard to meaningfully compare scores on the I-BAT across different patients (for further discussion, see de Beurs, Lange, Van Dyck, Blonk, & Koele, 1991).

A standardized BAT (S-BAT; e.g., Agras, Leitenberg, & Barlow, 1968) takes into consideration these limitations by providing a standardized situation (e.g., walking a certain distance), but only provides information about one situation. The standardized multitask BAT developed by de Beurs et al. (1991) improves on the S-BAT by assessing avoidance and fear related to a number of situations (i.e., taking a walk, shopping, and public transportation), thus providing a behavioral measure of agoraphobic avoidance reflecting the heterogeneity of agoraphobic fears. Panic induction procedures (e.g., hyperventilation, spinning in a chair) may also be used as a BAT.

It is also essential to assess subtle avoidance strategies, overprotective behaviors, and overreliance on safety cues that may be less obvious, such as always being sure to carry medication or water, wearing certain clothes, making sure to be with a safe person, avoiding caffeine or other substances, and distraction. These maladaptive coping strategies may be assessed by asking "Is there anything that you do or items you must carry with you to feel more comfortable in case of a panic attack?" A thorough assessment of agoraphobic avoidance and subtle avoidance or safety cues provides the information necessary for constructing a detailed exposure hierarchy for treatment.

Associated Features

Comorbidity.   PD commonly co-occurs with other Axis I disorders such as other anxiety disorders, depression, alcohol abuse, and hypochondriasis (e.g., Brown, Antony, & Barlow, 1995). Thus, it is important to conduct a comprehensive assessment so that any comorbidity is detected and may be taken into consideration when developing a treatment plan. Estimates indicate that for individuals with PD and agoraphobia, 51 to 91% have co-occurring disorders (for review, see Beck & Zebb, 1994). Comorbidity is typically assessed by an unstructured clinical interview or using semistructured interviews such as the ADIS-IV (Di Nardo et al., 1994).

Impairment.   It is helpful to assess the level of a patient's functional impairment given the significant impact that PD may have on emotional well-being, financial independence, and relationships (Antony, Roth, Swinson, Huta, & Devins, 1998). Useful self-report scales for assessing functional impairment include the Illness Intrusiveness Rating Scale (Devins et al., 1983) and the 36-Item Short-Form Health Survey (Ware & Sherbourne, 1992).

Course.   PD often takes a variable course. Fluctuations in chronicity and response to prior treatments are also factors that should be considered in the assessment (American Psychiatric Association, 1998).

Family Factors.   It is helpful to identify and assess factors related to the individual's family or social supports that are relevant to etiology and treatment (Antony & Swinson, 2000). Often, family members may engage in behaviors that accommodate an individual's anxiety symptoms (e.g., a spouse who does all the driving or shopping so that his or her partner with PD can avoid becoming fearful). These types of accommodating behaviors serve to maintain the symptoms of PD.

SUMMARY

A thorough assessment is essential for defining the targets for therapy, developing an individually tailored treatment plan, setting treatment goals, and measuring treatment progress and outcome. It is important to consider medical conditions and substances that may mimic panic symptoms. Determining whether panic attacks are uncued, assessing the focus of fear during a panic attack, and examining reasons for avoidance of situations are crucial to distinguishing PD from other anxiety disorders. Assessment of the nature and frequency of panic attacks and the core features of PD (interoceptive anxiety, panic cognitions, and agoraphobic avoidance) forms the basis for choosing treatment strategies, and periodic monitoring of these components provides indicators of treatment progress and outcome. Finally, comorbidity, levels of impairment, course, and family variables are also important factors to consider when developing and implementing treatment. Ideally, assessment should be multimodal, utilizing a combination of clinical interviews, self-report measures, self-monitoring diaries, and BATs.

REFERENCES

Agras, W. S., Leitenberg, H., & Barlow, D. H. (1968). Social reinforcement in the modification of agoraphobia. *Archives of General Psychiatry, 19*, 423–427.

American Psychiatric Association. (1998). *Practice guideline for the treatment of patients with panic disorder.* Washington, DC: Author.

American Psychiatric Association. (1994). *Diagnostic and statistical manual of mental disorders* (4th ed.). Washington, DC: Author.

Antony, M. M., & Barlow, D. H. (1996). Emotion theory as a framework for explaining panic attacks and panic disorder. In R. M. Rapee (Ed.), *Current controversies in the anxiety disorders* (pp. 55–76). New York: Guilford.

Antony, M. M., Roth, D., Swinson, R. P., Huta, V., & Devins, G. M. (1998). Illness intrusiveness in individuals with panic disorder, obsessive compulsive disorder, or social phobia. *Journal of Nervous and Mental Disease, 186*, 311–315.

Antony, M. M., & Swinson, R. P. (2000). *Phobic disorders and panic in adults: A guide to assessment and treatment.* Washington, DC: American Psychological Association.

Baker, S., Patterson, M., & Barlow, D. H. (in press). Panic disorder and agoraphobia. In M. M. Antony & D. H. Barlow (Eds.), *Handbook of assessment, treatment planning, and outcome evaluation: Empirically supported strategies for psychological disorders.* New York: Guilford.

Barlow, D. H. (in press). *Anxiety and its disorders: The nature and treatment of anxiety and panic* (2nd ed.). New York: Guilford.

Barlow, D. H., & Craske, M. G. (2000). *Mastery of your anxiety and panic III (client workbook).* San Antonio, TX: The Psychological Corporation.

Beck, J. G., & Zebb, B J. (1994). Behavioral assessment and treatment of panic disorder: Current status, future directions. *Behavior Therapy, 25*, 581–611.

Brown, T. A., Antony, M. M., & Barlow, D. H. (1995). Diagnostic comorbidity in panic disorder: Effect on treatment outcome and course of comorbid diagnoses following treatment. *Journal of Consulting and Clinical Psychology, 63*, 408–418.

Brown, T. A., & Cash, T. F. (1989). The phenomenon of panic in nonclinical populations: Further evidence and methodological considerations. *Journal of Anxiety Disorders, 3*, 139–148.

Brown, T. A., Di Nardo, P., & Barlow, D. H. (1994). *Anxiety Disorders Interview Schedule for DSM-IV.* San Antonio, TX: The Psychological Corporation.

Chambless, D. L., Caputo, G. C., Bright, P., & Gallagher, R. (1984). Assessment of fear of fear in agoraphobics: The Body Sensations Questionnaire and the Agoraphobic Cognitions Questionnaire. *Journal of Consulting and Clinical Psychology, 52*, 1090–1097.

Chambless, D. L., Caputo, G. C., Jasin, S. E., Gracely, E. J., & Williams, C. (1985). The Mobility Inventory for agoraphobia. *Behaviour Research and Therapy, 23*, 35–44.

Clark, D. (1986). A cognitive approach to panic. *Behaviour Research and Therapy, 24*, 461–470.

Clark, D. M., Salkovskis, P. M., Öst, L.-G., Breitholtz, E., Koehler, K. A., Westling, B. E., Jeavons, A., & Gelder, M. (1997). Misinterpretation of body sensations in panic disorder. *Journal of Consulting and Clinical Psychology, 65*, 203–213.

Clum, G. A., Broyles, S., Borden, J., & Watkins, P. L. (1990). Validity and reliability of the Panic Attack Symptoms and Cognitions Questionnaires. *Journal of Psychopathology and Behavioral Assessment, 12*, 233–245.

Dattilio, F. M., & Salas-Auvert, J. (2000). *Panic disorder: Assessment and treatment through a wide-angle lens.* Phoenix, AZ: Zeig, Tucker, & Co.

de Beurs, E., Chambless, D. L., & Goldstein, A. J. (1997). Measurement of panic disorder by a modified panic diary. *Depression and Anxiety, 6*, 133–139.

de Beurs, E., Lange, A., Van Dyck, R., Blonk, R., & Koele, P. (1991). Behavioral assessment of avoidance in agoraphobia. *Journal of Psychopathology and Behavioral Assessment, 13*, 285–300.

Devins, G. M., Blinik, Y. M., Hutchinson, T. A., Hollomby, D. J., Barre, P. E., & Guttman, R. D. (1983). The emotional impact of end-stage renal disease: Importance of patients' perceptions of intrusiveness and control. *International Journal of Psychiatry and Medicine, 13*, 327–343.

Di Nardo, P., Brown, T. A., & Barlow, D. H. (1994). *Anxiety Disorders Interview Schedule for DSM-IV (Lifetime Version).* San Antonio, TX: The Psychological Corporation.

First, M. B., Spitzer, R. L., Gibbon, M., & Williams, J. B. W. (1996). *Structured Clinical Interview for DSM-IV Axis I Disorders—Patient Edition (SCID-I/P, Version 2.0).* New York: Biometrics Research Department, New York State Psychiatric Institute.

Khawaja, N. G., & Oei, T. P. S. (1998). Catastrophic cognitions in panic disorder with and without agoraphobia. *Clinical Psychology Review, 18*, 341–365.

Khawaja, N. G., Oei, T. P. S., & Baglioni, A. J. (1994). Modification of the Catastrophic Cognitions Questionnaire (CCQ-M) for normals and patients: Exploratory and LISREL analyses. *Journal of Psychopathology and Behavioral Assessment, 16*, 325–342.

Mathews, A. M., Gelder, M., & Johnston, D. W. (1981). *Agoraphobia: Nature and treatment.* New York: Guilford.

Peterson, R. A., & Reiss, S. (1993). *Anxiety Sensitivity Index Revised test manual.* Worthington, OH: IDS Publishing Corporation.

Rapee, R. M., Craske, M. G., & Barlow, D. H. (1990). Subject-described features of panic attacks using self-monitoring. *Journal of Anxiety Disorders, 4*, 171–181.

Ware, J. E., & Sherbourne, C.D. (1992). The MOS 36-Item Short Form Health Survey (SF-36): Conceptual framework and item selection. *Medical Care, 30*, 473–481.

Chapter 9
Measures for Panic Disorder and Agoraphobia

Martin M. Antony

AGORAPHOBIC COGNITIONS QUESTIONNAIRE (ACQ) AND BODY SENSATIONS QUESTIONNAIRE (BSQ)

Original Citation

Chambless, D. L., Caputo, G. C., Bright, P., & Gallagher, R. (1984). Assessment of 'fear of fear' in agoraphobics: The Body Sensations Questionnaire and the Agoraphobic Cognitions Questionnaire. *Journal of Consulting and Clinical Psychology, 52,* 1090–1097.

Purpose

To measure "fear of fear." The ACQ measures fearful cognitions associated with panic attacks and agoraphobia. The BSQ measures the intensity of fear associated with particular physical symptoms of arousal.

Description

The ACQ and BSQ are among the most popular and well-researched instruments for assessing panic disorder and agoraphobia. They are useful in both research and clinical settings.

Martin M. Antony • Anxiety Treatment and Research Centre, St. Joseph's Healthcare, Hamilton, and Department of Psychiatry and Behavioural Neurosciences, McMaster University, Hamilton, Ontario L8N 4A6, Canada.

The ACQ is a 15-item self-report instrument in which patients rate the frequency of specific cognitions that occur when they are feeling anxious or frightened. Items 1 through 14 include cognitions that are often associated with panic disorder and agoraphobia. Item 15 provides a space to record and rate an optional "other" cognition. Each item is rated on a five-point scale ranging from 1 (thought never occurs) to 5 (thought always occurs when I am nervous).

The BSQ is an 18-item self-report instrument in which patients rate the extent to which they fear specific bodily sensations that occur when they are feeling anxious or frightened. Items 1 through 17 include bodily sensations that are often associated with anxiety, fear, and arousal. Item 18 provides a space to record and rate an optional "other" sensation. Each item is rated on a five-point scale ranging from 1 (not at all) to 5 (extremely).

Administration and Scoring

The ACQ and BSQ each take 5 to 10 minutes to complete. Typically, these scales are administered together, although they may also be used separately. The ACQ is scored by calculating the means for items 1 through 14. Alternatively, the ACQ can generate two subscales reflecting *loss of control* (the mean of items 6, 8, 9, 11–14) and *physical concerns* (the mean of items 1–5, 7, 10). Additional clinical information may be obtained by asking patients to circle their three most frequent panic-related thoughts after completing the instrument, although this is optional. The BSQ is scored by calculating the means for items 1 through 17. In addition, the clinician may ask patients to circle their three most distressing bodily sensations after completing the instrument, although this step is optional as is the case for the ACQ.

Psychometric Properties

Sample Scores and Norms.   Chambless et al. (1984) reported a mean score of 2.32 (*SD* = 0.66) on the ACQ for outpatients with agoraphobia. ACQ scores in a community sample (Bibb, 1988) were as follows: 14-item ACQ (mean = 1.60; *SD* = 0.46), ACQ loss of control subscale (mean = 1.89; *SD* = 0.70), ACQ physical concerns factor (mean = 1.31; *SD* = 0.33). The mean BSQ score in a group of outpatients with agoraphobia was 3.05 (*SD* = 0.86; Chambless et al., 1984). The mean BSQ score in a community sample was 1.80 (*SD* = 0.59).

Chambless and Gracely (1989) reported means and standard deviations for the ACQ and BSQ across groups of individuals with panic disorder, agoraphobia, depression, generalized anxiety disorder, obsessive compulsive disorder, or social phobia. However, for this study, the ACQ was not scored according to the standard instructions. Instead of calculating the average score for items in each subscale, the authors calculated sums for each subscale.

Reliability.   In a sample of outpatients with agoraphobia, Cronbach's alpha was .80 for the ACQ and .87 for the BSQ (Chambless et al., 1984), suggesting that both of these scales have good internal consistency. In addition, the ACQ and BSQ have both been found to have adequate stability and test–retest reliability (Arrindell, 1993; Chambless et al., 1984).

Validity.   There are several studies examining the factor structure of these scales (e.g., Arrindell, 1993b; Chambless et al., 2000), showing that the "fear of fear" construct is multidimensional in nature. The ACQ and BSQ have been shown to discriminate between individuals with panic disorder and agoraphobia, individuals with other anxiety disorders, and nonanxious individuals (Chambless & Gracely, 1989). In addition, Chambless, Beck, Gracely, and Grisham (2000) found evidence of construct validity in a study showing a significant relationship between feared sensations as measured by the BSQ and specific catastrophic thoughts as measured by the ACQ. There is also published evidence of concurrent validity and predictive validity for both scales (Arrindell, 1993a). The total scores on the BSQ and ACQ are correlated with one another ($r = .67$) in outpatients with agoraphobia (Chambless et al., 1984). Finally, the ACQ and BSQ are sensitive to changes following treatment, making them ideal for measuring outcome (Chambless et al., 1984).

Alternative Forms

The ACQ and BSQ have been translated into Dutch, German, French, Greek, Spanish, Swedish, Portuguese, and Mandarin.

Source

The ACQ and BSQ are reprinted in Appendix B of this volume. Additional information may be obtained from Dianne L. Chambless, Ph.D., Department of Psychology, University of North Carolina at Chapel Hill, Chapel Hill, NC 27599-3270, USA; (tel) 919-962-3989; (fax) 919-962-2537; (e-mail) chambles@email.unc.edu; (webpage) www.unc.edu/~chambless/questionnaires/index.html.

AGORAPHOBIC COGNITIONS SCALE (ACS)

Original Citation

Hoffart, A., Friis, S., & Martinsen, E. W. (1992). Assessment of fear of fear among agoraphobic patients: The Agoraphobic Cognitions Scale. *Journal of Psychopathology and Behavioral Assessment, 14*, 175–187.

Purpose

To measure fearful cognitions among individuals with panic disorder and agoraphobia.

Description

The ACS is a 10-item self-report questionnaire in which patients rate the intensity of various fearful cognitions. Each item is rated on a five-point scale ranging from 0 (not at all) to 4 (very much).

Administration and Scoring

The ACS takes 3 minutes to complete. Three subscale scores are generated as follows: *fear of bodily incapacitation* (mean of items 1–5), *fear of losing control* (mean of items 6, 7), and *fear of embarrassment* (mean of items 8–10).

Psychometric Properties

Sample Scores and Norms. Hoffart et al. (1992) reported means and standard deviations for each subscale across groups of individuals with agoraphobia, social phobia, generalized anxiety disorder, and no anxiety. For agoraphobic patients, the mean scores for the incapacitation, control, and embarrassment subscales were 1.87 (SD = 0.99), 1.72 (SD = 1.38), and 2.76 (SD = 0.95), respectively. The means for a nonanxious group were 0.34 (SD = 0.58), .92 (SD = 1.09), and 1.03 (SD = 0.97), respectively.

Reliability. In a sample of anxious and depressed outpatients, internal consistency (as indicated by Cronbach's alpha) for the incapacitation, control, and embarrassment subscales were .81, .63, and .74, respectively (Hoffart et al., 1992).

Validity. A factor analytic study supports the three-factor solution, although item 10 appears to correlate moderately with both the incapacitation and embarrassment subscales (Hoffart et al., 1992). Correlations among the three subscales range from .36 to .49 (Hoffart et al., 1992). Adequate criterion validity is suggested by significant correlations between subscale scores on the ACS and comparable subscale scores on the ACQ (Hoffart et al., 1992). The ACS is sensitive to changes following treatment (Hoffart et al., 1993; Hoffart & Martinsen, 1990).

Alternative Forms

The ACS is available in Norwegian.

Source

The ACS has been reprinted in Appendix B. Additional information may be obtained from the author, Asle Hoffart, Prof. Dr. Psychol, Research Institute, Modum Bads Nerve-sanatorium, N-3370, Vikersund, Norway; (tel) +47 32 78 97 00; (fax) +47 32 78 98 68; (e-mail) forskning@modum-bad.no.

AGORAPHOBIC SELF-STATEMENTS QUESTIONNAIRE (ASQ)

Original Citation

van Hout, W. J. P. J., Emmelkamp, P. M. G., Koopmans, P. C., Bögels, S. M., & Bouman, T. K. (in press). Assessment of self-statements in agoraphobic situations: Construction and psychometric evaluations of the Agoraphobic Self-Statements Questionnaire (ASQ). *Journal of Anxiety Disorders.*

Purpose

To measure positive and negative self-statements in agoraphobic situations.

Description

The ASQ is a 25-item self-report questionnaire in which patients rate the frequency of various positive and negative thoughts that occur during exposure to an anxiety-provoking situation. Each item is rated on a five-point scale ranging from 0 (never) to 4 (continuously).

Administration and Scoring

The ASQ takes 5 minutes to complete. Two subscale scores are generated as follows: *positive subscale* (mean of items 2, 5, 6, 11, 12, 16–18, 20, 21, 23, 24) and *negative subscale* (mean of items 1, 3, 4, 7–9, 10, 13–15, 19, 22, 25).

Psychometric Properties

Sample Scores and Norms. In the initial validation study (van Hout et al., in press), patients with panic disorder and agoraphobia reported more frequent positive and negative self-statements than did nonanxious controls. For patients, the mean scores for the negative and positive subscales were 1.95 (*SD* = 0.70) and 1.64 (*SD* = 0.51), respectively. The means for a non-anxious group were 0.35 (*SD* = 0.57) and 1.28 (*SD* = 1.0), respectively.

Reliability. In a sample of outpatients with panic disorder and agoraphobia, internal consistency (as indicated by Cronbach's alpha) was good for both subscales (.88 for the negative subscale and .87 for the positive subscale; van Hout et al., in press).

Validity. A confirmatory factor analysis supported the two-factor structure of this measure (van Hout et al., in press). Supporting the convergent and discriminant validity of this measure, the ASQ has been found to be significantly correlated with other measures of agoraphobic avoidance, catastrophic cognitions, and fear of bodily sensations, but not with measures of blood–injection–injury fear or depression (van Hout et al., in press). In addition, improvements following treatment of panic disorder and agoraphobia are associated with a decrease in the frequency of both negative self-statements (van Hout et al., in press; van Hout, Emmelkamp, & Scholing, 1994) and positive self-statements (van Hout et al., in press).

Alternative Forms

The ASQ is available in Dutch.

Source

The ASQ has been reprinted in a paper by van Hout et al. (in press) as well as in Appendix B. Additional information may be obtained from the author, Wiljo J.P.J. van Hout, Department of Clinical Psychology, University of Groningen, P.O. Box 30001, 9700 RB Groningen, The Netherlands; (tel) +31 50 363 7609; (fax) +31 50 363 7602; (e-mail) w.j.p.j.van.hout@ppsw.rug.nl.

ALBANY PANIC AND PHOBIA QUESTIONNAIRE (APPQ)

Original Citation

Rapee, R. M., Craske, M. G., & Barlow, D. H. (1994/1995). Assessment instrument for panic disorder that includes fear of sensation-producing activities: The Albany Panic and Phobia Questionnaire. *Anxiety, 1*, 114–122.

Purpose

To measure situational fears typically reported by people with agoraphobia and social phobia, as well as fear of activities that produce physical sensations (i.e., interoceptive fears).

Description

The APPQ is a 27-item self-report questionnaire that measures fear of situations and activities that are often avoided by people who suffer from agoraphobia and social phobia. Each item is rated on a nine-point scale ranging from 0 (no fear) to 8 (extreme fear).

Administration and Scoring

The APPQ takes 5 minutes to complete. Three subscale scores are generated as follows: *agoraphobia subscale* (sum of items 2, 11, 13, 14, 16, 18, 20, 25, 27), *social phobia subscale* (sum of items 1, 5, 8, 9, 12, 15, 21–24), and *interoceptive subscale* (sum of items 3, 4, 6, 7, 10, 17, 19, 26).

Psychometric Properties

Sample Scores and Norms. In a study of outpatients with panic disorder and moderate to severe agoraphobia, mean scores on the agoraphobia, social phobia, and interoceptive subscales were 12.8 (*SD* = 9.8), 13.1 (*SD* = 9.7), and 9.6 (*SD* = 9.2), respectively (Rapee, Craske, & Barlow, 1994/1995). Mean scores for outpatients with social phobia were 10.5 (*SD* = 11.6), 31.5 (*SD* = 13.2), and 3.8 (*SD* = 6.8), respectively (Rapee et al., 1994/1995). Mean scores for nonclinical controls were 3.5 (*SD* = 3.3), 5.3 (*SD* = 5.4), and 1.1 (*SD* = 1.9), respectively (Rapee et al., 1994/1995). Rapee et al. (1994/1995) also reported scores for individuals with panic disorder with only mild agoraphobia, panic disorder without agoraphobia, and a group of individuals with other anxiety disorders.

Reliability.   In a large sample of outpatients with anxiety disorders, internal consistency (as indicated by Cronbach's alpha) was good to excellent for each subscale (.90 for the agoraphobia subscale; .91 for the social phobia subscale; .87 for the interoceptive subscale; Rapee et al., 1994/1995). In addition, test–retest reliability was shown to be adequate for all three subscales in a sample of outpatients with panic disorder (Rapee et al., 1994/1995).

Validity.   A factor analysis supported the three-factor structure of the APPQ (Rapee et al., 1994/1995). In addition, correlations between the subscales of the APPQ and other measures of social anxiety and panic disorder-related symptoms are in the expected direction, with measures of social anxiety correlating highest with the social phobia subscale and panic-related measures correlating highest with the agoraphobia and interoceptive subscales (Rapee et al., 1994/1995). Furthermore, following cognitive–behavioral treatment for panic disorder, scores on all three subscales showed a significant decrease (Rapee et al., 1994/1995), suggesting that the APPQ is useful for measuring treatment outcome.

Finally, each of the APPQ subscales appears to be useful for distinguishing among various clinical groups. The interoceptive subscale distinguishes individuals with panic disorder and moderate to severe agoraphobia from individuals with social phobia or other anxiety disorders, as well as from nonclinical controls. The social phobia subscale distinguishes people with social phobia from people with panic disorder, people with other anxiety disorders, and nonclinical controls. The agoraphobia subscale distinguishes people with panic disorder and agoraphobia from people with social phobia, people with other anxiety disorders, and nonclinical controls (Rapee et al., 1994/1995).

Alternative Forms

A Spanish translation is available.

Source

The APPQ has been reprinted in a paper by Rapee et al. (1994/1995) as well as in Appendix B. Additional information may be obtained from the author, Ronald M. Rapee, Ph.D., Department of Psychology, Macquarie University, Sydney, NSW 2109, Australia; (tel) +61 2 9850 8032; (fax) +61 2 9850 8062; (e-mail) ron.rapee@mq.edu.au.

ANXIETY SENSITIVITY INDEX (ASI)

Original Citations

Peterson, R. A., & Reiss, S. (1993). *Anxiety Sensitivity Index Revised test manual.* Worthington, OH: IDS Publishing Corporation.

Reiss, S., Peterson, R. A., Gursky, D. M., & McNally, R. J. (1986). Anxiety sensitivity, anxiety frequency and the prediction of fearfulness. *Behaviour Research and Therapy, 24,* 1–8.

Purpose

To measure anxiety sensitivity (i.e., fear of anxiety-related symptoms).

Description

The ASI is a self-report questionnaire on which each of 16 items measuring fear of anxiety-related symptoms is rated by the patient. Each item is rated on a five-point scale ranging from 0 (very little) to 4 (very much). The ASI is one of the post popular and well-researched measures for panic disorder and related conditions. In fact, an entire book has recently been published on the topic of anxiety sensitivity (Taylor, 1999).

Administration and Scoring

The ASI can be administered in 3 to 5 minutes. It is scored by summing all 16 items. Possible scores range from 0 to 64, with higher scores reflecting higher levels of anxiety sensitivity.

Psychometric Properties

Sample Scores and Norms. Rapee, Brown, Antony, and Barlow (1992) reported means for the ASI across different anxiety disorder groups, as follows: panic disorder with mild or no agoraphobia, 36.4 ($SD = 10.3$); panic disorder with moderate or severe agoraphobia, 32.1 ($SD = 11.3$); generalized anxiety disorder, 28.6 ($SD = 10.6$); social phobia, 21.4 ($SD = 12.6$); specific phobia, 20.0 ($SD = 13.4$); obsessive-compulsive disorder, 27.2 ($SD = 13.4$). For nonclinical samples (averaging across 12 studies with more than 4500 participants), the mean score of the ASI was 19.1 ($SD = 9.11$; Peterson & Reiss, 1993). Additional data on clinical and nonclinical samples may be found in a number of sources (e.g., Peterson & Reiss, 1993; Taylor, Koch, & McNally, 1992).

Reliability. Across a number of studies, internal consistency (as indicated by Cronbach's alpha) appears to be good to excellent, ranging from .82 to .91 (Peterson & Reiss, 1993). In addition, test–retest reliability appears to be satisfactory, with correlations (rs) ranging from .71 to .75 (Peterson & Reiss, 1993).

Validity. The factor structure of the ASI has been a source of controversy in the literature, with some studies finding a single factor and other studies finding multiple factors (Peterson & Reiss, 1993). One of the most sophisticated studies, based on a series of exploratory and confirmatory factor analyses in a large clinical sample, found that the ASI has a single higher-order factor and three lower-order factors representing physical concerns, social concerns, and mental incapacitation concerns (Zinbarg, Barlow, & Brown, 1997). The ASI has been shown to have a satisfactory degree of criterion validity and construct validity (Peterson & Heilbronner, 1987; Peterson & Reiss, 1993; Reiss, Peterson, Gursky, & McNally, 1986). In addition, scores on the ASI are predictive of a number of panic-related variables such as response to panic induction challenges (e.g., Rapee et al., 1992) and the future development of uncued panic attacks (Schmidt, Lerew, & Jackson, 1999). Among the anxiety disorders, ASI scores tend to be most elevated in people with panic disorder, although they are also somewhat elevated in the other anxiety disorders as well (Taylor et al., 1992). Finally, the ASI is sensitive to the effects of treatment, showing significant decreases following cognitive–behavioral therapy for panic disorder (Hazen, Walker, & Eldridge, 1996).

Alternative Forms

The ASI has been translated into Spanish, Italian, Chinese, Dutch, German, and Hebrew, as well as other languages. In addition, a childhood version of the ASI has been published (Silverman, Fleisig, Rabian, & Peterson, 1991; Silverman, Ginsburg, & Goedhart, 1999). Several modified versions of the ASI have been reported in the literature. Apfeldorf, Shear, Leon, and Portera (1994) reported that a subset of items from the ASI (items 3, 4, 6, 10) is as effective as the full ASI for discriminating patients with panic disorder from patients without panic disorder. The authors called their abbreviated ASI the Brief Panic Disorder Screen (BPDS). In addition, Taylor and Cox (1998) developed an expanded 36-item version of the ASI (described elsewhere in this book) and a 23-item version of the ASI has recently been developed by the same authors (Cox & Taylor, 2000).

Source

The ASI is reprinted in Appendix B. The scale and manual are copyrighted and may be purchased from IDS Publishing Corporation, P.O. Box 389, Worthington, OH 43085, USA; (tel) 614-885-2323; (fax) 614-885-2323. The cost is $65 US plus shipping, which includes the test manual and 50 test forms.

ANXIETY SENSITIVITY INDEX–REVISED 36 (ASI-R-36)

Original Citation

Taylor, S., & Cox, B. J. (1998). An expanded Anxiety Sensitivity Index: Evidence for a hierarchic structure in a clinical sample. *Journal of Anxiety Disorders*, *12*, 463–483.

Purpose

To assess the dimensions of anxiety sensitivity (i.e., fear of anxiety-related symptoms).

Description

The ASI-R-36 is a self-report questionnaire in which each of 36 items measuring fear of anxiety-related symptoms is rated by the patient. Each item is rated on a five-point scale ranging from 0 (very little) to 4 (very much). This revision of the ASI was developed to more thoroughly measure the different dimensions underlying anxiety sensitivity. Ten items are from the original 16-item ASI and the remaining 26 items were developed for this revised version. Researchers may wish to include the missing 6 items from the original ASI (see Appendix B) so that total scores on the original ASI can be derived as well.

Administration and Scoring

The ASI-R-36 takes 5 minutes to complete. Six rationally derived subscale scores are generated as follows: *fear of cardiovascular symptoms* (sum of items 5, 7, 11, 19, 27, 33), *fear of respiratory symptoms* (sum of items 8, 13, 15, 16, 18, 26, 32), *fear of gastrointestinal symptoms* (sum of items 6, 9, 14, 25), *fear of publicly observable anxiety reactions* (sum of items 1, 3, 12, 20, 22, 24, 30, 35), *fear of dissociative and neurological symptoms* (sum of items 4, 17, 21, 23, 28, 29), and *fear of cognitive dyscontrol* (sum of items 2, 10, 31, 34, 36).

Psychometric Properties

Sample Scores and Norms.   Normative data are currently being collected, according to the authors.

Reliability.   In a mixed group of psychiatric outpatients (61% with a diagnosis of panic disorder with or without agoraphobia), internal consistency (as indicated by Cronbach's alpha) was good to excellent for each subscale (.88 for fear of cardiovascular symptoms; .91 for fear of respiratory symptoms; .80 for fear of gastrointestinal symptoms; .86 for fear of publicly observable anxiety reactions; .83 for fear of dissociative and neurological symptoms; .89 for fear of cognitive dyscontrol; Taylor & Cox, 1998). Data regarding test–retest reliability are not yet available.

Validity.   A factor-analytic study with a clinical sample found one higher-order factor and four lower order factors, corresponding to fear of cardiovascular symptoms, fear of respiratory symptoms, fear of publicly observable anxiety reactions, and fear of cognitive dyscontrol (Taylor & Cox, 1998). According to the authors, further data collection is currently under way to determine whether it might be more appropriate to score this instrument using four subscales rather than the original six.

At pretreatment, patients with panic disorder tended to score highest relative to patients with other anxiety disorders and individuals with other psychiatric disorders (Taylor & Cox, 1998). Each lower-order factor was significantly correlated with the Beck Anxiety Inventory (*r*s range from .35 to .60). Although each lower-order factor was also correlated with scores on the Beck Depression Inventory, the correlation was greatest for the cognitive dyscontrol factor. More validity data are currently being collected.

Alternative Forms

The ASI-36-R has been translated into Dutch and Spanish.

Source

The ASI-R-36 is reprinted in Appendix B. Additional information may be obtained from the author, Steven Taylor, Ph.D., Department of Psychiatry, University of British Columbia,

2255 Wesbrook Mall, Vancouver, BC, V6T 2A1, Canada; (tel) 604-822-7331; (fax) 604-822-7756; (e-mail) taylor@unixg.ubc.ca.

ANXIETY SENSITIVITY PROFILE (ASP)

Original Citation

Taylor, S., & Cox, B. J. (1998). Anxiety Sensitivity: Multiple dimensions and hierarchic structure. *Behaviour Research and Therapy, 36,* 37–51.

Purpose

To assess the cognitive aspects of anxiety sensitivity (i.e., beliefs about the dangerousness of various anxiety-related symptoms) and their multiple dimensions.

Description

The ASP is a self-report questionnaire containing 60 items that reflect particular physical sensations and other experiences that occur when an individual is anxious. The individual is asked to imagine experiencing each sensation and to rate the likelihood that the given feeling would lead to something bad happening, such as dying, going crazy, or being ridiculed. Each item is rated on a seven-point scale ranging from 1 (not at all likely) to 7 (extremely likely).

ADMINISTRATION AND SCORING

The ASP takes 10 minutes to complete. Six rationally derived subscale scores are generated as follows: *fear of cardiovascular symptoms* (sum of items 1, 6, 8, 14, 20, 31, 34, 42, 51, 55), *fear of respiratory symptoms* (sum of items 3, 15, 19, 21, 26, 30, 37, 45, 47, 59), *fear of gastrointestinal symptoms* (sum of items 4, 11, 16, 27, 28, 32, 40, 49, 50, 57), *fear of publicly observable anxiety reactions* (sum of items 10, 12, 23, 24, 33, 35, 38, 48, 53, 58), *fear of dissociative and neurological symptoms* (sum of items 5, 9, 17, 22, 29, 39, 43, 46, 52, 60), and *fear of cognitive dyscontrol* (sum of items 2, 7, 13, 18, 25, 36, 41, 44, 54, 56).

Psychometric Properties

Sample Scores and Norms. Normative data are currently being collected, according to the authors.

Reliability. In a group of university students, internal consistency (as indicated by Cronbach's alpha) was good to excellent for each subscale (.92 for fear of cardiovascular symptoms; .93 for fear of respiratory symptoms; .88 for fear of gastrointestinal symptoms; .89 for fear of publicly observable anxiety reactions; .89 for fear of dissociative and neurological symptoms; .94 for fear of cognitive dyscontrol; Taylor & Cox, 1998). Data regarding test–retest reliability are not yet available.

Validity. A factor-analytic study with a student sample found one higher-order factor and four lower-order factors, corresponding to fear of cardiovascular symptoms, fear of respiratory symptoms, fear of publicly observable anxiety reactions, and fear of cognitive dyscontrol (Taylor & Cox, 1998). According to the authors, further data collection is currently under way to determine whether it might be more appropriate to score this instrument using four subscales rather than the original six.

Each lower-order factor was significantly correlated with a measure of anxiety sensitivity (rs range from .41 to .57). In addition, these factors were significantly correlated with a trait measure of anxiety, although the magnitude of these correlations was small (rs range from .11 to .29). More validity data are currently being collected.

Alternative Forms

The ASP has been translated into Dutch and Spanish.

Source

The ASP is reprinted in a paper by Taylor and Cox (1998) and in Appendix B. Additional information may be obtained from the author, Steven Taylor, Ph.D., Department of Psychiatry, University of British Columbia, 2255 Wesbrook Mall, Vancouver, BC, V6T 2A1, Canada; (tel) 604-822-7331; (fax) 604-822-7756; (e-mail) taylor@unixg.ubc.ca.

BODY SENSATIONS INTERPRETATION QUESTIONNAIRE (BSIQ)

Original Citation

Clark, D. M., Salkovskis, P. M., Öst, L.-G., Breitholtz, E., Koehler, K. A., Westling, B. E., Jeavons, A., & Gelder, M. (1997). Misinterpretation of body sensations in panic disorder. *Journal of Consulting and Clinical Psychology, 65*, 203–213.

Purpose

To assess anxious misinterpretations associated with panic disorder and other anxiety-related conditions.

Description

The BSIQ is a self-report measure containing 27 ambiguous events presented in booklet form. It is a modified version of McNally and Foa's (1987) Interpretation Questionnaire. For each item, an event is described and the individual is asked the question "why?" In response, the individual describes, in his or her own words, the first interpretation for the event to enter his or her mind. Each event (along with space to record the individual's interpretation) is presented on a separate sheet of paper (about half the size of a standard 8½ × 11-inch page). After recording his or her interpretation of the event (in an open-ended fashion), the individual turns to the next page and reads a list of three possible interpretations for the event that was presented on the previous page. In each case, only one of the interpretations is negative. The other two are either both neutral or one is neutral and the other is positive.

The individual is instructed to rank the interpretations in order of how likely each would be to occur if he or she were in the situation (1 = most likely to come true; 2 = second most likely to come true; 3 = least likely to come true). Finally, after completing all 27 items, the individual returns to the start of the booklet and rates his or her beliefs regarding the likelihood of each interpretation being true (for each ambiguous event), using a nine-point scale ranging from 0 (not at all likely) to 8 (extremely likely).

The BSIQ generates four subscale scores representing interpretations about panic-related body sensations, social events, other external events (i.e., general worries), and other body symptoms (i.e., health anxiety concerns).

Administration and Scoring

The BSIQ takes 10 to 15 minutes to complete and 5 to 10 minutes to score. The items are grouped into four subscales (for each item, the "number" indicates the item number and the "letter" indicates which of the three interpretations is the catastrophic one): *panic body sensations scale* (items 1b, 6a, 8c, 14a, 19b, 22c, 25c), *social events scale* (items 3c, 5b, 9a, 12b, 15c, 18a, 21b, 26a), *external events scale* (2a, 7b, 11c, 16b, 20c, 24a), and *other symptoms scale* (4b, 10a, 13c, 17c, 23a, 27b).

For the ranking data, a score of 3, 2, or 1 is assigned depending on whether the catastrophic explanation is ranked first, second, or third (thus, larger scores reflect a tendency to rank the catastrophic interpretations as more probable). Then, mean ranking scores are calculated for each subscale. A mean negative belief rating is obtained by calculating the mean score for the negative explanations on each subscale. A mean neutral belief rating is obtained by calculating the mean for *both* of the neutral explanations on each subscale

Psychometric Properties

Sample Scores and Norms. For patients with panic disorder, mean ranking scores (possible range is 0–3) for each subscale are as follows: *panic body sensations* 2.2 (*SD* = 0.7), *general events* 1.9 (*SD* = 0.5), *social events* 1.9 (*SD* = 0.6), *other symptoms* 1.8 (*SD* = 0.7). Mean belief ratings for negative interpretations (possible range is 0–8) are *panic body sensations* 4.8 (*SD* = 1.0), *general events* 5.3 (*SD* = 1.1), *social events* 4.0 (*SD* = 1.8), *other symptoms* 4.0 (*SD* = 2.3). Mean belief ratings for neutral interpretations (possible range is 0–8) are *panic body sensations* 4.4 (*SD* = 2.4), *general events* 3.9 (*SD* = 1.8), *social events* 4.8 (*SD* = 1.2), *other symptoms* 5.2 (*SD* = 1.2). Clark et al. (1997) also provide norms for individuals with other anxiety disorders and for nonpatients.

Reliability. Clark et al. (1997) provide ratings of internal consistency (as indicated by Cronbach's alpha) for a brief version of the BSIQ (BBSIQ; see "Alternative Forms" below). The scales of the BBSIQ have satisfactory internal consistency (.86 for panic body sensation rankings; .90 for panic body sensation belief rankings; .74 for external event rankings; .80 for external even belief rankings). Data regarding internal consistency for the original BSIQ are not available. Data regarding test–retest reliability are not available for either the BSIQ or the BBSIQ.

Validity.   After controlling for state anxiety, individuals with panic disorder score significantly higher than individuals with other anxiety disorders on the panic body sensation subscale (based on both ranking and belief measures), but not on the other three subscales. Additional validity data have been collected using the brief version of the BSIQ (BBSIQ; see "Alternative Forms" below; Clark et al., 1997). In patients with panic disorder, the panic body sensation subscale is significantly correlated with the physical concerns factor on the ACQ ($r =$ .49), but not the social–behavioral consequences (i.e., loss of control) factor on the ACQ or state or trait anxiety as measured by the State–Trait Anxiety Inventory. The external event subscale of the BBSIQ is significantly correlated with the social–behavioral consequences (i.e., loss of control) factor on the ACQ as well as state and trait anxiety, but not with the physical concerns factor on the ACQ.

Alternative Forms

The BBSIQ consists of a subset of 14 items from the original BSIQ. Instead of four subscales, these are scored on two subscales: a *panic body sensations scale* (consisting of identical items from the original BSIQ) and an *external events scale* (consisting of items from the three remaining subscales on the BSIQ). The items that make up the BBSIQ are as follows (the corresponding item number from the original BSIQ is presented in parentheses): *panic body sensations scale* 2 (19), 3 (25), 5 (6), 8 (8), 11 (1), 12 (14), 14 (22); *external events scale* 1 (15), 4 (3), 6 (24), 7 (21), 9 (7), 10 (12), 13 (20). The BBSIQ has been translated into Swedish. Norms for the BBSIQ are provided in the paper by Clark et al. (1997).

Source

The instructions, BSIQ items, and interpretations are reprinted in Appendix B. However, it is to be noted that the complete set of items should not be presented all on the same page. Instead, items should be presented one at a time in the manner described earlier in the description of the instrument. Additional information may be obtained from the author, David M. Clark, Department of Psychology, Institute of Psychiatry, De Crespigny Park, Denmark Hill, London, SE5 8AF, United Kingdom; (tel) 44-20-7848-0245/0238; (fax) 44-020-7848-0591; (e-mail) d.clark@iop.kcl.ac.uk.

BODY VIGILANCE SCALE (BVS)

Original Citation

Schmidt, N. B., Lerew, D. R., & Trakowski, J. H. (1997). Body vigilance in panic disorder: Evaluating attention to bodily perturbations. *Journal of Consulting and Clinical Psychology, 65,* 214–220.

Purpose

To measure a tendency to attend to panic-related bodily sensations.

Description

The BVS is a four item self-report inventory designed to assess attentional focus to internal bodily sensations. The first three items assess degree of attentional focus, perceived sensitivity to changes in bodily sensations, and the average amount of time spent attending to bodily sensations. A fourth item provides separate ratings for attention to 15 different sensations that include all of the DSM-IV physical symptoms described for panic attacks as well as several additional symptoms. The scales and anchors used for rating each item differ slightly (see Appendix B).

Administration and Scoring

The BVS takes 3 to 5 minutes to administer. Item 3 is converted from a 0–100 point scale to a 0–10 point scale (e.g., 10 = 1, 20 = 2). For item 4, ratings for the 15 sensations are averaged to yield one overall score. The BVS total score is the sum of items 1–4.

Psychometric Properties

Sample Scores and Norms.   According to published data by Schmidt et al. (1997), the mean BVS scores for patients with panic disorder, patients with social phobia, and individuals from a community sample are 22.6 ($SD = 9.1$), 17.6 ($SD = 6.8$), and 18.3 ($SD = 8.5$), respectively. Data for additional normative groups and for individual items on the BVS are provided by Schmidt et al. (1997). Norms are based on an ethnically diverse sample.

Reliability.   The BVS has good internal consistency (Cronbach's alpha = .82) and adequate test–retest reliability across 5 weeks ($r = .58$) in patients with panic disorder (Schmidt et al., 1997). Reliability for other samples is provided by Schmidt et al. (1997).

Validity.   Schmidt et al. (1997) provide several sources of data supporting the validity of the BVS. Factor analyses in clinical and nonclinical samples suggest that the BVS measures a unitary construct. In addition, patients with panic disorder have significantly higher scores on the BVS than patients with social phobia or nonclinical controls. In patients with panic disorder, pretreatment BVS scores are significantly correlated with measures of anxiety sensitivity (i.e., fear of bodily sensation), anxiety, and depression, but not with measures of agoraphobic avoidance, panic attack frequency, or functional impairment. Patterns of correlations were slightly different at posttreatment for patients with panic disorder, and for individuals in a nonclinical sample. Finally, BVS scores tend to decrease following cognitive–behavioral treatment for panic disorder.

Source

The BVS is reprinted in the validation paper by Schmidt et al. (1997) as well as in Appendix B. Additional information may be obtained from the author, N. Brad Schmidt, Ph.D., Department of Psychology, Ohio State University, 245 Townshend Hall, Columbus, OH 43210, USA; (tel) 614-292-2687; (fax) 614-688-8261; (e-mail) schmidt.283@osu.edu; (webpage) http://anxiety.psy.ohio-state.edu/.

MOBILITY INVENTORY FOR AGORAPHOBIA (MI)

Original Citation

Chambless, D. L., Caputo, G. C., Jasin, S. E., Gracely, E. J., & Williams, C. (1985). The Mobility Inventory for Agoraphobia. *Behaviour Research and Therapy, 23*, 35–44.

Purpose

To measure the severity of agoraphobic avoidance and panic attacks.

Description

The MI is a self-report questionnaire that contains four parts. The first section provides a list of 26 different situations that are typically avoided by people with agoraphobia. There is also space to record and rate an optional "other" situation. Each item in this section is rated twice using a five-point scale ranging from 1 (never avoid) to 5 (always avoid). The first rating measures avoidance when accompanied and the second rating measures avoidance when alone. Typically, when researchers report scores on the MI, they are referring only to scores on part 1 of the instrument. The other sections of the MI are rarely used in research.

The second part of the MI requires that the individual circle the five items from part 1 that cause the greatest amount of concern or impairment. Part 3 contains three questions regarding (1) panic frequency in the past 7 days, (2) panic frequency in the past 3 weeks, and (3) severity of panic attacks during the past 7 days (using a five-point scale ranging from 1 [very mild] to 5 [extremely severe]). The fourth section of the MI asks the individual to provide the location and size of his or her safety zone, if relevant. For example, an individual's safety zone might be the area up to 2 miles from his or her home.

This most recent version of the MI is a slight revision of the original MI (as described by Chambless et al., 1985). The original version included only part 1, as well as a single question regarding panic frequency in the past 7 days.

Administration and Scoring

The MI takes 5 to 10 minutes to complete. When completing part 1, patients are encouraged to leave items blank if they are irrelevant to their lives. For example, if there are no subways in an individual's city or town, this item should be left blank. However, if more than five items are left blank, the author recommends that the questionnaire be considered invalid (D. L. Chambless, February 2000, personal communication).

Part 1 is scored by calculating the means for items 1 through 26, separately for *avoidance accompanied* and *avoidance alone*. Including item 27 when calculating the mean score is optional. Panic frequency is scored as a simple frequency count. The author recommends that researchers use nonparametric analyses (or conduct a log transformation before using parametric analyses), because responses on this item tend to be quite skewed (D. L. Chambless, February 2000, personal communication). Panic intensity is scored as per the individual's response. However, if the individual rates panic frequency as 0, panic intensity should be coded as missing, regardless of the response to this item.

Psychometric Properties

Sample Scores and Norms.   Chambless et al. (1985) reported mean scores on the MI for two samples of patients with agoraphobia. The means on the *avoidance alone* subscale for the two samples were 3.35 ($SD = 1.06$) and 3.30 ($SD = 0.99$). The means for the *avoidance accompanied* subscale for the two samples were 2.64 ($SD = 0.90$) and 2.41 ($SD = 0.70$). For a normal control sample, the means were 1.25 ($SD = 0.24$) and 1.07 ($SD = 0.08$) for the *avoidance alone* and *avoidance accompanied* subscales, respectively (Chambless et al., 1985). For individuals with social phobia, the corresponding means were 1.56 ($SD = 0.41$) and 1.35 ($SD = 0.27$), respectively, in one study (Chambless et al., 1985) and 2.17 ($SD = 0.77$) and 1.57 ($SD = 0.58$), respectively, in another study (Craske, Rachman, & Tallman, 1986). For patients with agoraphobia, the mean panic frequency (past 7 days) and mean panic intensity ratings were 3.07 ($SD = 3.88$; median = 2.11) and 3.19 ($SD = 1.00$; D. L. Chambless, February 2000, personal communication).

Reliability.   Internal consistency is excellent for both subscales in part 1, with Cronbach alphas ranging from .94 to .96 for the *avoidance alone* subscale and from .91 to .97 for the *avoidance accompanied* subscale (Chambless et al., 1985). Test–retest reliability is high for both subscales in part 1, with *r*s ranging from .89 to .90 for the *avoidance alone* subscale and from .75 to .86 for the *avoidance accompanied* subscale (Chambless et al., 1985).

Validity.   Two factor-analytic studies found that items from part 1 of the MI loaded on three factors, corresponding to public places, enclosed spaces, and open spaces (Arrindell, Cox, van der Ende, & Kwee, 1995; Cox, Swinson, Kuch, & Reichman, 1993). Another study found two factors, corresponding to public places and enclosed spaces (Kwon, Evans, & Oei, 1990). Scores on the *avoidance alone* and *avoidance accompanied* are significantly correlated with depression, trait anxiety, other measures of agoraphobia, and to a lesser extent with panic frequency (Chambless et al., 1985). The panic frequency ratings from the MI are significantly correlated ($r = .74$) with panic frequency ratings from a diary measure (de Beurs, Chambless, & Goldstein, 1997).

Individuals with agoraphobia score significantly higher on the MI subscales than do individuals from nonclinical and socially phobic samples (Chambless et al., 1985; Craske et al., 1986). In addition, Kinney and Williams (1988) reported that relative to measures of self-efficacy, scores on the MI (as well as on other self-report measures of agoraphobia) are only moderately correlated with actual avoidance during behavioral avoidance tests conducted in a naturalistic community setting. Finally, the MI measures of *avoidance alone*, *avoidance accompanied*, and panic frequency are all sensitive to change, showing significant reductions following treatment (Chambless et al., 1985).

Alternative Forms

The MI has been translated into Dutch, German, French, Greek, Spanish, Swedish, and Portuguese. Swinson, Cox, Shulman, Kuch, and Woszczyna (1992) reported findings based on a revision of the MI that included a third subscale. In addition to rating avoidance of various situations when alone and accompanied, ratings were also made for avoidance "without medication."

Source

The MI is reprinted in Appendix B. The latter version is a slight revision of the original (see description above). Additional information may be obtained from Dianne L. Chambless, Ph.D., Department of Psychology, University of North Carolina at Chapel Hill, Chapel Hill, NC 27599-3270, USA; (tel) 919-962-3989; (fax) 919-962-2537; (e-mail) chambles@email. unc.edu; (webpage) www.unc.edu/~chambless/questionnaires/index.html.

PANIC AND AGORAPHOBIA SCALE (PAS)

Original Citation

Bandelow, B. (1999). *Panic and Agoraphobia Scale (PAS)*. Seattle, WA: Hogrefe & Huber Publishers.

Purpose

To measure the severity of panic disorder with or without agoraphobia.

Description

The PAS was developed to measure changes in panic-related symptoms in psychological and pharmaceutical treatment trials, although it is appropriate for a broad range of clinical and research settings. The scale is available in both observer-rated and self-rated formats, each consisting of 13 items. Each item is rated on a five-point scale ranging from 0 to 4, with the specific descriptors and behavioral anchors differing from item to item (see Appendix B; Bandelow, 1995). Items ask about (1) panic attacks, (2) agoraphobic avoidance, (3) anticipatory anxiety, (4) disability and functional impairment, and (5) worries about health. Each of these areas generates a subscale score. In addition, the total score reflects overall severity. Ratings are based on the past week.

Administration and Scoring

Each version takes 5 to 10 minutes to complete. When using the self-administered version, the clinician should first explain what is meant by the terms *panic attack* and *agoraphobia*, although these terms are also defined on the scale. Before administering the observer-rated version, we strongly recommend consulting the manual (Bandelow, 1999), which provides detailed suggestions for rating each item. To obtain a total score on either the observer-rated or self-rated versions, all items (except item U, which assesses the percentage of panic attacks that are unexpected) are added together. Total scores can range from 0 to 52.

Subscale scores can be calculated by summing the appropriate items and dividing by the number of items in the subscale: *panic attacks* (sum of items A1, A2, A3 divided by 3), *agoraphobic avoidance* (sum of items B1, B2, B3 divided by 3), *anticipatory anxiety* (sum of items C1, C2 divided by 2), *disability* (sum of items D1, D2, D3 divided by 3), and *worries about health* (sum of items E1, E2 divided by 2). Item B2 in the self-rated version is scored as follows: 0 points = no situations inducing anxiety; 1 point = 1 situation; 2 points = 2 to 3 situations; 3 points = 4 to 8 situations; 4 points = more than 8 situations.

The following guidelines may be used for interpreting total scores from the observer-rated version: 0–6 = borderline or in remission; 7–17 = mild; 18–28 = moderate; 29–39 = severe; 40 points or more = very severe (Bandelow, 1999). The following guidelines may be used for interpreting total scores from the self-rated version: 0–8 = borderline or remission; 9–18 = mild; 19–28 = moderate; 29–39 = severe; 40 points or more = very severe (Bandelow, 1999).

Psychometric Properties

Sample Scores and Norms. Bandelow (1999) provides normative data for individual items on the PAS. With respect to total scores, the mean for patients suffering from panic disorder with or without agoraphobia was 23.6 (SD = 10.6) for the observer-rated version and 23.5 (SD = 10.3) for the self-rated version. Norms are not available for other clinical or nonclinical groups.

Reliability. Internal consistency is good for both versions, with a Cronbach's alpha of .85 for the observer-rated version and .86 for the self-rated version (Bandelow, 1999). Test–retest reliability (r = .73) and interrater reliability (r = .78) are both satisfactory for the observer-rated version (Bandelow, 1999).

Validity. Exploratory factor analysis of the observer-rated version generated three factors: (1) the panic attack items, (2) the agoraphobia and disability items, and (3) the anticipatory anxiety and health worry items (Bandelow, 1999). The factor structure was similar for the self-rated version. The PAS is significantly correlated with various measures of panic symptomatology, anxiety, and global impairment (rs range from .42 to .81; Bandelow, 1999). Finally, in an open trial of imipramine for panic disorder, the PAS showed good sensitivity to changes following treatment (Bandelow et al., 1998).

Alternative Forms

The PAS is available in 17 languages: Arabic, Danish, Dutch, English, French, German, Greek, Hebrew, Hungarian, Italian, Japanese, Portuguese, Russian, Serbocroat, Spanish, Swedish, and Turkish. Translations of the PAS are included in the manual.

Source

The observer-rated version of the PAS has been reprinted in a paper by Bandelow (1995) and the self-rated version is reprinted in Appendix B. Both versions are reprinted in the PAS manual (Bandelow, 1999). The scale and manual are copyrighted and may be purchased from Hogrefe & Huber Publishers (Seattle office), P.O. Box 2487, Kirkland, WA 98083-2487, USA; (tel order desk) 800-228-3749; (tel) 425-820-1500; (fax) 425-823-8324; Canadian office (tel) 416-482-6339; (website) www.hhpub.com. The complete test kit (including the manual, 50 copies of the observer-rated scale, and 50 copies of the self-rated scale) costs $79.50 US.

PANIC ATTACK QUESTIONNAIRE–REVISED (PAQ-R)

Original Citation

Cox, B. J., Norton, G. R., & Swinson, R. P. (1992). *Panic Attack Questionnaire–Revised.* Toronto, ON: Clarke Institute of Psychiatry.

Purpose

To provide detailed information on the phenomenology of panic attacks, including symptomatology, situational triggers, and coping styles.

Description

The PAQ-R is a revision of the Panic Attack Questionnaire (PAQ; Norton, Dorward, & Cox, 1986). This instrument provides descriptive ideographic information for clinical purposes as well quantitative data that can be used for research. For example, the PAQ and PAQ-R have been used extensively to identify individuals in nonclinical samples who experience panic attacks (Norton, Cox, & Malan, 1992; Norton, Pidlubny, & Norton, 1999) and to study the features of panic attacks in clinical samples (e.g., Cox, Endler, & Swinson, 1995; Cox, Swinson, Endler, & Norton, 1994).

The PAQ-R provides demographic data (e.g., sex, occupation), information about past treatment for various problems, family history of panic attacks, frequency of panic attacks during several periods, onset and course of panic attacks over time, rise time and duration of typical panic attacks, severity of panic symptoms, past history and future expectancy for having panic attacks in particular situations, perceived control and cognitive features of panic, functional impairment, suicidal ideation, and strategies for coping with panic attacks.

Administration and Scoring

The PAQ-R can be administered in 20 to 30 minutes, if the full version is used. Meaningful information can be reviewed in a few minutes. This instrument does not provide a score, although specific sections provide quantitative data.

Psychometric Properties

Sample Scores and Norms. Norms are available for particular sections of the PAQ and PAQ-R. Cox, Swinson, et al. (1994) reported the percentages of patients with panic disorder who experience each of 23 symptoms during their panic attacks. Similar data are available for the frequency of suicidal ideation and attempts in people with panic disorder (Cox, Direnfeld, Swinson, & Norton, 1994), the types of coping strategies used by patients (Cox, Endler, Swinson, & Norton, 1992), and the types of situations avoided (Cox et al., 1992).

Reliability and Validity. Although the PAQ and PAQ-R have not been subjected to systematic psychometric validation studies, many of the sections from these instruments were derived from other established measures and sources. For example, the descriptive questions regarding panic attacks map closely onto the diagnostic criteria in DSM-III-R and DSM-IV. Several of the situations used to determine situational fears were derived from the Fear Questionnaire. Finally, questions regarding suicide were similar to those asked in the Epidemiological Catchment Area Study.

In addition, there are data supporting the reliability and validity of particular sections of the PAQ and PAQ-R (in particular, internal consistency, construct validity, and factor structure). For example, Cox, Swinson, et al. (1994) studied the factor structure of 23 panic-related symptoms (as measured by the PAQ) in patients with panic disorder. Three reliable factors emerged: dizziness symptoms (Cronbach's alpha = .82), cardiorespiratory symptoms (Cronbach's alpha = .79), and cognitive symptoms (Cronbach's alpha = .81). In a study of undergraduate students who panic, a four-factor solution seemed to fit the data more closely (Whittal, Suchday, & Goetsch, 1994).

A potential limitation of the PAQ emerged in a study by Brown and Deagle (1992). Although many studies have used the PAQ to diagnose panic attacks in nonclinical samples, Brown and Deagle (1992) found that the PAQ often overestimated the frequency of panic attacks in a student sample, compared with a semistructured interview assessment of panic.

Source

The PAQ-R may be obtained from the author, Brian J. Cox, Ph.D., PZ-430 PsychHealth Centre, University of Manitoba, 771 Bannatyne Avenue, Winnepeg, Manitoba, R3E 3N4, Canada; (tel) 204-787-5166; (fax) 204-787-4879; (e-mail) coxbj@cc.umanitoba.ca.

PANIC DISORDER SEVERITY SCALE (PDSS)

Original Citation

Shear, M. K., Brown, T. A., Sholomskas, D. E., Barlow, D. H., Gorman, J. M., Woods, S. W., & Cloitre, M. (1992). *Panic Disorder Severity Scale (PDSS)*. Pittsburgh, PA: Department of Psychiatry, University of Pittsburgh School of Medicine.

Purpose

To assess panic disorder severity in patients who have already been diagnosed with panic disorder.

Description

The PDSS is a seven-item clinician-administered scale. Ratings for each item are made for the past month (other time periods are permitted, as long as the same period is used for each item). Items are rated on a five-point scale ranging from 0 (none or not present) to 4 (extreme, pervasive, near-constant symptoms, disabling/incapacitating). The dimensions assessed include panic attack frequency, distress during panic attacks, severity of anticipatory anxiety, fear and avoidance of agoraphobic situations, fear and avoidance of panic-related sensations, impairment in work functioning, and impairment in social functioning. Previous versions of this scale include the Cornell–Yale Panic Anxiety Scale (CY-PAS) and the Multicenter Panic-Anxiety Scale (MC-PAS).

Administration and Scoring

The PDSS takes 10 to 15 minutes to administer. The total score is the average of the scores for each of the seven items (scores may range from 0 to 4). The scale is sometimes scored by summing the ratings from the seven items (with scores ranging from 0 to 28), but norms are not available for this method of scoring.

Psychometric Properties

Sample Scores and Norms.   Among individuals with panic disorder and mild or no agoraphobia, the mean score on the PDSS is 1.59 ($SD = 0.43$). Means on the individual items are as follows: panic frequency 1.83 ($SD = 0.82$), panic distress 2.19 ($SD = 0.61$), anticipatory anxiety 1.94 ($SD = 0.75$), agoraphobic fear/avoidance 1.23 ($SD = 0.65$), interoceptive fear/avoidance 1.08 ($SD = 0.58$), work impairment/distress 1.29 ($SD = 0.98$), and social impairment/distress 1.55 ($SD = 0.82$; Shear et al., 1997).

Reliability.   Shear et al. (1997) studied the reliability of the PDSS in patients with panic disorder. Interrater reliability was high, with an intraclass correlation coefficient of .88 and interrater reliability for individual items ranging from .73 to .87. Internal consistency was low, with a Cronbach's alpha of .65.

Validity.   A confirmatory factor analysis found that a two-factor solution provided a better fit than a single-factor solution (Shear et al., 1997). Items 1 and 2 (panic frequency and distress) formed the first factor and the remaining items formed the second factor. As reported by Shear et al. (1997), individual items on the PDSS were most strongly correlated with other measures that assess a similar construct. For example, scores on the agoraphobia subscale of the Albany Panic and Phobia Questionnaire were more strongly correlated with item 4 (agoraphobic fear/avoidance) on the PDSS than any other item. Finally, the PDSS appears to be sensitive to change following treatment for panic disorder (Shear et al., 1997).

Alternative Forms

A modified "not diagnosed" version is available for cases in which the patient has not undergone a diagnostic interview and the clinician is not aware of whether the patient has ever experienced full or limited symptom panic attacks. In addition, a self-report version is in the final stages of development. More information about these versions may be obtained from the author, M. Katherine Shear, MD (see source information below).

Source

The PDSS is reprinted in Appendix B. Additional information may be obtained from the author, M. Katherine Shear, M.D., Anxiety Disorders Prevention Program, Western Psychiatric Institute and Clinic, University of Pittsburgh, 3811 O'Hara Street, Pittsburgh, PA 15213-2593, USA; (tel) 412-624-1340; (fax) 412-624-6644; (e-mail) shearmk@msx.upmc.edu.

PHOBIC AVOIDANCE RATING SCALE (PARS)

Original Citation

Hoffart, A., Friis, S., & Martinsen, E. W. (1989). The Phobic Avoidance Rating Scale: A psychometric evaluation of an interview-based scale. *Psychiatric Developments*, *1*, 71–81.

Purpose

To measure severity of agoraphobic avoidance.

Description

The PARS is a 13-item interview in which clinicians rate the extent to which an individual avoids each of 13 situations: 6 situations that are associated with avoidance in agoraphobia, 3 social situations, and 4 situations that are associated with avoidance in agoraphobia and certain specific phobias. Each item is rated on a five-point scale ranging from 0 (no avoidance) to 4 (avoids the situation regularly).

Administration and Scoring

The PARS can be administered in 10 to 15 minutes. Three subscale scores are generated as follows: *separation avoidance* (mean of items 1–6), *social avoidance* (mean of items 7–9), and *simple avoidance* (mean of items 10–13).

Psychometric Properties

Sample Scores and Norms. For agoraphobic patients, the mean scores for the *separation avoidance, social avoidance*, and *simple avoidance* subscales are 2.15 ($SD = 0.89$), 1.96 ($SD = 1.00$), and 1.47 ($SD = 1.06$), respectively (Hoffart et al., 1989). Norms for other groups (e.g., other anxiety disorders, depression with social phobia, depression without social phobia) are also provided by Hoffart et al. (1989).

Reliability. In a sample of anxious and depressed outpatients, internal consistency (as indicated by Cronbach's alpha) for the *separation avoidance, social avoidance*, and *simple avoidance* subscales were .88, .58, and .68, respectively (Hoffart et al., 1989). Interrater reliability coefficients for these subscales were .99, .95, and .99, respectively (Hoffart et al., 1989). Data regarding test–retest reliability are not available.

Validity. A factor-analytic study supports the three subscale structure of this scale (Hoffart et al., 1989). Correlations among the three subscales range from .25 to .54 (Hoffart et al., 1989). Adequate criterion validity is suggested by high correlations between the PARS subscales and a measure of agoraphobic avoidance, moderate correlations with a measure of general anxiety, and low correlations with measures of depression (Hoffart et al., 1989). In addition, individuals with agoraphobia tend to score higher than individuals with other anxiety disorders or depression on the *separation* and *simple* subscales, but differences were less robust for the *social* subscale (Hoffart et al., 1989). Finally, the PARS is sensitive to changes following cognitive–behavioral (Hoffart, 1995; Hoffart et al., 1989) and pharmacological treatment (Hoffart et al., 1993).

Alternative Forms

The PARS is available in Norwegian.

Source

The PARS is reprinted in the original article by Hoffart et al. (1989) and in Appendix B. Additional information may be obtained from the author, Asle Hoffart, Prof. Dr. Psychol, Research Institute, Modum Bads Nervesanatorium, N-3370, Vikersund, Norway; (tel) +47 32 78 97 00; (fax) +47 32 78 98 68; (e-mail) forskning@modum-bad.no.

TEXAS SAFETY MANEUVER SCALE (TSMS)

Original Citation

Kamphuis, J. H., & Telch, M .J. (1998). Assessment of strategies to manage or avoid perceived threats among panic disorder patients: The Texas Safety Maneuver Scale (TSMS). *Clinical Psychology and Psychotherapy, 5,* 177–186.

Purpose

To measure subtle within-situation avoidance behaviors (safety maneuvers) that occur in patients with panic disorder.

Description

The TSMS is a 50-item self-report questionnaire. In addition, four optional items are included for patients to record "other" safety behaviors. Each item is rated on a five-point scale measuring the extent to which people use particular subtle avoidance strategies to manage anxiety or panic. Ratings range from 0 (never to manage anxiety or panic) to 4 (always to manage anxiety or panic). To ensure that the avoidance is in fact related to anxiety and panic, a sixth option provides an opportunity for the individual to indicate whether he or she engages in the behavior, but not for the purpose of managing anxiety or panic. If this option is checked, the item is scored as if the patient never avoids (a score of 0 is assigned for the item). Note that in the original paper by Kamphuis and Telch (1998), there are minor errors in the scoring instructions for subscales, two of the reported subscale means, and in the numbering of items in the reprinted scale. These errors have been corrected for this book (Kamphuis, personal communication, August 30, 2000).

Administration and Scoring

The TSMS takes 5 to 10 minutes to complete. Six subscale scores are generated as follows: *agoraphobic avoidance* (sum of items 6–9, 35, 36, 37, 39, 40, 42), *relaxation techniques* (sum of items 47–50), and *stress avoidance* (sum of items 22–26), *somatic avoidance* (sum of items 28, 29, 31–34), *distraction techniques* (sum of items 10–15), *escape* (sum of items 19, 43–46). The remaining items (items 1–5, 16–18, 20, 21, 27, 30, 38, 41) are not used to generate subscale scores. A total score may be calculated by computing the sum of all 50 items.

Psychometric Properties

Sample Scores and Norms. In a psychometric study by Kamphuis and Telch (1998), mean total scores for individuals with panic disorder were as follows: total 78.43 (SD = 33.95); agoraphobic avoidance 18.28 (SD = 11.46); relaxation techniques 4.60 (SD = 4.37); stress avoidance 10.07 (SD = 5.19); somatic avoidance 10.71 (SD = 6.66); distraction techniques 9.70 (SD = 5.41); escape 8.38 (SD = 5.72). Norms are not available for other groups.

Reliability. In a study by Kamphuis and Telch (1998), internal consistency (as measured by Cronbach's alpha) was generally good to excellent: total .93; agoraphobic avoidance .90; relaxation techniques .88; stress avoidance .87; somatic avoidance .77; distraction techniques .82; escape .79.

Validity. Although the complete set of items in this scale was inductively generated by the authors, the final items in each subscale were based on an exploratory factor analysis. The TSMS and several of its subscales are significantly correlated with measures of general anxiety, anxiety sensitivity, agoraphobic avoidance, and depression. The specific pattern of correlations is provided in the original paper by Kamphuis and Telch (1998).

Source

The TSMS is reprinted in the original paper by Kamphuis and Telch (1998) with items numbered incorrectly and the corrected version is reprinted in Appendix B. Additional information may be obtained from the author, Jan H. Kamphuis, Ph.D., Department of Clinical Psychology, University of Amsterdam, Roetersstraat 15, 1018 WB Amsterdam, The Netherlands; (tel) 31-20-5256785/6810; (fax) 31-20-6391369; (e-mail) kp_kamphuis@macmail. psy.uva.nl; (webpage) www.psy.uva.nl.

BRIEF DESCRIPTIONS OF ADDITIONAL MEASURES

Acute Panic Inventory (API)

The API is a 17-item self-report questionnaire designed to measure paniclike responses to biological challenges and other stressful situations. The scale asks about several (but not all) of the DSM-IV panic attack symptoms as well as some additional symptoms. The items are reprinted in a paper by Dillon, Gorman, Liebowitz, Fyer, and Klein (1987).

Agoraphobia Scale (AS)

The AS is a 20-item self-report questionnaire designed to measure the severity of agoraphobic avoidance. The scale provides ratings of anxiety and avoidance for 20 different agoraphobic situations. The scale and psychometric properties are provided in a paper by Öst (1990). Additional information is available from the author, Lars-Göran Öst, Ph.D., Department of Psychology, Stockholm University, S-106, 91, Stockholm, Sweden; (tel) 46-8-163821; (fax) 46-8-166236; (e-mail) ost@psychology.su.se.

Autonomic Nervous System Questionnaire (ANS)

The ANS is a five-item self-report scale designed to screen for panic disorder in primary care settings. The scale and psychometric properties are provided in a paper by Stein et al. (1999). Additional information is available from the author, Murray Stein, MD, Department of Psychiatry (0985), University of California–San Diego, 9500 Gilman Drive, La Jolla, CA 92093-0985, USA; (tel) 858-622-6112; (fax) 858-450-1491; (e-mail) mstein@ucsd.edu.

Body Consciousness Questionnaire (BCQ)

The BCQ is a 15-item self-report scale designed to measure awareness of one's body. Three subscales are generated: *private body consciousness* (awareness of physical sensations), *public body consciousness* (beliefs regarding one's physical appearance), and *body competence* (beliefs about one's physical strength and coordination). Among these subscales, private body consciousness is the most theoretically relevant to the diagnosis of panic disorder. The scale items and psychometric properties are provided in a paper by Miller, Murphy, and Buss (1981).

Catastrophic Cognitions Questionnaire–Modified (CCQ-M)

The CCQ-M is a 21-item self-report scale designed to assess catastrophic cognitions associated with panic disorder and agoraphobia. The instrument generates three subscales: *emotional catastrophes*, *physical catastrophes*, and *mental catastrophes*. The CCQ-M is a revision of the Catastrophic Cognitions Questionnaire (Khawaja & Oei, 1992). The scale and psychometric properties are provided in a paper by Khawaja, Oei, and Baglioni (1994). Additional information may be obtained from the author, Tian P.S. Oei, Ph.D., School of Psychology, University of Queensland, QLD 4072, Australia; (tel) 61 7 3365 6449; (fax) 61 7 3365 4466; (e-mail) oei@psy.uq.edu.au.

Comprehensive Panic Profile (CPP)

The CPP is a self-administered questionnaire that provides a full-spectrum analysis of the principal features of panic disorder and agoraphobia (Clum, 1997). It consists of a measure of panic frequency as well as six scales that each measure a relevant dimension: the Panic Attack Symptom Scale (PASS; a 36-item measure of panic attack severity), the Panic Attack Cognitions Scale (PACS; a 25-item measure of cognitions associated with panic attacks), the Fear of Anxiety Scale (FAS; a 15-item scale for measuring fear of anxiety-related sensations and cognitions), the Avoidance Scale (AS; a 22-item measure of agoraphobic avoidance), the Coping Strategies Scale (CSS; a 28-item measure of panic-related coping strategies), and the Confidence in Coping Scale (CCS; a 10-item scale for measuring an individual's confidence in his or her ability to cope with panic attacks). In 1990, Clum, Broyles, Borden, and Watkins published a psychometric study on the PASS and PACS only. Additional information is available from the author, George A. Clum, Ph.D., Department of Psychology, Virginia Polytechnic Institute and State University, Blacksburg, VA 24061, USA; (tel) 540-231-5701; (fax) 540-231-3652; (e-mail) gclum@vt.edu.

Depersonalization–Derealization Inventory (DDI)

The DDI is a 28-item self-report scale designed to measure symptoms of depersonalization and derealization in people suffering from panic disorder. A manuscript (including the scale and its psychometric properties) is currently under review (Cox & Swinson, 2000). Additional information may be obtained from the author, Brian J. Cox, Ph.D., PZ-430 PsychHealth Centre, University of Manitoba, 771 Bannatyne Avenue, Winnepeg, Manitoba, R3E 3N4, Canada; (tel) 204-787-5166; (fax) 204-787-4879; (e-mail) coxbj@cc.umanitoba.ca.

Diagnostic Symptom Questionnaire–B (DSQ-B)

The DSQ-B is a brief self-report scale designed to measure panic attack symptoms during challenge and provocation procedures. Although the psychometric properties of this scale are not well-established, it remains one of the most commonly used scales for measuring panic attacks during challenges. The DSQ-B is an updated and expanded version of the Diagnostic Symptom Questionnaire (Sanderson, Rapee, & Barlow, 1989; Sanderson, Wetzler, & Asnis, 1994). Additional information may be obtained from the author, William C. Sanderson, Ph.D., Department of Clinical Psychology–GSAPP, Rutgers University, 152 Frelinghuysen Road, Piscataway, NJ 08854-8085, USA; (tel) 732-445-2272; (fax) 732-445-4888; (e-mail) wsanders @rci.rutgers.edu.

Discomfort Intolerance Scale (DIS)

The DIS is a five-item self-report scale designed to measure the extent to which individuals find it difficult to tolerate physical discomfort. The psychometric properties of this new scale have been presented at a scientific meeting (e.g., Fitzpatrick & Schmidt, 2000) and versions of the scale have been used in previous published studies (e.g., Schmidt & Cook, 1999; Schmidt & Lerew, 1998). Additional information may be obtained from the author, N. Brad Schmidt, Ph.D., Department of Psychology, Ohio State University, 245 Townshend Hall, Columbus, OH 43210, USA; (tel) 614-292-2687; (fax) 614-688-8261; (e-mail) schmidt.283 @osu.edu; (webpage) http://anxiety.psy.ohio-state.edu/.

National Institute of Mental Health Panic Questionnaire (NIMH PQ)

The NIMH PQ is a self-report questionnaire designed to obtain descriptive information about panic attacks and panic disorder. It was developed to be consistent with DSM-III-R criteria and contains 13 categories of questions, each with an average of 21 specific questions or probes (range of items per section is 3 to 81). A description of the scale and its psychometric properties is available in a paper by Scupi, Maser, and Uhde (1992).

Panic Appraisal Inventory (PAI)

The PAI is a 45-item self-report scale designed to measure panic-related cognitions using three subscales: anticipation of panic, panic consequences, and panic-coping. The scale was originally developed by Telch (1987). Psychometric properties have been published on both the original 35-item scale (Telch, Brouillard, Telch, Agras, & Taylor, 1989) and the current 45-item scale (Feske & de Beurs, 1997). Additional information may be obtained from the author, M. Telch, Ph.D., Department of Psychology, University of Texas, Austin, Mezes 330, Austin, TX 78712, USA; (tel) 512-471-3393; (fax) 512-471-5177; (e-mail) telch@psy.utexas.edu.

Panic-Associated Symptom Scale (PASS)

The PASS is a nine-item clinician-administered scale designed to measure the core symptoms of panic disorder (as defined in DSM-III-R), including the frequency and intensity of uncued panic attacks, cued panic attacks, and limited symptom attacks, as well as the severity of anticipatory anxiety and phobic avoidance. The scale and psychometric properties are provided in a paper by Argyle et al. (1990).

Panic Diary (PD)

The PD is a self-report diary that is used to record panic-related symptoms. In addition to reporting the features of each panic attack as it occurs, additional ratings (e.g., panic expectancy) are made on a daily basis. Psychometric properties have been published by de Beurs, Chambless, and Goldstein (1997). Additional information may be obtained from the author, Edwin de Beurs, Ph.D., Vrije Universiteit, Department of Psychiatry, Valeriusplein 9, 1075 BG Amsterdam, The Netherlands; (tel) +31 20 5736 534; (fax) +31205736 687; (e-mail) edwindb@pca-znw.nl.

Panic Disorder Self-Report (PDSR)

The PDSR is a self-report scale that is designed to diagnose panic disorder. Preliminary data on the psychometric properties of this scale have been presented (Newman, Zuelig, & Kachin, 1998) and a full manuscript has been submitted for publication. Additional information may be obtained from the author, Michelle G. Newman, Ph.D., Department of Psychology, Pennsylvania State University, 310 Moore Building, University Park, PA 16802-3103, USA; (tel) 814-863-1148; (fax) 814-863-7002; (e-mail) mgn1@psu.edu.

Self-Efficacy to Control a Panic Attack Questionnaire (SE-SCAQ)

The SE-SCAQ is a 25-item self-report scale designed to measure an individual's self-efficacy to control a panic attack when experiencing particular anxiety-provoking thoughts, when feeling certain uncomfortable sensations, and when exposed to particular situations. The instrument and its psychometric properties are described in a published abstract by Gauthier, Bouchard, Côté, Laberge, and French (1993), as well as in a recent review of panic-related measures (Bouchard, Pelletier, Gauthier, Côté, & Laberge, 1997). Additional information may be obtained from one of the authors, Stéphane Bouchard, Ph.D., Department of Psychoeducation, University of Québec at Hull, C.P. 1250, succursale B, Hull, Québec, J8X 3X7, Canada; (tel) 819-595-3900, ext. 2360; (fax) 819-595-2384; (e-mail) stephane—bouchard@uqah. uquebec.ca.

REFERENCES

Apfeldorf, W. J., Shear, M. K., Leon, A. C., & Portera, L. (1994). A brief screen for panic disorder. *Journal of Anxiety Disorders, 8.* 71–78.

Argyle, N., Deltito, J., Allerup, P., Maier, W., Albus, M., Nutzinger, D., Rasmussen, S., Ayuso, J. L., & Bech, P. (1991). The Panic-Associated Symptom Scale: Measuring the severity of panic disorder. *Acta Psychiatrica Scandinavica, 83*, 20–26.

Arrindell, W. A. (1993a). The fear of fear concept: Stability, retest artefact and predictive power. *Behaviour Research and Therapy, 31*, 507–518.

Arrindell, W. A. (1993b). The fear of fear concept: Evidence in favour of multidimensionality. *Behaviour Research and Therapy, 31*, 139–148.

Arrindell, W. A., Cox, B. J., van der Ende, J., & Kwee, M. G. T. (1995). Phobic dimensions-II: Cross-national confirmation of the multidimensional structure underlying the Mobility Inventory (MI). *Behaviour Research and Therapy, 33*, 711–724.

Bandelow, B. (1995). Assessing the efficacy of treatments for panic disorder and agoraphobia. II: The Panic and Agoraphobia Scale. *International Clinical Psychopharmacology, 10*, 73–81.

Bandelow, B. (1999). *Panic and Agoraphobia Scale (PAS) manual.* Seattle, WA: Hogrefe & Huber Publishers.

Bandelow, B., Brunner, E., Broocks, A., Beinroth, D., Hajak, G., Pralle, L., & Rüther, E. (1998). The use of the Panic and Agoraphobia Scale in a clinical trial. *Psychiatry Research, 77*, 43–49.

Bibb, J. L. (1988). *Parental bonding, pathological development, and fear of losing control among agoraphobics and normals.* Unpublished doctoral dissertation, American University, Washington, DC.

Bouchard, S., Pelletier, M.-H., Gauthier, J. G., Côté, G., & Laberge, B. (1997). The assessment of panic using self-report: A comprehensive survey of validated instruments. *Journal of Anxiety Disorder, 11*, 89–111.

Brown, T. A., & Deagle, E. A. (1992). Structured interview assessment of nonclinical panic. *Behavior Therapy, 23*, 75–85.

Chambless, D. L., Beck, A. T., Gracely, E. J., & Grisham, J. R. (2000). Relationship of cognitions to fear of somatic symptoms: A test of the cognitive theory of panic. *Depression and Anxiety, 11*, 1–9.

Chambless, D. L., & Gracely, E. J. (1989). Fear of fear and the anxiety disorders. *Cognitive Therapy and Research, 13*, 9–20.

Clum, G. A. (1997). *Manual for the Comprehensive Panic Profile.* Blacksburg, VA: Self-Change Systems.

Clum, G. A., Broyles, S., Borden, J., & Watkins, P. L. (1990). Validity and reliability of the Panic Attack Symptoms and Cognitions Questionnaires. *Journal of Psychopathology and Behavioral Assessment, 12*, 233–245.

Cox, B. J., Direnfeld, D. M., Swinson, R. P., & Norton, G. R. (1994). Suicidal ideation and suicide attempts in panic disorder and social phobia. *American Journal of Psychiatry, 151*, 882–887.

Cox, B. J., Endler, N. S., & Swinson, R. P. (1995). An examination of levels of agoraphobic severity in panic disorder. *Behaviour Research and Therapy, 33*, 57–62.

Cox, B. J., Endler, N. S., Swinson, R. P., & Norton, G. R. (1992). Situations and specific coping strategies associated with clinical and nonclinical panic attacks. *Behaviour Research and Therapy, 30*, 67–69.

Cox, B. J., & Swinson, R. P. (2000). *An instrument to assess depersonalization-derealization in panic disorder.* Manuscript submitted for publication

Cox, B. J., Swinson, R. P., Endler, N. S., & Norton, G. R. (1994). The symptom structure of panic attacks. *Comprehensive Psychiatry, 35*, 349–353.

Cox, B. J., Swinson, R. P., Kuch, K., & Reichman, J. T. (1993). Dimensions of agoraphobia assessed by the Mobility Inventory. *Behaviour Research and Therapy, 31*, 427–431.

Cox, B. J., & Taylor, S. (2000). *Robust dimensions of anxiety sensitivity: The ASI-R-23.* Manuscript submitted for publication.

Craske, M. G., Rachman, S. J., & Tallman, K. (1986). Mobility, cognitions, and panic. *Journal of Psychopathology and Behavioral Assessment, 8,* 199–210.

de Beurs, E., Chambless, D. L., & Goldstein, A. J. (1997). Measurement of panic disorder by a modified panic diary. *Depression and Anxiety, 6,* 133–139.

Dillon, D. J., Gorman, J. M., Liebowitz, M. R., Fyer, A. J., & Klein, D. F. (1987). Measurement of lactate-induced panic and anxiety. *Psychiatry Research, 20,* 97–105.

Feske, U., & de Beurs, E. (1997). The Panic Appraisal Inventory: Psychometric properties. *Behaviour Research and Therapy, 35,* 875–882.

Fitzpatrick, K. K., & Schmidt, N. B. (2000, November). *The Discomfort Intolerance Scale (DIS): Psychometric properties and clinical utility in patients with panic disorder.* Paper presented at the meeting of the Association for Advancement of Behavior Therapy, New Orleans, LA.

Gauthier, J., Bouchard, S., Côté, G., Laberge, B., & French, D. (1993). Development of two scales measuring self-efficacy to control panic attacks. *Canadian Psychology, 30,* 305.

Hazen, A. L., Walker, J. R., & Eldridge, G. D. (1996). Anxiety sensitivity and treatment outcome in panic disorder. *Anxiety, 2,* 34–39.

Hoffart, A. (1995). A comparison of cognitive and guided mastery therapy of agoraphobia. *Behaviour Research and Therapy, 33,* 423–434.

Hoffart, A., Due-Madsen, J., Lande, B., Gude, T., Bille, H., & Torgersen, S. (1993). Clomipramine in the treatment of agoraphobic inpatients resistant to behavioral therapy. *Journal of Clinical Psychiatry, 54,* 481–487.

Hoffart, A., & Martinsen, E. W. (1990). Exposure-based integrated vs. pure psychodynamic treatment of agoraphobic inpatients. *Psychotherapy, 27,* 210–218.

Khawaja, N. G., & Oei, T. P. S. (1992). Development of a catastrophic cognition questionnaire. *Journal of Anxiety Disorders, 6,* 305–318.

Khawaja, N. G., Oei, T. P. S., & Baglioni, A. J. (1994). Modification of the Catastrophic Cognitions Questionnaire (CCQ-M) for normals and patients: Exploratory and LISREL analyses. *Journal of Psychopathology and Behavioral Assessment, 16,* 325–342.

Kinney, P. J., & Williams, S. L. (1988). Accuracy of fear inventories and self-efficacy scales in predicting agoraphobic behavior. *Behaviour Research and Therapy, 26,* 513–518.

Kwon, S.-M., Evans, L., & Oei, T. P. S. (1990). Factor structure of the Mobility Inventory for Agoraphobia: A validation study with Australian samples of agoraphobic patients. *Journal of Psychopathology and Behavioral Assessment, 12,* 365–374.

McNally, R. J., & Foa, E. B. (1987). Cognition and agoraphobia: Bias in the interpretation of threat. *Cognitive Therapy and Research, 11,* 567–581.

Miller, L. C., Murphy, R., & Buss, A. H. (1981). Consciousness of body: Private and public. *Journal of Personality and Social Psychology, 41,* 397–406.

Newman, M. G., Zuelig, A. R., & Kachin, K. E. (1998, November). *The reliability and validity of the Panic Disorder Self-Report (PDSR): A new measure of panic disorder.* Paper presented at the meeting of the Association for Advancement of Behavior Therapy, Washington, DC.

Norton, G. R., Cox, B. J., & Malan, J. (1992). Nonclinical panickers: A critical review. *Clinical Psychology Review, 12,* 121–139.

Norton, G. R., Dorward, J., & Cox, B. J. (1986). Factors associated with panic attacks in nonclinical subjects. *Behavior Therapy, 17,* 239–252.

Norton, G. R., Pidlubny, S. R., & Norton, P. J. (1999). Prediction of panic attacks and related variables. *Behavior Therapy, 30,* 319–330.

Öst, L.-G. (1990). The Agoraphobia Scale: An evaluation of its reliability and validity. *Behaviour Research and Therapy, 28,* 323–329.

Peterson, R. A., & Heilbronner, R. L. (1987). The Anxiety Sensitivity Index: Construct validity and factor analytic structure. *Journal of Anxiety Disorders, 1,* 117–121.

Rapee, R. M., Brown, T. A., Antony, M. M., & Barlow, D. H. (1992). Response to hyperventilation and inhalation of 5.5% carbon dioxide-enriched air across the DSM-III-R anxiety disorders. *Journal of Abnormal Psychology, 101,* 538–552.

Sanderson, W. C., Rapee, R. M., & Barlow, D. H. (1989). The influence of an illusion of control on panic attacks induced via inhalation of 5.5% carbon dioxide-enriched air. *Archives of General Psychiatry, 46,* 157–162.

Sanderson, W. C., Wetzler, S., & Asnis, G. M. (1994). Alprazolam blockade of CO_2-provoked panic in patients with panic disorder. *American Journal of Psychiatry, 151,* 1220–1222.

Schmidt, N. B., & Cook, J. H. (1999). Effects of anxiety sensitivity on anxiety and pain during a cold pressor challenge in patients with panic disorder. *Behaviour Research and Therapy, 37,* 313–323.

Schmidt, N. B., & Lerew, D. R. (1998). Prospective evaluation of psychological risk factors as predictors of functional impairment during acute stress. *Journal of Occupational Rehabilitation, 8,* 199–211.

Schmidt, N. B., Lerew, D. R., & Jackson, R. J. (1999). Prospective evaluation of anxiety sensitivity in the pathogenesis of panic: Replication and extension. *Journal of Abnormal Psychology, 108,* 532–537.

Scupi, B. S., Maser, J. D., & Uhde, T. W. (1992). The National Institute of Mental Health Panic Questionnaire: An instrument for assessing clinical characteristics of panic disorder. *Journal of Nervous and Mental Disease, 180,* 566–572.

Shear, M. K., Brown, T. A., Barlow, D. H., Money, R., Sholomskas, D. E., Woods, S. W., Gorman, J. M., & Papp, L. A. (1997). Multicenter collaborative panic disorder severity scale. *American Journal of Psychiatry, 154,* 1571–1575.

Silverman, W. K., Fleisig, W., Rabian, B., & Peterson, R. A. (1991). Childhood anxiety sensitivity index. *Journal of Clinical Child Psychology, 20,* 162–168.

Silverman, W. K., Ginsburg, G. S., & Goedhart, A. W. (1999). Factor structure of the childhood anxiety sensitivity index. *Behaviour Research and Therapy, 37,* 903–917.

Stein, M. B., Roy-Byrne, P. P. McQuaid, J. R., Laffaye, C., Russo, J., McCahill, M. E., Katon, W., Craske, M., Bystritsky, A., Sherbourne, C. D. (1999). Development of a brief diagnostic screen for panic disorder in primary care. *Psychosomatic Medicine, 61,* 359–364.

Swinson, R. P., Cox, B. J., Shulman, I. D., Kuch, K., & Woszczyna, C. B. (1992). Medication use and the assessment of agoraphobic avoidance. *Behaviour Research and Therapy, 30,* 563–568.

Taylor, S. (1999). *Anxiety sensitivity: Theory, research, and treatment of the fear of anxiety.* Hillsdale, NJ: Erlbaum.

Taylor, S., & Cox, B. J. (1998). An expanded Anxiety Sensitivity Index: Evidence for a hierarchic structure in a clinical sample. *Journal of Anxiety Disorders, 12,* 463–483.

Taylor, S., Koch, W. J., & McNally, R. J. (1992). How does anxiety sensitivity vary across the anxiety disorders? *Journal of Anxiety Disorders, 6,* 249–259.

Telch, M. J. (1987). *The Panic Appraisal Inventory.* Unpublished manuscript, University of Texas.

Telch, M. J., Brouillard, M., Telch, C. F., Agras, W. S., & Taylor, C. B. (1989). Role of cognitive appraisal in panic-related avoidance. *Behaviour Research and Therapy, 27,* 373–383.

van Hout, W. J. P. J., Emmelkamp, P. M. G., & Scholing, A. (1994). The role of negative self-statements during exposure in vivo: A process study of eight panic disorder patients with agoraphobia. *Behavior Modification, 18,* 389–410.

Whittal, M. L., Suchday, S., & Goetsch, V. L. (1994). The Panic Attack Questionnaire: Factor analysis of symptom profiles and characteristics of undergraduates who panic. *Journal of Anxiety Disorders, 8,* 237–245.

Zinbarg, R. E., Barlow, D. H., & Brown, T. A. (1997). Hierarchical structure and general factor saturation of the Anxiety Sensitivity Index: Evidence and Implications. *Psychological Assessment, 9,* 277–284.

Chapter 10
Specific Phobia:
A Brief Overview and
Guide to Assessment

Martin M. Antony

Specific phobias are among the most prevalent of anxiety disorders, affecting about 11% of the general population (e.g., Kessler et al., 1994). *The Diagnostic and Statistical Manual of Mental Disorders* (DSM-IV; American Psychiatric Association, 1994) defines a specific phobia as marked and persistent fear that is excessive or unreasonable, and that is triggered by the presence of anticipation of a specific object or situation. DSM-IV defines five types of specific phobias: (1) *animal type*, which includes fears of animals such as spiders, snakes, dogs, cats, mice, and birds; (2) *natural environment type*, which includes fears of being near water, high places, and storms; (3) *blood–injection–injury type*, which includes fears of seeing blood, receiving injections or blood tests, and watching medical procedures; (4) *situational type*, which includes fears of situations such as driving, flying, elevators, enclosed places, and bridges; (5) *other type*, which includes fears of other situations, such as vomiting, choking, and loud sounds. To receive a diagnosis of specific phobia, an individuals fear must cause significant impairment in his or her functioning, or the person must be distressed about having the fear. In addition, the person must acknowledge that the fear is excessive and must avoid the feared stimulus or endure exposure with extreme distress.

This chapter provides a brief overview of the methods used to assess individuals with specific phobia. Included are suggestions regarding differential diagnosis, screening questions for specific phobias, suggestions regarding information to be assessed during a clinical interview, and recommendations for including behavioral assessments and self-report scales in the assessment process. The chapter ends with a brief section on the relationship between assessment, development of an effective treatment plan, and measurement of outcome. This

Martin M. Antony • Anxiety Treatment and Research Centre, St. Joseph's Healthcare, Hamilton, and Department of Psychiatry and Behavioral Neurosciences, McMaster University, Hamilton, Ontario L8N 4A6, Canada.

chapter is meant to highlight some of the most important issues that arise when assessing individuals with specific phobia. Readers who are interested in a more thorough discussion of these issues should consult relevant chapters by Antony and Swinson (2000) or McCabe and Antony (in press). All instruments mentioned in this chapter are described in Chapter 11 of this book, along with full citations.

DIFFERENTIAL DIAGNOSIS

A diagnosis of specific phobia is not assigned if an individual's fear is better accounted for by another DSM-IV disorder. For example, an individual who develops a fear of driving after a serious car accident would be given a diagnosis of posttraumatic stress disorder (PTSD) if all of the required symptoms of PTSD were present in addition to the fear of driving. An individual with social phobia who fears driving only because of the possibility of having his or her driving skills criticized by other drivers on the road would not receive an additional diagnosis of specific phobia if the fear were completely accounted for by the social phobia.

Specific phobias are sometimes difficult to distinguish from panic disorder and agoraphobia (PDA). This is particularly true for specific phobias of the situational type, which overlap considerably with the types of situations feared by individuals with PDA. Despite the similarities between PDA and situational specific phobias, these conditions also differ in important ways. First, individuals with specific phobias typically experience fear only when confronted with the phobic stimulus. In contrast, people with PDA tend to experience fear across a range of situations and also tend to experience uncued panic attacks, which are not triggered by any particular situations. Second, the focus of apprehension is often different in people with specific phobias versus people with PDA. For example, individuals with a specific phobia of flying are usually fearful of being in a plane crash, whereas individuals with PDA who fear flying are usually anxious about experiencing a panic attack and not being able to escape from the situation.

SCREENING QUESTIONS AND CLINICAL INTERVIEW

When screening for specific phobias, it is important to first assess the presence of fear associated with specific objects and situations. For example, a clinician might ask, "Do you feel fearful or uncomfortable when confronted by any of the following objects or situations: spiders, bugs, snakes, dogs, cats, birds, mice, storms, water, heights, the sight of blood or watching surgery, getting a blood test or injection, driving, flying, enclosed places (e.g., small rooms, tunnels, elevators), dental treatment, or other objects or situations?" This question should be followed up with additional questions to assess the intensity of the patient's fear during typical exposures, frequency of avoidance, degree to which the fear is excessive or out of proportion to the actual danger, and the extent to which the fear causes distress or functional impairment. Semistructured clinical interviews such as the Anxiety Disorders Interview Schedule for DSM-IV (Brown, Di Nardo, & Barlow, 1994; Di Nardo, Brown, & Barlow, 1994) and the Structured Clinical Interview for DSM-IV (First, Spitzer, Gibbon, & Williams, 1996) may be used to confirm the diagnosis of specific phobia.

Once the clinician has established that an individual has a specific phobia, additional questions can be used to identify the important clinical features associated with the individual's fear. Variables that should be assessed during the clinical interview include the etiology and course of the fear, the physical reactions experienced (e.g., panic attacks), history of fainting in the feared situation (this is an issue only for individuals with blood and injection phobias), types of fearful cognitions (e.g., fearful beliefs, predictions, cognitive biases), the extent to which the individual's fear is focused on symptoms of physical arousal (e.g., people who fear enclosed places are often fearful of experiencing breathlessness), situations that are avoided by the patient, patterns of subtle avoidance (e.g., distraction, relying on safety behaviors), variables that affect the individual's fear (e.g., for driving phobias—weather, amount of traffic, darkness, and so on), treatment history, family factors, and any associated medical problems. Identifying the clinical features of the patient's fear is essential for appropriate treatment planning.

SELF-REPORT SCALES

Chapter 11 reviews 26 measures for specific phobia, many of which are reprinted in Appendix B. Certain phobia types tend to be overrepresented among these available instruments. For example, although there are at least four measures of spider phobia, five measures of blood–injection–injury phobia, and six measures of dental phobia, measures of certain other common specific phobias (e.g., storms, water, driving, birds, cats) are not available. For other phobias (e.g., dogs, flying, heights, snakes), there are a small number of available measures, but they tend to be relatively old, or they have been subjected to very little research.

Screening Measures for Specific Phobias

Various versions of the Fear Survey Schedule (FSS) have been used to screen for specific phobias. Despite their popularity, the FSS is not ideal for this purpose. First, it contains questions about many situations that are not related to specific phobias (e.g., fears of arguing with parents, life after death). In addition, there is evidence that ratings on FSS items do not distinguish between the behavior of individuals with phobias and nonfearful controls on behavioral tests (Klieger & Franklin, 1993).

Measures for Animal Phobias

A number of scales are available for measuring symptoms of spider phobia. The Spider Questionnaire, Fear of Spiders Questionnaire, and Watts and Sharrock Spider Phobia Questionnaire are all appropriate for measuring severity of spider fear, although the latter two measures have the advantage of providing continuous Likert ratings for each item, rather than true/false ratings. The Spider Phobia Beliefs Questionnaire is useful for assessing an individual's beliefs about spiders and about his or her response to seeing spiders. The Snake Questionnaire (sometimes referred to in publications as the Snake Anxiety Questionnaire) is the only empirically supported scale for measuring severity of snake phobia. Finally, a new scale called the Dog Phobia Questionnaire appears to be a promising questionnaire for measuring the severity of dog phobias, although there are no published papers on this measure.

Measures for Natural Environment Phobias

The Acrophobia Questionnaire is the most frequently used measure for severity of fear and avoidance in situations involving heights. We are aware of no other instruments for measuring severity of natural environment phobias (e.g., storms, water) in adults.

Measures for Blood–Injection–Injury Phobias

Chapter 11 reviews several different scales for measuring the severity of blood–injection–injury fears. The Blood–Injection Symptom Scale is a brief measure that assesses symptoms of anxiety, faintness, and various physical sensations that occur during negative encounters with blood and injections. In contrast, the Medical Fear Survey and Mutilation Questionnaire assess the range of situations involving blood, injections, cutting, and medical procedures in which individuals experience fear or discomfort. Although it is considerably longer, the Medical Fear Survey has several advantages over the Mutilation Questionnaire, including ratings on a continuous Likert scale (instead of true/false ratings), evaluation of a broader range of situations, and the ability to generate subscale scores. Finally, the Threatening Medical Situations Inventory may be used to assess particular styles of coping with medical situations (e.g., a tendency to seek out versus avoid threat-related information).

Measures for Situational Phobias

Three published measures are suitable for assessing the features of claustrophobia (i.e., phobia of enclosed places), each with a somewhat different purpose. The Claustrophobia General Cognitions Questionnaire assesses the types of beliefs underlying an individual's claustrophobia. The Claustrophobia Situations Questionnaire assesses the range of situations avoided by individuals with claustrophobia. Finally, the Claustrophobia Questionnaire separately measures fears of claustrophobic situations involving a threat of suffocation, and fears of situations involving a threat of restriction.

The Fear of Flying Scale appears to be useful for measuring the severity of flying fear, although its psychometric properties have not yet been thoroughly researched. We are aware of no other empirically supported scales for assessing other specific phobias from the situational type.

Measures for Dental Phobia

Several options exist for measuring the severity of dental fear, the most popular of which are described in this section. The Dental Anxiety Inventory measures the overall severity of an individual's dental fear and is available in both extended (36-item) and brief (9-item) versions. The Dental Fear Survey provides information about the degree of avoidance associated with an individual's dental fear, the range of situations avoided by people who have dental phobias, and the types of anxiety sensations that are experienced during dental treatment. The Dental Cognitions Questionnaire assesses the types of fearful thoughts held by people with dental fears, including beliefs about dental treatment as well as beliefs about the anxiety symptoms that occur during dental treatment. The shortest measure for dental phobia is the Corah Dental Anxiety Scale, which has only 4 items and has been frequently used as a dental phobia severity measure.

Behavioral Approach Test

One of the most important tools for the assessment of specific phobias is the behavioral approach test (BAT; sometimes referred to as a behavioral avoidance test or a behavioral assessment test). The BAT involves assessing the features of a patient's phobia in the context of exposure to the phobic situation. Behavioral assessment provides the clinician with an opportunity to observe the patient's behaviors in the feared situation. Also, a BAT may provide a more accurate assessment of a patient's true response to the phobic situation because, unlike interviews, the findings are unlikely to be influenced by biases in retrospective recall, which are particularly problematic when a patient has not encountered the feared situation in a long time.

Antony and Swinson (2000) describe two types of BAT assessments: progressive BATs and selective BATs. In a *progressive BAT*, the clinician asks the patient to approach a feared situation gradually, measuring his or her response to the situation at each step. For example, steps for a BAT involving a spider phobia might involve looking at a spider from a distance, standing as close as possible to a spider in a jar, holding the jar, opening the jar, touching a spider with a pencil, and finally touching a spider with one's hand. The number of steps taken during the BAT is recorded. Other variables that can be assessed during the BAT include the fear level at each step (using a 0–100 point scale), anxious cognitions that occur during the exercise, subtle avoidance behaviors, and heart rate.

In a *selective BAT*, the clinician may select one or more situations from a patient's fear hierarchy and ask the individual to enter the situation(s). For example, an individual with a height phobia might be asked to climb a 6-foot ladder, stand by the railing on the second story of a shopping mall and look down, and ride to the sixth floor of a glass elevator while looking out. The measures taken during a selective BAT are similar to those discussed earlier and include such variables as subjective fear ratings (including expected fear levels before the exposure and actual fear ratings during the exposure), anxious cognitions, subtle avoidance behaviors, and heart rate.

Relationship between Assessment, Treatment Planning, and Outcome Evaluation

The information gathered during the assessment is useful for developing an effective treatment plan. For example, identifying the types of situations avoided by the individual and the variables that affect the patient's fear level while exposed to the phobic object or situation can help in the development of a hierarchy for use during exposure-based treatments (for a detailed description of empirically based treatments for specific phobia, see Antony, Craske, & Barlow, 1995; Antony & Swinson, 2000; Craske, Antony, & Barlow, 1997).

In addition to conducting a thorough assessment before treatment, the clinician should continue the assessment process throughout treatment to assess the patient's progress. In addition, if the patient agrees, it is often helpful to repeat some of the assessment measures (e.g., a BAT, self-report scales) at the end of treatment, to measure outcome, and periodically after treatment has ended, to measure the extent to which gains have been maintained.

SUMMARY AND CONCLUSIONS

This chapter provided a brief overview of the types of assessment strategies that are useful for evaluating individuals with specific phobias, including methods of screening for phobias, variables to assess during the initial clinical interview, self-report scales that can supplement information provided during the interview, and behavioral assessment strategies that provide an opportunity to observe the patient while he or she is exposed to the phobic situation. Finally, the importance of repeating parts of the assessment during and following treatment is discussed.

REFERENCES

American Psychiatric Association. (1994). *Diagnostic and statistical manual of mental disorders* (4th ed.). Washington, DC: Author.

Antony, M. M., Craske, M. G., & Barlow, D. H. (1995). *Mastery of your specific phobia, client manual.* San Antonio, TX: The Psychological Corporation.

Antony, M. M., & Swinson, R. P. (2000). *Phobic disorders and panic in Adults: A guide to assessment and treatment.* Washington, DC: American Psychological Association.

Brown, T. A., Di Nardo, P., & Barlow, D. H. (1994). *Anxiety Disorders Interview Schedule for DSM-IV.* San Antonio, TX: The Psychological Corporation.

Craske, M. G., Antony, M. M., & Barlow, D. H. (1997). *Mastery of your specific phobia (therapist guide).* San Antonio, TX: Psychological Corporation.

Di Nardo, P., Brown, T. A., & Barlow, D. H. (1994). *Anxiety Disorders Interview Schedule for DSM-IV (Lifetime Version).* San Antonio, TX: The Psychological Corporation.

First, M. B., Spitzer, R. L., Gibbon, M., & Williams, J. B. W. (1996). *Structured Clinical Interview for DSM-IV Axis I Disorders–Patient Edition (SCID-I/P, Version 2.0).* New York: Biometrics Research Department, New York State Psychiatric Institute.

Kessler, R. C., McGonagle, K. A., Zhao, S., Nelson, C. B., Hughes, M., Eshleman, S., Wittchen, H.-U., & Kendler, K. (1994). Lifetime and 12-month prevalence of DSM-III-R psychiatric disorders in the United States: Results from the National Comorbidity Survey. *Archives of General Psychiatry, 51,* 8–19.

Klieger, D. M., & Franklin, M. E. (1993). Validity of the Fear Survey Schedule in phobia research: A laboratory test. *Journal of Psychopathology and Behavioral Assessment, 15,* 207–217.

McCabe, R. E., & Antony, M. M. (in press). Specific and social phobia. In M. M. Antony & D. H. Barlow (Eds.), *Handbook of assessment, treatment planning, and outcome evaluation: Empirically supported strategies for psychological disorders.* New York: Guilford.

Chapter 11
Measures for Specific Phobia

Martin M. Antony

ACROPHOBIA QUESTIONNAIRE (AQ)

Original Citation

Cohen, D. C. (1977). Comparison of self-report and overt-behavioral procedures for assessing acrophobia. *Behavior Therapy, 8,* 17–23.

Purpose

To assess the severity of anxiety and avoidance related to common height situations.

Description

The AQ is a 40-item self-report questionnaire in which individuals rate their anxiety and avoidance relative to 20 different height-related situations. First, each of 20 items is rated on a seven-point anxiety scale ranging from 0 (not at all anxious; calm and relaxed) to 6 (extremely anxious). Then, the same 20 items are rated again with respect to avoidance, using a three-point scale ranging from 0 (would not avoid doing it) to 2 (would not do it under any circumstances).

Martin M. Antony • Anxiety Treatment and Research Centre, St. Joseph's Healthcare, Hamilton, and Department of Psychiatry and Behavioural Neurosciences, McMaster University, Hamilton, Ontario L8N 4A6, Canada.

Administration and Scoring

The AQ takes 5 minutes to administer. The scale is scored by separately computing the sum of the 20 anxiety ratings and the sum of the 20 avoidance ratings.

Psychometric Properties

Sample Scores and Norms. Cohen (1972) reported mean scores from a clinic sample of individuals with height phobias. The mean AQ anxiety and AQ avoidance scores were 61.30 (*SD* = 15.85) and 14.37 (*SD* = 5.70), respectively. These means are similar to pretreatment scores in a subsequent treatment study (Cohen, 1977). In a student sample, the means for the anxiety and avoidance scales were 27.10 (*SD* = 17.32) and 4.57 (*SD* = 4.17), respectively (Cohen, 1972). On average, scores on both subscales decreased by about half following behavioral treatment (Cohen, 1977).

Reliability. Spearman-Brown corrected split-half reliabilities for the AQ were *r* = .82 for the anxiety scale and *r* = .70 for the avoidance scale (Baker, Cohen, & Saunders, 1973). Test–retest reliability over 3 months was good for both scales (*r*s = .86 for anxiety and .82 for avoidance; Baker et al., 1973).

Validity. The avoidance and anxiety scales of the AQ correlated highly with one another (*r* = .73; Baker et al., 1973) and to a lesser degree with measures of general fear and personality functioning (*r*s range from .24 to .46). Correlations with scores on a behavioral test were moderate (Cohen, 1977). Convergent validity is unknown because there are no other established measures of height phobia severity for comparison. The AQ is sensitive to the effects of treatment (Baker et al., 1973; Bourque & Ladouceur, 1980; Cohen, 1977).

Source

The AQ is reprinted in Appendix B. Additional information may be obtained from the author, David Cohen, Ph.D., Department of Psychology, California State University, Bakersfield, CA 93311, USA; (tel) 661-664-2372; (fax) 661-665-6955; (e-mail) dcohen@csubak.edu.

BLOOD–INJECTION SYMPTOM SCALE (BISS)

Original Citation

Page, A. C., Bennett, K. S., Carter, O., Smith, J., & Woodmore, K. (1997). The Blood–Injection Symptom Scale (BISS). Assessing a structure of phobic symptoms elicited by blood and injections. *Behaviour Research and Therapy, 35,* 457–464.

Purpose

To measure anxiety, tension, and faintness related to blood and injections.

Description

The BISS is a 17-item self-report scale. By circling yes or no, respondents indicate which of 17 symptoms they have experienced during their worst experiences in a blood- or injection-related situation.

Administration and Scoring

The BISS takes 1 to 2 minutes to administer. Three subscales are generated as follows: *faintness subscale* (number of "yes" responses for items 3, 5–9, 12, 13, 17), *anxiety subscale* (number of "yes" responses for items 2, 4, 10, 14), *tension subscale* (number of "yes" responses for items 1, 11, 15, 16).

Psychometric Properties

Sample Scores and Norms. For a sample of individuals with blood-related fears, mean scores on the faintness, anxiety, and tension subscales were 3.89 ($SE = 0.33$), 1.74 ($SE = 0.17$), and 0.56 ($SE = 0.15$), respectively (Page et al., 1997). For a sample of individuals with injection-related concerns, mean scores on the faintness, anxiety, and tension subscales were 2.76 ($SE = 0.31$), 2.12 ($SE = 0.10$), and 0.81 ($SE = 0.20$), respectively (Page et al., 1997). The most extensive normative data available are on the author's webpage (www.psy.uwa.edu.au/ user/andrew/biss.htm).

Reliability. In the Page et al. (1997) study, internal consistency was variable, with a Cronbach's alpha of .86 for the total score and alphas ranging from .56 to .85 for the subscales. Hepburn and Page (1999) demonstrated moderate correlations between scores during two test trials (using a modified "state" version of the BISS), with *r*s ranging from .54 to .62 for the total score and the various subscales.

Validity. The final items selected for the BISS were derived from a factor analysis (Page et al., 1997). There are no published studies demonstrating convergent or predictive validity.

Alternative Forms

A *state* version of the BISS is available. This version includes more items in each subscale, some general severity items, and Likert-type scoring. More information is available on the BISS website (www.psy.uwa.edu.au/user/andrew/biss.htm).

Source

The BISS is reprinted in the original paper by Page et al. (1997) as well as in Appendix B. The scale and manual are also available on the author's website (www.psy.uwa.edu.au/user/ andrew/biss.htm). Additional information may be obtained from the author, Andrew C. Page, Ph.D., Department of Psychology, University of Western Australia, Nedlands, 6907, Australia, (tel) 61 8 9380 3577; (fax) 61 8 9380 2655; (e-mail) andrew@psy.uwa.edu.au.

CLAUSTROPHOBIA GENERAL COGNITIONS QUESTIONNAIRE (CGCQ) AND CLAUSTROPHOBIA SITUATIONS QUESTIONNAIRE (CSQ)

Original Citation

Febbraro, G. A. R. & Clum, G. A. (1995). A dimensional analysis of claustrophobia. *Journal of Psychopathology and Behavioral Assessment, 17,* 335–351.

Purpose

The CGCQ measures cognitions associated with claustrophobic situations. The CSQ measures anxiety and avoidance related to specific claustrophobic situations.

Description

The CGCQ is a 26-item self-report scale on which participants rate the likelihood of various fear-related outcomes that might occur in a claustrophobic situation. Each item is rated on a five-point scale ranging from 1 (not likely) to 5 (very likely). Before rating the items, the individual first lists several claustrophobic situations that are anxiety-provoking. At the end, there is space to record any other thoughts that occur in claustrophobic situations.

The CSQ is a self-report scale on which participants rate separately their fear and avoidance of 42 different enclosed or claustrophobic situations. Each item is rated on a five-point scale ranging from 1 (not anxious/never avoid) to 5 (extremely anxious/always avoid). At the end, there is space to record any other situations that are associated with anxiety or avoidance.

Administration and Scoring

The CGCQ takes 5 minutes to complete and generates three subscales: *fear of loss of control* (sum of items 2, 9, 12, 17, 20–22, 25, 26), *fear of suffocation* (sum of items 5, 7, 8, 10, 11, 13, 16, 23), and *fear of inability to escape* (sum of items 1, 4, 6, 14, 15, 18, 19, 24). Note that one item (item 3) did not load on any of the three factors.

The CSQ takes 5 to 10 minutes to complete and generates slightly different subscales for the anxiety and avoidance items. Two CSQ anxiety subscales are generated (based on a factor analysis of anxiety ratings): *fear of entrapment* (sum of items 1, 2, 4, 5, 7, 9, 11, 13–16, 18, 22, 24, 26, 27, 29, 30, 33) and *fear of physical confinement* (sum of items 3, 6, 8, 10, 17, 19–21, 23, 25, 34, 37, 38, 40–42). Note that seven items (items 12, 28, 31, 32, 35, 36, 39) did not load on either subscale.

Two CSQ avoidance subscales are generated (based on a factor analysis of avoidance ratings): *avoidance of crowds* (sum of items 3, 5, 7, 9, 11, 13–16, 18, 26, 28–31, 33, 36) and *avoidance of physical confinement* (sum of items 2, 4, 6, 8, 10, 12, 17, 19, 21–23, 24, 27, 38, 40). Note that ten items (items 1, 20, 25, 32, 34, 35, 37, 39, 41, 42) did not load on either subscale.

Psychometric Properties

All psychometric data are based on a sample of 94 individuals who reported fears of enclosed places (Febbraro & Clum, 1995). Twenty eight of these individuals met diagnostic criteria for claustrophobia (specific phobia), whereas the others received a range of different anxiety disorder diagnoses or no diagnosis.

Sample Scores and Norms. The mean CGCQ subscale scores for the heterogeneous sample described above were 16.20 (SD = 7.13) for the fear of loss of control subscale, 23.00 (SD = 7.53) for the fear of suffocation subscale, and 26.07 (SD = 6.60) for the fear of inability to escape subscale. The mean CSQ anxiety scores were 49.46 (SD = 15.33) for the fear of entrapment subscale and 37.41 (SD = 10.31) for the fear of physical confinement subscale. Mean CSQ avoidance scores were 36.02 (SD = 12.55) for avoidance of crowds and 49.55 (SD = 11.88) for avoidance of physical confinement.

Reliability. Internal consistency for the CGCQ subscales (as measured by Cronbach's alpha) was .88 for fear of loss of control, .88 for fear of suffocation, and .84 for fear of inability to escape. Internal consistency for the CSQ anxiety subscales was .94 for the fear of entrapment subscale and .87 for the fear of physical confinement subscale. Internal consistency for the CSQ avoidance subscales was .91 for avoidance of crowds and .88 for avoidance of physical confinement. Data on test–retest reliability are not available for either measure.

Validity. Subscales for both measures were determined by factor analysis. Subscale scores are all significantly correlated with one another, with rs ranging from .22 to .84. Data on convergent validity, discriminant validity, and treatment sensitivity are not available.

Source

The CGCQ and CSQ are reprinted in Appendix B. Additional information is available from the author, Greg A.R. Febbraro, Ph.D., Department of Psychology, Drake University, 2507 University Avenue, Des Moines, IA 50311, USA; (tel) 515-271-3964; (fax) 515-271-1925; (e-mail) greg.febbraro@drake.edu.

CLAUSTROPHOBIA QUESTIONNAIRE (CLQ)

Original Citation

Radomsky, A. S., Rachman, S., Thordarson, D. S., McIsaac, H. K., & Teachman, B. A. (in press). The Claustrophobia Questionnaire (CLQ). *Journal of Anxiety Disorders*.

Purpose

To assess claustrophobia and its component fears (fear of suffocation and fear of restriction).

Description

The CLQ is a 26-item self-report scale with subscales measuring fear of situations involving suffocation and restriction. Each item is rated on a five-point scale ranging from 0 (not at all anxious) to 4 (extremely anxious). Earlier versions of the CLQ (Rachman & Taylor, 1993) and its suffocation fear subscale (McNally & Eke, 1996; Taylor & Rachman, 1994) have been frequently used in the literature.

Administration and Scoring

The CLQ takes 5 to 10 minutes to complete. The *suffocation subscale* score is generated by computing the sum of the 14 suffocation subscale items. The *restriction subscale* score is generated by computing the sum of the 12 restriction subscale items. In addition, a total score can be generated by computing the sum of both subscale scores.

Psychometric Properties

All psychometric data reported below are based on the validation study by Radomsky, Rachman, Thordarson, McIsaac, and Teachman (in press).

Sample Scores and Norms. Mean scores for a group of claustrophobic students were 51.8 ($SD = 16.60$) for the total score, 23.8 ($SD = 8.4$) for the suffocation subscale, and 27.6 ($SD = 9.6$) for the restriction subscale. For a community sample of adults, mean scores were 28.9 ($SD = 19.4$) for the total score, 9.1 ($SD = 7.9$) for the suffocation subscale, and 19.9 ($SD = 12.8$) for the restriction subscale.

Reliability. Internal consistency is good to excellent, with Cronbach's alpha = .95 for the total scale, .85 for the suffocation subscale, and .96 for the restriction subscale. Test–retest reliability was high over 2 weeks, with $r = .89$ for the total CLQ score, $r = .89$ for the suffocation subscale, and $r = .77$ for the restriction subscale.

Validity. The CLQ items and subscales were determined by a factor analysis. The suffocation and restriction subscales are moderately intercorrelated ($r = .53$). The CLQ discriminates between those with claustrophobic fear and community controls. In addition, scores on the CLQ are predictive of fear responses in enclosed places, but not of fear responses to heights or snakes.

The CLQ total and subscale scores are significantly correlated with a measure of anxiety sensitivity (rs range from .27 to .33), but not with a measure of general anxiety or social anxiety. Although the total score and restriction subscale were significantly correlated with a measure of depression ($rs = .25$ and .26, respectively), the correlation between the suffocation subscale and a measure of depression was not quite significant ($r = .21$).

Source

The CLQ is reprinted in the validation study by Radomsky et al. (in press) as well as in Appendix B. Additional information may be obtained from the author, Adam Radomsky, Ph.D., Department of Psychology, Concordia University, 7141 Sherbrooke West, Montreal,

QC H4B 1R6, Canada; (tel) 514-848-2222; (fax) 514-848-4523; (e-mail) radomsky@vax2.
concordia.ca.

DENTAL ANXIETY INVENTORY (DAI)

Original Citation

Stouthard, M. E. A., Mellenbergh, G. J., & Hoogstraten, J. (1993). Assessment of dental
anxiety: A facet approach. *Anxiety, Stress, and Coping, 6,* 89–105.

Purpose

To measure severity of dental anxiety.

Description

The DAI is a self-report measures consisting of 36 fearful statements related to dental
situations. Items are rated on a five-point scale ranging from 1 (totally untrue) to 5 (completely
true). In addition, a nine-item brief version called the Short DAI (SDAI) is available. Items on
the SDAI (in order) include items 1, 6, 7, 14, 21, 22, 27, 29, and 35 from the DAI. The SDAI
items are rated on the same scale as that used on the DAI.

Administration and Scoring

The DAI takes 5 to 10 minutes to complete. A total score is generated by calculating the
sum of all 36 items. There are no reverse scored items and scores can range from 36 to 180. The
SDAI takes 3 to 5 minutes to complete. A total score is generated by calculating the sum of all
9 items. There are no reverse scored items and scores can range from 9 to 45.

Psychometric Properties

All psychometric data reported below are based on the initial validation study by
Stouthard, Mellenbergh, and Hoogstraten (1993). Additional data supporting this scale are
available in papers by Schuurs and Hoogstraten (1993) and Stouthard, Hoogstraten, and
Mellenbergh (1995).

Sample Scores and Norms.   The mean DAI score for a group of individuals known
to be anxious in dental situations is 130.5 (SD = 23.6). Mean DAI scores for a Dutch
community sample and a sample of Dutch dental patients were 66.9 (SD = 32.3) and 63.6
(SD = 29.1), respectively. Scores on the DAI tend to be lower after dental treatment than just
before or during dental treatment.

Reliability.   Internal consistency for the DAI is excellent, with Cronbach's alpha
ranging from .96 to .98 across four samples (Stouthard et al., 1993). Test–retest reliability was

also high (rs = .84 to .87 across two samples). In addition, a recent study by Aartman (1998) supports the reliability of the SDAI.

Validity. A factor analysis found that items load on three factors: general dental anxiety, fear of dentist's comments about teeth, and fear of drilling, extraction, and anesthesia. The DAI is highly correlated with the Corah Dental Anxiety Scale (rs = .82 and .69, in samples of students and dental patients, respectively). In addition, the correlation between the DAI score and a dentist's judgment regarding patients' anxiety was .38. The DAI distinguishes between individuals known to be anxious in dental situations and individuals known to be nonanxious. Finally, Aartman (1998) found support for the validity of the SDAI.

Alternative Forms

In addition to the English version, the DAI is available in Dutch, French, German, Italian, Norwegian, and Spanish. A manual is available in Dutch only. As reviewed earlier, a nine-item short version of the DAI (SDAI) is available.

Source

The 36-item DAI is reprinted in the validation study by Stouthard et al. (1995) and in Appendix B. The 9-item SDAI is reprinted in the validation paper by Stouthard et al. (1993) and can be derived from the DAI, as described earlier. Additional information is available from the author, Dr. Marlies E. A. Stouthard, Department of Social Medicine, Academic Medical Center, P.O. Box 22700, 1100 DE, Amsterdam, The Netherlands; (tel) +31 20 5664618; (fax) 31 20 6972316; (e-mail) m.e.stouthard@amc.uva.nl.

DENTAL COGNITIONS QUESTIONNAIRE (DCQ)

Original Citation

de Jongh, A., Muris, P., Schoenmakers, N., & Ter Horst, G. (1995). Negative cognitions of dental phobics: Reliability and validity of the Dental Cognitions Questionnaire. *Behaviour Research and Therapy, 33,* 507–515.

Purpose

To assess frequency and believability of negative cognitions related to dental treatment.

Description

The DCQ is a self-report measure containing 38 negative statements regarding dental treatment. For each item, the participant rates the percentage with which he or she believes the statement (0 = I don't believe this at all; 100 = I am absolutely convinced that this is true). In addition, each item is rated "yes" or "no" to indicate whether the thought tends to arise when the individual is about to undergo dental treatment.

Administration and Scoring

The DCQ takes 5 to 7 minutes to complete. There are no reverse-scored items. A total cognitions frequency scale is generated by calculating the number of yes responses (scores can range from 0 to 38). A believability score is generated by calculating the mean believability ratings for the 38 items (scores can range from 0 to 100).

Psychometric Properties

All psychometric data reported below are based on the initial validation study by de Jongh, Muris, Schoenmakers, and Ter Horst (1995), except for data regarding sensitivity for measuring treatment effects, which are based on a study by de Jongh, Muris, Ter Horst, et al. (1995).

Sample Scores and Norms.   In a sample of dental phobic individuals, the means for the DCQ frequency and believability scales were 22.5 (SD = 6.7) and 50.1 (SD = 16.3), respectively. In a student sample, the means for the DCQ frequency and believability scales were 9.8 (SD = 6.9) and 23.9 (SD = 16.4), respectively.

Reliability.   Internal consistency (Cronbach's alpha) in a student sample was .89 for the frequency scale and .95 for the believability scale. Test–retest reliability over a 5-week period was high, with r = .83.

Validity.   A factor analysis of the DCQ supports a single-factor structure. DCQ scores were significantly correlated with measures of state anxiety, trait anxiety, and worry (rs range from .22 to .36) and with a measure of dental anxiety (rs are .55 for the frequency scale and .36 for the believability scale). However, correlations between the DCQ scores and dental anxiety (as measured by the Corah Dental Anxiety Scale) were higher than correlations between the DCQ and either state or trait anxiety, supporting the discriminant validity of the scale. In addition, the DCQ distinguished individuals with dental phobia from nonphobic individuals. Finally, both scales from the DCQ appear to be sensitive to the effects of treatment (de Jongh, Muris, Ter Horst, et al., 1995).

Alternative Forms

In addition to an English language version, versions are available in Dutch, German, and Norwegian.

Source

The DCQ items are reprinted in the validation study by de Jongh et al. (1995) and the entire scale is reprinted in Appendix B. Additional information is available from the author,

Ad de Jongh, Ph.D., Department of Social Dentistry and Dental Health Education, Academic Centre for Dentistry, Louwesweg 1, 1066 EA Amsterdam, The Netherlands; (tel) +31 20 5188 232; (fax) +31 20 5188 233; (e-mail) adnicole@knoware.nl.

DENTAL FEAR SURVEY (DFS)

Original Citation

Kleinknecht, R. A., Klepac, R. K., & Alexander, L. D. (1973). Origins and characteristics of fear of dentistry. *Journal of the American Dental Association, 86,* 842–848.

Purpose

To assess dental avoidance, physiologic symptoms while in dental treatment, and fear of specific dental stimuli.

Description

The DFS is a 20-item self-report measure, although the original version had 27 items. Items 1 and 2 measure avoidance of dental situations; items 3 through 7 measure physiological symptoms while receiving dental treatment; items 8 through 19 measure fear, anxiety, or unpleasantness associated with various dental situations; item 20 provides a global rating of dental fear. Items 1 through 7 are rated on a five-point scale ranging from 1 (never) to 5 (nearly every time). Items 8 through 20 are rated on a five-point scale ranging from 1 (no fear) to 5 (extreme fear).

Administration and Scoring

The DFS takes between 2 and 5 minutes to complete. The instrument is scored by calculating the sum of all 20 items. Higher scores reflect more severe dental fear. Scores may range from 20 to 100. Some studies have also reported subscale scores.

Psychometric Properties

Sample Scores and Norms.   The mean DFS score for dental phobic individuals was 75.8 (*SD* = 12.9) in one study (Moore, Berggren, & Carlsson, 1991) and 76.6 (*SD* = 14.3) in another study (Johansson & Berggren, 1992). The mean DFS score for a large student sample was 38.6 (*SD* = 13.9; McGlynn, McNeil, Gallagher, & Vrana, 1987).

Reliability.   In a large student sample, internal consistency was excellent (Cronbach's alpha = .95) and test–retest reliability was good (*r* = .88; McGlynn et al., 1987).

Validity.   Factor-analytic studies have tended to find three factors representing (1) patterns of dental avoidance and anticipatory anxiety (8 items), (2) fear associated with particular procedures and stimuli (6 items), and (3) physical arousal symptoms during dental treatment (5 items; Kleinknecht, McGlynn, Thorndike, & Harkavy, 1984; McGlynn et al., 1987). In a study by Kleinknecht and Bernstein (1978), scores on the DFS were found to be more strongly related to other self-report measures than behavioral indicators of fear. However, scores on the DFS were predictive of missed or canceled appointments. The DFS is sensitive to the effects of treatment (Moore et al., 1991; Moore & Brødsgaard, 1994).

Alternative Forms

Versions of the DFS are available in English, Spanish, Korean, Portuguese (Brazil), Chinese, Swedish, Dutch, Japanese, and Hebrew.

Source

The DFS is reprinted in Appendix B. Additional information may be obtained from the author, Ronald A. Kleinknecht, Ph.D., College of Arts and Sciences, Western Washington University, Bellingham, WA 98225, USA; (tel) 360-650-3763; (fax) 360-650-6809; (e-mail) ronald.kleinknecht@wwu.edu.

FEAR OF SPIDERS QUESTIONNAIRE (FSQ)

Original Citation

Szymanski, J., & O'Donohue, W. (1995). Fear of Spiders Questionnaire. *Journal of Behavior Therapy and Experimental Psychiatry, 26*, 31–34.

Purpose

To assess the severity of spider phobia.

Description

The FSQ is a self-report measure comprised of 18 fearful statements regarding spiders. Each item is rated on an eight-point scale ranging from 0 (totally disagree) to 7 (totally agree).

Administration and Scoring

The FSQ can be administered in 5 minutes. It is scored by adding up the scores from each of the 18 items. Total scores can range from 0 to 126.

Psychometric Properties

Sample Scores and Norms.   The mean FSQ score for a group of spider phobic individuals was 89.1 (*SD* = 19.6) before treatment and 39.9 (*SD* = 25.4) after treatment (Muris & Merckelbach, 1996). The mean score for nonphobic controls is 3.0 (*SD* = 7.8; Muris & Merckelbach, 1996).

Reliability.   Internal consistency is generally excellent, with Cronbach's alphas ranging from .88 to .97 across studies and samples (Muris & Merckelbach, 1996; Szymanski & O'Donohue, 1995). The stability of the FSQ over time is excellent, with a 3-week test–retest correlation of .91 in a nonclinical sample (Muris & Merckelbach, 1996).

Validity.   A factor analysis found two uncorrelated factors representing avoidance/help seeking (items 1, 6, 8, 10, 12, 14, 15, 17) and fear of harm (items 2–5, 7, 9, 11, 13, 16, 18; Szymanski & O'Donohue, 1995). In addition, the FSQ differentiates between individuals with and without spider phobias and is sensitive to the effects of treatment (Muris & Merckelbach, 1996; Szymanski & O'Donohue, 1995). The FSQ is significantly correlated with scores on the Spider Questionnaire as well as ratings during a behavioral avoidance test (Muris & Merckelbach, 1996; Szymanski & O'Donohue, 1995). Finally, compared with the Spider Questionnaire, the FSQ appears to be more sensitive for measuring fear in the nonphobic range (Muris & Merckelbach, 1996).

Source

The FSQ items are reprinted in the validation study by Szymanski and O'Donohue (1995) and the full scale is reprinted in Appendix B. Additional information is available from the author, William T. O'Donohue, Ph.D., Department of Psychology, University of Nevada–Reno, Reno, NV 89557, USA; (tel) 775-784-8072; (fax) 775-784-1869; (e-mail) wto@unr.edu.

FEAR SURVEY SCHEDULE (FSS)

Original Citations

Geer, J. H. (1965). The development of a scale to measure fear. *Behaviour Research and Therapy, 3,* 45–53.

Wolpe, J., & Lang, P. J. (1964). A Fear Survey Schedule for use in behaviour therapy. *Behaviour Research and Therapy, 2,* 27–30.

Purpose

To identify the specific objects and situations that an individual fears.

Description

Several different fear survey schedules have been published and researched since the 1950s. The first of these, developed by Akutagawa (1956), was a survey of 50 items representing commonly occurring fears. Although the scale was never adopted widely, it was used in at least one published study by Lang and Lazovik (1963) to measure outcome following behavior therapy. In 1965, Geer published a second Fear Survey Schedule (FSS-II) patterned after the original scale by Akutagawa. This 51-item scale was designed as a research tool and was empirically derived from an original item pool of 111 items. Wolpe and Lang (1964) published a third Fear Survey Schedule (FSS-III) based on an early version of Geer's scale. Unlike the FSS-II, the 72-item FSS-III was designed to be used in clinical settings. A revised and extended version of the FSS-III, with 108 items, was published in 1969 (Wolpe & Lang, 1969). Although there have been other fear survey schedules developed over the years, the FSS-II and FSS-III remain the most popular versions.

The FSS-II and FSS-III are self-report instruments containing lists of objects and situations. Participants are instructed to rate their fear of each item. Items on the FSS-II are rated on a seven-point scale ranging from 0 (none) to 6 (terror). Items on the FSS-III are rated on a five-point scale ranging from 0 (not at all) to 4 (very much).

The FSS-II and FSS-III have been used extensively over the past few decades to identify individuals who may be suffering from phobias, to assess severity of fears, and to evaluate outcome following treatment. In addition to including items that are related to common specific phobias (e.g., injections, airplanes), these scales also include items related to social phobia (e.g., speaking in public), agoraphobic situations (e.g., crowds), and situations that are not typically associated with fear in people with phobic disorders (e.g., noise of vacuum cleaners, sirens, ugly people, nude men and women, and parting from friends). Therefore, as noted in a review by Antony and Swinson (2000), the FSS is not an ideal scale for assessing fears in people with specific phobias. There is a need for the development of an updated fear survey schedule that more closely reflects the types of situations and objects feared by people with specific phobias.

Administration and Scoring

The FSS-II and FSS-III are scored by adding up the scores on all items. For the FSS-II, scores can range from 51 to 357. For the FSS-III, scores can range from 0 to 288 (for the 72-item version) or from 0 to 432 (for the 108-item version). Higher scores indicate greater fear. Given that a total fear score is often of little value, either clinically or from a research perspective, it may be more useful to examine ratings on particular items that are of interest, rather than obtaining a total score.

Psychometric Properties

Sample Scores and Norms.   Mean scores on the FSS-II for nonclinical samples of men and women are 75.78 (SD = 33.84) and 100.16 (SD = 36.11), respectively (Geer, 1965). Mean scores on the FSS-III for nonclinical samples of men and women are 144.63 (SD = 32.28) and 164.23 (SD = 33.91), respectively (Grossberg & Wilson, 1965). On both versions of the FSS, women tend to score significantly higher than men (Geer, 1965; Grossberg & Wilson, 1965). Several studies also report scores for particular clinical groups.

Reliability. Internal consistency of the FSS-II is high ($r = .94$, using the Kuder–Richardson Formula 20; Geer, 1965). Internal consistency of the FSS-III is also high, with a Cronbach's alpha of .95 (Arrindell, 1980).

Validity. There have been numerous factor analytic studies of the FSS-II and FSS-III, with somewhat different patterns of results (e.g., Arrindell, 1980; Arrindell, Pickersgill, Merckelbach, Ardon, & Cornet, 1991; Bates, 1971; Hallam & Hafner, 1978; Landy & Gaupp, 1971; Meikle & Mitchell, 1974; Rubin, Katkin, Weiss, & Efran, 1968; Wilson & Priest, 1968). Although some studies have found that particular anxiety disorder groups have unique response patterns on the FSS (e.g., Stravynski, Basoglu, Marks, Sengun, & Marks, 1995), others have found that FSS factors do not discriminate well among patients from various anxiety disorder groups (e.g., Beck, Carmin, & Henninger, 1998).

The FSS-II is correlated with a number of anxiety scales, but not with introversion or extroversion (Geer, 1965). Correlations with social desirability are significant, but relatively low (Geer, 1965). Items on the FSS-III do not discriminate between fearful and nonfearful individuals assessed during a behavioral assessment test (Klieger & Franklin, 1993). However, FSS-III scores have been shown to decrease following behavioral treatment for specific phobias (e.g., Öst, 1989; Öst, Fellenius, & Sterner, 1991)

Alternative Forms

The FSS-II and FSS-III have been translated into a number of languages. In addition, several FSS measures for children have been published (e.g., Gullone & King, 1992; Ollendick, 1983; Scherer & Nakamura, 1968)

Source

The FSS-II items are reprinted in the original validation paper by Geer (1965). The complete scale is reprinted in Appendix B. The 72-item FSS-III is reprinted in the original paper by Wolpe and Lang (1964). The 108-item FSS-III scale (Wolpe & Lang, 1969) and manual (Wolpe & Lang, 1977) are sold through the Educational and Industrial Testing Service (EdiTS), P.O. Box 7234, San Diego, CA 92167, USA; (tel) 800-416-1666 or 619-222-1666; (fax) 619-226-1666; (e-mail) edits@k-online.com; (website) www.edits.net. The cost for the manual and 25 forms is $13.25 US.

MEDICAL FEAR SURVEY (MFS)

Original Citation

Kleinknecht, R. A., Thorndike, R. M., & Walls, M. M. (1996). Factorial dimensions and correlates of blood, injury, injection and related medical fears: Cross validation of the Medical Fear Survey. *Behaviour Research and Therapy, 34,* 323–331.

Purpose

To assess five dimensions of medically related fear.

Description

The MFS is a 50-item self-report scale that assesses the severity of medical fears. Each item is rated on a five-point scale ranging from 0 (no fear or concern at all) to 4 (terror).

Administration and Scoring

The MFS takes 5 minutes to complete. Scores are obtained for five subscales (each with ten items) as follows: *injections and blood draws* (sum of items 1, 6, 16, 20, 24, 27, 31, 34, 45, 47), *sharp objects* (sum of items 2, 3, 7, 15, 21, 26, 29, 32, 42, 44), *examinations and symptoms as intimation of illness* (sum of items 4, 8, 13, 17, 22, 28, 37, 39, 43, 48), *blood* (sum of items 5, 9, 10, 19, 23, 25, 33, 35, 40, 49), *mutilation* (sum of items 11, 12, 14, 18, 30, 36, 38, 41, 46, 50).

Psychometric Properties

Sample Scores and Norms. Subscale means for a sample of undergraduate students were reported by Kleinknecht, Kleinknecht, Sawchuk, Lee, and Lohr (1999) as follows: *injections* —males = 6.86 (SD = 5.70), females = 10.74 (SD = 7.73); *sharp objects*—males = 2.47 (SD = 3.05), females = 6.10 (SD = 5.38); *examinations and symptoms*—males = 5.93 (SD = 4.08), females = 8.12 (SD = 5.04); *blood*—males = 2.34 (SD = 3.74), females = 6.21 (SD = 6.44); *mutilation*—males = 10.75 (SD = 6.56), females = 18.17 (SD = 8.31). Females tend to score significantly higher than males on all subscales (Kleinknecht et al., 1999). Normative data are not currently available for clinically diagnosed individuals with blood, injection, or other medical phobias.

Reliability. Internal consistency is good to excellent for each subscale, with Cronbach alphas ranging from .84 to .94 across subscales and samples (Kleinknecht et al., 1999). Test–retest reliability has not yet been established.

Validity. Subscales of the MFS were derived by factor analysis (Kleinknecht, Thorndike, & Walls, 1996). The MFS is significantly correlated with several other measures of blood, injection, and injury phobia (rs range from .73 to .88; Kleinknecht et al., 1999). The correlations between the MFS and a measure of trait anxiety are moderately low, though significant (rs range from .26 to .30; Kleinknecht et al., 1999). Finally, most of the MFS scales are moderately correlated with anxiety sensitivity (Kleinknecht et al., 1999). Sensitivity to change following treatment has not yet been reported.

Alternative Forms

Translations are currently being developed in Mexico, Portugal, and Spain.

Source

The MFS is reprinted in Appendix B. Additional information may be obtained from the author, Ronald A. Kleinknecht, Ph.D., College of Arts and Sciences, Western Washington University, Bellingham, WA 98225, USA; (tel) 360-650-3763; (fax) 360-650-6809; (e-mail) ronald.kleinknecht@wwu.edu.

MUTILATION QUESTIONNAIRE (MQ)

Original Citation

Klorman, R., Hastings, J. E., Weerts, T. C., Melamed, B. G., & Lang, P. J. (1974). Psychometric description of some specific-fear questionnaires. *Behavior Therapy*, *5*, 401–409.

Purpose

To assess the verbal–cognitive component of mutilation and blood/injury fear.

Description

The MQ is a 30-item self-report scale. Each item is a fearful or nonfearful statement related to blood, injury, or mutilation. Participants rate each item as true or false.

Administration and Scoring

The MQ takes 5 minutes to complete. The instrument is scored by assigning a "1" to each true response and a "0" to each false response. Then, items 5, 9, 14, 18, 21, and 28 are reverse-scored and the items are added up. Scores can range from 0 to 30.

Psychometric Properties

Sample Scores and Norms.   Öst, Sterner, and Fellenius (1989) reported mean MQ scores before and after treatment for three different groups of individuals with blood phobia. Pretreatment means ranged from 17.70 to 20.60 (*SD*s ranged from 3.2 to 5.3). Following treatment, means ranged from 10.0 to 11.5 (*SD*s ranged from 3.7 to 5.4). Means for various other groups are provided elsewhere (e.g., Fredrikson, 1983; Kleinknecht, 1992; Kleinknecht & Thorndike, 1990).

Reliability.   Internal consistency is fair to good, as indicated by Cronbach's alphas ranging from .77 to .86 across various nonclinical samples (Kleinknecht & Thorndike, 1990).

Validity.   A two-factor solution emerged for the MQ in a study by Kleinknecht and Thorndike (1990). One factor was labeled "repulsion and revulsion of blood, injury, and mutilation" and the other was labeled "fear of bodily damage." The MQ is significantly correlated with blood and injury-related items from the Fear Survey Schedule and is predictive of a history of fainting in situations involving blood and injury (Kleinknecht & Thorndike, 1990). MQ scores are also related to a tendency to avoid blood and injury-related situations (Kleinknecht & Lenz, 1989) and to show greater levels of arousal in response to mutilation-related slides (Klorman, Weissberg, & Wiesenfeld, 1977). Finally, several studies have shown that the MQ is sensitive to the effects of treatment (e.g., Öst et al., 1989, 1991; Öst, Lindahl, Sterner, & Jerremalm, 1984).

Alternative Forms

The MQ has been translated into a number of languages.

Source

The MQ is reprinted in Appendix B. Additional information may be obtained from the author, Rafael Klorman, Ph.D., Clinical and Social Sciences in Psychology, University of Rochester, Meliora Hall, RC Box 270266, Rochester, NY 14627-0266, USA; (tel) 716-275-2595; (fax) 716-273-1100; (e-mail) klorman@psych.rochester.edu.

SNAKE QUESTIONNAIRE (SNAQ)

Original Citation

Klorman, R., Hastings, J. E., Weerts, T. C., Melamed, B. G., & Lang, P. J. (1974). Psychometric description of some specific-fear questionnaires. *Behavior Therapy*, *5*, 401–409.

Purpose

To assess the verbal–cognitive component of snake fear.

Description

The SNAQ is a 30-item self-report scale. Each item is a fearful or nonfearful statement related to snakes. Participants rate each item as true or false. This scale has also been referred to as the Snake Anxiety Questionnaire in some studies (e.g., Klieger, 1987, 1994).

Administration and Scoring

The SNAQ takes 5 minutes to complete. The instrument is scored by assigning a "1" to each true response and a "0" to each false response. Then, items 6, 12, 16, 17, 20, 25, 27, and 28 are reverse-scored and the items are added up. Scores can range from 0 to 30.

Psychometric Properties

Sample Scores and Norms.   Fredrikson (1983) reported that the mean score on the SNAQ for a group of individuals with snake phobias was 24.44 ($SD = 2.95$). In the same study, means for male and female college students were 5.80 ($SD = 3.82$) and 9.06 ($SD = 6.09$), respectively.

Reliability.   Estimates of internal consistency (based on Kuder–Richardson Formula 20) were high, ranging from .78 to .90 across samples and studies (Fredrikson, 1983; Klorman, Hastings, Weerts, Melamed, & Lang, 1974). Test–retest reliability for the SNAQ (administered 1 year apart) was high, with $r = .84$ (Fredrikson, 1983).

Validity.   The SNAQ discriminates those with snake phobias from those with spider phobias and from nonphobic students (Fredrikson, 1983). In addition, scores on the SNAQ were correlated with aversiveness ratings while watching slides depicting snakes (Fredrikson, 1983). The SNAQ is also sensitive to the effects of treatment (Öst, 1978).

However, Klieger (1987) reported that the relationship between scores on the SNAQ and a tendency to avoid a caged snake during a behavioral test was not strong (in fact, for males there was no relationship between these variables). Although the SNAQ was adequately sensitive for identifying individuals with no fear of snakes, it was not particularly sensitive for identifying individuals who were fearful of snakes. In other words, the SNAQ tends to yield false positives. A significant number of individuals who reported fearing snakes were able to approach a caged snake during a behavioral test.

Alternative Forms

The SNAQ has been translated into several languages (e.g., Swedish).

Source

The SNAQ is reprinted in Appendix B. Additional information may be obtained from the author, Rafael Klorman, Ph.D., Clinical and Social Sciences in Psychology, University of Rochester, Meliora Hall, RC Box 270266, Rochester, NY 14627-0266, USA; (tel) 716-275-2595; (fax) 716-273-1100; (e-mail) klorman@psych.rochester.edu.

SPIDER PHOBIA BELIEFS QUESTIONNAIRE (SBQ)

Original Citation

Arntz, A., Lavy, E., van den Berg, G., & van Rijsoort, S. (1993). Negative beliefs of spider phobics: A psychometric evaluation of the Spider Phobia Beliefs Questionnaire. *Advances in Behaviour Research and Therapy, 15*, 257–277.

Purpose

To measure fearful beliefs about spiders and about one's reaction to seeing spiders.

Description

The SBQ is a 78-item self-report scale. Items 1 through 42 measure the strength of fearful beliefs regarding spiders. Items 43 through 78 measure the strength of fearful beliefs about one's reaction to encountering a spider. All items are rated on a 0–100 point scale, where 0 = I do not believe it at all (0%) and 100 = I absolutely believe it (100%).

Administration and Scoring

The SBQ takes 10 to 15 minutes to complete. The measure is scored by calculating the mean ratings for the *spider-related beliefs subscale* (items 1 through 42) and the *self-related beliefs subscale* (items 43 through 78). There are no reverse-scored items.

Psychometric Properties

Sample Scores and Norms.   Mean scores for the spider-related beliefs subscale in a group of patients with a specific phobia of spiders were 48.76 (17.74) before treatment and 10.15 (13.69) after treatment (Arntz, Lavy, van den Berg, & van Rijsoort, 1993). In the same sample, mean scores for the self-related beliefs subscale were 49.79 (18.72) before treatment and 8.00 (13.15) following treatment.

Reliability.   Internal consistency (as measured by Cronbach's alpha) was excellent for both the spider-related ($\alpha = .94$) and self-related ($\alpha = .94$) subscales (Arntz et al., 1993). Test–retest reliability was acceptable, with $r = .68$ for the spider-related beliefs subscale and $r = .71$ for the self-related beliefs subscale (Arntz et al., 1993).

Validity.   Exploratory factor analyses found that the spider-related beliefs could be grouped into five meaningful factors and the self-related beliefs could be grouped into four factors (with three items not being included). Scoring instructions and psychometric data on these nine subscales are provided by Arntz et al. (1993). The SBQ differentiates between untreated individuals with spider phobia and individuals without spider phobia (Arntz et al., 1993). In addition, the SBQ is sensitive to the effects of treatment. In fact, posttreatment scores were not significantly different than scores from a nonphobic sample (Arntz et al., 1993). Finally, Rodriguez, Craske, Mineka, and Hladek (1999) found that increases in phobic cognitions (as measured by the SBQ) following treatment of spider phobia were predictive of subsequent return of fear.

Alternative Forms

The SBQ is available in English and Dutch.

Source

The SBQ items are reprinted in the validation study by Arntz, et al. (1993). The entire scale is reprinted in Appendix B. Additional information may be obtained from the author, Arnoud Arntz, Ph.D., Department of Medical, Clinical, and Experimental Psychology, Maastricht University, P.O. Box 616, 6200 MD, Maastricht, The Netherlands; (tel) 31-43-388-1606; (fax) 31-43-388-4155; (e-mail) arnoud.arntz@mp.unimaas.nl.

SPIDER QUESTIONNAIRE (SPQ)

Original Citation

Klorman, R., Hastings, J. E., Weerts, T. C., Melamed, B. G., & Lang, P. J. (1974). Psychometric description of some specific-fear questionnaires. *Behavior Therapy, 5,* 401–409.

Purpose

To assess the verbal–cognitive component of spider fear.

Description

The SPQ is a 31-item self-report scale. Each item is a fearful or nonfearful statement related to spiders. Participants rate each item as true or false.

Administration and Scoring

The SPQ takes 5 minutes to complete. The instrument is scored by assigning a "1" to each true response and a "0" to each false response. Then, items 6, 12, 14, 16, 17, 20, 25, 27, and 28 are reverse-scored and the items are added up. Scores can range from 0 to 31.

Psychometric Properties

Sample Scores and Norms. Fredrikson (1983) reported that the mean score on the SPQ for a group of individuals with spider phobias was 23.76 (*SD* = 3.80). Muris and Merckelbach (1996) reported that the mean SPQ scores for spider phobic individuals before and after treatment were 23.2 (*SD* = 2.9) and 14.0 (*SD* = 6.8). In the Fredrikson (1983) study, means for college students ranged from 3.80 to 5.02 (*SD*s ranged from 3.42 to 4.88).

Reliability. Internal consistency ratings have been inconsistent. Muris and Merckelbach (1996) reported Cronbach's alpha of .62 before treatment and .90 after treatment. Studies using Kuder–Richardson Formula 20 to calculate internal consistency have tended to yield higher reliability coefficients (Fredrikson, 1983; Klorman, Hastings, Weerts, Melamed, & Lang, 1974). Scores on the SPQ are stable over 3 weeks (r = .94; Muris & Merckelbach, 1996) and over 1 year (r = .87; Fredrikson, 1983), indicating excellent test–retest reliability.

Validity. The SPQ discriminates those with spider phobias from those with snake phobias (Fredrikson, 1983) and from nonphobic individuals (Fredrikson, 1983; Muris & Merckelbach, 1996). In addition, scores on the SPQ were correlated with aversiveness ratings while watching slides depicting spiders (Fredrikson, 1983) as well as with other measures of spider-related fear and avoidance (Muris & Merckelbach, 1996). Finally, the SPQ is sensitive to the effects of treatment (Hellström & Öst, 1995; Muris & Merckelbach, 1996; Öst, 1978, 1996).

Alternative Forms

The SPQ has been translated into several languages (e.g., Dutch, Swedish). In addition, a version for children (SPQ-C; Kindt, Brosschot, & Muris, 1996) has been developed.

Source

The SPQ is reprinted in Appendix B. Additional information may be obtained from the author, Rafael Klorman, Ph.D., Clinical and Social Sciences in Psychology, University of Rochester, Meliora Hall, RC Box 270266, Rochester, NY 14627-0266, USA; (tel) 716-275-2595; (fax) 716-273-1100; (e-mail) klorman@psych.rochester.edu.

BRIEF DESCRIPTIONS OF ADDITIONAL MEASURES: SPECIFIC PHOBIA

Corah Dental Anxiety Scale (CDAS)

The CDAS is a four-item self-report scale designed to measure severity of trait dental anxiety (Corah, 1969). This scale is sometimes referred to as the Dental Anxiety Scale (DAS). Over the years, several modifications and revisions have been published including the five-item Modified Dental Anxiety Scale (MDAS; Humphris, Morrison, & Lindsay, 1995) and the four-item Dental Anxiety Scale–Revised (Ronis, 1994). The CDAS and the DAS-R are both reprinted in validation papers by Ronis and colleagues (Ronis, 1994; Ronis, Hansen, & Antonakos, 1995). The MDAS is reprinted in a validation paper by Humphris et al. (1995). The CDAS and its modifications have been very popular among researchers who study dental anxiety.

Dental Fear Interview (DFI)

The DFI is a 10-item clinician-administered interview for assessing the severity of dental fear. The interview and its psychometric properties are available in the validation paper by Vrana, McNeil, and McGlynn (1986). Additional information may be obtained from the author, Daniel W. McNeil, Ph.D., Department of Psychology, West Virginia University, 114 Oglebay, Morgantown, WV 26506-6040, USA; (tel) 304-293-2001, ext. 622; (fax) 304-293-6606; (e-mail) dmcneil@wvu.edu.

Dog Phobia Questionnaire (DPQ)

The DPQ is a 27-item self-report scale for measuring the severity of dog phobia. The scale is still in development, although preliminary findings have been presented by the authors (Hong & Zinbarg, 1999). Additional information may be obtained from the author, Richard E. Zinbarg, Ph.D., Richard E. Zinbarg, Ph.D., Department of Psychology, Northwestern University, 2029 Sheridan Road, Evanston, IL 60208-2710, USA; (tel) 847-467-2290; (fax) 847-491-7859; (e-mail) zinbarg@northwestern.edu.

Fear of Flying Scale (FFS)

The FFS is a 21-item self-report measure for assessing fear associated with various aspects of flying. The scale was originally developed by Björn Helge Johnsen, Leif Brenne, Dagfinn Berntzen, Trond Haug, Kenneth Hugdahl, and K. Gunnar Götestam. It is described in a paper by Haug et al. (1987). Additional information may be obtained from K. Gunnar Götestam, Norwegian University of Science and Technology, Trondheim (NTNU), Department of Psychiatry and Behavioural Medicine, P.O. Box 3008 Lade, NO-7441 Trondheim, Norway; (tel) +47 7386 4600; (fax) 47 7386 4910; (e-mail) gotestam@medisin.ntnu.no.

Sheffield Dental Phobia Scale (SDPS)

This scale is a 12-item self-report measure for assessing the psychological and social impact of having severe dental anxiety. The items for the scale are reprinted in the validation study by Kent, Rubin, Getz, and Humphris (1996), although the title of the scale is not mentioned in the article. Additional information may be obtained from the author, Gerry Kent, Ph.D., Department of Psychology, University of Sheffield, Sheffield, S10 2PT, United Kingdom; (tel) 44-144-22-26527; (fax) 44-144-276-6515; (e-mail) g.kent@sheffield.ac.uk.

Medical Avoidance Survey (MAS)

The MAS is a 21-item self-report scale designed to measure avoidance of medical situations. The scale is described in a paper by Kleinknecht et al. (1996). The MAS is still in the final stages of development. Additional information may be obtained from the author, Ronald A. Kleinknecht, Ph.D., College of Arts and Sciences, Western Washington University, Bellingham, WA 98225, USA; (tel) 360-650-3763; (fax) 360-650-6809; (e-mail) ronald.kleinknecht@wwu.edu.

Origins Questionnaire (OQ)

The OQ is a 16-page self-report questionnaire that assesses an individual's history with respect to a phobic object or situation (Menzies & Clarke, 1993). It is designed to determine the etiology of an individual's phobia. Additional information may be obtained from the author, Ross G. Menzies, Ph.D., Department of Behavioural Sciences, Faculty of Health Sciences, University of Sydney, P.O. Box 170, 1825 East Street, Room G103, Lidcombe, NSW 2141, Australia; (tel) +61 2 9351 9283; (fax) +61 2 9351 9540; (e-mail) r.menzies@cchs.usyd.edu.au.

Phobia Origins Questionnaire (POQ)

The POQ is a nine-item self-report questionnaire that assesses an individual's history of experiencing various etiologically relevant events in the context of a feared object or situation. The POQ was originally described in a paper by Öst and Hugdahl (1981) and its psychometric properties have been reported in recent papers by Kheriaty, Kleinknecht, and Hyman (1999) and Menzies, Kirkby, and Harris (1998). Additional information is available from the author, Lars-Göran Öst, Ph.D., Department of Psychology, Stockholm University, S-106, 91, Stockholm, Sweden; (tel) 46-8-163821; (fax) 46-8-166236; (e-mail) ost@psychology.su.se.

Retrospective Childhood and Current Adult Fear Survey (RCCAFS)

The RCCAFS is a self-report scale for adults that lists 80 objects and situations that are often feared. Respondents indicate whether they ever feared the stimulus, the earliest age when the fear started (if relevant), the current intensity of the fear, and the age at which the fear stopped (if relevant). The scale was originally developed by Reichler, Sylvester, and Hyde (1983) and its psychometric properties were reported in a paper by Mann, Sylvester, and Chen (1996). Additional information is available from the author, Carrie Sylvester, M.D., Northwestern University Medical School, Child and Adolescent Psychiatry, Children's Memorial Hospital, 2300 Children's Plaza, #10, Chicago, IL 60614-3394, USA; (tel) 773-880-4833; (fax) 773-880-4066; (e-mail) csylvester@childrensmemorial.org.

Threatening Medical Situations Inventory (TMSI)

The TMSI was developed to measure cognitive confrontation (monitoring) and cognitive avoidance (blunting) responses to medical threat. The measure presents respondents with four threatening medical scenarios, each followed randomly by three monitoring and three blunting responses. The respondent rates the likelihood (on a five-point scale) that he or she would respond to the situation in each of the ways listed if the threatening medical situation were actually encountered. A sample item is provided in the validation study by van Zuuren, de Groot, Mulder, and Muris (1996). Additional information may be obtained from the author, Dr. Florence J. van Zuuren, Department of Clinical Psychology, University of Amsterdam, Roetersstraat 15, 1018 WB, Amsterdam, The Netherlands; (tel) 31-20-5256717; (fax) 31-20-6391369; (e-mail) kp_zuuren@macmail.psy.uva.nl.

Watts and Sharrock Spider Phobia Questionnaire (WS-SPQ)

The WS-SPQ is a self-report scale on which respondents indicate (with a "yes" or "no") whether they agree with 43 statements about spiders. In some reports the acronym for this scale has been WS and in others it has been referred to as the SPQ, not to be confused with the Spider Questionnaire (SPQ; Klorman et al., 1974). Three subscales are generated to measure vigilance, preoccupation, and avoidance of spiders, respectively. In addition, five items assess factual knowledge about spiders and five other items do not load on any particular factor. The scale items are reprinted in the validation study by Watts and Sharrock (1984). Data on an expanded version of this scale are reported by Barker and Edelmann (1987).

REFERENCES

Aartman, I. H. A. (1998). Reliability and validity of the short version of the Dental Anxiety Interview. *Community Dentistry and Oral Epidemiology, 26,* 350–354.

Akutagawa, D. (1956). *A study in construct validity of the psychoanalytic concept of latent anxiety and test of a projection distance hypothesis.* Unpublished doctoral dissertation, University of Pittsburgh.

Antony, M. M., & Swinson, R. P. (2000). *Phobic disorders and panic in adults: A guide to assessment and treatment.* Washington, DC: American Psychological Association.

Arrindell, W. A. (1980). Dimensional structure and psychopathology correlates of the Fear Survey Schedule (FSS-III) in a phobic population: A factorial definition of agoraphobia. *Behaviour Research and Therapy, 18,* 229–242.

Arrindell, W. A., Pickersgill, M. J., Merckelbach, H., Ardon, A. M., & Cornet, F. C. (1991). Phobic dimensions: III. Factor analytic approaches to the study of common phobic fears: An updated review of findings obtained with adult subjects. *Advances in Behaviour Research and Therapy, 13,* 73–130.

Baker, B. L., Cohen, D. C., & Saunders, J. T. (1973). Self-directed desensitization for acrophobia. *Behaviour Research and Therapy, 11,* 79–89.

Barker, H. J., & Edelmann, R. J. (1987). Questionnaire dimension of spider phobia: A replication and extension. *Personality and Individual Differences, 8,* 737–739.

Bates, H. D. (1971). Factorial structure and MMPI correlates of a Fear Survey Schedule in a clinical population. *Behaviour Research and Therapy, 9,* 355–360.

Beck, J. G., Carmin, C. N., & Henninger, N. J. (1998). The utility of the Fear Survey Schedule-III: An extended replication. *Journal of Anxiety Disorders, 12,* 177–182.

Bourque, P., & Ladouceur, R. (1980). An investigation of various performance-based treatments with acrophobics. *Behaviour Research and Therapy, 18,* 161–170.

Cohen, D. C. (1972). *Personality predictors and the outcome of varieties of desensitization.* Unpublished doctoral dissertation, Harvard University, Cambridge, MA.

Convergent validity of the Phobia Origins Questionnaire (POQ): A review of the evidence. *Behaviour Research and Therapy, 36,* 1081–1089.

Corah, N. L. (1969). Development of a dental anxiety scale. *Journal of Dental Research, 48,* 596.

de Jongh, A., Muris, P., Ten Horst, G. T., van Zuuren, F., Schoenmakers, N., & Makkes, P. (1995). One session cognitive treatment of dental phobia: Preparing dental phobics for treatment by restructuring negative cognitions. *Behaviour Research and Therapy, 33,* 947–954.

Fredrikson, M. (1983). Reliability and validity of some specific fear questionnaires. *Scandinavian Journal of Psychology, 24,* 331–334.

Grossberg, J. M., & Wilson, H. K. (1965). A correlational comparison of the Wolpe–Lang Fear Survey Schedule and Taylor Manifest Anxiety Scale. *Behaviour Research and Therapy, 3,* 125–128.

Gullone, E., & King, N. J. (1992). Psychometric evaluation of a revised fear survey schedule for children and adolescents. *Journal of Child Psychology and Psychiatry, 33,* 987–998.

Hallam, R. S., & Hafner, R. J. (1978). Fears of phobic patients: Factor analyses of self-report data. *Behaviour Research and Therapy, 16,* 1–6.

Haug, T., Brenne, L., Johnsen, B. H., Berntzen, D., Götestam, K. G., & Hugdahl, K. (1987). The three-systems analysis of fear of flying: A comparison of a consonant vs. a non-consonant treatment method. *Behaviour Research and Therapy, 25,* 187–194.

Hellström, K., & Öst, L.-G. (1995). One-session therapist directed exposure vs. two forms of manual directed self-exposure in the treatment of spider phobia. *Behaviour Research and Therapy, 33,* 959–965.

Hepburn, T., & Page, A. C. (1999). Effects of images about fear and disgust upon responses to blood–injury phobic stimuli. *Behavior Therapy, 30,* 63–77.

Hong, N. N., & Zinbarg, R. E. (1999, November). *Assessing the fear of dogs: The Dog Phobia Questionnaire.* Paper presented at the meeting of the Association for Advancement of Behavior Therapy, Toronto, ON.

Humphris, G. M., Morrison, T., & Lindsay, S. J. E. (1995). The Modified Dental Anxiety Scale: Validation and United Kingdom norms. *Community Dental Health, 12,* 143–150.

Johansson, P., & Berggren, U. (1992). Assessment of dental fear: A comparison of two psychometric instruments. *Acta Odontologica Scandinavica, 50,* 43–49.

Kent, G., Rubin, G., Getz, T., & Humphris, G. (1996). Development of a scale to measure the social and psychological effects of severe dental anxiety: Social attributes of the Dental Anxiety Scale. *Community Dentistry and Oral Epidemiology, 24,* 394–397.

Kheriaty, E., Kleinknecht, R. A., & Hyman, I. E. (1999). Recall and validation of phobia origins as a function of a structured interview versus the Phobia Origins Questionnaire. *Behavior Modification, 23,* 61–78.

Kindt, M., Brosschot, J. F., & Muris, P. (1996). Spider Phobia Questionnaire for Children (SPQ-C): A psychometric study and normative data. *Behaviour Research and Therapy, 34,* 277–282.

Kleinknecht, R. A. (1992). The Mutilation Questionnaire for assessing blood/injury fear and phobia. *The Behavior Therapist, 15,* 66–67.

Kleinknecht, R. A., & Bernstein, D. A. (1978). The assessment of dental fear. *Behavior Therapy, 9,* 626–634.

Kleinknecht, R. A., Kleinknecht, E. E., Sawchuk, C., Lee, T., & Lohr, J. (1999). The Medical Fear Survey: Psychometric properties. *The Behavior Therapist, 22,* 109–119.

Kleinknecht, R. A., & Lenz, J. (1989). Blood/injury fear, fainting, and avoidance of medically related situations: A family correspondence study. *Behaviour Research and Therapy, 27,* 537–547.

Kleinknecht, R. A., McGlynn, F. D., Thorndike, R. M., & Harkavy, J. (1984). Factor analysis of the dental fear survey with cross-validation. *Journal of the American Dental Association, 108,* 59–61.

Kleinknecht, R. A., & Thorndike, R. M. (1990). The Mutilation Questionnaire as a predictor of blood/injury fear and fainting. *Behaviour Research and Therapy, 28,* 429–437.

Kleinknecht, R. A., Thorndike, R. M., & Walls, M. M. (1996). Factorial dimensions and correlates of blood, injury, injection and related medical fears: Cross validation of the Medical Fear Survey. *Behaviour Research and Therapy, 34,* 323–331.

Klieger, D. M. (1987). The Snake Anxiety Questionnaire as a measure of ophidiophobia. *Educational and Psychological Measurement, 47,* 449–459.

Klieger, D. M. (1994). A new approach to the measurement of ophidiophobia. *Personality and Individual Differences, 16,* 505–508.

Klieger, D. M., & Franklin, M. E. (1993). Validity of the Fear Survey Schedule in phobia research: A laboratory test. *Journal of Psychopathology and Behavioral Assessment, 15,* 207–217.

Klorman, R., Weissberg, R. P., & Wiesenfeld, A. (1977). Individual differences in fear and autonomic reactions to affective stimulation. *Psychophysiology, 14,* 45–51.

Landy, F. J., & Gaupp, L. A. (1971). A factor analysis of the FSS-III. *Behaviour Research and Therapy, 9,* 89–93.

Lang, P. J., & Lazovik, A. D. (1963). The experimental desensitization of an animal phobia. *Journal of Abnormal and Social Psychology, 66,* 519–525.

Mann, B. J., Sylvester, C. E., & Chen, R. (1996). Reliability and validity of the Retrospective Childhood and Current Adult Fears Survey (RCCAFS). *Journal of Anxiety Disorders, 10,* 59–72.

McGlynn, F. D., McNeil, D. W., Gallagher, S. L., & Vrana, S. (1987). Factor structure, stability, and internal consistency of the Dental Fear Survey. *Behavioral Assessment, 9,* 57–66.

McNally, R., & Eke, M. (1996). Anxiety sensitivity, suffocation fear, and breath-holding duration as predictors of response to carbon dioxide challenge. *Journal of Abnormal Psychology, 105,* 146–149.

Meikle, S., & Mitchell, M. C. (1974). Factor analysis of the Fear Survey Schedule with phobics. *Journal of Clinical Psychology, 30,* 44–46.

Menzies, R. G., & Clarke, J. C. (1993). The etiology of fear of heights and its relationship to severity and individual response patterns. *Behaviour Research and Therapy, 31,* 355–365.

Menzies, R. G., Kirkby, K., & Harris, L. M. (1998). The convergent validity of the Phobia Origins Questionnaire (POQ): A review of the evidence. *Behaviour Research and Therapy, 36,* 1081–1089.

Moore, R., Berggren, U., & Carlsson, S. G. (1991). Reliability and clinical usefulness of psychometric measures in a self-referred population of odontophobics. *Community Dentistry and Oral Epidemiology, 19,* 347–351.

Moore, R., & Brødsgaard, I. (1994). Group therapy compared with individual desensitization for dental anxiety. *Community Dentistry and Oral Epidemiology, 22,* 258–262.

Muris, P., & Merckelbach, H. (1996). A comparison of two spider phobia questionnaires. *Journal of Behavior Therapy and Experimental Psychiatry, 27,* 241–244.

Ollendick, T. H. (1983). Reliability and validity of the revised Fear Survey for Children (FSSC-R). *Behaviour Research and Therapy, 21,* 395–399.

Öst, L.-G. (1978). Fading vs. systematic desensitization in the treatment of snake and spider phobia. *Behaviour Research and Therapy, 16,* 379–389.

Öst, L.-G. (1989). One-session treatment for specific phobias. *Behaviour Research and Therapy, 27,* 1–7.

Öst, L.-G. (1996). One-session group treatment for spider phobia. *Behaviour Research and Therapy, 34,* 707–715.

Öst, L.-G., Fellenius, J., & Sterner, U. (1991). Applied tension, exposure in vivo, and tension-only in the treatment of blood phobia. *Behaviour Research and Therapy, 29,* 561–574.

Öst, L.-G., Lindahl, I.-L., Sterner, U., & Jerremalm, A. (1984). Exposure in vivo vs. applied relaxation in the treatment of blood phobia. *Behaviour Research and Therapy, 22,* 205–216.

Öst, L.-G., Sterner, U., & Fellenius, J. (1989). Applied tension, applied relaxation, and the combination in the treatment of blood phobia. *Behaviour Research and Therapy, 27,* 109–121.

Öst, L.-G., & Hugdahl, D. (1981). Acquisition of phobias and anxiety response patterns in clinical patients. *Behaviour Research and Therapy, 19,* 439–447.

Rachman, S., & Taylor, S. (1993). Analyses of claustrophobia. *Journal of Anxiety Disorders, 7,* 281–291.

Reichler, R. J., Sylvester, C. E., & Hyde, T. S. (1983). *The Retrospective Childhood and Current Adult Fears Survey.* Department of Psychiatry, Northwestern University, Chicago.

Rodriguez, B. I., Craske, M. G., Mineka, S., & Hladek, D. (1999). Context-specificity of relapse: Effects of therapist and environmental context on return of fear. *Behaviour Research and Therapy, 37,* 845–862.

Ronis, D. L. (1994). Updating a measure of dental anxiety: Reliability, validity, and norms. *Journal of Dental Hygiene, 68,* 228–233.

Ronis, D. L., Hansen, C. H., & Antonakos, C. L. (1995). Equivalence of the original and revised Dental Anxiety Scales. *Journal of Dental Hygiene, 69,* 270–272.

Rubin, B. M., Katkin, E. S., Weiss, B. W., & Efran, J. (1968). Factor analysis of a Fear Survey Schedule. *Behaviour Research and Therapy, 6,* 65–75.

Scherer, M. W., & Nakamura, C. Y. (1968). A fear survey schedule for children (FSS-FC): A factor analytic comparison with manifest anxiety (CMAS). *Behaviour Research and Therapy, 6,* 173–182.

Schuurs, A. H. B., & Hoogstraten, J. (1993). Appraisal of dental anxiety and fear questionnaires: A review. *Community Dentistry and Oral Epidemiology, 21,* 329–339.

Stouthard, M. E. A., Hoogstraten, J., & Mellenbergh, G. J. (1995). A study on the convergent and discriminant validity of the Dental Anxiety Inventory. *Behaviour Research and Therapy, 33,* 589–595.

Stravynski, A., Basoglu, M., Marks, M., Sengun, S., & Marks, I. M. (1995). The distinctiveness of phobias: A discriminant analysis of fears. *Journal of Anxiety Disorders, 9,* 89–101.

Taylor, S., & Rachman, S. J. (1994). Klein's suffocation theory of panic. *Archives of General Psychiatry, 51,* 505–506.

van Zuuren, F. J., de Groot, K. I., Mulder, N. L., & Muris, P. (1996). Coping with medical threat: An evaluation of the Threatening Medical Situations Inventory (TMSI). *Personality and Individual Differences, 21,* 21–31.

Vrana, S., McNeil, D. W., & McGlynn, F. D. (1986). A structured interview for assessing dental fear. *Journal of Behavior Therapy and Experimental Psychiatry, 17,* 175–178.

Watts, F. N., & Sharrock, R. (1984). Questionnaire dimensions of spider phobia. *Behaviour Research and Therapy, 22,* 575–580.

Wilson, G. D., & Priest, H. F. (1968). The principal components of phobic stimuli. *Journal of Clinical Psychology, 24,* 191.

Wolpe, J., & Lang, P. J. (1969). *Fear Survey Schedule.* San Diego: Educational and Industrial Testing Service.

Wolpe, J., & Lang, P. J. (1977). *Manual for the Fear Survey Schedule.* San Diego: Educational and Industrial Testing Service.

Chapter 12
Social Phobia: A Brief Overview and Guide to Assessment

Susan M. Orsillo and Charity Hammond

Social phobia, defined by the presence of significant and enduring fear of social or performance situations, is a commonly occurring, chronic, and significantly impairing disorder that frequently goes untreated (Magee, Eaton, Wittchen, McGonagle, & Kessler, 1996). Results from a recent epidemiological study, the National Comorbidity Survey, indicate that social phobia is the most common anxiety disorder, and the third most common psychological disorder in the population. About 13.3% of adults (11.1% of men and 15.5% of women) meet criteria for social phobia at some point in their lives, and the lifetime prevalence of social phobia has increased significantly in recent cohorts (except for those with exclusive fears of public speaking; Heimberg, Stein, Hiripi, & Kessler, 2000; Magee et al., 1996).

This chapter will provide a clinical description of social phobia and a brief overview of some issues that are relevant to its assessment. For more detailed reviews of the assessment of social phobia see Antony and Swinson (2000), Beidel and Turner (1998), Heimberg, Liebowitz, Hope, and Schneier (1995), Hofmann and Barlow (in press), Hofmann and DiBartolo (2001), and Stein (1995). All instruments mentioned in this chapter are described elsewhere in this book, along with full citations.

CLINICAL DESCRIPTION

Social phobia is characterized by intense and persistent fear of social situations in which scrutiny and embarrassment could occur. Exposure to feared situations almost always results

Susan M. Orsillo and Charity Hammond • National Center for PTSD–Women's Health Sciences Division, Boston VA Healthcare System, and Boston University School of Medicine, Boston, Massachusetts 02130.

in an intense anxiety response that may include full-blown panic attacks. Social situations are typically avoided, although a client may force him- or herself to endure a social situation despite extreme distress. Significant anticipatory anxiety about upcoming social situations is common. To be diagnosed with social phobia, the adult client must recognize that the fear is excessive and the fear and/or avoidance must cause marked distress or significantly interfere with the client's life functioning (American Psychiatric Association {APA}, 1994).

The types of situations feared by clients with social phobia typically fall into two domains: social interactional and performance. Social interactional situations include initiating or maintaining casual conversations, meeting new people, dating, speaking to authority figures, and being assertive. Performance situations include public speaking, writing (e.g., making out a check), eating or using a restroom while others are present, or performing in front of others (e.g., playing sports or participating in a concert or recital). Social phobia can be specified as general when the client's social fears are present in most social situations (APA, 1994).

Approximately one third of people with lifetime social phobia report experiencing only speaking fears, whereas the remaining two thirds report at least one additional social fear (Kessler, Stein, & Berglund, 1998). Those with pure speaking fears experience social phobia that is less chronic, less impairing, and less highly comorbid with other disorders (Kessler et al., 1998).

ASSESSMENT STRATEGIES

Depending on the purpose of the assessment, a number of approaches are available to evaluate symptoms of social phobia. A comprehensive assessment will often include a clinical interview, the administration of a clinician rating scale and self-report measures, and behavioral and cognitive assessment. Associated features of social phobia may also be assessed, and issues related to differential diagnosis considered.

Clinical Interview

The assessment process itself is a phobic situation for many clients with social phobia. Social interactional fears may make it difficult for the client to fully describe his or her current symptoms in an interview, and performance-based fears can be activated when a client is asked to complete questionnaires. Although these fears can make assessment challenging, they also provide an opportunity for the clinician to directly observe the client in a naturalistic, fear-eliciting situation.

The chronic avoidance pattern of clients with social phobia can also negatively impact the assessment process. Given that social phobia is often associated with an early onset (Magee et al., 1996), clients may be unaware of the severely restricted lifestyle they have created as a way to avoid social situations that are anxiety provoking (Beidel & Turner, 1998). Thus, it may be difficult for them to identify situations they avoid. For instance, a client may not report avoidance of parties and dating if she views her behavior as simply reflecting her preference for a "quiet life." It may also be difficult for clients to rate the intensity of fear they might experience in a situation that they have avoided for a long period of time. A client might underrate his fear of public speaking if he has not been exposed to a performance situation in over a decade.

Subtle forms of avoidance related to social phobia should also be assessed in the clinical interview. Clients may engage in behavior such as wearing turtlenecks to cover blushing, eating in restaurants with dim lighting, talking only to safe people, or drinking before a party as a means of increasing their comfort level in social situations (Antony, 1997). A newly developed, but as yet unpublished measure, the Social Coping Scale (reviewed in Chapter 13), assesses safety behaviors related to social anxiety and may be a helpful adjunct to this part of the clinical interview.

Clinician Rating Scales

The Liebowitz Social Anxiety Scale and the Brief Social Phobia Scale are clinician-rated measures of social phobia reviewed in Chapter 13. Both scales assess fear and avoidance separately, although the independence of the two constructs has not been established with either measure. These rating scales do not yield a diagnosis, but they can be helpful in identifying a range of situations that are problematic for the client, they can be helpful in the creation of a fear and avoidance hierarchy, and they are sensitive to changes associated with treatment.

Self-Report Measures

There are a number of self-report measures (reviewed in Chapter 13) that provide useful information about the nature and extent of social fears associated with social phobia. The Social Avoidance and Distress Scale and Fear of Negative Evaluation Scale were developed before the diagnostic criteria for social phobia, and do not seem to have strong diagnostic utility, but they continue to be widely used as measures of social anxiety. The Social Phobia and Social Interaction Anxiety Scales and the Social Phobia and Anxiety Inventory have been psychometrically evaluated and they each appear to contribute uniquely to the assessment of social phobia (Ries et al., 1998). Although each of these measures has relative merits, none of them provides a DSM-IV diagnosis of social phobia, and estimates of diagnostic utility have been somewhat low. However, the Social Phobia Inventory is a new scale that seems to have promising diagnostic utility, and two unpublished scales, the Inventory of Social Interactions and the Social Phobia Questionnaire, both assist in the assignment of a DSM-IV diagnosis.

Cognitive Assessment Strategies

Given the theoretical importance of cognitive processes in the development and maintenance of social phobia, cognitive assessment is an important component of social phobia assessment (Heimberg, 1994). A number of methods exist for assessing cognitions associated with social phobia (Arnkoff & Glass, 1989; Elting & Hope, 1994; Heimberg, 1994). Some of the most common methods include (1) thought listing (having the client write down thoughts that occurred during a specified period), (2) think-aloud or articulated thought tasks (requiring the client to speak thoughts aloud while performing a role-play or other task), and (3) structured self-statement measures (questionnaires that assess the presence of certain thoughts). The Social Interaction Self-Statement Test and the Self-Statements during Public Speaking Scale can be used for this purpose. Measures of irrational beliefs, attributions, self-focused attention, schemata, and expectations can also be used as adjunct measures (Arnkoff & Glass, 1989). Finally, experimental paradigms such as the modified Stroop task and the visual dot probe can be used to assess attentional processes (Elting & Hope, 1994), although these methods may not be readily available to most clinicians.

Behavioral Assessment Test (BAT)

BATs are an integral component of social phobia assessment in that they can allow for a concurrent examination of self-reported, behavioral, and psychophysiological reactions to a feared situation. In a typical BAT, the client is instructed to participate in a situation that elicits social fear. Subjective units of discomfort scale (SUDS) ratings can be taken during a phase of anticipatory anxiety, and throughout the BAT. Behavioral manifestations of anxiety and social skill can be observed and coded. Psychophysiological responses such as heart rate and blood pressure can also be monitored.

Standardized BATs include conversations with same- and opposite-sex strangers and an impromptu speech given to a small audience (McNeil, Ries, & Turk, 1995). Individualized BATs tailored to the client's most feared situations can also be used (e.g., Heimberg, Hope, Dodge, & Becker, 1990), although their unique nature makes comparisons across clients difficult. Given that virtually all clients experience fear in an impromptu speech task, this is a BAT that can easily be used with all clients and that has been demonstrated to be reliable (Beidel, Turner, Jacob, & Cooley, 1989). Although it is helpful to have confederates as audience members for the speech task, if that is not feasible, the clinician may use a video camera to record the patient giving his or her speech.

Fydrich, Chambless, Perry, Buergener, and Beazley (1998) developed a rating system for the behavioral assessment of social skills (modified from previous versions developed by Trower, Bryant, & Argyle, 1978, and Turner, Beidel, Dancu, & Keys, 1986) to yield ratings of social performance among clients diagnosed with social phobia. This rating system includes five categories (gaze, vocal quality, speech length, discomfort, and conversation flow) that can be evaluated based on a videotaped role-play. The Social Phobia Rating Scale was found to have very good interrater reliability and internal consistency and good convergent and divergent validity. Further, individuals diagnosed with social phobia received significantly less positive ratings than participants in an anxious and a normal control group (Fydrich et al., 1998). The behavioral anchors for the social performance rating scale are reprinted in the original citation.

Self-Monitoring

A number of self-monitoring techniques are frequently used in the ongoing assessment of social phobia. Diary sheets can be individually designed to assess whatever domains of functioning are of interest to the clinician. Clients might be asked to monitor any events that involve exposure to a socially feared situation or that result in the onset of social anxiety. A typical diary might require the client to note the time and date of the event, details about the nature of the event (e.g., my boss criticized my report; I was called on in class; I thought about my upcoming date), and the level of anxiety experienced on a Likert scale. Additional information such as thoughts, physiological symptoms, and behavioral responses can also be collected for each event.

Summary of Assessment Methods

The best assessment of social phobia will include a combination of the above-mentioned strategies that fit the clinician's conceptualization of social phobia and his or her assessment question of interest. Turner, Beidel, and Wolff (1994) demonstrated that assessment indices, including responses to self-report measures, independent evaluator ratings, and behavioral performance data, could be combined to yield a valid composite index of functioning that reflects treatment gains.

Associated Features

A number of constructs have been identified as related to social phobia that may also be important targets of assessment. Individuals diagnosed with social phobia frequently are self-conscious, perfectionistic, and overly sensitive to criticism and negative evaluation (Antony & Swinson, 2000). Thus, measures such as the Self-Consciousness Scale and the Frost Multidimensional Perfectionism Scale may be useful. Clients with social phobia may underachieve in school or at work because of their fear and avoidance of speaking in front of others or to individuals in authority. It is not uncommon for individuals with social phobia (specifically generalized type) to have few friends, to remain outside of a committed relationship, and to have a relatively small support network. Thus, assessment of quality of life factors can be important.

A number of disorders are commonly comorbid with social phobia suggesting the importance of a full diagnostic interview. Clients with social phobia may use substances (such as alcohol) as a way of managing their anxiety. Strong associations exist between lifetime social phobia and the mood disorders (Kessler, Stang, Wittchen, Stein, & Walters, 1999) and between social phobia, generalized type and avoidant personality disorder (Schneier, Spitzer, Gibbon, Fyer, & Liebowitz, 1991). Further, symptoms of social avoidance and social anxiety are present across a number of other psychological disorders, including the other anxiety disorders, the mood disorders, schizoid personality disorder, body dysmorphic disorder, bulimia nervosa, and anorexia nervosa. Thus, a semistructured diagnostic interview can assist in differential diagnosis.

REFERENCES

American Psychiatric Association. (1994). *Diagnostic and statistical manual of mental disorders* (4th ed.). Washington, DC: Author.

Antony, M. M. (1997). Assessment and treatment of social phobia. *Canadian Journal of Psychiatry*, 42, 826–834.

Antony, M. M., & Swinson, R. P. (2000). *Phobic disorders and panic in adults: A guide to assessment and treatment.* Washington, DC: American Psychological Association.

Arnkoff, D. B., & Glass, C. R. (1989). Cognitive assessment in social anxiety and social phobia. *Clinical Psychology Review*, 9, 61–74.

Beidel, D. C., & Turner, S. M. (1998). *Shy children, phobic adults: Nature and treatment of social phobia.* Washington, DC: American Psychological Association.

Beidel, D. C., Turner, S. M., Jacob, R. G., & Cooley, M. R. (1989). Assessment of social phobia: Reliability of an impromptu speech task. *Journal of Anxiety Disorders*, 3, 149–158.

Elting, D. T., & Hope, D. A. (1994). Cognitive assessment. In R. G. Heimberg, M. R. Liebowitz, D. A. Hope, & F. R. Schneier (Eds.), *Social phobia: Diagnosis, assessment, and treatment* (pp. 232–258). New York: Guilford.

Fydrich, T., Chambless, D. L., Perry, K. J., Buergener, F., & Beazley, M. B. (1998). Behavioral assessment of social performance: A rating system for social phobia. *Behaviour Research and Therapy*, 36, 995–1010.

Heimberg, R. G. (1994). Cognitive assessment strategies and the measurement of outcome of treatment for social phobia. *Behaviour Research and Therapy, 32,* 269–280.

Heimberg, R. G., Hope, D. A., Dodge, C. S., & Becker, R. E. (1990). DSM-III-R subtypes of social phobia: Comparison of generalized social phobics and public speaking phobics. *Journal of Nervous and Mental Disease, 178,* 172–179.

Heimberg, R. G., Liebowitz, M. R., Hope, D. A., & Schneier, F. R. (Eds.). (1995). *Social phobia: Diagnosis, assessment, and treatment.* New York: Guilford.

Heimberg, R. G., Stein, M. B., Hiripi, E., & Kessler, R. C. (2000). Trends in the prevalence of social phobia in the United States: A synthetic cohort analysis of changes over four decades. *European Psychiatry, 15,* 29–37.

Hofmann, S. G., & Barlow, D. H. (in press). Social phobia (social anxiety disorder). In D. H. Barlow (Ed.), *Anxiety and its disorders: The nature and treatment of anxiety and panic.* New York: Guilford.

Hofmann, S. G., & DiBartolo, P. M. (2001). *From social anxiety to social phobia: Multiple perspectives.* Boston: Allyn & Bacon.

Kessler, R. C., Stang, P., Wittchen, H. U., Stein, M., & Walters, E. E. (1999). Lifetime comorbidities between social phobia and mood disorders in the U.S. National Comorbidity Survey. *Psychological Medicine, 29,* 555–567.

Kessler, R. C., Stein, M. B., & Berglund, P. A. (1998). Social phobia subtypes in the National Comorbidity Survey. *American Journal of Psychiatry, 155,* 613–619.

Magee, W. J., Eaton, W. W., Wittchen, H. U., McGonagle, K. A., & Kessler, R. C. (1996). Agoraphobia, simple phobia, and social phobia in the National Comorbidity Survey. *Archives of General Psychiatry, 53,* 159–168.

McNeil, D. W., Ries, B. J., & Turk, C. (1994). Behavioral assessment: Self-report, physiology and overt behavior. In R. G. Heimberg, M. R. Liebowitz, D. A. Hope, & F. R. Schneier (Eds.), *Social phobia: Diagnosis, assessment, and treatment* (pp. 202–231). New York: Guilford.

Ries, B. J., McNeil, D. W., Boone, M. L., Turk, C. L., Carter, L. E., & Heimberg, R. G. (1998). Assessment of contemporary social phobia verbal report instruments. *Behaviour Research and Therapy, 36,* 983–994.

Schneier, F. R., Spitzer, R. L., Gibbon, M., Fyer, A. J., & Liebowitz, M. (1991). The relationship of social phobia subtypes and avoidant personality disorder. *Comprehensive Psychiatry, 32,* 496–502.

Stein, M. B. (Ed.). (1995). *Social phobia: Clinical and research perspectives.* Washington, DC: American Psychiatric Press.

Trower, P., Bryant, B., & Argyle, M. (1978). *Social skills and mental health.* Pittsburgh, PA: University of Pittsburgh Press.

Turner, S. M., Beidel, D. C., Dancu, C. V., & Keys, D. J. (1986). Psychopathology of social phobia and comparison to avoidant personality disorder. *Journal of Abnormal Psychology, 95,* 389–394.

Turner, S. M., Beidel, D. C., & Wolff, P. L. (1994). A composite measure to determine improvement following treatment for social phobia: The Index of Social Phobia Improvement. *Behaviour Research and Therapy, 32,* 471–476.

Chapter 13
Measures for Social Phobia

Susan M. Orsillo

BRIEF SOCIAL PHOBIA SCALE (BSPS)

Original Citation

Davidson, J. R. T., Potts, N. L. S., Richichi, E. A., Ford, S. M., Krishnan, R. R., Smith, R. D., & Wilson, W. (1991). The Brief Social Phobia Scale. *Journal of Clinical Psychiatry, 52*, 48–51.

Purpose

To assess fear, avoidance, and physiological arousal associated with social phobia.

Description

The BSPS is an 18-item observer-rated scale designed to assess symptoms of social phobia. It consists of three subscales: *fear, avoidance,* and *physiological arousal.* Part I includes seven social situations that are rated for fear on a five-point scale ranging from 0 (none) to 4 (extreme = incapacitating and/or very painfully distressing) and avoidance on a five-point scale ranging from 0 (never—0%) to 4 (always—100%). In Part II, the respondent is asked to rate the severity of four physiological symptoms one might experience in a social situation on a five-point scale from 0 (none) to 4 (extreme = incapacitating and/or very painfully distressing). The time period used for rating is the previous week; if no exposure has occurred during that period, the respondent is asked to imagine how he or she would feel if

Susan M. Orsillo • National Center for PTSD–Women's Health Sciences Division. Boston VA Healthcare System, and Boston University School of Medicine, Boston, Massachusetts 02130.

exposed to the situations now. The authors of the scale recommend that it be administered following a semistructured interview that allows the clinician to gain some familiarity with the patient's symptoms.

Administration and Scoring

The BSPS takes 5 to 15 minutes to administer. A total score can be calculated by summing all of the items. Subscale scores can be derived by summing the ratings for *fear, avoidance,* and *physiological arousal.*

Psychometric Properties

The original citation of the BSPS included psychometric data for a very small sample of patients (Davidson et al., 1991). Below we report data primarily from a much larger sample of 275 patients who were seeking treatment for social phobia (Davidson et al., 1997).

Sample Means and Norms. The mean total score for a sample of 275 patients seeking treatment for social phobia was 41.61 (*SD* = 9.81; Davidson et al., 1997). In the same sample, the mean scores for each of the subscales were 17.16 (*SD* = 4.30) for *fear,* 17.17 (*SD* = 5.30) for *avoidance* and 7.28 (*SD* = 3.26) for *physiological arousal.*

Reliability. Internal consistency for the total scale was .81 (Davidson et al., 1997). Cronbach's alphas for the individual subscales were .60 for *physiological arousal,* .70 for *fear,* and .78 for *avoidance* (Davidson et al., 1997).

Test–retest over 1 week on patients who showed no improvement between screening and baseline on an independent measure was .91 for the total score (Davidson et al., 1997). Test–retest reliability was .87 for *fear,* .90 for *avoidance,* and .77 for *physiological arousal* (Davidson et al., 1997).

Validity. A factor analysis of the BSPS yielded six factors (Davidson et al., 1997). The strongest included both fear and avoidance items reflecting generalized social phobia (Davidson et al., 1997). Factor 2 was comprised of physiological symptoms, factor 3 was comprised of performance-based situations, factor 4 represented speaking in public, factor 5 was fear and avoidance of social gatherings, and factor 6 loaded highest on speaking with strangers (Davidson et al., 1997).

The correlations between the total score of another interview measure of social phobia and the total score, *fear* subscale, and *avoidance* subscale for the BSPS were strong and significant (*r*s ranging from .70 to .72); however, the *physiological* scale was not associated with this measure (*r* = .04; Davidson et al., 1997). Similarly, the total score, *fear* subscale, and *avoidance* subscale for the BSPS were moderately associated with a self-report measure of social phobia (*r*s ranging from .43 to .51), whereas the *physiological* subscale was not (*r* = .03; Davidson et al., 1997). Total and subscale scores on the BSPS were moderately, but significantly, associated with another interviewer-based measure of anxiety (*r*s ranging from .15 to .34; Davidson et al., 1997).

The total score, *fear* and *avoidance* subscales were significantly associated with a measure of disability in the domains of work, social-life, and family-life/home responsibilities (*rs* ranging from .22 to .55), whereas scores on the *physiological* subscale were unrelated to these measures (Davidson et al., 1997).

Patients who showed improvement by clinician rating demonstrated a significant decrease in total BSPS score whereas nonresponders did not (Davidson et al., 1997). Further, those patients who received drug treatment versus placebo showed a significant decrease on their BSPS total score, *fear*, *avoidance*, and *physiological* subscales (Stein, Fyer, Davidson, Pollack, & Wiita, 1999). In contrast, the *avoidance* and *physiological arousal* subscales did not change as a function of drug treatment (Davidson et al., 1997).

Alternative Forms

A computerized version of the BSPS, yielding similar sample scores and good internal consistency, is described in Kobak et al. (1998).

Source

The BSPS is reprinted in the original article and in Appendix B. Additional information about the scale can be obtained by contacting Jonathan R. T. Davidson, M.D., Department of Psychiatry, Duke University Medical Center, Box 3812, Durham, NC 27710, USA; (tel) 919-684-2880; (fax) 919-684-8866; (e-mail) tolme@acpub.duke.edu.

FEAR OF NEGATIVE EVALUATION (FNE) AND SOCIAL AVOIDANCE AND DISTRESS SCALE (SADS)

Original Citation

Watson, D., & Friend, R. (1969). Measurement of social-evaluative anxiety. *Journal of Consulting and Clinical Psychology, 33*, 448–457.

Purpose

To measure distress and avoidance in social situations and concerns with social-evaluative threat.

Description

The FNE and the SADS were developed together to measure two constructs reflecting social-evaluative anxiety. The FNE consists of 30 items referring to expectation and distress related to negative evaluation from others. The SADS consists of 28 items measuring distress in, and avoidance of, social situations. Each of the items is rated as "true" or "false." No time period is designated for determining the presence or absence of a symptom. The scales are more appropriate for assessing social anxiety than social phobia per se.

Administration and Scoring

The SADS and FNE take 10 to 15 minutes each to administer. On the SADS, the respondent scores one point for each of the following items that are rated "true" (2, 5, 8, 10, 11, 13, 14, 16, 18, 20, 21, 23, 24, 26) and one point for each of the following items that are rated "false" (1, 3, 4, 6, 7, 9, 12, 15, 17, 19, 22, 25, 27, 28). On the FNE, the respondent scores one point for each of the following items that are rated "true" (2, 3, 5, 7, 9, 11, 13, 14, 17, 19, 20, 22, 24, 25, 28, 29, 30) and one point for each of the following items that are rated "false" (1, 4, 6, 8, 10, 12, 15, 16, 18, 21, 23, 26, 27). Higher scores reflect more anxiety.

Psychometric Properties

Sample Means and Norms. Among the development sample of 297 college students, the mean on the SADS was 11.2 for females and 8.24 for males (Watson & Friend, 1969). The mean on the FNE was 13.97 for males and 16.1 for females (Watson & Friend, 1969). The mean total score for a sample of 265 patients seeking treatment for an anxiety disorder was 14.3 (*SD* = 8.7) for males and 14.9 (*SD* = 8.4) for females on the SADS and 17.3 (*SD* = 7.6) for males and 17.8 (*SD* = 8.2) for females on the FNE (Oei, Kenna, & Evans, 1991). Patients with a diagnosis of social phobia scored an average of 20.7 (*SD* = 5.1) on the SADS and 21.9 (*SD* = 5.8) on the FNE (Oei et al., 1991).

Reliability. In a sample of college students, the internal consistency of the SADS was excellent; Kuder–Richardson Formula 20 yielded a correlation of .94 (Watson & Friend, 1969). Internal consistency for the FNE using Kuder–Richardson Formula 20 was excellent ranging from .94 to .96 (Watson & Friend, 1969). Similar results were obtained in a sample of patients with anxiety disorders (Oei et al., 1991).

Test–retest over a 1-month period for college students was found to range from .68 to .79 on the SADS and from .78 to .94 on the FNE (Watson & Friend, 1969).

Validity. A factor analysis on the items comprising the SADS and FNE supported the independence of the two scales (Oei et al., 1991). All but two items loaded on the expected factors. Further, the two scales are moderately, but significantly, correlated with each other (r = .40; Oei et al., 1991).

Turner, McCanna, and Beidel (1987) found that although patients diagnosed with social phobia scored higher than those with other anxiety disorders, the only significant difference was between those diagnosed with social phobia and those diagnosed with simple phobia. Similar results were found on the FNE. These authors concluded that the SADS and FNE lack specificity for social phobia (Turner et al., 1987). However, patients in this study who were diagnosed with social phobia had lower mean scores on the FNE than other groups of patients with social phobia (Heimberg, Hope, Rapee, & Bruch, 1988).

The SADS and FNE have been shown to differentiate between individuals diagnosed with various anxiety disorders. For instance, a group of individuals diagnosed with social phobia scored significantly higher on the SADS than a group of individuals diagnosed with simple phobia or panic disorder (Oei et al., 1991). Further, a group of individuals diagnosed with social phobia scored significantly higher on the FNE than a group of individuals diagnosed with simple phobia (Oei et al., 1991). However, the SADS could not differentiate those with social phobia from those with generalized anxiety disorder (GAD) or panic disorder with agoraphobia (Oei et al., 1991). Further, the FNE could not differentiate individuals with social phobia from those with GAD, panic disorder, or panic disorder with agoraphobia (Oei et al., 1991).

Some experimental validity for the SADS and FNE has been obtained using college students. For instance, students who scored high on the SADS reported that they were less interested than controls in returning to be in an experiment, particularly if they were in a group discussion condition (Watson & Friend, 1969). Winton, Clark, and Edelmann (1995) demonstrated that individuals scoring high on the FNE were biased toward identifying others' facial expressions as negative.

Across three college samples, the FNE was significantly correlated with measures of anxiety (.60), social-evaluative anxiety (.47), social approval (.77) and less strongly with measures of locus of control (.18) and achievement anxiety (.28; Watson & Friend, 1969). The SADS was significantly correlated with measures of audience sensitivity (.76), anxiety (.54), social-evaluative anxiety (.45), and less so with achievement anxiety (.18; Watson & Friend, 1969).

Among a sample of patients diagnosed with a variety of anxiety disorders, the SADS and FNE were moderately, but significantly, correlated with measures of anxiety (rs range from .50 to .70), depression (rs range from .42 to .56), and general distress (rs range from .49 to .55; Cox, Ross, Swinson, & Direnfeld, 1998; Turner et al., 1987).

The FNE has been shown to be one of the most sensitive social phobia treatment outcome measures following cognitive–behavioral group therapy (Cox et al., 1998; Heimberg et al., 1990).

Alternative Forms

A Hindi version of the SADS (Sheikh & Kaushik, 1990) and Japanese versions of the FNE and SADS (Ishikawa, Sasaki, & Hukui, 1992) have been developed. A recalibration of the scale to a five-point Likert scale was preliminarily developed by Gillock, Carmin, Klocek, and Raja (1999). A brief version of the FNE was developed by Leary (1983a) and has been found to be highly correlated with the original scale. Items that correlated .50 and higher with the scale total were selected and the response format was changed from true/false to a five-point scale. The brief FNE demonstrated very good internal consistency, test–retest reliability, and validity (Leary, 1983a).

Source

The SADS and FNE are reprinted in the original articles and in Appendix B. Additional information about the scales can be obtained by contacting David Watson, Ph.D., Psychology Department, University of Hawaii, Honolulu, HI 96822, USA; (tel) 808-956-8414; (fax) 808-956-4700.

LIEBOWITZ SOCIAL ANXIETY SCALE (LSAS)

Original Citation

Liebowitz, M. R. (1987). Social phobia. *Modern Problems in Pharmacopsychiatry, 22,* 141–173.

Purpose

To assess the full range of performance and social difficulties reported by individuals with social phobia.

Description

The LSAS is a widely used 24-item interviewer-rated instrument that assesses fear and avoidance of particular situations in people with social phobia. The LSAS consists of two subscales that measure difficulty with *social interaction* (11 items) and *performance* (13 items) situations. Respondents are asked to rate fear on a four-point scale ranging from 0 (none) to 3 (severe) and avoidance on a four-point scale ranging from 0 (never) to 3 (usually—67–100%) to represent their symptom severity during the past week. Clinical judgment is applied in assigning the final ratings.

Administration and Scoring

The LSAS takes 20 to 30 minutes to administer. It produces a number of indices: *total fear* (sum fear ratings on all 24 items), *fear of social interaction* (sum of fear ratings for items 5, 7, 10–12, 15, 18, 19, 22–24), *fear of performance* (sum of fear ratings for items 1–4, 6, 8, 9, 13, 14, 16, 17, 20, 21), *total avoidance* (sum of avoidance ratings on all 24 items), *avoidance of social interaction* (sum of avoidance ratings for items 5, 7, 10–12, 15, 18, 19, 22–24), *avoidance of performance* (sum of avoidance ratings for items 1–4, 6, 8, 9, 13, 14, 16, 17, 20, 21), and *total fear and avoidance* (sum of total fear and total avoidance scores).

Psychometric Properties

The majority of the psychometric data available on the LSAS is from a paper describing a sample of 382 patients diagnosed with social phobia who participated in one of a number of treatment outcome studies (Heimberg et al., 1999). Unless otherwise cited, all of the data described below are from this source.

Sample Means and Norms. Mean scores on the LSAS for the full sample were 67.2 (SD = 27.5) for the total score, 35.5 (SD = 13.6) for total fear, 16.9 (SD = 7.7) for fear of social interaction, 18.6 (SD = 6.8) for fear of performance, 31.6 (SD = 14.5) for total avoidance, 15.7 (SD = 8.2) for avoidance of social interaction, and 16.0 (SD = 7.3) for avoidance of performance.

Reliability. Cronbach's alpha for the LSAS total score was .96. The alpha coefficients ranged from .81 to .92 for the fear subscales and from .83 to .92 for the avoidance subscales. Total fear and total avoidance scores were highly correlated (.91) suggesting that these subscales may not adequately assess independent constructs, at least in clinical samples. This finding was replicated by Cox et al. (1998).

Validity. An exploratory factor analysis was conducted on the LSAS (Safren et al., 1999). Separate factor analyses of fear and avoidance scores yielded a similar four-factor solution: (1) social interaction, (2) public speaking, (3) observation by others, and (4) eating and drinking in public.

Correlations between scores on the LSAS and other measures support the convergent validity of this measure (Heimberg et al., 1999). LSAS total score was significantly associated with a clinician severity rating from a structured clinical interview (.52), and a number of self-report measures of social anxiety (rs ranging from .49 to .73). Further, additional specific relationships were established. The LSAS fear of social interaction was significantly correlated with another measure of social interactional anxiety (.76), but less closely associated with a measure of social performance anxiety (.50). In contrast, the LSAS fear of performance subscale was more closely associated with a measure of social performance anxiety (.65) than with a measure of social interactional anxiety (.52). These relationships were even stronger in a subsample of patients posttreatment, likely because of the increased variance of scores in that sample.

Discriminant validity for the LSAS was also assessed by examining its relationship with measures assessing depression. In a posttreatment subsample (chosen for its variability), the LSAS was only moderately associated with measures of depression (rs ranging from .52 to .56). Further, in 9 out of 12 instances, correlations between the LSAS and measures of social anxiety were significantly higher than those between the LSAS and measures of depression.

The treatment sensitivity of the LSAS has also been demonstrated in a number of studies (e.g., Baldwin, Bobes, Stein, Scharwaechter, & Faure, 1999; Bouwer & Stein, 1998; Heimberg et al., 1999; Lott et al., 1997). However, using a self-report version of the LSAS, Cox et al. (1998) found that the performance-avoidance subscale showed good treatment sensitivity, but that the social interaction-fear subscale did not.

Alternative Forms

The LSAS has been translated into a French version that was validated by Yao et al. (1999) and a Spanish version that was validated by Bobes et al. (1999). A computer-administered version of the scale was highly associated with the interviewer-administered version (Kobak et al., 1998).

Source

The LSAS is reprinted in the original article and in Appendix B. To obtain more information about the measure, contact Michael R. Liebowitz, M.D., New York State Psychiatric Institute (Unit 120), Columbia University, 722 West 168th Street, New York, NY 10032, USA; (tel) 212-543-5366; (fax) 212-923-2417; (e-mail) liebowitz@nyspi.cpmc.columbia.edu.

SELF-STATEMENTS DURING PUBLIC SPEAKING SCALE (SSPS)

Original Citation

Hofmann, S. G., & DiBartolo, P. M. (2000). An instrument to assess self-statements during public speaking: Scale development and preliminary psychometric properties. *Behavior Therapy, 31,* 499–515.

Purpose

To measure cognitions associated with public speaking.

Description

The SSPS is a 10-item self-report questionnaire that assesses fearful thoughts that typically arise during public speaking. It consists of two 5-item subscales, the *positive self-statements* (SSPS-P) and *negative self-statements* (SSPS-N). The respondent is asked to rate the degree to which he or she agrees with each item on a six-point scale ranging from 0 (if you do not agree at all) to 5 (if you agree extremely with the statement). An earlier state-version of the measure was entitled "Cognitions During the Talk Scale."

Administration and Scoring

Each subscale of the SSPS takes 5 minutes to administer. A score on the SSPS-P is derived by summing items 1, 3, 5, 6, 9. The score on the SSPS-N is derived by summing items 2, 4, 7, 8, 10.

Psychometric Properties

Psychometric data are reported in a multistudy, multisample paper by Hofmann and DiBartolo (2000).

Sample Means and Norms. In two samples of undergraduate students, the mean score on the SSPS-P ranged from 15.4 to 15.8 and the SSPS-N ranged from 7.1 to 7.9. Among a sample of patients seeking treatment for social phobia, the mean SSPS-P score was 13.4 (*SD* = 6.0) and the mean SSPS-N score was 12.3 (*SD* = 6.3).

Reliability. Internal consistency in two college undergraduate samples ranged from .75 to .84 for the SSPS-P and from .83 to .86 on the SSPS-N. Similar findings were derived from a clinical sample. Further, the two subscales were correlated between −.45 and −.69. Three-month test–retest reliability in a sample of patients awaiting treatment for social phobia was .78 for the SSPS-P subscale and .80 for the SSPS-N subscale.

Validity. A factor analysis was conducted with a preliminary version of the measure in a sample of college students. Although five factors emerged, the first two accounted for 51% of the variance. Thus, only items (10) loading on those two factors were retained. A factor analysis on these 10 items confirmed the structure and the two factors accounted for 61.1% of the variance. This factor structure was replicated in another sample of students recruited from a different college and in a clinical sample.

Individuals diagnosed with social phobia scored significantly higher on the SSPS-N and significantly lower on the SSPS-P than college students. Further, scores on the SSPS-N decreased significantly among patients diagnosed with social phobia from pre- to posttreatment. An increase in scores on the SSPS-P following treatment was not significant.

Correlations between the subscales of the SSPS and other measures within a college sample support the convergent validity of the measure. Both subscales were significantly correlated most strongly with a measure of fear of public speaking (SSPS-P $r = -.58$; SSPS-N $r = .67$). Both the SSPS-P and the SSPS-N were also significantly associated with measures of social anxiety (rs range from $-.29$ to $-.34$ and from $.37$ to $.49$, respectively). Scores on the SSPS-N were significantly correlated with both negative ($.48$) and positive ($-.32$) subscales on a self-evaluation measure, and scores on the SSPS-P were significantly correlated with scores on a positive ($.35$) and a negative ($-.18$) self-evaluation measure.

The utility of the SSPS was examined in a small sample of female college students participating in an experimental paradigm. Female students who scored high on the SSPS-N reported lower expectations for their success in a public speaking task, reported more anxiety during the task, and less satisfaction with their performance than low SSPS-N scorers.

Alternative Forms

The SSPS has been translated into Spanish and German.

Source

The SSPS is reprinted in Appendix B. To obtain more information about the measure, contact Stefan G. Hofmann, Ph.D., Department of Psychology, Boston University, 648 Beacon St, 6th Floor, Boston, MA 02215, USA; (tel) 617-353-9610; (fax) 617-353-9609; (e-mail) shofmann@bu.edu.

SOCIAL INTERACTION SELF-STATEMENT TEST (SISST)

Original Citation

Glass, C. R., Merluzzi, T. V., Biever, J. L., & Larsen, K. H. (1982). Cognitive assessment of social anxiety: Development and validation of a self-statement questionnaire. *Cognitive Therapy and Research, 6*, 37–55.

Purpose

To measure positive and negative thoughts associated with social anxiety.

Description

The SISST is one of the most widely used self-report measures for cognitive assessment of social phobia (Elting & Hope, 1995). It is a 30-item scale designed to measure the frequency of positive (facilitative) and negative (debilitative) self-statements that arise before, during, or after a social interaction. Items were empirically derived on the basis of judges' ratings from a larger pool of potential items generated from participants who listed thoughts while imagining difficult social situations. The SISST can be used in relation to a role-played social interaction or respondents can be asked to complete the measure with a recent interaction in mind. The frequency of each item is rated on a five-point scale ranging from 1 (hardly ever) to 5 (very often). Some of the items are worded for men who have completed an interaction with a woman. However, pronouns can be varied so that the SISST can be used in reference to interactions with either men or women, in same-sex as well as in different-sex conversations, and for interactions that involve more than one person.

Administration and Scoring

The SISST can be administered in 5 to 10 minutes. Subscale scores are calculated by adding the numerical responses for the subscales: *positive (facilitative) thoughts* (SISST-P; sum of items 2, 4, 6, 9, 10, 12–14, 17, 18, 24, 25, 27, 28, 30) and *negative (debilitative) thoughts* (SISST-N; sum of items 1, 3, 5, 7, 8, 11, 15, 16, 19–23, 26, 29).

Psychometric Properties

Sample Scores and Norms. Socially anxious female students obtained a mean score of 38.88 ($SD = 9.93$) on the SISST-N and 49.62 ($SD = 7.39$) on the SISST-P (Glass et al., 1982). In contrast, female students with low levels of social anxiety obtained a mean score of 33.32 ($SD = 8.27$) on the SISST-N and 54.95 ($SD = 7.05$) on the SISST-P (Glass et al., 1982). In a small clinical sample, individuals diagnosed with social phobia obtained a mean score of 54.75 ($SD = 12.68$) on the SISST-N and 36.21 ($SD = 11.44$) on the SISST-P (Dodge, Hope, Heimberg, & Becker, 1988).

Reliability. Item–total scale correlations in a college sample ranged from .58 to .77 for SISST-N items and from .45 to .75 for SISST-P items (Glass et al., 1982). Cronbach's alphas derived from student samples ranged from .85 to .89 for the SISST-P and were .91 for the SISST-N (Osman, Markway, & Osman, 1992; Zweig & Brown, 1985). Split-half reliability was .73 for the SISST-P scores and .86 for the SISST-N scores within a college sample (Glass et al., 1982).

Test–retest reliability ranged from .72 to .76 for scores on the SISST-N and from .73 to .89 for scores on the SISST-P among college students presented with the same written social situation (Zweig & Brown, 1985). Similar test–retest reliability was demonstrated for students who received contextually different test stimuli (Zweig & Brown, 1985).

Validity. A factor analysis conducted on a college sample revealed a four-factor solution, with 60.9% of the variance loading on the first factor, self-deprecation (Glass et al., 1982). The second factor reflected positive anticipation, the third fear of negative evaluation, and the fourth coping. A factor analysis on a larger college sample yielded a two-factor solution that was fairly consistent with rationally derived positive and negative subscales (Osman et al., 1992).

Several studies have demonstrated expected group differences on the SISST. For instance, students with high levels of social anxiety scored significantly higher on SISST-N and significantly lower on SISST-P than did students with low levels of social anxiety (Glass et al., 1982; Zweig & Brown, 1985). In a treatment-seeking sample, patients with more social interactional anxiety scored significantly higher than those with more specific public-speaking phobia on the SISST-N (Dodge et al., 1988).

The SISST appears to have good convergent validity, particularly for the negative subscale. Scores on the SISST-P were significantly, positively correlated with a measure of social skill (*r*s ranging from .71 to .77) and negatively correlated with a measure of anxiety (*r*s ranging from −.52 to −.76) in three samples of college students (Glass et al., 1982). Scores on the SISST-N were significantly associated with measures of social anxiety (*r*s range from .25 to .74; Glass et al., 1982; Osman et al., 1992; Zweig & Brown, 1985). In some samples, the relationship between social anxiety and SISST-P was less robust (e.g., Osman et al., 1992; Zweig & Brown, 1985). Further, SISST-N scores were moderately, but significantly, correlated with behavioral ratings of social skill and anxiety (*r*s range from .23 to .32) in college students whereas SISST-P scores were not (*r*s range from .03 to .18; Glass et al., 1982).

There is some evidence that scores on the SISST-N are related to general psychological distress (*r*s range from .35 to .59; Osman et al., 1992). However, scores on the SISST seem to be unrelated to social desirability (e.g., Zweig & Brown, 1985).

In a treatment-seeking sample, scores on the SISST-N were correlated with self-report measures of social anxiety, fear of negative evaluation, general anxiety, and fear of public speaking (*r*s range from .39 to .78; Dodge et al., 1988; Ries et al., 1998). SISST-P scores were only indirectly related to these measures (Dodge et al., 1988). The percentage of negative thoughts elicited using a thought-listing task was significantly associated with scores on the SISST-N (Dodge et al., 1988). However, scores on the SISST were not associated with clinicians' ratings of phobic severity or physiological reactivity (Dodge et al., 1988). A more recent study found that clinicians' ratings of global impairment were significantly correlated with both the negative (.32 to .38) and positive (−.35 to −.41) subscales of the SISST (Beazley, Glass, Chambless, & Arnkoff, in press).

Some support for the treatment sensitivity of the SISST has been established (e.g., Turner, Beidel, & Jacob, 1994; Heimberg et al., 1990).

Alternative Forms

A French version of the SISST was developed and validated by Yao et al. (1998). The measure has also been translated into Spanish (Caballo, 1993).

Source

The SISST is reprinted in the original article and in Appendix B. More information about the instrument can be obtained by contacting Carol R. Glass, Ph.D., Department of Psychology, Catholic University of America, Washington, DC 20064, USA; (tel) 202-319-5759; (fax) 202-319-6263; (e-mail) glass@cua.edu.

SOCIAL PHOBIA AND ANXIETY INVENTORY (SPAI)

Original Citations

Turner, S. M., Beidel, D. C., Dancu, C. V., & Stanley, M. A. (1989). An empirically derived inventory to measure social fears and anxiety: The Social Phobia and Anxiety Inventory. *Psychological Assessment, 1,* 35–40.

Turner, S. M., Beidel, D. C., & Dancu, C. V. (1996). *SPAI: Social Phobia and Anxiety Inventory.* North Tonawanda, NY: Multi-Health Systems.

Purpose

To measure severity of symptoms associated with social anxiety and social phobia.

Description

The SPAI is a 45-item self-report questionnaire that was empirically developed to be a specific measure of social phobia. It measures the somatic, cognitive, and behavioral aspects of social phobia across a variety of situations and settings. Each item is rated for frequency on a seven-point scale ranging from 0 (never) to 6 (always). There is no specific time period for which respondents rate the occurrence of symptoms. The SPAI consists of two subscales: *social phobia* and *agoraphobia*.

Administration and Scoring

The SPAI can be administered in 20 to 30 minutes. Subscale scores are calculated by summing the items that constitute each subscale. A difference score (which was initially referred to in the literature as the total score) is obtained by subtracting the *agoraphobia* subscale score from the *social phobia* subscale score. The difference score is thought to be a purer measure of social phobia in that the *agoraphobia* subscale serves as a suppressor variable to control for symptoms of social anxiety that are best conceptualized as part of agoraphobia. A score of 39 or higher on the *agoraphobia* subscale may indicate the presence of panic disorder. Additional cutoff scores are suggested in the manual and the original article for clinical and student samples.

Psychometric Properties

Sample Scores and Norms.   Percentile scores for the total sample, and by racial identity, are available for a large community sample (Gillis, Haaga, & Ford, 1995). In a clinical sample, the mean score for individuals diagnosed with social phobia was 94.0 (Turner, Beidel, Dancu, & Stanley, 1989). Ries et al. (1998) found that individuals diagnosed with generalized social phobia obtained a mean difference score of 96.5 (SD = 19.4), a comorbid generalized social phobia and avoidant personality group obtained a mean score of 116.6 (SD = 17.0), and the speech phobia group obtained a mean score of 75.8 (SD = 26.8). Socially anxious college students had a mean score of 72.2 (SD = 20.4) compared with 32.7 (SD = 21.3) for nonanxious students (Turner, Beidel, et al., 1989). Mean difference scores ranging from 56 to 58 have been found in student and community samples (Osman et al., 1996). Additional normative information is available from the manual.

Reliability.   Both subscales of the SPAI have been shown to be internally consistent with Cronbach's alpha ranging from .94 to .96 for the *social phobia* subscale and .85 to .86 for the *agoraphobia* subscale (Osman et al., 1996; Turner, Beidel, et al., 1989). Test–retest reliability on the difference score over 2 weeks in a sample of college students was .86 (Turner, Beidel, et al., 1989).

Validity.   A confirmatory factor analysis was conducted with a sample of college students (Turner, Stanley, Beidel, & Bond, 1989). The results, for the most part, supported the two-factor solution and were replicated in a sample of individuals meeting diagnostic criteria for social phobia. Further, the two-factor solution was replicated in a student and community sample (Osman, Barrios, Aukes, & Osman, 1995; Osman et al., 1996). An exploratory factor analysis conducted with a sample of college students utilizing only the social phobia items was conducted that resulted in a five-factor solution yielding the following factors: Individual Social Interaction, Somatic and Cognitive, Group Interaction, Avoidance, Focus of Attention (Turner, Stanley, et al., 1989). This five-factor model was, for the most part, replicated in a college sample by Osman et al. (1995). However, in the sample of individuals with social phobia, an exploratory factor analysis yielded a slightly different solution. The majority of the items loaded on the first factor, labeled Social Phobia, and two other smaller factors, Somatic and Avoidance, were obtained (Turner, Stanley, et al., 1989). Finally, Turner, Stanley, et al. (1989) conducted a Q factor analysis with a mixed student and patient sample, in which participants, rather than item scores, are used to determine the factor structure of the measure. A three-factor model, Social Anxiety, Agoraphobia, and Mixed Anxiety, provided the best fit.

College students with a diagnosis of social phobia scored significantly higher on the social phobia, agoraphobia, and the difference score than those without the diagnosis (Beidel, Turner, Stanley, & Dancu, 1989). Patients with a diagnosis of social phobia scored significantly higher than those with panic disorder with or without agoraphobia and those with obsessive-compulsive disorder (Turner, Beidel, et al., 1989). Generalized social phobics scored significantly higher than those with speech phobia (Ries et al., 1998).

The SPAI difference score has been shown to be significantly correlated with other self-report measures of social anxiety (rs range from .41 to .77; Beidel, Turner, & Cooley, 1993; Cox et al., 1998; Herbert, Bellack, & Hope, 1991; Osman et al., 1995, 1996; Ries et al., 1998). Correlations are slightly higher between these measures and the SPAI *social phobia* subscale. SPAI difference scores were moderately, but significantly, associated with distress in social situations derived from daily monitoring forms (.43 to .47; Beidel, Borden, Turner, & Jacob, 1989; Beidel, Turner, et al., 1989). A cognitive score derived from the SPAI was moderately associated with self-monitored frequency of (.23 to .36), and distress related to (.30 to .36) disturbing thoughts (Beidel, Borden, et al., 1989; Beidel, Turner, et al., 1989). Further, an SPAI item that assesses anticipatory somatic response was significantly correlated with pulse rate (.43) during a public-speaking task (Beidel, Borden, et al., 1989). Scores on the SPAI behavioral avoidance factor were associated with the time participants spoke before escaping the public-speaking task (−.33; Beidel, Borden, et al., 1989), and self-reported entry into anxiety-producing situations (.31; Beidel, Turner, et al., 1989). However, in another sample, scores on the SPAI were not associated with time spent in a behavioral assessment test (Ries et al., 1998). Scores on the difference scale were also significantly correlated with discomfort ratings during a behavioral test (.47) and with an impromptu speech (.64; Herbert et al., 1991). Difference scores were significantly correlated with several measures of anxiety during a role-play (.64 to .84; Rodebaugh, Chambless, Terrill, Floyd, & Uhde, 2000).

Correlations between the SPAI completed by participants and completed by someone who knew them well was .63 (Beidel, Turner, et al., 1989).

Some evidence of discriminant validity is available for the SPAI. In one sample, although measures of social anxiety were associated with the *social phobia* subscale and difference scores, they were not significantly associated with the score on the *agoraphobia* subscale (rs ranging from .03 to .43; Herbert et al., 1991). The difference score was only moderately correlated with measures of agoraphobia (.15 to .32), blood/injury phobia (.12 to .47), and general psychological distress (.21 to .50; Herbert et al., 1991; Osman et al., 1996). Further, the difference score is not associated with a measure of social desirability (Osman et al., 1995).

A score of 60 on the SPAI resulted in 41.4% false negatives and 8.9% false positives in a college sample (Turner, Beidel, et al., 1989). In a clinical sample, a score of 90 yielded a false negative rate of 38.1% and a false positive rate of 16.7 to 20.0%, depending on the diagnosis (Turner, Beidel, et al., 1989). In a discriminant function analysis with clinical and student samples, the SPAI correctly classified 74 to 77% of the socially phobic individuals (Beidel, Turner, et al., 1989; Turner, Beidel, et al., 1989).

Treatment sensitivity has been well established with the SPAI (e.g., Beidel et al., 1993; Cox et al., 1998; Ries et al., 1998; Taylor et al., 1997).

Alternative Forms

A well-validated version of the SPAI designed to assess childhood social fears has been developed (Beidel, Turner, & Fink, 1996). This measure is also available through Multi-Health Systems (see below). The SPAI has been translated into several languages including South American Portuguese, Icelandic, Canadian French, U.S. Spanish, and Swedish. It has been validated in an adolescent Spanish sample (Olivares, García-López, Hidalgo, Turner, & Beidel, 1999). The SPAI has also been translated into Dutch (Bögels & Reith, 1999).

Source

The SPAI is published by Multi-Health Systems Inc., 908 Niagara Falls Blvd., North Tonawanda, NY 14120-2060, USA; (tel) 800-456-3003 (USA) or 800-268-6011 (Canada); (fax) 416-424-1736; (webpage) www.mhs.com. The SPAI complete kit, which includes a manual and 25 scoring forms, costs $55.00 US. Additional information about the SPAI can be obtained by contacting Samuel Turner, Ph.D., Maryland Center for Anxiety Disorders, Department of Psychology, University of Maryland, College Park, MD 20742, USA; (tel) 301-405-0232; (fax) 301-405-8154.

SOCIAL PHOBIA INVENTORY (SPIN)

Original Citation

Connor, K. M., Davidson, J. R. T., Churchill, L. E., Sherwood, A., Foa, E., & Wesler, R. H. (2000). Psychometric properties of the Social Phobia Inventory (SPIN). *British Journal of Psychiatry, 176*, 379–386.

Purpose

To assess fear, avoidance, and physiological arousal associated with social phobia.

Description

The SPIN is a 17-item questionnaire designed to assess symptoms of social phobia. Each item contains a symptom that is rated by the respondent based on how much he or she was bothered by the symptom during the prior week on a five-point scale ranging from 0 (not at all) to 4 (extremely). It consists of three subscales: *fear, avoidance,* and *physiological arousal.*

Administration and Scoring

The SPIN takes 10 minutes to administer. A total score can be calculated by summing all the items and subscale scores can be derived by summing the ratings for *fear*, *avoidance*, and *physiological arousal*.

Psychometric Properties

Psychometric data are derived from a large sample of healthy volunteers, psychiatric outpatients without social phobia, and patients with social phobia who participated in one of three clinical trials (Connor et al., 2000).

Sample Means and Norms. The mean pretreatment score for the social phobia group was 41.1 (*SD* = 10.2). The mean score for the nonpsychiatric control group was 12.1 (*SD* = 9.3).

Reliability. Internal consistency for the total scale ranged from .82 to .94 across the groups. Cronbach's alphas for the individual subscales ranged from .68 to .79 for *fear*, .71 to .81 for *avoidance*, and .57 to .73 for *physiological arousal*.

Test–retest reliability in a subsample of patients who showed no improvement between two visits was .78 to .89 for the total score.

Validity. A factor analysis yielded five factors. Factor 1 represented fear and avoidance of talking to strangers and in social gatherings. Factor 2 included items about criticism and embarrassment. Factor 3 contained physiological items. Factor 4 included fear and avoidance of people in authority. Factor 5 reflected avoiding being the center of attention and fear of public speaking.

Patients diagnosed with social phobia scored significantly higher on the SPIN than did nonpsychiatric controls.

SPIN total scores have been shown to be moderately, but significantly, correlated with interviewer ratings of social phobia (*r*s ranging from .55 to .92). Further, the SPIN subscale scores were significantly correlated with an interviewer rating of fear (*r*s ranging from .61 to .82), avoidance (*r*s ranging from .47 to .62), and physiological response (*r*s ranging from .62 to .66). For the patients with social phobia, posttreatment SPIN scores were significantly correlated with clinical global impression severity (.70).

Discriminant validity was established via correlations between the SPIN and a measure of blood–injury phobia (.34) and a measure of disability (.33) which were smaller. Further, scores on the SPIN were not found to be significantly associated with a measure of general health.

A cutoff score of 19 distinguished between patients with and without social phobia with a diagnostic efficiency of 79%.

Treatment sensitivity has also been established with the SPIN.

Source

The SPIN can be obtained from Kathryn M. Connor, M.D., Box 3812, Duke University Medical Center, Durham, NC 27710, USA; (tel) 919-684-5849; (fax) 919-684-8866; (e-mail) kathryn.connor@duke.edu.

SOCIAL PHOBIA SCALE (SPS) AND SOCIAL INTERACTION ANXIETY SCALE (SIAS)

Original Citation

Mattick, R. P. & Clarke, J. C. (1998). Development and validation of measures of social phobia scrutiny fear and social interaction anxiety. *Behaviour Research and Therapy, 36,* 455–470.

Purpose

The purpose of the SPS is to assess fears of being scrutinized during routine activities. The purpose of the SIAS is to assess fears of more general social interaction.

Description

The SPS and SIAS are widely used measures that were originally developed in an unpublished form in 1989. The SPS contains 20 items that are rated on a five-point scale ranging from 0 (not at all characteristic or true of me) to 4 (extremely characteristic or true of me). Items describe situations involving being observed by others while engaged in activities such as eating or writing. The original version of the SIAS consists of 19 items, but many studies use a 20-item version that is identical to the original except for the addition of one item (item 5 in the version reprinted in Appendix B). Items on the SIAS describe cognitive, affective, and behavioral reactions to interactional situations. Items are rated on a five-point scale ranging from 0 (not at all characteristic or true of me) to 4 (extremely characteristic or true of me).

Administration and Scoring

The SPS and SIAS each take 5 minutes to self-administer. The SPS is scored by taking the sum of all of the items. The SIAS is scored by reverse coding the positively worded items (items 8 and 10 on the 19-item scale, items 5, 9, and 11 on the 20-item scale).

Psychometric Properties

Sample Scores and Norms.   Individuals diagnosed with social phobia had a mean score of 40.0 (*SD* = 16.0) on the SPS and 24.6 (*SD* = 16.4) on the 19-item version of the SIAS (Mattick & Clarke, 1998). Participants from the community had a mean score of 14.4 on the SPS (*SD* = 11.2) and 18.8 (*SD* = 11.8) on the 19-item version of the SIAS (Mattick & Clarke, 1998). Mean scores for students and individuals diagnosed with agoraphobia and simple phobia can be found in Mattick and Clarke (1998). Heimberg, Mueller, Holt, Hope, and Liebowitz (1992) reported mean scores of 32.8 (*SD* =14.9) on the SPS and 49.0 (*SD* = 15.6) on the 20-item version of the SIAS for a sample of individuals diagnosed with social phobia. The mean scores for a community sample were 12.5 (*SD* = 11.5) on the SPS and 19.9 (*SD* = 14.2) on the 20-item version of the SIAS (Heimberg et al., 1992).

Reliability.   Cronbach's alphas for both scales have suggested high internal consistency for both the SPS (.87 to .94) and the SIAS (.86 to .94) across a variety of clinical, community, and student samples (Heimberg et al., 1992; Mattick & Clarke, 1998; Osman, Gutierrez, Barrios, Kopper, & Chiros, 1998). Test–retest reliability over 4 to 12 weeks has also been found to be quite high for both the SPS (rs range from .66 to .93) and the SIAS (rs range from .86 to .92; Heimberg et al., 1992; Mattick & Clarke, 1998).

Validity.   Factor analysis was conducted on a large sample of individuals diagnosed with social phobia (Mattick & Clarke, 1998). The SPS contained three factors: general scrutiny concern, specific fears, and fear of being viewed as ill or losing control in front of others. In the same sample, a factor analysis on the SIAS supported the notion that the measure taps into a unitary construct of social interactional fear (Mattick & Clarke, 1998).

A confirmatory factor analysis was conducted on a clinical sample to empirically test the assumption that the SPS and SIAS measure two specific dimensions of social anxiety (Safren, Turk, & Heimberg, 1998). The results did not support the two-factor model. Instead, the data were best accounted for by a three-factor model: interaction anxiety, being observed by others, and fear that others will notice anxiety symptoms. However, hierarchical factor analysis suggested that these three factors all load on a single, higher-order factor, social anxiety. A somewhat similar three-factor model obtained from a college student sample was described by Habke, Hewitt, Norton, and Asmundson (1997) but this model yielded a poor fit in a confirmatory factor analysis conducted by Osman et al. (1998). Instead, Osman et al. (1998) found that the two-factor model provided good fit in two independent samples. Further research is needed to reconcile these conflicting findings.

Patients diagnosed with social phobia scored significantly higher than those with agoraphobia, undiagnosed students, and community participants on both the SPS and the SIAS (Heimberg et al., 1992; Mattick & Clarke, 1998). Further, individuals with agoraphobia scored significantly higher than those diagnosed with simple phobia (Mattick & Clarke, 1998). In another large clinical sample, individuals diagnosed with social phobia scored significantly higher on the SIAS than those with any other anxiety disorder or nonanxious participants (Brown et al., 1997). On the SPS, patients with social phobia scored significantly higher than all other groups with the exception of patients diagnosed with panic disorder with agoraphobia. However, high scores on both measures by patients diagnosed with panic disorder with agoraphobia seem to be accounted for by a comorbid social phobia diagnosis (Brown et al., 1997).

Correlational data also provide some support for the convergent and discriminant validity of the SPS and SIAS. Other measures of social anxiety have been shown to be significantly associated with both the SPS (.64 to .75) and the SIAS (.66 to .81; Cox et al., 1998; Habke et al., 1997; Heimberg et al., 1992; Mattick & Clarke, 1998; Ries et al., 1998). Somewhat smaller correlations emerged between measures of general anxiety and the SPS (.42 to .57) and SIAS (.45 to .58), depression and the SPS (.54) and SIAS (.47), and locus of control and the SPS (.31) and SIAS (.30; Mattick & Clarke, 1998). Further, neither scale was significantly associated with a measure of social desirability (Mattick & Clarke, 1998).

There is also some evidence that the SPS and SIAS seem to measure different, though related, constructs. Both Heimberg et al. (1992) and Brown et al. (1997) demonstrated the SPS was more strongly related to measures of anxiety about performance or being observed by others, whereas the SIAS was more strongly associated with measures of social interaction anxiety.

Using one standard deviation above the mean derived from a community sample ($\geq$34 for the SAIS and $\geq$24 for the SPS) to determine caseness, Heimberg et al. (1992) correctly classified 82% of the social phobia group by the SIAS and 73% of the social phobia group by the SPS (Heimberg et al., 1992). The overall efficiency of these cutoff scores in a mixed group of anxiety-disordered patients was 73% for the SPS and 75% for the SIAS (Brown et al., 1997). When a criterion score was required on both measures, the overall efficiency rate was 77% (Brown et al., 1997).

The SIAS and SPS have both been shown to be sensitive to treatment (e.g., Cox et al., 1998; Mattick & Peters, 1988; Mattick, Peters, & Clarke, 1989; Ries et al., 1998).

Source

Items from SPS and SIAS are published in the original article and the scales are reprinted in Appendix B. More information about the measures can be obtained by contacting Richard P. Mattick, M.D., National Drug and Alcohol Research Centre, University of New South Wales, Sydney, NSW 2052, Australia; (tel) 61-2-9398-9333; (fax) 61-2-9399-7143; (e-mail) r.mattick@unsw.edu.au.

BRIEF DESCRIPTIONS OF ADDITIONAL MEASURES

Fear of Intimacy Scale (FIS)

The FIS is a 35-item self-report scale developed to measure fear of intimacy, or the inhibited capacity to exchange personally important thoughts and feelings with significant others (Descutner & Thelen, 1991). The measure is reprinted in the original article (Descutner & Thelen, 1991). Additional psychometric properties are examined in Doi and Thelen (1993).

Interaction Anxiousness Scale (IAS)

The IAS is a 15-item self-report questionnaire designed to measure dispositional social anxiety. It was constructed to measure only the affective component of social anxiety (Leary & Kowalski, 1993). The measure is reprinted in the original article (Leary, 1983b). Psychometric properties of the English (Leary & Kowalski, 1993) and the Spanish (Sanz, 1994) version have been examined. More information on the scale can be obtained from Mark Leary, Ph.D., Department of Psychology, Wake Forest University, Winston-Salem, NC 27109, USA; (tel) 336-758-5750; (fax) 336-758-4733; (e-mail) leary@wfu.edu.

Inventory of Interpersonal Situations (IIS)

The IIS is a 35-item self-report measure designed to assess social anxiety. It provides both a frequency and a discomfort score. The English version of the questionnaire is reprinted in a paper by van Dam-Baggen and Kraaimaat (1999), which also examines psychometric properties of the scale. French, German, and Turkish versions of the scale are available. The copyright is held by Swets Test Publishers, Heereweg 347, 2160 CA Lisse, the Netherlands (phone +31 252 435 375, fax +31 252 415 888, webpage www.swets.nl/stp). For more information about the IIS, contact Rien van Dam-Baggen, Ph.D., Department of Clinical

Psychology, University of Amsterdam, the Netherlands; (tel) 31-20-525-6817; (fax) 31-20-639-1369; (e-mail) dambaggen@psy.uva.nl.

Inventory of Social Interactions (ISI)

The ISI is a self-report scale currently under development designed to assess social phobia according to DSM-IV criteria. Preliminary research suggests that the ISI has good internal consistency, convergent validity, and discriminant validity. This measure has not been published to date. More information can be found at the website, nas.psy.uga.edu/SCALES. html or by contacting Nader Amir, Ph.D., Department of Psychology, University of Georgia, Athens, GA 30606, USA; (tel) 706-542-1173; (fax) 706-542-8048; (e-mail) amir@egon. psy.uga.edu.

Personal Report of Confidence as a Speaker (PRCS)

The PRCS was originally developed by Gilkinson (1942) as a 104-item self-report measure of fear of public speaking. Paul (1966) developed a 30-item short form of the measure that may be used as a screening or treatment outcome measure. Some psychometric data are available in Daly (1978). Normative data by ethnicity and gender are available in Phillips, Jones, Rieger, and Snell (1997).

Self-Consciousness Scale (SCS)

The SCS is a 23-item self-report questionnaire that measures public and private self-consciousness and social anxiety (Fenigstein, Scheier, & Buss, 1975). Hope and Heimberg (1988) found that public, but not private, self-consciousness was related to self-report and observer ratings of social anxiety. A Turkish version of the SCS scale has been developed and validated (Ruganci, 1995). More information about the scale can be obtained by contacting Arnold Buss, Department of Psychology, University of Texas, Austin, TX 78712, USA.

Shyness and Sociability Scales

A nine-item self-report shyness scale and five-item self-report sociability scale were developed by Cheek and Buss (1981). A German version of the scale is available (Czeschlik & Nuerk, 1995).

Social Anxiety Sensitivity Index (SASI)

The SASI is a 25-item self-report questionnaire currently under development that is designed to measure sensitivity of fear of social interactions. Preliminary research supports the measure's internal consistency, convergent, divergent, and predictive validity. This measure has not been published to date. More information can be found at the website, nas.psy.uga.edu/ SCALES.html or by contacting Nader Amir, Ph.D., Department of Psychology, University of Georgia, Athens, GA 30606, USA; (tel) 706-542-1173; (fax) 706-542-8048; (e-mail) amir@ egon.psy.uga.edu.

Social Cognitions Questionnaire (SCQ)

The SCQ is a 22-item self-report measure developed to assess cognitions associated with social anxiety and social phobia. The measure taps into three dimensions: negative self-beliefs, fear of performance failure, and fear of negative evaluation. In preliminary research, the SCQ has been shown to have excellent internal consistency, good convergent validity, and adequate discriminant validity. This measure has not been published to date. For more information, or to obtain a copy of the measure, contact Adrian Wells, Ph.D., Department of Clinical Psychology, University of Manchester, Rawnsley Building, Manchester Royal Infirmary, Manchester, United Kingdom; (tel) 44-161-276-5387; (fax) 44-161-273-2135; (e-mail) adrian.wells@man.ac.ak.

Social Coping Scale (SCS)

The SCS is a 28-item self-report questionnaire that assesses safety behaviors associated with social anxiety. The scale has been shown to have excellent test–retest reliability and good convergent and discriminant validity, and to be sensitive to changes with treatment. Sample items include "I only go to those social events where I know what to expect" and "I tend to steer the conversation towards the other person." The SCS is currently under development and can be obtained by contacting Deborah Dobson, Ph.D., Department of Psychology, Foothills Medical Centre, 1403-29 Street NW, Calgary, AB, T2N 2T9, Canada; (tel) 403-670-4804; (fax) 403-670-2060; (e-mail) ddobson@ucalgary.ca.

Social Phobia Questionnaire (SPQ)

The SPQ is a 15-item self-report questionnaire designed to directly assess social phobia according to DSM-IV criteria. It assesses fear and avoidance of a number of social situations as well as level of severity, distress, and impairment in functioning. Preliminary data suggest that the SPQ has high test–retest reliability, good convergent and discriminant validity, and that it can differentiate individuals with social phobia from controls. The SPQ is not currently published, but it can be obtained by contacting Michelle G. Newman, Ph.D., Department of Psychology, Pennsylvania State University, 310 Moore Building, University Park, PA 16802-3103, USA; (tel) 814-863-1148; (fax) 814-863-7002; (e-mail) mgn1@psu.edu.

Social Reticence Scale (SRS)

The SRS is a 22-item self-report measure of shyness. It has been shown to have good internal consistency, test–retest reliability, and convergent validity (Jones & Russell, 1982).

Speaking Extent and Comfort Scale (SPEACS)

The SPEACS is a 20-item self-report scale designed to measure four aspects of conversational experience: frequency and comfort of talking generally and about the self (Lyons & Spicer, 1999). The measure has been shown to have good test–retest reliability and convergent validity. Internal consistency on the scale was quite low, which the authors interpret as reflecting the tendency for people to approach conversations in situationally specific ways. The SPEACS was not developed in a clinical context and thus its clinical utility is unknown. The measure is reprinted in the original citation (Lyons & Spicer, 1999).

Stanford Shyness Survey

The Stanford Shyness Survey was developed by Zimbardo in 1977. Shortened versions of the measure were developed by Pilkonis (1977) and Maroldo, Eisenreich, and Hall (1979).

REFERENCES

Baldwin, D., Bobes, J., Stein, D., Scharwaechter, I., & Faure, M. (1999). Paroxetine in social phobia/social anxiety disorder: Randomized, double-blind, placebo-controlled study. *British Journal of Psychiatry, 175,* 120–126.

Beazley, M. B., Glass, C. R., Chambless, D. L., & Arnkoff, D. B. (in press). Cognitive self-statements in social phobia: A comparison across three types of social situations. *Cognitive Therapy and Research.*

Beidel, D. C., Borden, J. W., Turner, S. M., & Jacob, R. G. (1989). The Social Phobia and Anxiety Inventory: Concurrent validity with a clinic sample. *Behaviour Research and Therapy, 27,* 573–576.

Beidel, D. C., Turner, S. M., & Cooley, M. R. (1993). Assessing reliable and clinically significant change in social phobia: Validity of the Social Phobia and Anxiety Inventory. *Behaviour Research and Therapy, 31,* 331–337.

Beidel, D. C., Turner, S. M., & Fink, C. M. (1996). Assessment of childhood social phobia: Construct, convergent, and discriminative validity of the Social Phobia and Anxiety Inventory for Children (SPAI-C). *Psychological Assessment, 8,* 235–240.

Beidel, D. C., Turner, S. M., Stanley, M. A., & Dancu, C. V. (1989). The Social Phobia and Anxiety Inventory: Concurrent and external validity. *Behavior Therapy, 20,* 417–427.

Bobes, J., Badia, X., Luque, A., Garcia, M., Gonzalez, M. P., & Dal-Re, R. (1999). Validation of the Spanish version of the Liebowitz Social Anxiety Scale, social anxiety and distress scale and Sheehan disability inventory for the evaluation of social phobia. *Medical Clinics, 112,* 530–538.

Bögels, S. M., & Reith, W. (1999). Validity of two questionnaires to assess social fears: The Dutch Social Phobia and Anxiety Inventory and the Blushing, Trembling, and Sweating Questionnaire. *Journal of Psychopathology and Behavioral Assessment, 21,* 51–66.

Bouwer, C., & Stein, D. J. (1998). Use of the selective serotonin reuptake inhibitor citalopram in the treatment of generalized social phobia. *Journal of Affective Disorders, 49,* 79–82.

Brown, E. J., Turovsky, J., Heimberg, R. G., Juster, H. R., Brown, T. A., & Barlow, D. H. (1997). Validation of the Social Interaction Anxiety Scale and the Social Phobia Scale across the anxiety disorders. *Psychological Assessment, 9,* 21–27.

Caballo, V. E. (1993). Relationships among some behavioral and self-report measures of social skills. *Psicologia Conductual, 1,* 69–91.

Cheek, J. M., & Buss, A. H. (1981). Shyness and sociability. *Journal of Personality and Social Psychology, 41,* 330–339.

Cox, B. J., Ross, L., Swinson, R. P., & Direnfeld, D. M. (1998). A comparison of social phobia outcome measures in cognitive–behavioral group therapy. *Behavior Modification, 22,* 285–297.

Czeschlik, T., & Nuerk, H. C. (1995). Shyness and sociability: Factor structure in a German sample. *European Journal of Psychological Assessment, 11,* 122–127.

Daly, J. (1978). The assessment of social-communicative anxiety via self-reports: A comparison of measures. *Communication Monographs, 45,* 204–218.

Davidson, J. R. T., Miner, C. M., De Veaugh-Geiss, J., Tupler, L. A., Colket, J. T., & Potts, N. L. S. (1997). The Brief Social Phobia Scale: A psychometric evaluation. *Psychological Medicine, 27,* 161–166.

Descutner, C. J., & Thelen, M. H. (1991). Development and validation of Fear of Intimacy Scale. *Psychological Assessment, 3,* 218–225.

Dodge, C. S., Hope, D. A., Heimberg, R. G., & Becker, R. E. (1988). Evaluation of the Social Interaction Self-Statement Test with a social phobic population. *Cognitive Therapy and Research, 12,* 211–222.

Doi, S. C., & Thelen, M. H. (1993). The Fear of Intimacy Scale: Replication and extension. *Psychological Assessment, 5,* 377–383.

Elting, D. T., & Hope, D. A. (1995). Cognitive assessment. In R. G. Heimberg, M. R. Liebowitz, D. A. Hope, & F. R. Schneier (Eds.), *Social phobia: Diagnosis, assessment, and treatment* (pp. 232–258). New York: Guilford.

Fenigstein, A., Scheier, M. F., & Buss, A. H. (1975). Public and private self-consciousness: Assessment and theory. *Journal of Consulting and Clinical Psychology, 43,* 522–527.

Gilkinson, H. (1942). Social fears as reported by students in college speech classes. *Speech Monographs, 9,* 131–160.

Gillis, M. M., Haaga, D. A., & Ford, G. T. (1995). Normative values for the Beck Anxiety Inventory, Fear Questionnaire, Penn State Worry Questionnaire, and Social Phobia and Anxiety Inventory. *Psychological Assessment, 7,* 450–455.

Gillock, K., Carmin, C., Klocek, J., & Raja, S. (1999, March). *Recalibrating two measures of social phobia: Social Avoidance and Distress Scale and Fear of Negative Evaluation Scale.* Poster session presented at the meeting of the Anxiety Disorders Association of America, San Diego, CA.

Habke, A. M., Hewitt, P. L., Norton, G. R., & Asmundson, G. (1997). The Social Phobia and Social Interaction Anxiety Scales: An exploration of the dimensions of social anxiety and sex differences in structure and relations with pathology. *Journal of Psychopathology and Behavioral Assessment, 19,* 21–39.

Heimberg, R. G., Dodge, C. S., Hope, D. A., Kennedy, C. R., Zollo, L. J., & Becker, R. E. (1990). Cognitive-behavioral group treatment for social phobia: Comparison with a credible placebo. *Cognitive Therapy and Research, 14,* 1–23.

Heimberg, R. G., Hope, D. A., Rapee, R. M., & Bruch, M. A. (1988). The validity of the Social Avoidance and Distress Scale and the Fear of Negative Evaluation Scale with social phobic patients. *Behaviour Research and Therapy, 26,* 407–410.

Heimberg, R. G., Horner, K. J., Juster, H. R., Safren, S. A., Brown, E. J., Schneier, F. R., & Liebowitz, M. R. (1999). Psychometric properties of the Liebowitz Social Anxiety Scale. *Psychological Medicine, 29,* 199–212.

Heimberg, R. G., Mueller, G. P., Holt, C. S., Hope, D. A., & Liebowitz, M. R. (1992). Assessment of anxiety in social interaction and being observed by others: The Social Interaction Anxiety Scale and the Social Phobia Scale. *Behavior Therapy, 23,* 53–73.

Herbert, J. D., Bellack, A. S., & Hope, D. A. (1991). Concurrent validity of the Social Phobia and Anxiety Inventory. *Journal of Psychopathology and Behavioral Assessment, 13,* 357–368.

Hope, D. A., & Heimberg, R. G. (1988). Public and private self-consciousness and social phobia. *Journal of Personality Assessment, 52,* 626–639.

Ishikawa, R., Sasaki, K., & Hukui, I. (1992). Standardization of Japanese version of FNE and SADS. *Japanese Journal of Behavior Therapy, 18,* 10–17.

Jones, W. H., & Russell, D. (1982). The Social Reticence Scale: An objective instrument to measure shyness. *Journal of Personality Assessment, 46,* 6.

Kobak, K. A., Schaettle, S. C., Greist, J. H., Jefferson, J. W., Katzelnick, D. J., & Dottl, S. L. (1998). Computer-administered rating scales for social anxiety in a clinical drug trial. *Depression and Anxiety, 7,* 97–104.

Leary, M. R. (1983a). A brief version of the Fear of Negative Evaluation Scale. *Personality and Social Psychology Bulletin, 9,* 371–375.

Leary, M. R. (1983b). Social anxiousness: The construct and its measurement. *Journal of Personality Assessment, 47,* 66–75.

Leary, M. R., & Kowalski, R. M. (1993). The Interaction Anxiousness Scale: Construct and criterion-related validity. *Journal of Personality Assessment, 61,* 136–146.

Lott, M., Greist, J. H., Jefferson, J. W., Kobak, K. A., Katzelnick, D. J., Katz, R. J., & Schaettle, S. C. (1997). Brofaromine for social phobia: A multicenter, placebo-controlled, double-blind study. *Journal of Clinical Psychopharmacology, 17,* 255–260.

Lyons, A. L., & Spicer, J. (1999). A new measure of conversational experience: The Speaking Extent and Comfort Scale (SPEACS). *Assessment, 6,* 189–202.

Maroldo, G. K., Eisenreich, B. J., & Hall, P. (1979). Reliability of a modified Stanford shyness survey. *Psychological Reports, 44,* 706.

Mattick, R. P., & Peters, L. (1988). Treatment of severe social phobia: Effects of guided exposure with and without cognitive restructuring. *Journal of Consulting and Clinical Psychology, 56,* 251–260.

Mattick, R. P., Peters, L., & Clarke, J. C. (1989). Exposure and cognitive restructuring for severe social phobia: A controlled study. *Behavior Therapy, 20,* 3–23.

Oei, T. P., Kenna, D., & Evans, L. (1991). The reliability, validity, and utility of the SAD and FNE scales for anxiety disorder patients. *Personality and Individual Differences, 12,* 111–116.

Olivares, J., García-López, L. J., Hidalgo, M. D., Turner, S. M., & Beidel, D. C. (1999). The Social Phobia and Anxiety Inventory: Reliability and validity in an adolescent Spanish population. *Journal of Psychopathology and Behavioral Assessment, 21,* 67–78.

Osman, A., Barrios, F. X., Aukes, D., & Osman, J. R. (1995). Psychometric evaluation of the Social Phobia and Anxiety Inventory in college students. *Journal of Clinical Psychology, 51,* 235–243.

Osman, A., Barrios, F. X., Haupt, D., King, K., Osman, J. R., & Slavens, S. (1996). The Social Phobia and Anxiety Inventory: Further validation in two nonclinical samples. *Journal of Psychopathology and Behavioral Assessment, 18*, 35–47.

Osman, A., Gutierrez, P. M., Barrios, F. X., Kopper, B. A., & Chiros, C. E. (1998). The Social Phobia and Social Interaction Anxiety Scales: Evaluation of psychometric properties. *Journal of Psychopathology and Behavioral Assessment, 20*, 249–264.

Osman, A., Markway, K., & Osman, J. R. (1992). Psychometric properties of the Social Interaction Self-Statement Test in a college sample. *Psychological Reports, 71*, 1171–1177.

Paul, G. (1966). *Insight versus desensitization in psychotherapy: An experiment in anxiety reduction.* Palo Alto, CA: Stanford University Press.

Phillips, G. C., Jones, G. E., Rieger, E. J., & Snell, J. B. (1997). Normative data for the Personal Report of Confidence as a Speaker. *Journal of Anxiety Disorders, 11*, 215–220.

Pilkonis, P. A. (1977). Shyness, public and private, and its relationship to other measures of social behavior. *Journal of Personality, 45*, 585–595.

Ries, B. J., McNeil, D. W., Boone, M. L., Turk, C. L., Carter, L. E., & Heimberg, R. G. (1998). Assessment of contemporary social phobia verbal report instruments. *Behaviour Research and Therapy, 36*, 983–994.

Rodebaugh, T. L., Chambless, D. L., Terrill, D. R., Floyd, M., & Uhde, T. (2000). Convergent, discriminant, and criterion-related validity of the Social Phobia and Anxiety Inventory. *Depression and Anxiety, 11*, 10–14.

Ruganci, R. N. (1995). Private and public self-consciousness subscales of the Fenigstein, Scheier, and Buss self-consciousness scale: A Turkish translation. *Personality and Individual Differences, 18*, 279–282.

Safren, S. A., Heimberg, R. G., Horner, K. J., Juster, H. R., Schneier, F. R., & Liebowitz, M. R. (1999). Factor structure of social fears: The Liebowitz Social Anxiety Scale. *Journal of Anxiety Disorders, 13*, 253–270.

Safren, S. A., Turk, C. L., & Heimberg, R. G. (1998). Factor structure of the Social Anxiety Scale and the Social Phobia Scale. *Behaviour Research and Therapy, 36*, 443–453.

Sanz, J. (1994). The Spanish version of the Interaction Anxiousness Scale: Psychometric properties and relationship with depression and cognitive factors. *European Journal of Psychological Assessment, 10*, 129–135.

Sheikh, K., & Kaushik, S. S. (1990). Hindi adaptation of Social Avoidance and Distress Scale. *Journal of Personality and Clinical Studies, 6*, 237–241.

Stein, M. B., Fyer, A. J., Davidson, J. R. T., Pollack, M. H., & Wiita, B. (1999). Fluvoxamine treatment of social phobia (social anxiety disorder): A double-blind, placebo-controlled study. *American Journal of Psychiatry, 156*, 756–760.

Taylor, S., Woody, S., McLean, P. D., & Koch, W. J. (1997). Sensitivity of outcome measures for treatments of generalized social phobia. *Assessment, 4*, 181–191.

Turner, S. M., Beidel, D. C., Cooley, M. R., Woody, S. R., & Messer, S. C. (1994). A multi-component behavioral treatment for social phobia: Social effectiveness therapy. *Behaviour Research and Therapy, 32*, 381–390.

Turner, S. M., Beidel, D. C., Dancu, C. V., & Stanley, M. A. (1989). An empirically derived inventory to measure social fears and anxiety: The Social Phobia and Anxiety Inventory. *Psychological Assessment, 1*, 35–40.

Turner, S. M., Beidel, D. C., & Jacob, R. G. (1994). Social phobia: A comparison of behavior therapy and atenolol. *Journal of Consulting and Clinical Psychology, 62*, 350–358.

Turner, S. M., McCanna, M., & Beidel, D. C. (1987). Validity of the Social Avoidance and Distress and Fear of Negative Evaluation Scales. *Behaviour Research and Therapy, 25*, 113–115.

Turner, S. M., Stanley, M. A., Beidel, D. C., & Bond, L. (1989). The Social Phobia and Anxiety Inventory: Construct validity. *Journal of Psychopathology and Behavioral Assessment, 11*, 221–234.

van Dam-Baggen, R., & Kraaimaat, F. (1999). Assessing social anxiety: The Inventory of Interpersonal Situations. *European Journal of Psychological Assessment, 15*, 25–38.

Winton, E. C., Clark, D. M., & Edelmann, R. J. (1995). Social anxiety, fear of negative evaluation, and the detection of negative emotion in others. *Behaviour Research and Therapy, 33*, 193–196.

Yao, S. N., Cottraux, J., Mollard, E., Albuisson, E., Note, I., Jalencques, I., Fanget, F., Robbe-Grillet, P., Dechassey, M., Ektmedjian, N., Bouvard, M., & Coudert, A. J. (1998). The French version of the Social Interaction Self-Statement Test (SISST): A validation and sensitivity study in social phobics. *Behavioural and Cognitive Psychotherapy, 26*, 247–259.

Yao, S. N., Note, I., Fanget, F., Albuisson, E., Bouvard, M., Jalenques, I., & Cottraux, J. (1999). Social anxiety in social phobics: Validation of Liebowitz's Social Anxiety Scale-French version. *Encephale, 25*, 429–435.

Zimbardo, P. G. (1977). *Shyness: What it is, what to do about it.* Reading, MA: Addison–Wesley.

Zweig, D. R., & Brown, S. D. (1985). Psychometric evaluation of a written stimulus presentation format for the Social Interaction Self-Statement Test. *Cognitive Therapy and Research, 9*, 285–295.

Chapter 14
Generalized Anxiety Disorder: A Brief Overview and Guide to Assessment

Lizabeth Roemer and Eden Medaglia

Generalized anxiety disorder (GAD) is centrally defined in the DSM-IV (American Psychiatric Association, 1994) by excessive worry and anxiety about multiple topics that occurs more days than not for at least 6 months. The worry (and anxiety) is found to be difficult to control, and is associated with three (or more) of the following six symptoms: muscle tension, restlessness/feeling keyed up or on edge, difficulty concentrating/mind going blank, being easily fatigued, irritability, and sleep disturbance.

GAD was initially introduced in DSM-III (American Psychiatric Association, 1980) as a residual category (i.e., only assigned when criteria for other anxiety disorders were not met), but has since undergone numerous empirically based revisions (e.g., Brown, Barlow, & Liebowitz, 1994; Marten et al., 1993). For instance, in DSM-III-R (American Psychiatric Association, 1987), *worry* was identified as the central defining feature of GAD, and a host of associated somatic features were specified. In DSM-IV, the pervasiveness and uncontrollability of worry were emphasized, whereas the unrealistic nature of worry was dropped from the definition. A particularly important change in DSM-IV was a refinement of the associated features, eliminating the autonomic arousal symptoms (e.g., accelerated heart rate, sweaty palms) that tend to be associated with many other anxiety disorders, but are less frequent among individuals with GAD (Marten et al., 1993). In fact, the number of associated features required for the diagnosis was decreased from 6 (out of 18) in DSM-III-R to 3 (out of 6) in DSM-IV.

Lizabeth Roemer and Eden Medaglia • Department of Psychology, University of Massachusetts at Boston, Boston, Massachusetts 02125.

Table 1. Targets of Assessment in GAD

Worry
Beliefs about worry (positive and negative)
Intolerance of uncertainty
Anxiety (cognitive and somatic)
Associated features (e.g., tension, trouble sleeping)
Comorbid symptoms (e.g., social anxiety, panic symptoms, depressive symptoms,
   other phobic anxiety and avoidance, medical conditions, substance use)
Desired goals/values, areas of behavioral inaction
Emotional avoidance

This chapter provides a brief overview of elements thought to be clinically (and diag-
nostically) beneficial in the assessment of GAD, as well as suggested strategies for assessing
these elements. We recommend that these strategies be used prior to and throughout the course
of treatment to assess changes in GAD symptomatology and associated features. Table 1
provides a summary of the features that should be assessed. All instruments mentioned in this
chapter are described elsewhere in this book, along with full citations. Those instruments not
reviewed in the subsequent chapter on measures of GAD (Chapter 15) are described in the
chapter on measures of anxiety and related constructs (Chapter 7).

ASSESSING WORRY AND FACTORS ASSOCIATED WITH ITS MAINTENANCE

Assessment of GAD necessarily begins with assessment of its central defining feature,
worry. Much theoretical and empirical work has been devoted to understanding the nature and
function of worry over the past decade (for thorough reviews, see Borkovec, 1994; Borkovec,
Hazlett-Stevens, & Diaz, 1999; Wells, 1995). Worry is defined as primarily a verbal-linguistic
(as opposed to imaginal) activity focused on the generation of potential future catastrophes
(Borkovec, 1994). As such, worry is closely identified with the cognitive component of
anxiety.

Research and theorizing on the function of worry has highlighted several potential factors
that may maintain worry. First, worry may serve an emotionally avoidant function: Worry is
associated with decreased physiological arousal in response to phobic stimuli (e.g., Borkovec
& Hu, 1990) and may therefore be negatively reinforcing because it reduces uncomfortable
somatic arousal (Borkovec, 1994). However, worry also interferes with habituation of anxious
responding after repeated exposure to phobic stimuli (Borkovec & Hu, 1990). In other words,
worry leads to initial somatic relief, but long-term maintenance of anxious responding.

Other functions of worry have been suggested in studies that identified several positive
beliefs about worry that are commonly endorsed by chronic worriers (e.g., Borkovec et al.,
1999; Cartwright-Hatton & Wells, 1997; Davey, Tallis, & Capuzzo, 1996). Individuals with
GAD often report believing that worry is motivating, prepares them for the worst, facilitates
problem-solving, makes avoidance of catastrophes possible, and effectively distracts them
from other difficulties. Further, individuals with GAD report high levels of intolerance of
uncertainty (Freeston, Rhéaume, Letarte, Dugas, & Ladouceur, 1994). Thus, worry may be
maintained in part because the prediction of potential future (negative) events gives an illusion
of certainty.

Finally, several researchers have pointed out that worry may be maintained in part because attempts to stop worrying paradoxically increase the frequency of this activity. Attempts to control or suppress cognitive activity can be unsuccessful and instead lead to increases in target thoughts (e.g., Roemer & Borkovec, 1993; Wegner, 1994; Wells, 1995), although research findings on the effects of thought suppression have been somewhat inconsistent (for a review, see Purdon, 1999).

Thus, important worry-related elements to assess in GAD include: (1) the occurrence, frequency, controllability, and pervasiveness of worry and (2) factors associated with the maintenance of worry, which may include the emotion/arousal reduction function of worry, positive beliefs about the function of worry, and unsuccessful attempts to control or suppress worry.

Tools for Assessing Worry and Its Maintaining Factors

The Anxiety Disorders Interview Schedule for DSM-IV (Brown, Di Nardo, & Barlow, 1994; Di Nardo, Brown, & Barlow, 1994) and the GAD Questionnaire provide examples of questions for assessing the features of worry. It is important to be aware that although many clients will use the word "worry" to describe their cognitive activity or describe themselves as "worriers," some may use other words such as "concern" or "apprehension" to describe the same activity (e.g., "I find I am often concerned about bad things happening," "I can't stop thinking about possible catastrophes"). Also, it is important to carefully assess the frequency of worry. An individual with GAD may believe so strongly in the functionality of worry that he or she cannot readily see the ways in which the worry is excessive or interferes with functioning. Asking about other people's responses to the individual's level of worry can sometimes help to ascertain whether the worry is in fact excessive. Finally, it is important to assess the topics about which the individual typically worries. Individuals with GAD will often indicate that they worry about "everything." The question "Do you worry excessively about minor things?" has been found to effectively discriminate individuals with GAD from those with other anxiety disorders (Barlow, 1988).

The Penn State Worry Questionnaire is a commonly used self-report measure that assesses intensity (but not content) of pathological worry. In addition, one may want to use the Worry Domains Questionnaire (WDQ) to assess worry topics, although supplementing it with the Anxious Thoughts Inventory (see Chapter 7) may be advised because the WDQ does not include assessment of health-related worries. A worry scale has also been developed specifically for older adults (Wisocki, 1988).

In addition, several self-monitoring forms for worry have been developed, which are useful both for initial assessment, and particularly as an awareness/intervention tool throughout treatment. Craske, Barlow, and O'Leary (1992) describe a Worry Record in which clients record the intensity and topic of worry, associated symptoms, an event description, and a thought record each time their anxiety increases. Borkovec and Roemer (1994) describe the use of a daily diary in which level of anxiety is recorded four times throughout the day, with descriptions of events for times of high anxiety. Finally, Borkovec and colleagues (1999) describe the use of a Worry Outcome Diary in which clients record specific negative predictions weekly and then go back to assess whether the outcome was as negative as they had predicted and how well they coped with it.

Potential maintaining factors for worry should ideally be assessed during a clinical interview to identify the idiosyncratic function of an individual's worries. In addition, several self-report measures have been developed to assess factors that may be relevant. Positive beliefs about worry are assessed in the Why Worry Questionnaire, Consequences of Worrying Scale, and Meta-Cognitions Questionnaire (see Chapter 7). Attempts to control worry or other negative thoughts, along with general negative beliefs about worry and other negative thoughts (which are likely to motivate attempts to control worry) are assessed in several measures, primarily found in Chapter 7: the Meta-Cognitions Questionnaire, Thought Control Questionnaire, White Bear Suppression Inventory, Anxious Thoughts Inventory, Acceptance and Action Questionnaire, and Consequences of Worrying Scale (in Chapter 15). Finally, a scale for assessing level of intolerance of uncertainty has also been developed (Chapter 15; Freeston et al., 1994).

ASSESSING GENERAL ANXIETY

In addition to assessing worry and the factors that maintain it, assessment of GAD typically includes an assessment of general anxiety severity. In choosing a measure for assessing anxiety in conjunction with GAD, it is important to keep in mind that measures heavily loaded with arousal symptoms of anxiety (e.g., the Beck Anxiety Inventory) are unlikely to provide an accurate assessment of anxiety levels in these individuals. As noted earlier, GAD is not frequently associated with symptoms such as accelerated heart rate and trembling or shaking. Instead it is associated with symptoms such as muscle tension or feeling keyed up or on edge. In addition, given that GAD is highly comorbid with major depression, measures that are confounded with depression (e.g., the State–Trait Anxiety Inventory) may not be ideal. On the other hand, measures such as the Depression Anxiety Stress Scales, with a separate stress/tension component (which has been found to be significantly higher among individuals with GAD versus other anxiety disorders except OCD; Brown, Chorpita, Korotitsch, & Barlow, 1997), and measures that specifically assess the cognitive as well as the somatic aspect of anxiety (e.g., the Trimodal Anxiety Questionnaire) may be particularly useful for the assessment of anxiety among individuals diagnosed with GAD. In addition, the Hamilton Anxiety Rating Scale and the Clinical Anxiety Scale (both reprinted in Appendix B) contain interview questions that specifically assess the associated symptoms of GAD (e.g., restlessness, muscle tension).

ASSESSING COMORBID CONDITIONS AND DIFFERENTIAL DIAGNOSIS

GAD is associated with high levels of comorbidity (Brown & Barlow, 1992). Also, because worry (anxious apprehension) is common across the anxiety disorders (Barlow, in press), differential diagnosis is often a challenge. Thus, assessment of an individual who presents with symptoms of GAD must include assessment of other anxious and depressive symptoms to ensure that both primary and secondary treatment targets are accurately identified.

In terms of differential diagnosis with other anxiety disorders, a diagnosis of GAD requires excessive worry focused on several topics, which are not confined to the features of other Axis I disorders (e.g., phobic situations associated with other anxiety disorders). Thus, an individual with GAD may report excessive worry about performance in social situations (similar to individuals with social phobia), but would also report excessive worry about other topics such as health or finances. Differential diagnosis with depression is also challenging because the two share overlapping features: high levels of negative affect and cognitive rumination. Careful history taking is advised and a GAD diagnosis is appropriate if symptoms of GAD (e.g., excessive worry) occur in the absence of depressive episodes and if the onset of GAD precedes the onset of major depression (Borkovec & Roemer, 1994).

Similar to the relationship between GAD and other anxiety disorders, if worries are solely about health-related concerns, a diagnosis of hypochondriasis should be considered. In addition, GAD-like symptoms may be directly caused by the presence of a real medical condition such as hyperthyroidism. Before assigning a diagnosis of GAD in such cases, it must be established that the symptoms of GAD preceded the onset of the medical condition or that the GAD symptoms persisted even after the medical condition was appropriately treated. Otherwise, a diagnosis of anxiety disorder due to a general medical condition might be appropriate.

Even after an appropriate diagnosis of GAD has been made following these considerations, assessment of comorbid symptoms remains important. GAD is often associated with comorbid diagnoses of social phobia, panic disorder, and major depressive disorder (Brown & Barlow, 1992); therefore, assessment of social anxiety, occurrence of panic attacks, and depressive symptoms is highly recommended (for descriptions of measures, see Chapters 9 and 13, this volume, and the depression volume by Nezu, Ronan, Meadows, & McClure, 2000). Also, research and theory suggest that anxiety often leads to depression (e.g., see Alloy, Kelly, Mineka, & Clements, 1990) so that continued assessment of depressive symptoms throughout treatment is advised. As with all disorders, medical complaints and substance use should also be assessed.

NATURE OF AVOIDANCE IN GAD

A major difference between GAD and the other anxiety disorders is the absence of clear phobic avoidance in this disorder. Individuals diagnosed with GAD commonly engage in daily activities without any obvious avoidance of feared situations. However, GAD is associated with high levels of procrastination (Borkovec et al., 1999), and it may be that excessive worry and catastrophizing constricts behavior in ways that are less obvious (Roemer & Orsillo, in press). For instance, individuals with GAD may avoid engaging in pleasurable activities due to beliefs that failure to work and to worry continuously will lead to negative outcomes. Similarly, individuals with GAD may avoid pursuing certain goals such as career advancement or social connectedness, for fear of imagined negative outcomes in these arenas. Thus, comprehensive assessment of GAD may be enhanced by identification of desired or valued goals and activities, coupled with assessment of factors that interfere with accomplishment of those goals, so as to identify salient areas of behavioral inaction (e.g., Hayes, Strosahl, & Wilson, 1999).

Finally, as noted earlier, GAD seems to be characterized by emotional avoidance. Worry is proposed to be negatively reinforced by the reduction of somatic arousal (Borkovec, 1994) and individuals who report having GAD symptoms also report worrying to distract themselves from more distressing topics (Borkovec & Roemer, 1995). Thus, assessment of the tendency to avoid emotional arousal, for instance with the Acceptance and Action Questionnaire or Affective Control Scale (see Chapter 7), may also be beneficial. A clinical interview may help identify the idiosyncratic nature of an individual's tendency to avoid intense emotional states. Because GAD is associated with difficulty relaxing (e.g., feeling keyed up or on edge, muscle tension), it is important to assess avoidance of both negative and positive emotions. Individuals with GAD may avoid pleasant, relaxing states for fear that such states leave them unprepared for potential future catastrophes.

OTHER CONSIDERATIONS

In addition to the considerations reviewed earlier and summarized in Table 1, clinicians should also attend to cultural and developmental issues in their assessment of individuals with GAD. Friedman (this volume) reviews general cultural considerations in assessing anxiety; unfortunately, very little cultural research has addressed GAD in particular. Beck and Stanley (this volume) provide an overview of particular issues in assessing anxiety among older adults; Stanley and Averill (1999) provide a more extensive discussion specific to GAD among older adults. Finally, other resources address the nature of worry and GAD in children (Silverman & Ginsburg, 1995; Vasey & Daleiden, 1994).

REFERENCES

Alloy, L. B., Kelly, K. A., Mineka, S., & Clements, C. M. (1990). Comorbidity of anxiety and depressive disorders: A helplessness–hopelessness perspective. In J. D. Maser & C. R Cloninger (Eds.). *Comorbidity of mood and anxiety disorders* (pp. 499–544). Washington,. DC: American Psychiatric Press.

American Psychiatric Association. (1980). *Diagnostic and statistical manual of mental disorders* (3rd. ed.). Washington, DC: Author.

American Psychiatric Association. (1987). *Diagnostic and statistical manual of mental disorders* (3rd ed., rev.). Washington, DC: Author.

American Psychiatric Association. (1994). *Diagnostic and statistical manual of mental disorders* (4th ed.). Washington, DC: Author.

Barlow, D. H. (1988). *Anxiety and its disorders: The nature and treatment of anxiety and panic.* New York: Guilford.

Barlow, D. H. (in press). *Anxiety and its disorders: The nature and treatment of anxiety and panic* (2nd ed.). New York: Guilford.

Borkovec, T. D. (1994). The nature, functions, and origins of worry. In G. C. L. Davey & F. Tallis (Eds.), *Worrying: Perspectives on theory, assessment, and treatment* (pp. 5–34). New York: Wiley.

Borkovec, T. D., Hazlett-Stevens, H., & Diaz, M. L. (1999). The role of positive beliefs about worry in generalized anxiety disorder and its treatment. *Clinical Psychology and Psychotherapy, 6,* 126–138.

Borkovec, T. D., & Hu, S. (1990). The effect of worry on cardiovascular response to phobic imagery. *Behaviour Research and Therapy, 28,* 69–73.

Borkovec, T. D., & Roemer, L. (1994). Generalized anxiety disorder. In R. T. Ammerman & M. Hersen (Eds.), *Handbook of prescriptive treatments for adults* (pp. 261–281). New York: Plenum Press.

Borkovec, T. D., & Roemer, L. (1995). Perceived functions of worry among generalized anxiety disorder subjects: Distraction from more emotionally distressing topics? *Journal of Behavioral Therapy and Experimental Psychiatry, 26,* 25–30.

Brown, T. A., & Barlow, D. H. (1992). Comorbidity among anxiety disorders: Implications for treatment and DSM-IV. *Journal of Consulting and Clinical Psychology, 60,* 835–844.

Brown, T. A., Barlow, D. H., & Liebowitz, M. R. (1994). The empirical basis of generalized anxiety disorder. *American Journal of Psychiatry, 151,* 1272–1280.

Brown, T. A., Chorpita, B. F., Korotitsch, W., & Barlow, D. H. (1997). Psychometric properties of the Depression Anxiety Stress Scales (DASS) in clinical samples. *Behaviour Research and Therapy, 35,* 79–89.

Brown, T. A., Di Nardo, P., & Barlow, D. H. (1994). *Anxiety Disorders Interview Schedule for DSM-IV.* San Antonio, TX: The Psychological Corporation.

Cartwright-Hatton, S., & Wells, A. (1997). Beliefs about worry and intrusions: The Meta-Cognitions Questionnaire and its correlates. *Journal of Anxiety Disorders, 11,* 279–296.

Craske, M. G., Barlow, D. H., & O'Leary, T. (1992). *Mastery of your anxiety and worry.* San Antonio, TX: The Psychological Corporation.

Davey, G. C. L., Tallis, F., & Capuzzo, N. (1996). Beliefs about the consequences of worrying. *Cognitive Therapy and Research*, *20*, 499–520.

Di Nardo, P., Brown, T. A., & Barlow, D. H. (1994). *Anxiety Disorders Interview Schedule for DSM-IV (Lifetime Version)*. San Antonio, TX: The Psychological Corporation.

Freeston, M. H., Rhéaume, J., Letarte, H., Dugas, M. J., & Ladouceur, R. (1994). Why do people worry? *Personality and Individual Differences*, *17*, 791–802.

Hayes, S. C., Strosahl, K. D., & Wilson, K. G. (1999). *Acceptance and commitment therapy: An experiential approach to behavior change*. New York: Guilford.

Marten, P. A., Brown, T. A., Barlow, D. H., Borkovec, T. D., Shear, K. M., & Lydiard, R. B. (1993). Evaluation of the ratings comprising the associated symptom criterion of DSM-III-R Generalized Anxiety Disorder. *Journal of Nervous and Mental Disease*, *181*, 676–682.

Nezu, A. M., Ronan, G. F., Meadows, E. A., & McClure, K. S. (2000). *Practitioner's guide to empirically based measures of depression*. New York: Kluwer Academic/Plenum Publishers.

Purdon, C. (1999). Thought suppression and psychopathology. *Behaviour Research and Therapy*, *37*, 1029–1054.

Roemer, L., & Borkovec, T. D. (1993). Worry: Unwanted cognitive experience that controls unwanted somatic experience. In D. M. Wegner & J. Pennebaker (Eds.), *Handbook of mental control* (pp. 220–238). Englewood Cliffs, NJ: Prentice–Hall.

Roemer, L., & Orsillo, S. M. (in press). Expanding our conceptualization of and treatment for generalized anxiety disorder: Integrating mindfulness/acceptance-based approaches with existing cognitive-behavioral models. *Clinical Psychology: Science and Practice*.

Roemer, L., Orsillo, S. M., & Barlow, D. H. (in press). Generalized Anxiety Disorder. In D. H. Barlow, *Anxiety and its disorders: The nature and treatment of anxiety and panic* (2nd ed.). New York: Guilford.

Silverman, W. K., & Ginsburg, G. S. (1995). Specific phobia and generalized anxiety disorder. In J. S. March (Ed.) *Anxiety disorders in children and adolescents* (pp. 151–180). New York: Guilford.

Stanley, M. A., & Averill, P. M. (1999). Strategies for treating generalized anxiety in the elderly. In M. Duffy et al. (Eds.), *Handbook of counseling and psychotherapy with older adults.* (pp. 511–525). New York: Wiley.

Vasey, M. W., & Daleiden, E. L. (1994). Worry in children. In G. Davey & F. Tallis (Eds.), *Worrying: Perspectives on theory, assessment and treatment* (pp. 185–207). New York: Wiley.

Wegner, D. M. (1994). Ironic processes of mental control. *Psychological Review*, *101*, 34–52.

Wells, A. (1995). Meta-cognition and worry: A cognitive model of generalized anxiety disorder. *Behavioural and Cognitive Psychotherapy*, *23*, 301–320.

Wisocki, P. A. (1988). Worry as a phenomenon relevant to the elderly. *Behavior Therapy*, *19*, 369–379.

Chapter 15
Measures for Generalized Anxiety Disorder

Lizabeth Roemer

CONSEQUENCES OF WORRYING SCALE (COWS)

Original Citation

Davey, G. C. L., Tallis, F., & Capuzzo, N. (1996). Beliefs about the Consequences of Worrying. *Cognitive Therapy and Research, 20*, 499–520.

Purpose

To measure the degree to which individuals hold various beliefs about the consequences of worry.

Description

The COWS is a relatively recent, 29-item, factor analytically derived, self-report questionnaire that assesses the degree to which individuals believe a range of consequences apply to their worry. It contains three negative consequences subscales (disrupting performance, exaggerating the problem, and causing emotional distress) as well as two positive consequences subscales (motivational influence and helping analytical thinking). Each item presents a possible consequence of worry and is followed by a five-point Likert-type response

Lizabeth Roemer • Department of Psychology, University of Massachusetts at Boston, Boston, Massachusetts 02125.

scale representing how much that consequence describes the individual when he or she worries.

Administration and Scoring

The COWS can be administered in 5 to 10 minutes. A score for each subscale is obtained by summing responses to items comprising that scale. The *disrupting performance* subscale is comprised of items 1, 4–6, 12, 16, 23, 27; the *exaggerating the problem* subscale is comprised of items 11, 15, 18, 20, 26; the *causes emotional distress* subscale is comprised of items 7, 10, 14, 19; the *motivates* scale consists of items 8, 9, 13, 22, 24, 29; the *helps analytical thinking* subscale consists of items 2, 3, 17, 21, 25, 28. *Total negative consequences* and *total positive consequences* scores can be derived by summing the subscales within each factor (listed in the description).

Psychometric Properties

All psychometric data for the COWS to date have been derived from an unselected undergraduate sample (Davey et al., 1996).

Sample Means and Norms. No published norms are available.

Reliability. All scales have good to acceptable internal consistency (αs ranging from .72 to .87). Internal consistency of the larger factors (negative and positive consequences) is indicated by significant correlation among the subscales within each factor (rs ranging from .71 to .82). Test–retest reliability has not been reported.

Validity. Convergent validity for the COWS is suggested by the finding of significant moderate correlations between all three negative consequences subscales and several measures of psychopathology, e.g., the State–Trait Anxiety Inventory (rs between .55 and .58), Penn State Worry Questionnaire (rs between .44 and .57), Worry Domains Questionnaire (rs between .46 and .50), and Beck Depression Inventory (rs between .46 and .50). Further support for the utility of both the negative and positive subscales is evident from the finding that high scores on both higher-order factor scales were associated with significantly greater levels of pathological worry as assessed by the PSWQ. The scale has yet to be validated on a clinical sample.

Source

The COWS is reprinted in the original article and in Appendix B. For more information, contact Graham C. L. Davey, Ph.D., Professor of Psychology, School of Cognitive and Computing Sciences, University of Sussex, Falmer, Brighton, BN1 9RH, United Kingdom; (tel): 44 1273 678485; (fax) 44 1273 671320; (e-mail) grahamda@cogs.susx.ac.uk.

GENERALIZED ANXIETY DISORDER QUESTIONNAIRE (GADQ) AND GENERALIZED ANXIETY DISORDER QUESTIONNAIRE–IV (GADQ-IV)

Original Citations

GADQ: Roemer, L., Borkovec, M., Posa, S., & Borkovec, T. D. (1995). A self-report diagnostic measure of generalized anxiety disorder. *Journal of Behavior Therapy and Experimental Psychiatry, 26*, 345–350.

GADQ-IV: Newman, M. G., Zuellig, A. R., Kachin, K. E., & Constantino, M. J. (2001). *The reliability and validity of the GAD-Q-IV: A revised self-report measure of generalized anxiety disorder.* Manuscript submitted for publication.

Purpose

To provide a self-report diagnostic assessment of GAD.

Description

The original GADQ was a 10-item self-report measure that was designed to assess DSM-III-R criteria for GAD. Although this measure demonstrated adequate validity (Roemer et al., 1995), it is based on outdated diagnostic criteria. A revised version, the GADQ-IV, has recently been developed (Newman et al., 2001) and initial, unpublished data suggest it is a promising screening device for GAD. Items on this scale correspond to DSM-IV criteria for GAD. Thus, they assess presence of worry, its excessiveness and uncontrollability, duration, presence of six associated symptoms, as well as degree of interference and distress associated with worry on nine-point Likert-type response scales. Participants are also asked to list the topics they worry about.

Administration and Scoring

The GADQ-IV can be administered in three to four minutes. It can be scored as a continuous measure or as a dichotomous diagnostic tool. To use it as a continuous measure, for items 1–4, and 6, all positive responses are coded as 1 whereas all negative responses are coded as 0. For item 5, the total number of individual worries listed is tallied. For item 7, the total number of checked items is tallied. Items 8 and 9 are scored as the number that was circled. All values are summed to calculate a total score. The maximum possible score is 33. In order to meet diagnostic criteria for GAD, the individual must answer yes to items 1–3, and 6; must indicate three or more worry topics on item 5; must report three or more symptoms in response to item 7, and must score 4 or more on item 8 or 9.

Psychometric Properties

The psychometric properties reported here are taken from an unpublished manuscript (Newman et al., 2001).

Sample Means and Norms. Newman et al. (2001) reported a mean total score of 19.93 (SD = 7.84) in a sample of individuals with GAD diagnosed by a semistructured interview compared with a mean of 2.34 (SD = 4.69) among nonanxious controls. In an unselected college sample, the mean was 5.27 (SD = 6.87).

Reliability. The GADQ-IV has demonstrated good internal consistency (α = .84) and good 2-week test–retest reliability (r = .81) in a college sample.

Validity. Both convergent and discriminant validity have been demonstrated for the GADQ-IV in the finding of strong correlations with the Penn State Worry Questionnaire (r = .63) and a measure of trait anxiety (r = .58) but more modest correlations with measures of depression (r = .23) or dysfunctional attitudes (r = −.24) in a college sample. Most importantly, the GADQ-IV's validity is supported by comparisons between GADQ-IV diagnoses and clinician-administered Anxiety Disorder Interview Schedule (ADIS-IV) diagnoses in a sample of treatment-seeking individuals diagnosed with GAD, social phobia, or panic disorder, and a nonanxious comparison group. The GADQ-IV showed a specificity of 97% and a sensitivity of 69%. Diagnoses made by GADQ-IV yielded a 17% false positive rate and a 7.6% false negative rate. The degree of concordance between GADQ-IV and ADIS-IV diagnoses (κ = .70) was higher than that reported between independent assessors for this disorder (Barlow & DiNardo, 1991). Overall predictive power of the questionnaire was 91%. Validity of the use of a continuous score for the GADQ-IV was supported by the finding that individuals diagnosed with GAD by ADIS-IV interview scored significantly higher on the GADQ-IV than those diagnosed with either social phobia or panic disorder, as well as nonanxious controls.

Alternative Forms

A French self-report diagnostic measure for GAD, the Worry and Anxiety Questionnaire, has been developed by another group of researchers (Dugas, Freeston, Lachance, Provencher, & Ladouceur, 1995).

Source

The GADQ-IV is reprinted in Appendix B. For more information, contact Michelle G. Newman, Ph.D., Department of Psychology, 310 Moore Building, Penn State University, University Park, PA 16802, USA; (tel) 814-863-1148; (fax) 814-865-7002; (e-mail) mgn1@psu.edu.

INTOLERANCE OF UNCERTAINTY SCALE (IUS)

Original Citation

Freeston, M. H., Rhéaume, J., Letarte, H., Dugas, M. J., & Ladouceur, R. (1994). Why do people worry? *Personality and Individual Differences, 17,* 791-802.

Purpose

To assess the degree to which an individual has difficulty tolerating uncertainty, a factor associated with GAD.

Description

The IUS is a 27-item measure designed to assess several aspects of intolerance of uncertainty: the emotional and behavioral consequences of being uncertain, how being uncertain reflects on a person's character, the expectation that the future will be predictable, frustration when it is not, attempts to control the future, and all-or-nothing responses in uncertain situations (Freeston et al., 1994). Difficulty tolerating uncertainty has been theoretically and empirically linked to GAD. The scale was initially developed in French but an English version has also been validated. Items consist of statements that describe how people may react to the uncertainties of life and respondents indicate on a five point Likert-type scale how characteristic each statement is of them.

Administration and Scoring

The IUS can be administered in 3 to 4 minutes. It is scored by summing all responses. Possible scores range from 27 to 135.

Psychometric Properties

Sample Means and Norms.   Ladouceur et al. (2000) reported a mean score of 87.08 (SD = 21.08) for a sample of individuals diagnosed with GAD by semistructured interview, whereas Freeston et al. (1994) reported a mean of 43.8 (SD = 10.8) for a nonanxious college sample.

Reliability.   The IUS demonstrates excellent internal consistency for both the French (α = .91; Freeston et al., 1994) and English (α = .95; Buhr & Dugas, 2000) versions in college student samples. It also demonstrates adequate 5-week test–retest reliability for the French (r = .78; Dugas, Freeston, & Ladouceur, 1997) and English (r = .74; Buhr & Dugas, 2000) versions in college samples.

Validity.   Freeston et al. (1994) demonstrated convergent validity for the IUS in that it was significantly correlated with measures of worry (rs = .57 and .63) and of trait anxiety (r = .57). The significant relationship with worry remained even when degree of anxiety and depression was partialled out, supporting the specificity of the measure. A similar specific relationship has been found with the English version of the scale (Buhr & Dugas, 2000). In addition, the IUS has been found to significantly discriminate a GAD clinical sample from nonanxious controls (Dugas, Gagnon, Ladouceur, & Freeston, 1998). Finally, IUS scores were significantly reduced following cognitive–behavioral treatment of GAD patients and these reductions were maintained at follow-up (Ladouceur et al., 2000).

Source

The IUS is reprinted in Appendix B. For information regarding the English version, contact Michel Dugas, Ph.D., Department of Psychology, Concordia University, 7141 Sherbrooke St., West Montreal, Quebec, H4B 1R6, Canada; (tel) 514-848-2215; (fax) 514-848-4523; (e-mail) dugas@vax2.concordia.ca.

PENN STATE WORRY QUESTIONNAIRE (PSWQ)

Original Citation

Meyer, T. J., Miller, M. L., Metzger, R. L., & Borkovec, T. D. (1990). Development and validation of the Penn State Worry Questionnaire. *Behaviour Research and Therapy*, *28*, 487–495.

Purpose

To measure trait worry.

Description

The PSWQ is a widely used 16-item self-report questionnaire that assesses an individual's general tendency to worry excessively. It was designed specifically to assess the intensity and excessiveness of worry without reference to specific content of the worries. Each item presents a statement and is followed by a five-point Likert-type response scale representing how typical the individual feels the statement is of him or her.

Administration and Scoring

The PSWQ can be administered in 3 minutes. Scoring consists of reverse-scoring items 1, 3, 8, 10, and 11 and then summing all 16 items. Possible scores range from 16 to 80, with higher scores reflecting higher levels of worry.

Psychometric Properties

Sample Means and Norms.   The following means (and standard deviations) have been reported in the literature (Molina & Borkovec, 1994): GAD patients—67.66 (SD = 8.86); nonanxious selected groups—44.27 (SD = 11.44); unselected groups—47.65 (SD = 12.99). In a normative community sample matched to the U.S. national census, a score of 41 fell at the 50th percentile, whereas a score of 51 fell at the 80th percentile (Gillis, Haaga & Ford, 1995). A study of older adults revealed a slightly lower mean for GAD clients—59.9 (SD = 11.5; Beck, Stanley, & Zebb, 1995).

Reliability.   The PSWQ is associated with good to very good internal consistency (αs ranging from .86 to .93 across clinical and college samples; Molina & Borkovec, 1994). In addition, adequate to good test–retest reliability has been demonstrated in college samples (rs ranging from .74 to .93 across periods ranging from 2 to 10 weeks; Molina & Borkovec, 1994).

Validity. As expected, the PSWQ is moderately correlated with two other worry measures, the Student Worry Scale ($r = .59$) and the Worry Domains Questionnaire ($r = .67$; Davey, 1993). These latter scales assess content-specific normal worry and thus are associated with both constructive and pathological worry, whereas the PSWQ is only associated with the latter. Among student samples, the PSWQ is moderately correlated with measures of anxiety (rs range from .40 to .74) and less strongly correlated with depression ($r = .36$), but within GAD samples, these relationships are weaker, suggesting that worry is a distinct construct among a clinically anxious sample (Molina & Borkovec, 1994). The construct validity of the scale is further supported by the finding of a stronger association between the PSWQ and the cognitive scale of the Cognitive Somatic Anxiety Questionnaire ($r = .70$) than between the PSWQ and the somatic scale ($r = .55$; Meyer, Miller, Metzger, & Borkovec, 1990). Perhaps most relevant to its clinical use, PSWQ scores have been found to be significantly higher among individuals with GAD than among any other anxiety disorder group (Brown, Antony, & Barlow, 1992). Finally, PSWQ scores have been shown to be sensitive to change in that they are significantly reduced following cognitive–behavioral treatment for GAD (Borkovec & Costello, 1993).

Alternative Forms

The PSWQ has been translated into Chinese, Dutch, French, German, Greek, Italian, Spanish, and Thai. A child and adolescent version has been developed (Chorpita, Tracey, Brown, Collica, & Barlow, 1997), as has a weekly assessment version that allows for measurement of change across brief time periods (Stöber & Bittencourt, 1998).

Source

The PSWQ is reprinted in the original article and in Appendix B. For more information, contact T. D. Borkovec, Ph.D., Department of Psychology, Penn State University, University Park, PA 16802, USA; (tel) 814-863-1725; (fax) 814)-865-7002; (e-mail) tdb@psu.edu.

WHY WORRY SCALE (WW AND WW-II)

Original Citation

Freeston, M. H., Rhéaume, J., Letarte, H., Dugas, M. J., & Ladouceur, R. (1994). Why do people worry? *Personality and Individual Differences, 17,* 791-802.

Purpose

To measure the reasons people worry.

Description

The original Why Worry Scale was a 20-item self-report measure of the reasons that individuals engage in worry (i.e., perceived positive consequences of worry). The scale has recently been revised (the Why Worry-II) to reflect more recent research on the cognitions that underlie worry. The new scale consists of 25 items, five in each of the following subscales: worry aids in problem-solving, worry helps to motivate, worrying protects the individual from negative emotions in the event of a negative outcome, the act of worrying itself prevents negative outcomes, and worry is a positive personality trait. For both scales, respondents indicate how characteristic each statement is of them on a five-point Likert-type scale.

Administration and Scoring

The WW and WW-II each take 3 to 4 minutes to administer. The WW is scored by summing responses to all items, and a total score can similarly be obtained for the WW-II. In addition, subscale scores can be calculated for the WW-II by summing the responses to items within each subscale: *aids in problem-solving*—items 3, 5, 9, 14, 21; *motivates*—items 8, 15, 16, 18, 19; *protects from negative emotions in the event of a negative outcome*—items 2, 4, 13, 22, 23; *prevents negative outcomes*—items 6, 11, 17, 20, 24; and *positive personality trait*—items 1, 7, 10, 12, 25.

Psychometric Properties

Psychometric data for the WW are taken from the original article and two subsequent studies, all of which used the French version of the scale in a college sample. The data for the WW-II are taken from a very recent study, also in a college sample, using the English version, which has not yet been published.

Sample Means and Norms.   Freeston et al. (1994) reported a mean of 32.8 (SD = 7.9) for a nonanxious college sample and a mean of 43.3 (SD = 7.9) for a group of students diagnosed GAD by self-report questionnaire. Ladouceur, Blais, Freeston, and Dugas (1998) reported a mean of 46.9 (SD = 22.5) for a group of individuals who met diagnostic criteria for GAD by structured clinical interview. No norms have been reported for the WW-II.

Reliability.   Freeston et al. (1994) report good internal consistency for the WW (α = .87). Holowka, Dugas, Francis, and Laugesen (2000) report excellent internal consistency for the total WW-II (α = .93) and adequate to good internal consistency for the five subscales (αs .71 to .84). Test–retest reliability has not been reported for either scale.

Validity.   Both scales have demonstrated convergent validity in the form of significant correlations with the PSWQ that remain even when controlling for trait levels of depression and anxiety. In addition, the WW-II is significantly more highly correlated with the positive consequences subscale of the COWS (which assesses the same construct, r = .65) than it is with measures of worry, depression, or anxiety. Freeston et al. (1994) found that students diagnosed with GAD by self-report displayed significantly higher scores on the WW than did participants who only reported somatic anxiety symptoms, whereas the latter group reported significantly higher scores than did a nonanxious group. Similarly, individuals diagnosed with

GAD by clinical interview or by self-report reported higher total WW scores than did those who did not meet criteria for GAD (Ladouceur et al., 1998) and WW scores discriminated a group of individuals diagnosed with GAD from a nonclinical sample (Dugas et al., 1998). The WW-II has not yet been investigated in a clinical sample and confirmation of its factor structure is currently under investigation.

Alternative Forms

Both scales are available in French and English. An alternative version of the WW-II is also available in a structured interview format (Structured Interview on Beliefs about Worry) and is currently under further psychometric investigation (Dr. Dugas can also be contacted for more information about this scale).

Source

The WW-II is reprinted in Appendix B. For more information about the WW, contact Mark Freeston, Ph.D., Head of Research and Training, Newcastle Cognitive and Behavioural Therapies Centre, Plummer Court, Carliol Place, Newcastle, NE1 6UR, United Kingdom; (tel) 44 191 219 6284; (fax) 44 191 219 6282. For information regarding the English version of the WW-II, contact Michel Dugas, Ph.D., Department of Psychology, Concordia University, 7141 Sherbrooke St., West Montreal, Quebec, H4B 1R6; Canada; (tel) 514-848-2215; (fax) 514-848-4523; (e-mail) dugas@vax2.concordia.ca.

WORRY DOMAINS QUESTIONNAIRE (WDQ)

Original Citation

Tallis, F., Eysenck, M., & Mathews, A. (1992). A questionnaire for the measurement of nonpathological worry. *Personality and Individual Differences*, *13*, 161–168.

Purpose

To measure nonpathological worry.

Description

The WDQ is a 25-item self-report questionnaire that assesses the degree to which an individual worries about five specific domains: relationships, lack of confidence, aimless future, work, and financial. The measure was designed to assess content-specific worry in a normative population. Items were acquired from a large community sample and cluster analyses were performed on ratings from a second sample so as to identify worry domains. Each item presents a particular worry topic and is followed by a five-point Likert-type response scale representing how much the individual worries about the topic.

Administration and Scoring

The WDQ can be completed in 4 minutes. Each item is given a score of 0 for a response of "not at all," 1 for a response of "a little," and so on. A total score is calculated by adding each item score. In addition, separate domain scores are calculated by totaling the items that comprise each domain: *relationships*—4, 16, 19, 21, 23; *lack of confidence*—2, 10, 15, 18, 20; *aimless future*—3, 5, 8, 13, 22; *work*—6, 14, 17, 24, 25; and *financial*—1, 7, 9, 11, 12.

PSYCHOMETRIC PROPERTIES

Sample Means and Norms. An overall mean of 40.03 (*SD* = 19.8) has been reported for a small sample of individuals with GAD (Tallis, Davey, & Bond, 1994). An overall mean of 26.6 (*SD* = 13.0) is reported for a student sample, and 23.1 (*SD* = 13.4) is the reported mean for a working sample.

Reliability. The WDQ is associated with excellent overall internal consistency (α = .91) and adequate to good internal consistency for the subscales (αs ranging from .72 to .88) in nonclinical samples (Stöber, 1998). In addition, good test–retest reliability has been demonstrated in college samples for overall scores and for four of the five subscales (all *rs* > .80, except for Work, *r* = .71; Stöber, 1998).

Validity. As expected, the WDQ is moderately correlated with two other worry measures, the Student Worry Scale (*r* = .68) and the Worry Domains Questionnaire (*r* = .67; Davey, 1993). Unlike the PSWQ, the WDQ is associated with constructive, as well as pathological, worry. Convergent validity is demonstrated by the finding of moderate correlations between self- and peer-report versions of the WDQ (*r* = .49; Stöber, 1998). Studies have found the WDQ to be significantly correlated with trait anxiety (*r* = .71). In addition, the WDQ shows a significant relationship with both active cognitive coping (*r* = .26) and avoidance coping (*r* = .30) that is independent of trait anxiety. Thus, as noted above, the scale assesses both negative and positive aspects of worry (Tallis et al., 1994). Studies exploring the factor structure of the WDQ have yielded inconsistent findings. One supported the validity of the five factors (Joorman & Stöber, 1997), whereas a second suggested that some items on the scale are misplaced and that a health worry domain should be added (van Rijsoort, Emmelkamp, & Vervaeke, 1999). In fact, both sets of authors comment that health concerns are overlooked in the WDQ, perhaps because health worries are less characteristic of normal than pathological worry. van Rijsoort and colleagues provide a revised version of the WDQ that adds this domain. A health worry subscale is also included in the Anxious Thoughts Inventory described elsewhere in this volume. The authors of the WDQ suggest including it in clinical assessment to determine areas of worry to target in treatment, but suggest including the PSWQ as a measure of general pathological worry as well (Tallis et al., 1994).

Alternative Forms

The WDQ has been translated into French. As noted above, a revised version is available in which a health worry domain is added and some items are reclassified (van Rijsoort et al., 1999).

Source

The WDQ is reprinted in the original paper by Tallis et al. (1994) and in Appendix B.

WORRY SCALE FOR OLDER ADULTS (WS)

Original Citation

Wisocki, P. A. (1988). Worry as a phenomenon relevant to the elderly. *Behavior Therapy*, *19*, 369–379.

Purpose

To measure the extent to which older adults worry about events commonly associated with aging, as well as the frequency of those worries.

Description

The WS is a 35-item self-report questionnaire that assesses an individual's degree of worry in three content areas: social, financial, and health. It was designed specifically to assess the extent of worry among older adults. Each item lists a potential topic of worry and is followed by a five-point Likert-type response scale representing how frequently the individual worries about this topic (ranging from "never" to "much of the time [more than 2 times a day])."

Administration and Scoring

The WS can be administered in 5 to 10 minutes. Each item is given a score of 0 for "never," 1 for "rarely," and so on, and scores are summed to obtain a total score. Subscale totals are calculated by summing items in each subscale (*finances*: 1–5; *health*: 6–22; *social conditions*: 23–35). Possible total scores range from 0 to 140, with higher scores reflecting more frequent worry.

Psychometric properties

Sample Means and Norms. The following means (and standard deviations) have been reported in the literature (Stanley, Beck, & Zebb, 1996): for individuals with GAD, total score—35.4 (SD = 20.9), social—13.2 (SD = 9.5), finances—4.1 (SD = 3.6), health—18.3 (SD = 10.5); for nonanxious controls, total score—11.0 (SD =10.4), social—4.0 (SD = 4.3), finances—1.1 (SD = 1.7), health—6.0 (SD = 5.8). Unselected community samples of active older adults have yielded total mean scores ranging from 10.4 to 17.4, whereas samples of homebound older adults have found mean scores ranging from 17.3 to 23.7 (Wisocki, 1994).

Reliability. The WS total score is associated with excellent overall internal consistency in both GAD (α = .93) and nonanxious (α = .94) individuals and adequate to very good internal consistency for its subscales in both populations (αs ranging from .76 to .91; Stanley, Beck, & Zebb, 1996). The scale demonstrates fair 2- to 4-week test–retest reliability ($r = .69$), although test–retest reliability for the health subscale is low ($r = .58$; Stanley, Beck, & Zebb, 1996).

     Validity. Convergent validity for the WS has been demonstrated by significant correlations between the scale and measures of anxiety (rs ranging from .54 to .63) and depression (rs from .50 to. 78; Wisocki, 1988; Wisocki, Handen, & Morse, 1986). The WS was also significantly correlated with trait anxiety within both a GAD ($r = .40$) and a nonanxious ($r = .57$) sample (Stanley, Beck, & Zebb, 1996). Older adults diagnosed with GAD using a structured interview scored significantly higher on the WS than did a community sample of older adults (Stanley, Beck, & Zebb, 1996) and WS scores decreased significantly from posttreatment to follow-up after cognitive–behavioral intervention (Stanley, Beck, & Glassco, 1996). Finally, in a discriminant function analysis, the social scale of the WS significantly differentiated older adults with GAD from nonanxious controls (Beck, Stanley, & Zebb, 1996).

Alternative Forms

     The WS has been translated into French, Spanish, and Hebrew. A revised, expanded version is now available from the author. This 88-item scale has three additional subscales—personal concerns, family concerns, and world issues. Its psychometric properties are currently under investigation.

Source

     The WS is reprinted in the original article and in Appendix B. Although the full title is that shown in Appendix B, typically the questionnaire is administered under the title "The Worry Scale." For more information, contact Dr. Patricia A. Wisocki, Psychology Department, University of Massachusetts, Amherst, MA 01003, USA; (tel) 413-545-1359; (fax) 413-545-0996; (e-mail) wisocki@psych.umass.edu.

BRIEF DESCRIPTIONS OF ADDITIONAL MEASURES

Generalized Anxious Temperament Scale (GATS)

     The GATS is a relatively new, 26-item self-report measure that assesses the continuum of lifelong generally anxious temperament. The scale is preprinted in an article that presents an argument for considering GAD as an extreme form of a normal personality disposition called "generalized anxious temperament" (Akiskal, 1998). The author indicates that this scale is under development. For more information, contact Hagop S. Akiskal, MD, Veterans Affairs Medical Center, Psychiatry Service 116A, 3350 La Jolla Village Drive, San Diego, CA 92161, USA; (tel) 619-552-8585, ext. 2226; (fax) 619-534-8598; (e-mail) hakiskal@ucsd.edu.

Student Worry Scale (SWS)

The SWS is a 10-item self-report measure that assesses frequency of worry about 10 content areas that were identified by college students as topics about which they worry. The scale, along with its initial psychometric properties, is described in the original article (Davey, Hampton, Farrell, & Davidson, 1992) and is compared with other measures of worry in a subsequent article (Davey, 1993). For more information, contact Graham C. L. Davey, Ph.D., Professor of Psychology, School of Cognitive and Computing Sciences, University of Sussex, Falmer, Brighton, BN1 9RH, United Kingdom; (tel): 44 1273 678485; (fax) 44 1273 671320; (e-mail) grahamda@cogs.susx.ac.uk.

REFERENCES

Akiskal, H. S. (1998). Toward a definition of generalized anxiety disorder as an anxious temperament type. *Acta Psychiatrica Scandinavica, 98*(Suppl. 393), 66–73.

Barlow, D. H., & DiNardo, P. A. (1991). The diagnosis of generalized anxiety disorder: Development, current status, and future direction. In R. M. Rapee & D. H. Barlow (Eds.), *Chronic anxiety: Generalized anxiety disorder and mixed anxiety-depression* (pp. 95–118). New York: Guilford.

Beck, J. G., Stanley, M. A., & Zebb, B. J. (1995). Psychometric properties of the Penn State Worry Questionnaire in older adults. *Journal of Clinical Geropsychology, 1,* 33–42.

Beck, J. G., Stanley, M., & Zebb, B. (1996). Characteristics of generalized anxiety disorder in older adults: A descriptive study. *Behaviour Research and Therapy, 34,* 225–234.

Borkovec, T. D., & Costello, E. (1993). Efficacy of applied relaxation and cognitive–behavioral therapy in the treatment of generalized anxiety disorder. *Journal of Consulting and Clinical Psychology, 61,* 611–619.

Brown, T. A., Antony, M. M., & Barlow, D. H. (1992). Psychometric properties of the Penn State Worry Questionnaire in a clinical anxiety disorders sample. *Behaviour Research and Therapy, 30,* 33–37.

Buhr, K., & Dugas, M. (2000, November). *Validation of the English version of the Intolerance of Uncertainty Scale.* Paper presented at the annual meeting of the Association for Advancement of Behavior Therapy, New Orleans.

Chorpita, B. F., Tracey, S. A., Brown, T. A., Collica, T. J., & Barlow, D. H. (1997). Assessment of worry in children and adolescents: An adaptation of the Penn State Worry Questionnaire. *Behaviour Research and Therapy, 35,* 569–581.

Davey, G. C. L. (1993). A comparison of three worry questionnaires. *Behaviour Research and Therapy, 31,* 51–56.

Davey, G. C. L., Hampton, J., Farrell, J., & Davidson, S. (1992). Some characteristics of worrying: Evidence for worrying and anxiety as separate constructs. *Personality and Individual Differences, 13,* 133–147.

Dugas, M. J., Freeston, M. H., Lachance, S., Provencher, M., & Ladouceur, R. (1995, July). *The Worry and Anxiety Questionnaire: Initial validation in nonclinical and clinical samples.* Paper presented at the World Congress of Behavioural and Cognitive Therapies, Copenhagen.

Dugas, M. J., Freeston, M. H., & Ladouceur, R. (1997). Intolerance of uncertainty and problem orientation in worry. *Cognitive Therapy and Research, 21,* 593–606.

Dugas, M. J., Gagnon, F., Ladouceur, R., & Freeston, M. (1998). Generalized anxiety disorder: A preliminary test of a conceptual model. *Behaviour Research and Therapy, 36,* 215–226.

Gillis, M. M., Haaga, D. A. F., & Ford, G. T. (1995). Normative values for the Beck Anxiety Inventory, Fear Questionnaire, Penn State Worry Questionnaire, and Social Phobia and Anxiety Inventory. *Psychological Assessment, 7,* 450–455.

Holowka, D. W., Dugas, M. J., Francis, K., & Laugesen, N. (2000, November). *Measuring beliefs about worry: A psychometric evaluation of the Why Worry Questionnaire.* Paper presented at the Annual Meeting of the Association for Advancement of Behavior Therapy, New Orleans.

Joormann, J., & Stöber, J. (1997). Measuring facets of worry: A LISREL analysis of the Worry Domains Questionnaire. *Personality and Individual Differences, 23,* 827–837.

Ladouceur, R., Blais, F., Freeston, M. H., & Dugas, M. J. (1998). Problem solving and problem orientation in generalized anxiety disorder. *Journal of Anxiety Disorders, 12,* 139–152.

Ladouceur, R., Dugas, M. J., Freeston, M. H., Léger, E., Gagnon, F., & Thibodeau, N. (2000). Efficacy of a new cognitive–behavioral treatment for generalized anxiety disorder: Evaluation in a controlled clinical trial. *Journal of Consulting and Clinical Psychology, 68,* 957–964.

Meyer, T. J., Miller, M. L., Metzger, R. L., & Borkovec, T. D. (1990). Development and validation of the Penn State Worry Questionnaire. *Behaviour Research and Therapy, 28,* 487–495.

Molina, S., & Borkovec, T. D. (1994). The Penn State Worry Questionnaire: Psychometric properties and associated characteristics. In G. C. L. Davey & F. Tallis (Eds.), *Worrying: Perspectives on theory, assessment, and treatment* (pp. 265–283). New York: Wiley.

Stanley, M., Beck, J. G., & Glassco, J. D. (1996). Treatment of generalized anxiety disorder in older adults: A preliminary comparison of cognitive behavioral and supportive approaches. *Behavior Therapy, 27,* 565–581.

Stanley, M., Beck, J. G., & Zebb, B. (1996). Psychometric properties of four anxiety measures in older adults. *Behaviour Research and Therapy: Behavioral Assessment, 34,* 827–838.

Stöber, J. (1998). Reliability and validity of two widely-used worry questionnaires: Self-report and self-peer convergence. *Personality and Individual Differences, 24,* 887–890.

Stöber, J., & Bittencourt, J. (1998). Weekly assessment of worry: An adaptation of the Penn State Worry Questionnaire for monitoring changes during treatment. *Behaviour Research and Therapy, 30,* 33–37.

Tallis, G., Davey, G. C. L., & Bond, A. (1994). The Worry Domains Questionnaire. In G. C. L. Davey & F. Tallis (Eds.), *Worrying: Perspectives on theory, assessment, and treatment* (pp. 287–292). New York: Wiley.

van Rijsoort, S., Emmelkamp, P., & Vervaeke, G. (1999). The Penn State Worry Questionnaire and the Worry Domains Questionnaire: Structure, reliability, and validity. *Clinical Psychology and Psychotherapy, 6,* 297–307.

Wisocki, P. A. (1994). The experience of worry among the elderly. In G. C. L. Davey & F. Tallis (Eds.), *Worrying: Perspectives on theory, assessment, and treatment* (pp. 247–261). New York: Wiley.

Wisocki, P. A., Handen, B., & Morse, C. (1986). The Worry Scale as a measure of anxiety among homebound and community active elderly. *The Behavior Therapist, 5,* 91–95.

Chapter 16
Obsessive-Compulsive Disorder: A Brief Overview and Guide to Assessment

Laura J. Summerfeldt

OVERVIEW AND ASSESSMENT OF OBSESSIVE-COMPULSIVE DISORDER

Overview of the Disorder

Obsessive-compulsive disorder (OCD) is an anxiety disorder characterized by (1) obsessions—intrusive and distressing thoughts, urges, or impulses, (2) compulsions—repetitive and/or highly ritualized overt or covert behaviors usually aimed at decreasing the distress caused by obsessions, and (3) often but not invariably, avoidance of stimuli that trigger obsessions. Lifetime prevalence of OCD is currently thought to be about 2.5%, with the disorder typically following a chronic waxing and waning course (American Psychiatric Association, 1994).

General Comments Regarding Assessment

Goals of assessment are determined by the needs and theoretical orientation of the clinician or researcher, and the treatment modalities being considered. Depending on these, a range of variables may warrant assessment, including environmental/familial, neuropsy-

Laura J. Summerfeldt • Department of Psychology, Trent University, Peterborough, Ontario K9J 7B8, Canada.

Table 1. Summary of Challenges
in Assessment of OCD

Overlap and/or comorbidity
Heterogeneity of symptom content
Upsetting and/or embarrassing symptom content
Symptom shift and multiplicity
Clinical features affecting response style
   Compulsive avoidance
   Obsessional exactness and doubt
Lack of insight
Multiple aspects of "severity"

chological, cognitive, and personality factors (see Table 1). A clinically useful review of such assessment targets can be found elsewhere (see Taylor, Thordarson, & Söchting, in press). Ascertainment of the nature and severity of the OCD symptoms themselves, however, is always crucial. This is the focus of the present chapter.

Issues in the Assessment of OCD

An important distinction must be made between screening for the possibility of OCD (i.e., diagnosis) versus assessment of its nature and severity once the diagnosis has been established. Although the two are interrelated, this chapter will focus on the second issue. The chapter's purpose is to review crucial practical, clinical, and conceptual issues the clinician should be aware of when assessing OCD symptoms. The psychometric features of available assessment instruments are discussed in several well-written reviews (e.g., Taylor, 1995, 1998), as well as later in the present volume. This chapter will instead provide an overview of challenges to be met in the assessment of OCD symptoms and discuss their implications for (1) efforts at assessment and case formulation and (2) identifying a good assessment instrument.

Overlap and Comorbidity: The Issue of Discriminant Validity

When ascertaining the severity or nature of a client's OCD symptoms, as with any other form of assessment, one must be aware of the assessment instrument's discriminant validity. That is, is the measure uniquely sensitive to OCD symptoms, or is it also tapping into other disorders? Because so many other experiences and behaviors can have the overt appearance of obsessions or compulsions, this is a particularly important issue in the assessment of OCD. This issue is further complicated if these other conditions are coexisting with the OCD. The task then becomes determining which symptoms belong with which disorder. Challenges to differential diagnosis often complicate efforts to measure the severity of OCD.

Obsessions. As indicated in Table 2, many painful and recurrent cognitions may be described as "obsessions" by the sufferer but are not obsessions according to DSM-IV criteria. This distinction may be difficult for the inexperienced interviewer. Furthermore, clumsily worded items on standardized measures of OCD can sometimes erroneously capture these experiences. For example, the original Padua Inventory (PI; Sanavio, 1988) was revised from 60 to 39 items (Burns, Keortge, Formea, & Sternberger, 1996) in part to address its

Table 2. Conditions with
Overlapping Features

Often mistaken for obsessions
    Depressive ruminations
    Jealous ruminations
    Worry
    Fantasy
Often mistaken for compulsions
    Tics
    Impulsive hair pulling, skin picking
    Other impulsive behaviors (e.g., shopping, gambling)
    Habits (e.g., nail biting)
    Compulsive sexual behavior

inclusion of several items that tapped worry rather than obsessions (e.g., "I invent doubts and problems about most of the things I do").

Compulsions. Repetitive, irresistible, stereotyped behaviors are found in disorders other than OCD, as shown in Table 2. In part because of this, some researchers and clinicians maintain that several disparate conditions may be part of a common family—known as the "obsessive-compulsive spectrum." Conventional members of this spectrum include tricho-tillomania, body dysmorphic disorder, and tic-related disorders (e.g.,Tourette's disorder). These conditions bear keeping in mind when assessing the presence and severity of compulsions in OCD, because their symptoms can be topographically similar. Useful guidelines for differentiating among OCD and spectrum conditions can be found in Black (1998).

Comorbidity is common in OCD (see Antony, Downie, & Swinson, 1998). When assessing OCD, it is important that the instrument being used is at least *more* sensitive to OCD symptoms than to symptoms of other disorders. This is not always the case. Many self-report measures of OCD are highly correlated with severity of depression. This may be in part because of the known covariation of the two disorders, but it also may be because some measures are insufficiently uniquely sensitive to OCD. The Compulsive Activity Checklist (CAC), for example, has been found to be almost as highly correlated with measures of depression as it is with measures of OC symptoms (Foa, Steketee, Kozak, & Dugger, 1987). As another example, determining the source of "compulsive" avoidance behaviors is often difficult, as they often arise from many conditions often comorbid with OCD (e.g., agoraphobia). Such ambiguity about the source of symptoms may be a particular problem with self-report measures, which do not permit clarification by the clinician. Table 3 provides a list of DSM-IV conditions that are sometimes difficult to distinguish from OCD.

Heterogeneity of Symptom Content

Diversity of symptoms in OCD is one of the greatest challenges to its assessment, and one of the principal flaws in many assessment tools. Measures of OCD should provide information about two things: the nature/content of the symptoms and their severity. The first issue is important, as each case of OCD can look very different: An individual can present in an almost limitless number of ways.

Table 3. Other Diagnostic
Categories to Consider

Normal intrusive thoughts and "compulsive" behaviors
Generalized anxiety disorder
Psychotic disorder
Paraphilias (pedophilia)
Specific phobia
Other "spectrum" disorders (e.g., body dysmorphic disorder)

Idiosyncratic Expression. While it may well be possible to summarize symptoms in terms of their predominant theme (e.g., "contamination," or "checking"), within each category there are a variety of possible forms of expression. Someone with predominant "checking compulsions" may physically check appliances, review documents for errors, silently check over their day by mentally imaging their activities, check by touching, looking, asking others, or check that they haven't caused accidents to happen, acted on impulse, or misheard something someone said. Functionally, it may be "checking," but the way that it becomes manifest for the individual may be highly idiosyncratic.

It is a challenge for a single measure to accommodate all of these different symptom manifestations, especially when it is simultaneously trying to ascertain the severity of each symptom. Inadequate content validity regarding symptoms is one of the greatest flaws in commonly used measures for OCD. Most content-based measures do not have the ability to capture idiosyncratic symptoms; many fail even in representing basic categories of symptoms. While most measures access the most traditionally recognized OC symptoms (e.g., overt checking and cleaning compulsions), many neglect those that are less frequently reported, or are less easily discerned. For example, obsessions and covert compulsions (e.g., mental checking, counting, mental rituals) are neglected in several popular measures, including the CAC, the PI, and the Maudsley Obsessive-Compulsive Inventory (MOCI). Ironically, such symptoms, being less easily identifiable by an observer, should receive added attention in a sensitive measurement instrument.

Upsetting and/or Embarrassing Content of Symptoms

Many OCD symptoms are objectively peculiar and some are more ego-dystonic than others. Patients are often reluctant to disclose "crazy" symptoms, and the majority of individuals with OCD do not seek help. There may be many reasons for this, including embarrassment and/or the fear that others will consider them dangerous. Without the clarification and guidance of an empathic interviewer (e.g., if there is exclusive reliance on self-report), upsetting and/or embarrassing symptoms may go unreported. These themes may not be easily disclosed even if the individual has grasped that they are by definition experienced as intrusive (that is, they have recognized that these are not a reflection of themselves).

To ensure accuracy of reporting, extra work may have to be done by the clinician to educate patients about the nature of obsessions and their role in provoking compulsions. The use of the Yale–Brown Obsessive Compulsive Scale (Y-BOCS; Goodman, Price, Rasmussen, Mazure, Delgado, et al., 1989; Goodman, Price, Rasmussen, Mazure, Fleishmann, et al., 1989; Goodman, Rasmussen, et al., 1989) structured interviewer-rated checklist is particularly effective (1) in putting the patient at ease by demonstrating that symptoms are often reported and (2) by permitting tailored probing by the interviewer to detect unique or subjectively disturbing symptoms.

Symptom Shift and Multiplicity

OC symptoms shift over time. Individuals rarely maintain the same constellation of symptoms over the course of the illness (Rettew, Swedo, Leonard, Lenane, & Rapoport, 1992). In addition, patients differ in the variety of symptoms they experience: Some may have a few symptom themes, others many (see Antony et al., 1998; Summerfeldt, Richter, Antony, & Swinson, 1999). These issues pose a problem for measures that confound variety of symptoms with severity. Patients who have multiple symptoms may be incorrectly assessed as having more severe OCD even if symptoms are mild, whereas patients who have few symptoms may be assessed as having mild OCD although these symptoms are severe.

Symptom shift and multiplicity have clear implications for measurement. Particularly when tracking OCD over time and comparing severity of symptoms (1) among different individuals or (2) at different points in time in the same individual, a measure is needed that provides comparable severity ratings independent of both the *content* of symptoms and the *number* of symptoms. The easiest solution to both needs is to use a content free severity measure (i.e., the Y-BOCS).

Clinical Features Affecting Response Style

Clinical features integral to OCD may by their very nature influence accurate assessment.

Compulsive Avoidance. Compulsions are one way of undoing the distress caused by obsessions. Another common strategy in OCD is avoidance of the cues that prompt obsessions in the first place. This may even be true of words/items in an assessment instrument. In our center we are accustomed to the anxiety provoked by OCD assessments. Individuals have stated that they spend much of their time trying to avoid thinking about these upsetting things; having to focus on them, even as part of a clinical assessment, is horrible. Thus, avoidance of threatening/unpleasant cues contained in measures of symptoms may lead to underreporting.

Obsessional Exactness and Doubt. A common feature of OCD is doubt, which in some cases extends to many experiences. If left to her or his own devices and "open recall" (e.g., filling out a self-report measure without guidance), the individual may go into torments over whether she or he is recalling experiences, or comprehending the question, accurately. Rereading/rewriting compulsions may actually become manifest in response to self-report instruments. Relatedly, in some cases a symptomatic need for exactness may extend to the physical completion of the question. Although questionnaires with a range of response options (i.e., five-point) are more reliable, in some cases of OCD the cost of the increased decisions required may outweigh the psychometric advantages. A criticism of the MOCI, for example, is its binary (true/false) format versus the Likert format (0–5) of the PI. Its benefit, however, is that the OCD patient only has to commit to a "true" or a "false"; the leeway for decision-making is smaller.

These clinical features of OCD have several practical implications, particularly for self-report assessment methods. They include: (1) procrastination and anxiety about assessment, (2) slowed responding, and (3) potential for contaminated responses. Clinicians experienced in this area are familiar with the corrected, revised, and multiply qualified appearance of questionnaires returned by individuals with OCD. Such data are of little empirical value, in terms of providing a reliable quantification of symptoms.

Lack of Insight

Insight in OCD exists on a continuum. The patient can have greater or lesser insight not only into the reasonableness of his or her obsessions or compulsions, but, perhaps more importantly, whether behaviors in fact are symptoms, and what they might be symptoms of. This is related to the issue of ego-dystonicity. Symptoms, particularly compulsions, can become manifest in ways that the individual may never have considered a "symptom" (e.g., need for reassurance, prayers). Clinician's guidance may be crucial in their initial ascertainment.

Multiple Aspects of Severity

Content validity also pertains to the idea of severity: Is a measure including items that tap into all possible ways the disorder can impact on the individual? Severity can include such issues as time consumed, amount of subjective distress or disturbance, and functional interference. Most measures of OCD do not address this issue, tapping into only one or perhaps two facets of severity. One strength of a recent self-report measure—the Obsessive-Compulsive Inventory (Foa, Kozak, Salkovskis, Coles, & Amir, 1998)—is its inclusion of both frequency and distress indices.

SUMMARY AND RECOMMENDATIONS

In short, clinicians need to be aware of several practical, clinical, and conceptual issues germane to the accurate assessment of OCD symptoms. Their implications for choosing an assessment tool are summarized in Table 4. These points particularly apply to first-time assessment of symptoms, that is, in a "naive" OCD sufferer. To date, only one scale has attempted to address all of these points—the interviewer-rated Y-BOCS. Initially designed to detect changes in symptoms in medication trials, the Y-BOCS continues to be regarded as the gold standard in OCD measurement. Although a self-report version is gaining in popularity, the author would encourage clinicians—for reasons discussed throughout this chapter—to regard the time required for an initial interviewer-rated Y-BOCS as a worthwhile investment,

Table 4. Implications for an Assessment Instrument for OCD Symptoms

Avoids primary use of self-report in the absence of guidance, particularly in the form of questionnaires
Allows for comprehensive ascertainment of wide range of symptoms
Permits rating of severity independent of *number* or *type* of symptoms
Sensitive to multiple aspects of severity, including time spent, distress felt, and functional impairment

particularly if a reliable and valid self-report measure, such as the revised PI, is administered simultaneously. The clinician's guidance may be less necessary in subsequent assessments.

REFERENCES

American Psychiatric Association. (1994). *Diagnostic and statistical manual of mental disorders* (4th ed.). Washington, DC: Author.

Antony, M. M., Downie, F., & Swinson, R. P. (1998). Diagnostic issues and epidemiology in obsessive-compulsive disorder. In R. P. Swinson, M. M. Antony, S. Rachman, & M. A. Richter (Eds.), *Obsessive-compulsive disorder: Theory, research, and treatment* (pp. 3–32). New York: Guilford.

Black, D. W. (1998). Recognition and treatment of obsessive-compulsive spectrum disorders. In R. P. Swinson, M. M. Antony, S. Rachman, & M. A. Richter (Eds.), *Obsessive-compulsive disorder: Theory, research, and treatment* (pp. 426–458). New York: Guilford.

Burns, G. L., Keortge, S. G., Formea, G. M., & Sternberger, L. G. (1996). Revision of the Padua Inventory for obsessive compulsive disorder symptoms: Distinctions between worry, obsessions, and compulsions. *Behaviour Research and Therapy, 34*, 163–173.

Foa, E. B., Kozak, M. J., Salkovskis, P. M., Coles, M. E., & Amir, N. (1998). The validation of a new obsessive-compulsive disorder scale: The Obsessive-Compulsive Inventory. *Psychological Assessment, 10*, 206–214.

Foa, E. B., Steketee, G., Kozak, M., & Dugger, D. (1987). Effects of imipramine on depression and obsessive-compulsive symptoms. *Psychiatry Research, 21*, 123–136.

Goodman, W. K., Price, L. H., Rasmussen, S. A., Mazure, C., Delgado, P., Heninger, G. R., & Charney, D. S. (1989). The Yale–Brown Obsessive Compulsive Scale. II. Validity. *Archives of General Psychiatry, 46*, 1012–1016.

Goodman, W. K., Price, L. H., Rasmussen, S. A., Mazure, C., Fleishmann, R. L., Hill, C. L., Heninger, G. R., & Charney, D. S. (1989). The Yale–Brown Obsessive Compulsive Scale. I. Development, use, and reliability. *Archives of General Psychiatry, 46*, 1006–1011.

Goodman, W. K., Rasmussen, S. A., Price, L. H., Mazure, C., Heninger, G. R., & Charney, D. S. (1989). *Manual for the Yale–Brown Obsessive Compulsive Scale (revised)*. New Haven: Connecticut Mental Health Center.

Rettew, D. C., Swedo, S. E., Leonard, H. L., Lenane, M. C., & Rapoport, J. L. (1992). Obsessions and compulsions across time in 79 children and adolescents with obsessive-compulsive disorder. *Journal of the American Academy of Child and Adolescent Psychiatry, 31*, 1050–1056.

Sanavio, E. (1988). Obsessions and compulsions: The Padua Inventory. *Behaviour Research and Therapy, 26*, 169–177.

Summerfeldt, L. J., Richter, M. A., Antony, M. M., & Swinson, R. P. (1999). Symptom structure in obsessive-compulsive disorder: A confirmatory factor-analytic study. *Behaviour Research and Therapy, 37*, 297–311.

Taylor, S. (1995). Assessment of obsessions and compulsions: Reliability, validity, and sensitivity to treatment effects. *Clinical Psychology Review, 15*, 261–296.

Taylor, S. (1998). Assessment of obsessive-compulsive disorder. In R. P. Swinson, M. M. Antony, S. Rachman, & M. A. Richter (Eds.), *Obsessive-compulsive disorder: Theory, research, and treatment* (pp. 229–257). New York: Guilford.

Taylor, S., Thordarson, D. S., & Söchting, I. S. (in press). Assessment, treatment planning, and outcome evaluation for obsessive-compulsive disorder. In M. M. Antony & D. H. Barlow (Eds.), *Handbook of assessment, treatment planning, and outcome evaluation: Empirically supported strategies for psychological disorders*. New York: Guilford.

Chapter 17
Measures for Obsessive-Compulsive Disorder

Martin M. Antony

COMPULSIVE ACTIVITY CHECKLIST (CAC)

Original Citations

Freund, B., Steketee, G. S., & Foa, E. B. (1987). Compulsive Activity Checklist (CAC): Psychometric analysis with obsessive-compulsive disorder. *Behavioral Assessment, 9*, 67–79.

Purpose

To measure impairment in daily activities due to obsessive-compulsive symptoms.

Description

There are many different versions of the CAC in the literature, and several different names have been used for this instrument. In addition, some investigators have tended to use it as a self-report instrument, whereas others have used it as an interview-based scale. The original version was a 62-item assessor-rated scale, developed by Richard Hallam and first reported by Philpott (1975). This version was initially known as the Obsessive Compulsive Interview Checklist. Subsequent names for this instrument have included the Compulsion

Martin M. Antony • Anxiety Treatment and Research Centre, St. Joseph's Healthcare, Hamilton, and Department of Psychiatry and Behavioural Neurosciences, McMaster University, Hamilton, Ontario L8N 4A6, Canada.

Checklist (Marks, Stern, Mawson, Cobb, & MacDonald, 1980) and eventually the CAC (Mawson, Marks, & Ramm, 1982), which is currently the most commonly used name. The specific items and the length of the scale have varied considerably across studies. For example, Freund, Steketee, and Foa (1987) published data on a 38-item version; Cottraux, Bouvard, Defayolle, and Messy (1988) published an 18-item version; Steketee and Freund (1993) published a 28-item revision of the 38-item scale (called the CAC-R). This section will focus primarily on the Freund et al. (1987) 38-item CAC, and to a lesser extent on the 28-item CAC-R (although preliminary data suggest that this version may be preferable to the 38-item version; Steketee & Freund, 1993).

The Freund et al. (1987) CAC is a 38-item instrument that can be administered as either an interviewer-rated scale or a self-rated scale. Each item is rated on a four-point scale, ranging from 0 (no problem with activity) to 3 (unable to complete or attempt activity). The possible range of scores is 0 to 114.

Steketee and Freund (1993) revised the CAC by deleting items that did not differentiate individuals with OCD from those without OCD, as well as items with low item–total correlations, and items that failed to load on factors relating to OCD symptoms. The resulting CAC-R is a 28-item self-report scale. For the 28-item version, items 7 and 8 were combined (i.e., "using a toilet to urinate or defecate"), and items 20, 24, 27, 30–32, 34, 35, and 37 were deleted. In addition, the wording of a few items was changed (e.g., for item 21, the word "spigots" was changed to "faucets").

Administration and Scoring

The CAC can be administered in 5 minutes. The total score is calculated by summing all of the items. In addition, subscales can be calculated as follows: washing subscale (sum of items 2–14, 16–20, 31–36), checking subscale (sum of items 1, 15, 21–30, 37, 38). Higher scores reflect greater impairment.

Psychometric Properties

Sample Scores and Norms.   Sample scores for various OCD-related groups were provided by Freund et al. (1987). The mean total CAC score for a group of individuals with OCD was 43.66 (SD = 18.94). For individuals with primarily washing rituals, means on the washing and checking subscales were 33.24 (SD = 13.68) and 12.00 (SD = 7.68), respectively. For individuals with primarily checking rituals, means on the washing and checking subscales were 8.95 (SD = 5.59) and 16.48 (SD = 9.44), respectively.

Reliability.   In a sample of individuals with OCD, internal consistency (as measured by Cronbach's alpha) was excellent for the total score (α = .91) as well as for the washing (α = .93) and checking (α = .89) subscales (Frend et al., 1987). In a student sample, internal consistency was found to be good for the total score (α = .86) and fair for the subscales (α = .78 for both subscales; Sternberger & Burns, 1990a). However, a subsequent study by Steketee and Freund (1993) found that nine items had low item–total correlations (less than .40) in an OCD patient sample. Interrater reliability was low when the scale was completed by two interviewers (r = .62), either on the same day or after an average of 37 days (r = .63). However, interrater reliability was excellent when the CAC was completed once by an interviewer and once by the patient (r = .94) on the same day (Freund et al., 1987).

Validity.   A factor analysis supported the subscales of the CAC, although items 16 and 32 did not load strongly on their respective factors (Freund et al., 1987). A discriminant function analysis correctly classified 84% of individuals with OCD (compared with non-anxious controls) based on their CAC total scores (Steketee & Freund, 1993). In addition, the CAC correctly identified OCD patients as having primarily checking or washing rituals 85% of the time (Freund et al., 1987). Individuals with OCD scored significantly higher than nonanxious controls and individuals with other anxiety disorders on all but nine items (Steketee & Freund, 1993).

Freund et al. (1987) found that the CAC was positively correlated with measures of OCD symptomatology, fear, and functional impairment, but not with measures of depression, anxiety, neuroticism, or general psychopathology. In contrast, Sternberger and Burns (1990a) found significant correlations between the CAC and all nine subscales of the SCL-90 (rs range from .14 to .38). Correlations between the CAC and the Maudsley Obsessional Compulsive Inventory are lower than might be expected, with rs ranging from .29 to .33 across two studies (Freund et al., 1987; Sternberger & Burns, 1990a). Finally, the CAC appears to be sensitive to changes following treatment (Freund et al., 1987).

Alternative Forms

As reviewed earlier, there are various versions of the CAC, with different numbers of items. There is a French version containing 18 items (Cottraux et al., 1988).

Source

The CAC has been reprinted in several sources including the original citation (Freund et al., 1987) and in Appendix B. The CAC-R is reprinted in a paper by Steketee and Freund (1993). Further information on the CAC may be obtained from the author, Blanche V. Freund, Ph.D., Brief Therapy Center, 276 NE 27th St., Miami, FL 33137, USA; (tel) 305-573-1733; (fax) 305-576-2355; (e-mail) freunddrblanche@aol.com. Information regarding the CAC-R may be obtained from the author, Gail Steketee, Ph.D., Boston University School of Social Work, 264 Bay State Road, Boston, MA 02215, USA; (tel) 617-353-3750; (fax) 617-353-5612; (e-mail) steketee@bu.edu.

FROST INDECISIVENESS SCALE (FIS)

Original Citation

Frost, R. O., & Shows, D. L. (1993). The nature and measurement of compulsive indecisiveness. *Behaviour Research and Therapy, 31*, 683–692.

Purpose

To measure problems with decision-making and indecisiveness.

Description

The FIS is a 15-item self-report instrument in which patients rate the extent to which they agree with statements regarding a tendency to be indecisive. Each item is rated on a five-point scale ranging from 1 (strongly disagree) to 5 (strongly agree).

Administration and Scoring

The FIS can be administered in 3 to 5 minutes. In early research a total score was calculated by reversing scores on items 2, 3, 5, 6, 8, and 9, and then summing all 15 items. Higher scores reflect more indecisiveness. More recent scoring uses two factorially derived subscales reflecting *fears about decision-making* (sum of items 1, 4, 7, 10–15) and *positive decision-making* (sum of items 2, 3, 5, 6, 8, 9). In these most recent scoring instructions, no items are reverse scored.

Psychometric Properties

Sample Scores and Norms.   In a study by Steketee, Frost, and Kyrios (2001), mean scores on the *fears about decision-making* subscale (Fears) were 29.5 (*SD* = 8.9) for self-identified compulsive hoarders, 22.7 (*SD* = 5.6) for patients with OCD, and 18.1 (*SD* = 5.9) for community controls. Mean scores on the *positive decision-making* subscale (Positive) were 19.0 (*SD* = 6.1) for hoarders, 17.7 (*SD* = 5.2) for patients with OCD, and 17.4 (*SD* = 4.5) for community controls.

Reliability.   Internal consistency (Cronbach's alpha) of the FIS total score was .90 in a student sample (Frost & Shows, 1993). Internal consistency was .89 for the Fears subscale and .83 for the Positive subscale in a community sample (Steketee et al., 2001).

Validity.   Total scores on the FIS are correlated with the tendency to hoard possessions (Frost & Gross, 1993; Frost & Shows, 1993), as well as with measures of obsessive-compulsive symptomatology and certain dimensions of perfectionism (Frost & Shows, 1993; Gayton, Clavin, Clavin, & Broida, 1994). With respect to OCD symptoms, the FIS appears to be significantly correlated with measures of compulsive checking and doubting (is range from .29 to .41), but not with measures of compulsive washing (*r*s range from .02 to .09), at least in a nonclinical sample (Frost & Shows, 1993). The Fears subscale correlated significantly (*r* = .40) with the Y-BOCS total score, whereas the Positive subscale did not in a large community and clinical sample (Steketee et al., 2001). Compulsive hoarders had significantly higher Fears subscale scores than nonhoarding OCD patients who had significantly higher Fears subscale scores than community controls. There were no differences in levels of Positive Decision-Making among these three groups (Steketee et al., 2001). The Fears subscale was also strongly correlated with measures of depression and anxiety; the Positive subscale was moderately and negatively correlated with these measures (Steketee et al., 2001).

Alternative Forms

The FIS has been translated into Portuguese.

Source

The FIS items are reprinted in Frost and Shows (1993) and the entire scale is reprinted in Appendix B. Additional information is available from the author, Randy O. Frost, Ph.D., Department of Psychology, Smith College, Northampton, MA 01063, USA; (tel) 413-585-3911; (fax) 413-585-3786; (e-mail) rfrost@smith.edu.

MAUDSLEY OBSESSIONAL COMPULSIVE INVENTORY (MOC OR MOCI)

Original Citation

Hodgson, R. J., & Rachman, S. (1977). Obsessive compulsive complaints. *Behaviour Research and Therapy*, *15*, 389–395.

Purpose

To measure obsessional-compulsive complaints.

Description

The MOC is a 30-item self-report instrument in which patients rate items as either true or false. Items are related to particular obsessive-compulsive behaviors and rituals. Scores can range from 0 to 30.

Administration and Scoring

The MOC takes 5 minutes to administer. The instrument is scored by assigning a "1" to each true response and a "0" to each false response. Then, items 5, 9, 11, 13, 15–17, 19, 21–25, 27, and 29 are reverse-scored and the items are added up. In addition to the total score (sum of all 30 items), subscale scores can be calculated as follows: *checking subscale* (sum of items 2, 6, 8, 14, 15, 20, 22, 26, 28), *cleaning subscale* (sum of items 1, 4, 5, 9, 13, 17, 19, 21, 24, 26, 27), *slowness subscale* (sum of items 2, 4, 8, 16, 23, 25, 29), and *doubting subscale* (sum of items 3, 7, 10–12, 18, 30). Because the subscales were determined by a factor analysis, and some items loaded on multiple factors, some items appear in more than one subscale. In addition, items 2 and 8 load negatively on the slowness subscale (e.g., individuals who report more slowness are *less* likely to get nasty thoughts and have difficulty getting rid of them), although these items are not scored any differently than the other items in that subscale.

Psychometric Properties

Sample Scores and Norms. Richter, Cox, and Direnfeld (1994) reported means on the MOC in a group of patients diagnosed with OCD according to DSM-III-R. The mean total score was 13.67 (*SD* = 6.01). Means on the subscales were as follows: *checking* 4.73 (*SD* = 2.15), *washing* 3.40 (*SD* = 3.29), *doubting* 4.80 (*SD* = 2.41), *slowness* 2.63 (*SD* = 1.59). Total scale means for obsessional patients (mean = 18.86; *SD* = 4.92) were also provided by Hodgson and Rachman (1977), although participants in the sample were not diagnosed according to formalized criteria (DSM-III was not yet published). The mean total score for a student sample was 6.32 (*SD* = 3.92; Dent & Salkovskis, 1986).

Reliability.   In a study by Richter et al. (1994), internal consistency (as measured by Cronbach's alpha) was good for the total score (α = .85), cleaning subscale (α = .87), and doubting subscale (α = .86), and low for the checking subscale (α = .63) and slowness subscale (α = .45). In contrast, Emmelkamp, Kraaijkamp, and van den Hout (1999) found internal consistency to be low in a sample of patients with OCD, both for the total MOC (α = .70) and for the subscales (αs = .47 to .62), even after deleting two items with low item total correlations (items 9 and 14). Stability is moderate to high, with test–retest reliability coefficients ranging from .69 (Sternberger & Burns, 1990a) to .84 (Emmelkamp et al., 1999).

Validity.   The subscales of the MOC are empirically supported by a factor analysis reported in the original paper (Hodgson & Rachman, 1977) and a confirmatory factor analysis by Emmelkamp et al. (1999). However, some studies have found slightly different factors (e.g., Sternberger & Burns, 1990a). The total score on the MOC is significantly correlated with a broad range of psychopathology measures (e.g., all six subscales on the SCL-90), although correlations with other OCD measures appear to be particularly strong (Emmelkamp et al., 1999; Sternberger & Burns, 1990a). In a nonclinical sample, high scorers on the MOC were more likely than low scorers to report symptoms of OCD and GAD on a structured diagnostic interview, but no more likely to report symptoms of social anxiety or specific phobia (Sternberger & Burns, 1990b). In addition, the MOC distinguished patients with OCD from patients with eating disorders, other anxiety disorders, and nonanxious controls, but not from patients suffering from depression (Emmelkamp et al., 1999). Finally, the MOC is sensitive to the effects of treatment, but not as sensitive as patient ratings of change on individually tailored target symptoms (Emmelkamp et al., 1999).

Source

The MOC has been reprinted in several sources including the original citation (Hodgson & Rachman, 1977) and in Appendix B. Additional information is available from Dr. S. Rachman, Department of Psychology, University of British Columbia, 2136 West Mall, Vancouver, BC, V6T 1Z4, Canada; (tel) 604-822-5861; (fax) 604-822-6075; (e-mail) rachman @unixg.ubc.ca.

OBSESSIVE COMPULSIVE INVENTORY (OCI)

Original Citation

Foa, E. B., Kozak, M. J., Salkovskis, P. M., Coles, M. E., & Amir, N. (1998). The validation of a new obsessive compulsive disorder scale: The Obsessive-Compulsive Inventory. *Psychological Assessment, 10*, 206–214.

Purpose

To measure the severity of obsessive-compulsive symptoms.

Description

The OCI is a 42-item self-report instrument in which patients rate separately the frequency of particular obsessions and compulsions and the distress created by these symptoms. Frequency of each symptom is rated on a five-point scale ranging from 0 (never) to 4 (almost always). Distress for each symptom is rated on a five-point scale ranging from 0 (not at all) to 4 (extremely). Scores for frequency and distress can each range from 0 to 168.

Administration and Scoring

The OCI takes 10 to 15 minutes to administer. The instrument is scored by summing the items to obtain separate scores for frequency and distress. There are no reverse-scored items. In addition to generating a total score, scores for seven separate subscales can be calculated as follows: *washing* (mean of items 2, 4, 8, 21, 22, 27, 38, 42); *checking* (mean of items 3, 7, 9, 10, 19, 24, 31, 32, 40); *doubting* (mean of items 26, 37, 41); *ordering* (mean of items 14, 15, 23, 29, 35); *obsessing* (mean of items 1, 12, 13, 17, 20, 28, 30, 33); *hoarding* (mean of items 6, 11, 34); *neutralizing* (mean of items 5, 16, 18, 25, 36, 39).

Psychometric Properties

In addition to a validation study in several clinical groups (Foa et al., 1998), Simonds, Thorpe, and Elliott (2000) examined the psychometric properties of the OCI in a nonclinical sample. This section, however, emphasizes the findings from the Foa et al. study, which are likely to be more relevant to clinical practice.

Sample Scores and Norms.   Foa et al. (1998) report means for a number of different groups, including individuals with OCD, generalized social phobia, PTSD, and nonanxious controls. For a sample of individuals with OCD, the mean total score for the distress ratings was 66.33 ($SD = 31.9$). For nonanxious controls, the mean total on the distress ratings was 25.25 ($SD = 20.8$). For individuals with OCD and nonanxious controls, the mean total scores for the frequency ratings were 66.36 ($SD = 29.4$) and 34.15 ($SD = 21.2$), respectively. A cutoff score of 40 for the distress scale allowed for correct identification of 80% of participants with OCD (from a larger group of individuals with anxiety disorders and nonanxious controls; Foa et al., 1988).

Foa et al. (1998) also reported mean scores on each of the seven subscales. For the distress ratings, the subscale means for the OCD sample were as follows: *washing* 1.44 ($SD = 1.3$); *checking* 1.51 ($SD = 0.9$); *doubting* 1.84 ($SD = 1.3$); *ordering* 1.87 ($SD = 1.2$); *obsessing* 1.79 ($SD = 1.1$); *hoarding* 1.24 ($SD = 1.3$); *mental neutralizing* 1.38 ($SD = 1.0$). For the frequency ratings, the subscale means for the OCD sample were as follows: *washing* 1.44 ($SD = 1.4$); *checking* 1.51 ($SD = 0.9$); *doubting* 2.01 ($SD = 1.1$); *ordering* 1.87 ($SD = 1.1$); *obsessing* 1.67 ($SD = 0.8$); *hoarding* 1.22 ($SD = 1.1$); *mental neutralizing* 1.49 ($SD = 0.9$). Subscale means for other diagnostic groups and for nonanxious controls are available in Foa et al. (1998).

Reliability.   As reported by Foa et al. (1998), internal consistency for the entire scale was excellent in a sample of OCD patients (Cronbach's alphas = .92 for the distress ratings and .93 for the frequency ratings). Internal consistency for the individual subscales varied somewhat, with αs across subscales ranging from .68 to .94 for the distress ratings, and from .72 to .96 for the frequency ratings. Internal consistency was highest for the washing subscale (distress and frequency ratings) and lowest for the obsessing subscale (distress ratings) and mental neutralizing subscale (frequency ratings). Test–retest reliability for the total score was satisfactory in the OCD sample (r = .87 for the distress ratings and .84 for the frequency ratings; Foa et al., 1998). Test–retest reliability coefficients were comparable in a nonanxious control group and for most of the individual subscales.

Validity.   Patients with OCD score significantly higher (based on OCI totals on both the distress and frequency scales) than individuals with PTSD, social phobia, and nonanxious controls (Foa et al., 1998). In addition, each of the seven subscales (except for hoarding) differentiates individuals with OCD from individuals from these other groups, for both distress and frequency ratings. For the hoarding subscale, individuals with OCD scored higher than some, but not all comparison groups, and showed slightly different patterns for distress and frequency ratings (Foa et al., 1998).

In patients with OCD, Foa et al. (1998) reported that the OCI is significantly correlated with CAC total scores (r = .65), MOC scores (r = .68), Y-BOCS total scores (r = .23), Y-BOCS compulsion scores (r = .25), but not the Y-BOCS obsession scores (r = .14). The OCI is also significantly correlated with measures of anxiety and depression.

Alternative Forms

According to Foa et al. (1998) a revision of the OCI is planned to improve the discriminant validity of the hoarding subscale. In addition, the authors are planning to develop a brief version of the scale.

Source

The OCI is reproduced in Appendix B. Additional information may be obtained from the author, Edna B. Foa, Ph.D., Center for the Study and Treatment of Anxiety, University of Pennsylvania, School of Medicine, 3535 Market Street, 6th floor, Philadelphia, PA 19104, USA; (tel) 215-746-3327; (fax) 215-746-3311; (e-mail) foa@mail.med.upenn.edu.

OVERVALUED IDEAS SCALE (OVIS)

Original Citation

Neziroglu, F., McKay, D., Yaryura-Tobias, J. A., Stevens, K. P., & Todaro, J. (1999). The Overvalued Ideas Scale: Development, reliability and validity in obsessive-compulsive disorder. *Behaviour Research and Therapy, 37*, 881–902.

Purpose

To measure strength of belief in obsessive-compulsive disorder and related disorders, such as body dysmorphic disorder and hypochondriasis.

Description

The OVIS is a 10-item interview-based scale. The instrument begins with an open-ended question asking the individual to record the most prominent OCD-related belief that has been present in the past week. Next, there are 10 items that measure different facets related to the strength of the belief. Each item is rated on a 10-point scale ranging from 1 to 10. Each item has slightly different descriptors anchoring the 10-point scale (see Appendix B).

Administration and Scoring

The OVIS takes 5 to 10 minutes to administer. It should be administered by an experienced clinician, because an initial pilot study suggested that the scale is unreliable when administered as a self-report instrument (Neziroglu et al., 1999). The scale is scored by taking the mean of the individual's ratings on the 10 items. Scores can range from 1 to 10.

Psychometric Properties

Sample Scores and Norms. The mean score on the OVIS for a sample of individuals with OCD was 4.6 (SD = 3.1; range = 1.6 to 8.7; Neziroglu et al., 1999).

Reliability. The internal consistency of the OVIS was found to be good, as indicated by a coefficient of .85 (Neziroglu et al., 1999). Stability was also found to be high, with test–retest reliability and interrater reliability (r) coefficients of .80 and .81, respectively (Neziroglu et al., 1999).

Validity. OVIS scores are significantly correlated with another measure of overvalued ideation (i.e., item 11 of the Y-BOCS), measures of OCD symptomatology, anxiety, and depression (Neziroglu et al., 1999). Thus, although convergent validity was demonstrated for the OVIS, the scale appears to lack discriminant validity (Neziroglu et al., 1999). Finally, the OVIS is a significant predictor of outcome following intensive behavioral treatment for OCD and body dysmorphic disorder (Neziroglu, Stevens, Yaryura-Tobias, & McKay, in press).

Alternative Forms

The OVIS has been translated into Portuguese, Spanish, French, and Italian.

Source

The OVIS is reprinted in the original article by Neziroglu et al. (1999) and in Appendix B. Additional information can be obtained from the author, Fugen Neziroglu, Ph.D., Bio-

Behavioral Institute, Department of Biopsychosocial Research, 935 Northern Blvd., Great Neck, NY 10021-5304, USA; (tel) 516-487-7116; (fax) 516-829-1731; (e-mail) neziroglu @aol.com.

PADUA INVENTORY–WASHINGTON STATE UNIVERSITY REVISION (PI-WSUR)

Original Citation

Burns, G. L., Keortge, S. G., Formea, G. M., & Sternberger, L. G. (1996). Revision of the Padua Inventory of Obsessive Compulsive Disorder Symptoms: Distinctions between worry, obsessions and compulsions. *Behaviour Research and Therapy, 34*, 163–173.

Purpose

To measure obsessions and compulsions.

Description

There are three published versions of the Padua Inventory (PI), all three of which are self-report scales. The original PI (Sanavio, 1988) contains 60 items, the Padua Inventory Revised (PI-R; van Oppen, Hoekstra, & Emmelkamp, 1995) contains 41 items, and PI-WSUR (Burns, Keortge, Formea, & Sternberger, 1996) contains 39 items. The PI-R and PI-WSUR are subsets of items from the original PI. On all three versions, items describing obsessive and compulsive symptoms are rated on a five-point scale ranging from 0 (not at all) to 4 (very much). For the PI-WSUR, the total score can range from 0 to 156.

PI and its revised versions contain items to measure both obsessions and compulsions, whereas some other OCD measures (e.g., the CAC and the MOC) have tended to emphasize the measurement of compulsions only. In addition, there is evidence that PI revisions have improved psychometric properties, relative to the original PI. For example, the PI-WSUR does a better job at discriminating OCD symptoms from worry. Researchers interested in the PI may want to consider using the entire 60-item scale and deriving one or both revised versions as appropriate.

The remainder of this review focuses primarily on the PI-WSUR, which has recently gained considerable popularity (e.g., Taylor, 1998). Readers interested in the PI-R should consult the validation paper by van Oppen, Hoekstra, and Emmelkamp (1995). For information on the original PI, there are numerous psychometric papers in addition to the original validation paper by Sanavio (1988). Most of these are validation studies in nonclinical samples (e.g., Kyrios, Bhar, & Wade; 1996; Mancini, Gragnani, Orazi, & Pietrangeli, 1999; McDonald & de Silva, 1999; Sternberger & Burns, 1990c; van Oppen, 1992).

Administration and Scoring

The PI-WSUR takes 10 minutes to administer and 5 minutes to score. The total score is calculated by computing the sum of all 39 items. In addition, scores for five subscales may be computed as follows: *contamination obsessions and washing compulsions subscale* (COWC; sum of items 1–10); *dressing/grooming compulsions subscale* (DRGRC; sum of items 11–13); *checking compulsions subscale* (CHCK; sum of items 14–23); *obsessional thoughts of harm to self/others subscale* (OTAHSO; sum of items 24–30); *obsessional impulses to harm self/others subscale* (OITHSO; sum of items 31–39).

Psychometric Properties

Sample Scores and Norms.   In a sample of individuals with OCD ($n = 15$), Burns et al. (1996) obtained total and subscale scores for the PI-WSUR. Means were as follows: total score 54.93 ($SD = 16.72$); COWC subscale 13.87 ($SD = 7.96$); DRGRC subscale 5.20 ($SD = 4.61$); CHCK subscale 19.87 ($SD = 9.69$); OTAHSO subscale 10.00 ($SD = 5.01$); OITHSO subscale 6.00 ($SD = 3.87$). The total score for a large normative sample was 21.78 ($SD = 16.33$). Mean scores on each subscale in the normative sample are reported by Burns et al. (1996).

Reliability.   Based on findings from a normative sample, Burns et al. (1996) reported that internal consistency for the PI-WSUR total scores was excellent (Cronbach's $\alpha = .92$). For the subscales, internal consistency was fair to good, with αs ranging from .77 (OTAHSO subscale) to .88 (CHCK subscale). Test–retest reliability was .76 for the total score and ranged from .61 (OTAHSO subscale) to .84 (OITHSO subscale) for the subscales (Burns et al., 1996).

Validity.   Much of the validity data on the PI-WSUR has focused on demonstrating that the PI-WSUR differentiates between OCD symptoms and worry, as measured by the Penn State Worry Questionnaire (PSWQ). Although the PI-WSUR subscales and total score are significantly correlated with scores on the PSWQ (rs range from .08 to .37), each item on the PI-WSUR is more strongly correlated with its own subscale and with the total score on the PI-WSUR than with the PSWQ (Burns et al., 1996). In addition, although the PI shares 34% of its variance with the PSWQ (Freeston et al., 1994), the PI-WSUR shares only 12% of its variance with the PSWQ (Burns et al., 1996). Finally, a factor-analytic study supports the subscale structure of the PI-WSUR, as well as the ability of the instrument to discriminate OCD symptoms from worry (Burns et al., 1996).

In addition to data on the discrimination of OCD symptoms and worry by the PI-WSUR, studies on the other versions of the PI have examined other types of validity. For example, the PI-R has been shown to be sensitive to the effects of treatment (van Oppen, Emmelkamp, van Balkom, & van Dyck, 1995) and also to discriminate between people with OCD from people with other anxiety disorders and from normal controls (van Oppen, Hoekstra, & Emmelkamp, 1995). Both the PI and the PI-R correlate significantly with other measures of OCD, but also with measures of anxiety, depression, and other forms of psychopathology (van Oppen, 1992; van Oppen, Hoekstra, & Emmelkamp, 1995).

Alternative Forms

The 39-item PI-WSUR has been translated into Spanish and German. The original 60-item PI is available in English, Italian, Dutch, French, German, Greek, Hurdu (Pakistan), Japanese, and Spanish. As discussed earlier, there is also a 41-item revision of the PI (van Oppen, Hoekstra, & Emmelkamp, 1995), which is a subset of items from the original 60-item PI.

Source

The PI-WSUR is reprinted in Appendix B. Additional information may be obtained from the author, G. Leonard Burns, Ph.D., Psychology Department, Washington State University, Pullman, WA 99164-4820; (tel) 509-335-8229; (fax) 509-335-5043; (e-mail) glburns@mail. wsu.edu. The 60-item PI was reprinted in the original paper by Sanavio (1988) and in a compilation of measures by Shear et al. (2000). Information regarding the original PI may be obtained from the author, Ezio Sanavio, Dipartimento di psicologia generale, via Venezia 8, 35131, Padova, Italy; (fax) +49 8276600; (e-mail) sanavio@ux1.unipd.it. An English version of the original PI may also be purchased from Nfer Nelson, Darville House, 2 Oxford Road East, Windsor, Berkshire, SL4 1DF, United Kingdom, (tel) +44 1753 858961; (fax) +44 1753 856830.

RESPONSIBILITY ATTITUDE SCALE (RAS) AND RESPONSIBILITY INTERPRETATIONS QUESTIONNAIRE (RIQ)

Original Citation

Salkovskis, P. M., Wroe, A. L., Gledhill, A., Morrison, N., Forrester, E., Richards, C., Reynolds, M., & Thorpe, S. (2000). Responsibility attitudes and interpretations are characteristic of obsessive compulsive disorder. *Behaviour Research and Therapy, 38,* 347–372.

Purpose

To measure responsibility-related beliefs as they apply to obsessive-compulsive disorder.

Description

According to Salkovskis's cognitive theory of obsessions (Salkovskis, 1985, 1998), OCD is associated with a tendency to interpret one's cognitive intrusions (i.e., obsessions) as indicating possible responsibility for causing harm to oneself or others. Compulsions and neutralizing behaviors are hypothesized to be driven, in part, by a desire to prevent harm from occurring. The RAS and RIQ are designed to measure responsibility beliefs that are believed to contribute to the maintenance of OCD.

The RAS is a 26-item self-report scale designed to assess general attitudes, assumptions, and beliefs about responsibility. Each item describes a general belief about responsibility that the individual rates according to how much he or she agrees with the statement. Items are rated on a seven-point scale ranging from 1 (totally agree) to 7 (totally disagree).

The RIQ is a 22-item self-report scale designed to assess the frequency of and belief in specific interpretations regarding intrusive thoughts about possible harm. In the first part (section F), individuals rate the frequency with which they experienced 22 specific responsibility-related ideas during periods when they were bothered by intrusive thoughts, impulses, or images in the previous 2 weeks. Items are divided into two sections: F1 (high-responsibility items) and F2 (low-responsibility items). Each item is rated using a five-point scale, ranging from 0 (idea never occurred) to 4 (idea always occurred when I had worrying intrusive thoughts). In the second part (section B), the individual rates the extent to which he or she believed in each of the 22 responsibility-related ideas during the previous 2 weeks. Again, items are divided into two sections: B1 (high-responsibility items) and B2 (low-responsibility items). For the belief subscales, each item is rated on a scale ranging from 0 (I did not believe this idea at all) to 100 (I was completely convinced this idea was true).

Administration and Scoring

The RAS and RIQ each take 5 to 10 minutes to complete. To score the RAS, first assign a score for each item as follows: 1 = totally agree; 2 = agree very much; 3 = agree slightly; 4 = neutral; 5 = disagree slightly; 6 = disagree very much; 7 = totally disagree. The total score on the RAS is the mean of all 26 items.

The RIQ generates four subscales. An F1 score is computed by calculating the means of the 16 items in section F1. An F2 score is computed by calculating the means of the 6 items in section F2. A B1 score is computed by calculating the means of the 16 items in section B1. A B2 score is computed by calculating the means of the 6 items in section B2. Scores for the F1 and F2 subscales can range from 0 to 4. Scores for the B1 and B2 subscales can range from 0 to 100.

Psychometric Properties

Sample Scores and Norms.   In a validation study by Salkovskis et al. (2000), mean scores on the RAS were 4.69 (SD = 1.01) for individuals with OCD, 4.0 (SD = 0.92) for individuals with other anxiety disorders, and 3.48 (SD = 1.01) for nonclinical controls. On the RIQ, the mean frequency scores for the high-responsibility interpretations were 1.94 (SD = 0.87) for individuals with OCD, 1.04 (SD = 0.85) for individuals with other anxiety disorders, and 0.67 (SD = 0.61) for nonclinical controls. The mean belief scores for the high-responsibility interpretations were 49.46 (SD = 15.76) for individuals with OCD, 27.91 (SD = 25.56) for individuals with other anxiety disorders, and 15.76 (SD = 17.52) for nonclinical controls. Means were not reported for either the frequency or belief scores on the low responsibility interpretations, due to low test–retest reliability on these subscales (Salkovskis et al., 2000).

Reliability.   In a mixed sample of anxious and nonanxious participants, test–retest reliability was high for the RAS over a 2-week period (r = .94). Internal consistency for the RAS was excellent, with a Cronbach's alpha of .92 (Salkovskis et al., 2000). In a mixed sample of anxious and nonanxious participants, test–retest reliability coefficients were .90 for the frequency of high-responsibility interpretations, .69 for the frequency of low-responsibility interpretations, .80 for the belief in the high-responsibility interpretations, and .22 for the belief in the low-responsibility interpretations. Internal consistency for all four subscales of the RIQ was good to excellent with Cronbach's alphas ranging from .86 to .93. (Salkovskis et al., 2000).

Validity.   In the validation study by Salkovskis et al. (2000), individuals with OCD scored significantly higher on the RAS than did individuals with other anxiety disorders and nonclinical controls. The RAS was significantly correlated with scores on other OCD-related measures, with rs ranging from .54 to .57. These correlations were essentially unchanged when the effects of anxiety and depression were partialed out. A regression analysis confirmed that the RAS is a primary predictor of obsessionality, but not of anxiety or depression (Salkovskis et al., 2000).

For the RIQ, validity data were only analyzed for the frequency of and beliefs regarding high-responsibility interpretations because of the low test–retest reliabilities for the low-responsibility interpretations. Both high-responsibility interpretation subscales were higher among individuals with OCD than among individuals with other anxiety disorders and nonclinical controls. Both subscales were significantly correlated with other measures of OCD symptomatology, although these correlations were smaller (but still significant) when the effects of anxiety and depression were partialed out (Salkovskis et al., 2000). A regression analysis confirmed that the RIQ is a primary predictor of obsessionality, but not of anxiety or depression (Salkovskis et al., 2000).

Source

The RAS and RIQ are both reprinted in the source article by Salkovskis et al. (2000), and in Appendix B. Additional information may be obtained from the author, Paul Salkovskis, Ph.D., Department of Psychology, Institute of Psychiatry, De Crespigny Park, Denmark Hill, London, SE5 8AF, United Kingdom; (tel) 44-20-7848-5039; (fax) 44-020-7848-0591; (e-mail) p.salkovskis@iop.kcl.ac.uk.

THOUGHT–ACTION FUSION SCALE (TAF SCALE)

Original Citation

Shafran, R., Thordarson, D. S., & Rachman, S. (1996). Thought–action fusion in obsessive compulsive disorder. *Journal of Anxiety Disorders, 10*, 379–391.

Purpose

To measure a cognitive distortion associated with obsessive-compulsive disorder.

Description

The construct of thought–action fusion (TAF) has two components: (1) the belief that thinking about an unacceptable or disturbing event will make it more likely to happen (e.g., "if I think about harming a loved one, I will be more likely to do it") and (2) the belief that having an unacceptable thought is almost the moral equivalent to carrying out the unacceptable action (e.g., "thinking about harming a loved one is almost just as bad as actually doing so"; Shafran, Thordarson, & Rachman, 1996). TAF has been hypothesized to contribute to beliefs about responsibility and has been theoretically and empirically linked to OCD (Rachman & Shafran, 1998).

The TAF Scale is a 19-item self-report questionnaire that measures three types of TAF: fusion of thoughts and actions regarding issues of morality, fusion of thoughts and actions regarding causing harm to others, and fusion of thoughts and actions regarding causing harm to oneself. Each item is scored on a five-point scale ranging from 0 (strongly disagree) to 4 (strongly agree).

Administration and Scoring

The TAF Scale takes 5 to 10 minutes to administer. The instrument is scored by adding up the items in each of three subscales: *moral* (sum of items, 1, 3, 4, 6, 8, 10, 11, 13, 15, 17–19); *likelihood-others* (sum of items 2, 5, 7, 9); *likelihood-self* (sum of items 12, 14, 16). No items are reverse-scored.

Psychometric Properties

Sample Scores and Norms. Shafran et al. (1996) report means for an obsessional sample and a community adult sample. Mean scores for the obsessional sample were 20.03 (SD = 13.17) on the moral subscale, 4.77 (SD = 4.74) on the likelihood-other subscale, and 4.41 (SD = 2.09) on the likelihood-self subscale. Mean scores for the community sample were 12.74 (SD = 11.13) on the moral subscale, 1.03 (SD = 2.14) on the likelihood-other subscale, and 2.09 (SD = 2.49) on the likelihood-self subscale.

Reliability. Internal consistency for the TAF subscales was good to excellent, with Cronbach's alphas ranging from .85 to .96 across obsessional and nonanxious groups (Shafran et al., 1996). Test–retest reliability is not available.

Validity. Although a three-factor solution (consistent with the three subscales of the TAF Scale) emerged in two nonanxious samples, a two-factor solution, including a "moral" factor and a likelihood factor (including items from both the likelihood-other and likelihood-self subscales), emerged for an obsessional sample (Shafran et al., 1996). Individuals in the obsessional sample scored higher than adults in a community sample on all three TAF subscales. However, for all subscales except the likelihood-other subscale, differences between the obsessional sample and a student sample were nonsignificant. In a group of obsessional individuals, all three TAF subscales were significantly correlated with measures of OCD checking (rs ranged from .31 to .38) and depression (rs ranged from .33 to .42). Only the likelihood-other subscale was significantly (although weakly) correlated with OCD cleaning (r = .18).

Source

The TAF Scale is reprinted in the original validation paper by Shafran et al. (1996) and in Appendix B. Additional information may be obtained from the author, Roz Shafran, Ph.D., Oxford University Department of Psychiatry, Warneford Hospital, Oxford, OX3 7JX, United Kingdom; (tel) +44 1865 226 479; (fax) +44 1865 226 244; (e-mail) roz.shafran@psych.ox.ac.uk.

YALE–BROWN OBSESSIVE COMPULSIVE SCALE (Y-BOCS)

Original Citations

Goodman, W. K., Price, L. H., Rasmussen, S. A., Mazure, C., Delgado, P., Heninger, G. R., & Charney, D. S. (1989). The Yale–Brown Obsessive Compulsive Scale: II. Validity. *Archives of General Psychiatry, 46,* 1012–1016.

Goodman, W. K., Price, L. H., Rasmussen, S. A., Mazure, C., Fleischmann, R. L., Hill, C. L., Heninger, G. R., & Charney, D. S. (1989). The Yale–Brown Obsessive Compulsive Scale: I. Development, use, and reliability. *Archives of General Psychiatry, 46,* 1006–1011.

Purpose

To measure the severity and types of symptoms in obsessive-compulsive disorder.

Description

The Y-BOCS is a 10-item clinician-administered semistructured interview that measures the severity of obsessions and compulsions. Each item is rated on a five-point scale ranging from 0 to 4, and is anchored by slightly different descriptors, although generally a 0 reflects no symptoms and a 4 reflects extremely severe symptoms. The Y-BOCS generates ratings of severity for obsessions and compulsions, as well as an overall rating of severity. In addition to the official 10 items, the authors developed 9 additional investigational items that measure insight, avoidance, indecisiveness, perceived responsibility, slowness, pervasive doubting, global severity, global improvement, and the clinician's impressions regarding the reliability of the ratings obtained. However, these additional items are rarely used and are not included in the scoring of either the total or subscale scores.

The interview is usually preceded by a 64-item clinician-administered checklist that asks about the presence of various obsessions and compulsions, both currently and in the past. Items on the checklist are checked if present and left blank if absent. Once identifying the pattern of current symptoms, the most prominent symptoms (including the most prominent obsessions, compulsions, and avoidance behaviors) are recorded on a target symptom list. The Y-BOCS interview is administered after the target symptoms have been identified. In Appendix B, we have included the most recent, expanded version of the checklist, taken from the Revised Y-BOCS that is currently in development.

Administration and Scoring

The Y-BOCS takes 30 minutes to administer and can take longer if the symptom checklist is used to obtain detailed symptom information. Subsequent administrations usually become quicker. A total score on the Y-BOCS is obtained by calculating the sum of items 1 through 10. Subscale scores are obtained for obsessions (sum of items 1–5) and compulsions (sum of items 6–10). The total Y-BOCS score can range from 0 to 40 and the total subscale scores can range from 0 to 20.

Psychometric Properties

Sample Scores and Norms. Goodman, Price, Rasmussen, Mazure, Fleischmann, et al. (1989) reported the mean Y-BOCS scores for a sample of OCD patients seen by four raters. Averaging across the four raters, the mean total Y-BOCS score was 21.9 ($SD = 8.0$) and the means for the obsessions and compulsions subscales were 10.7 ($SD = 4.0$) and 11.2 ($SD = 4.0$), respectively. These means are comparable to those found in other studies. Generally, for participation in pharmaceutical trials with OCD patients, a cutoff of 16 or higher is used to determine eligibility (Shear et al., 2000).

Reliability. In the original study by Goodman, Price, Rasmussen, Mazure, Fleischmann, et al. (1989), internal consistency was high for the total Y-BOCS scale, with Cronbach's alphas ranging from .88 to .91 across four raters. A subsequent study by Woody, Steketee, and Chambless (1995) found lower levels of internal consistency, with alphas of .69 for the total scale, .77 for the obsessions subscale, and .51 for the compulsions subscale. Several of the items in the compulsions subscale (items 6, 8, and 9) had particularly low correlations with the entire compulsions subscale. Despite the mixed internal consistency findings, the Y-BOCS has consistently been found to have excellent interrater reliability (e.g., Goodman, Price, Rasmussen, Mazure, Fleischmann, et al., 1989; Woody et al., 1995). Test–retest reliability at 1-week intervals also appears to be excellent (Kim, Dysken, & Kuskowski, 1990).

Validity. Factor analyses of 10 Y-BOCS items have consistently supported a two-factor structure for the Y-BOCS, although they have been inconsistent regarding which items belong in which factors. An initial study by McKay, Danyko, Neziroglu, and Yaryura-Tobias (1995) supported the distinction between obsessions and compulsions, whereas subsequent studies have found that factors are best defined by other dimensions (e.g., Amir, Foa, & Coles, 1997; McKay, Neziroglu, Stevens, & Yaryura-Tobias, 1998). A factor analysis of the symptom checklist found four main groupings (obsessions/checking, symmetry/ordering, contamination/cleaning, and hoarding), with considerable heterogeneity within factors and overlap across factors (Summerfeldt, Richter, Antony, & Swinson, 1999).

The total and subscale scores on the Y-BOCS have generally been found to correlate significantly with other measures of OCD symptomatology, but also with measures of anxiety and depression (Goodman, Price, Rasmussen, Mazure, Delgado, et al., 1989; Richter et al., 1994; Woody et al., 1995). Finally, the Y-BOCS is sensitive to change following cognitive–behavioral and pharmacological treatments for OCD (Goodman, Price, Rasmussen, Mazure, Delgado, et al., 1989; van Oppen, Emmelkamp, et al., 1995; Woody et al., 1995). In fact, the Y-BOCS has become the gold standard for measuring symptom improvement in OCD treatment studies (Shear et al., 2000).

Alternative Forms

A self-report version of the Y-BOCS (recently updated by Baer, 2000) has been shown to have good psychometric properties (Steketee, Frost, & Bogart, 1996; Warren, Zgourides, & Monto, 1993), as has a computerized version (Rosenfeld, Dar, Anderson, Kobak, & Greist (1992). In addition, modified versions of the Y-BOCS have been developed for a number of populations including children with OCD (Scahill et al., 1997), individuals with body dysmorphic disorder (Phillips et al., 1997), individuals who shop compulsively (Monahan, Black, &

Gabel, 1996), and individuals with trichotillomania (Stanley, Prather, Wagner, Davis, & Swann, 1993).

Finally, a new version of the Y-BOCS is in development. Goodman, Rasmussen, and Price (1999) are in the final stages of developing an official second edition of the Y-BOCS. This scale retains the basic structure of the original, but there are several important changes. First, item 4 (resistance against obsessions) has been replaced with an item measuring "obsession-free interval." Second, items 1 and 6 are scored on a six-point scale instead of a five-point scale, as was the case in the original Y-BOCS. Third, the Revised Y-BOCS includes expanded assessment of avoidance behaviors. Finally, the symptom checklist has been expanded and modified to be more consistent with types of symptoms reported by patients with OCD. The Revised Y-BOCS has 12 items, including 5 that measure the severity of obsessions, 5 that measure severity of compulsions, 1 that measures avoidance, and 1 that measures insight.

Source

The Y-BOCS has been reprinted in Appendix B. We have also included the most recent, expanded version of the symptom checklist (from the Revised Y-BOCS). The self-report version of the Y-BOCS is reprinted in Baer (2000). Further information on the Y-BOCS may be obtained from the author, Wayne K. Goodman, M.D., Department of Psychiatry, University of Florida, Brain Institute Room L4-1000, P.O. Box 100256, Gainesville, FL 32610-0256, USA; (tel) 352-392-3681; (fax) 352-392-9887; (e-mail) wkgood@psych.med.ufl.edu.

BRIEF DESCRIPTIONS OF ADDITIONAL MEASURES: OBSESSIVE-COMPULSIVE DISORDER

Brown Assessment of Beliefs Scale (BABS)

The BABS is a seven-item clinician-administered scale designed to assess delusional beliefs and degree of insight in OCD and other psychiatric disorders. Only the first six items are included in the total score. A description of the scale and its psychometric properties is available in the original validation paper by Eisen et al. (1998). Further information may be obtained from the author, Jane L. Eisen, M.D., Department of Psychiatry, Brown University Medical School, Butler Hospital, 345 Blackstone Blvd., Providence, RI 02906, USA, (tel) 401-455-6243; (fax) 401-455-6442; (e-mail) jane_eisen@brown.edu.

Hamburg Obsession/Compulsion Inventory–Short Form (HOCI-S)

The HOCI-S is a 72-item, true/false, self-report scale designed to assess symptoms of OCD. The instrument generates six subscales: *checking, cleaning, arranging things, counting/ touching/speaking, thoughts of words/pictures*, and *thoughts about doing harm to oneself or others*. The HOCI-S is a revision of the 188-item Hamburg Obsession/Compulsion Inventory (Zaworka, Hand, Lünenschloss, & Jauernig, 1983). The psychometric properties of the HOCI-S are provided in a paper by Klepsch, Zaworka, Hand, Lünenschloss, and Jauernig (1991).

Interpretations of Intrusions Inventory (III)

The III is a new 31-item self-report scale for measuring interpretations of recently occurring obsessive thoughts. Three subscales are generated: *importance of thoughts*, *control of thoughts*, and *responsibility*. The psychometric properties of the III are available in a recent paper by the Obsessive Compulsive Cognitions Working Group (in press) and the items are reprinted in a recent chapter by Taylor, Kyrios, and Thordarson (in press). Further information may be obtained by contacting Gail Steketee, Ph.D., Boston University School of Social Work, 264 Bay State Road, Boston, MA 02215, USA; (tel) 617-353-3750; (fax) 617-353-5612; (e-mail) steketee@bu.edu.

Leyton Obsessional Inventory (LOI)

The LOI uses a card sorting procedure to obtain yes/no replies to 69 questions regarding obsessional symptoms. The scale is also sometimes administered in a self-report questionnaire format. The instrument generates two subscales: *obsessive symptoms* and *obsessive personality traits*. The LOI items, instructions for completing the scale, and psychometric properties of the LOI are provided in a paper by Cooper (1970) as well as in a compilation of scales by Schutte and Malouff (1995).

National Institute of Mental Health Global Obsessive-Compulsive Scale (NIMH-GOCS)

The NIMH-GOCS is a single-item clinician-rated scale for assessing OCD severity (Insel et al., 1983). Scores range from 1 (no difficulty) to 15 (most severe). Despite its popularity in pharmacotherapy treatment research, the psychometric properties of the NIMH-GOCS have not been well studied.

National Institute of Mental Health Obsessive-Compulsive Rating Scale (NIMH-OC)

The NIMH-OC is a brief clinician-rated scale for assessing OCD severity. Although this is a popular scale in pharmaceutical trials, its psychometric properties are not well established. Versions with eight items (see Pato & Pato, 1991) and four items (see Rapoport, Elkins, & Mikkelsen, 1980) have been reported in the literature.

Obsessive Beliefs Questionnaire (OBQ)

The OBQ is a new 87-item self-report scale for measuring dysfunctional assumptions held by people with OCD. Six subscales are generated: *overestimation of threat*, *tolerance of uncertainty*, *importance of thoughts*, *control of thoughts*, *responsibility*, and *perfectionism*. The psychometric properties of the OBQ are available in a recent paper by the Obsessive Compulsive Cognitions Working Group (in press) and the items are reprinted in a recent chapter by Taylor et al. (in press). Further information may be obtained by contacting Gail Steketee, Ph.D., Boston University School of Social Work, 264 Bay State Road, Boston, MA 02215, USA; (tel) 617-353-3750; (fax) 617-353-5612; (e-mail) steketee@bu.edu.

Saving Inventory-Revised (SI)

The SI is an unpublished 26-item self-report scale designed to measure symptoms of compulsive hoarding, compulsive acquisition, and related symptoms (Frost, Steketee, & Kyrios, 1999). This scale is a revision of the Hoarding Scale (Frost & Gross, 1993). Additional information may be obtained from the author, Randy O. Frost, Ph.D., Department of Psychology, Smith College, Northampton, MA 01063, USA; (tel) 413-585-3911; (fax) 413-585-3786; (e-mail) rfrost@science.smith.edu.

Self-Rated Scale for Obsessive-Compulsive Disorder (SRS)

The SRS is a 35-item self-report scale for measuring symptoms of OCD. The items and psychometric properties of this scale are provided in a validation study by Kaplan (1994).

Symmetry, Ordering, and Arranging Questionnaire (SOAQ)

The SOAQ is a new 20-item self-report measure that assesses ordering, arranging, and need for symmetry and exactness in the placement of objects. The psychometric properties were described in a presentation by Radomsky and Rachman (2000) and a manuscript is currently being prepared for publication. Additional information may be obtained from the author, Adam Radomsky, Ph.D., Department of Psychology, Concordia University, 7141 Sherbrooke West, Montreal, QC, H4B 1R6, Canada; (tel) 514-848-2222; (fax) 514-848-4523; (e-mail) radomsky@vax2.concordia.ca.

Vancouver Obsessional Compulsive Inventory (VOCI)

The VOCI is a new 55-item self-report scale for measuring obsessions and compulsions. This scale is a revision of the popular Maudsley Obsessional Compulsive Inventory (MOC). Six subscales are generated: *contamination, checking, obsessions, hoarding, indecisiveness/ perfection/concern over mistakes*, and *routine/counting/slowness*. The psychometric properties of the VOCI were presented at an international conference (Thordarson, Radomsky, Rachman, Shafran, & Sawchuk, 1997) and a manuscript is now in preparation for publication. Further information may obtained by contacting Dana S. Thordarson, Ph.D., Department of Psychiatry, University of British Columbia, 2255 Wesbrook Mall, Vancouver, BC, V6T 2A1, Canada; (tel) 604-822-8030; (fax) 604-822-7756; (e-mail) danat@unixg.ubc.ca.

BRIEF DESCRIPTIONS FOR OBSESSIVE-COMPULSIVE SPECTRUM DISORDER MEASURES

Body Dysmorphic Disorder Diagnostic Module (BDD Diagnostic Module)

The BDD Diagnostic Module is a brief clinician-administered interview for diagnosing body dysmorphic disorder. Versions are available for adolescents and adults. The psychometric properties of the BDD Diagnostic Module were presented at a conference by Phillips, Atala, and Pope (1995). A copy of the instrument and any additional information may be obtained from the author, Katharine A. Phillips, M.D., Butler Hospital, 345 Blackstone Blvd., Providence, RI 02906, USA; (tel) 401-455-6490; (fax) 401-455-6539; (e-mail) Katharine _Phillips@brown.edu; (webpage) www.butler.org/bdd/.

Body Dysmorphic Disorder Examination (BDDE)

The BDDE is designed to measure symptoms of body dysmorphic disorder and negative body image. The scale is available in a semistructured interview format (33 items) and a self-report format (26 items). The psychometric properties of the BDDE were reported in a validation study by Rosen and Reiter (1996). A copy of the instrument and any additional information may be obtained from the author, James C. Rosen, Ph.D., Department of Psychology, University of Vermont, Burlington, VT 05405, USA; (tel) 802-656-2680; (e-mail) james.rosen@uvm.edu.

Body Dysmorphic Disorder Questionnaire (BDDQ)

The BDDQ is a four-item self-report scale designed to screen for the presence of body dysmorphic disorder. Versions are available for adolescents and adults. The psychometric properties of the BDDQ were presented at a conference by Phillips et al. (1995). A copy of the instrument and any additional information may be obtained from the author, Katharine A. Phillips, M.D., Butler Hospital, 345 Blackstone Blvd., Providence, RI 02906, USA; (tel) 401-455-6490; (fax) 401-455-6539; (e-mail) Katharine_Phillips@brown.edu; (webpage) www.butler.org/bdd/.

Massachusetts General Hospital (MGH) Hairpulling Scale

The MGH Hairpulling Scale is a seven-item self-report instrument for assessing severity of repetitive hair pulling and trichotillomania. The development and psychometric properties of the scale are described in two papers by the authors (Keuthen et al., 1995; O'Sullivan et al., 1995). The instrument is reprinted in a paper by Keuthen et al. (1995). Additional information may be obtained from the author, Nancy J. Keuthen, Ph.D., Trichotillomania Clinic and Research Unit, Department of Psychiatry, Massachusetts General Hospital–East Building, 149 13th Street, 9th floor, Charlestown, MA 02129-2060; (tel) 617-726-4074; (fax) 617-726-4078; (e-mail) keuthen@psych.mgh.harvard.edu.

NIMH Trichotillomania Severity Scale (NIMH-TSS) and Trichotillomania Impairment Scale (NIMH-TIS)

The NIMH-TSS is a five-item clinician-rated measure for assessing the severity of trichotillomania (Swedo et al., 1989). The NIMH-TIS provides a single rating of impairment caused by hair pulling (Swedo et al., 1989). Both scales were derived from the Y-BOCS. The psychometric properties of these scales were reported in a paper by Stanley, Breckenridge, Snyder, and Novy (1999). Additional information may be obtained from the author, Susan

Swedo, M.D., Child Psychiatry, NIMH, 10 Center Drive MSC 1381, Building 10, Room 4N222, Bethesda, MD 20892-1381, USA; (tel) 301-496-3501; (fax) 301-480-8348; (e-mail) swedos@irp.nimh.nih.gov.

Psychiatric Institute Trichotillomania Scale (PITS)

The PITS is a six-item clinician-rated measure for assessing the features and severity of trichotillomania. The scale is reprinted in a paper by the authors (Winchel et al., 1992). In addition, the psychometric properties of scale were reported in a recent paper by another group of researchers (Stanley et al., 1999). Additional information may be obtained from the author, Dr. Barbara Stanley; New York State Psychiatric Institute, Unit 42, 1051 Riverside Drive, New York, NY 10032, USA; (tel) 212-543-5918; (fax) 212-543-6017; (e-mail) bstanley@neuron. cpmc.columbia.edu.

Yale–Brown Obsessive Compulsive Scale Modified for Body Dysmorphic Disorder (BDD-YBOCS)

The BDD-YBOCS is a 12-item clinician-administered interview for assessing the severity of body dysmorphic disorder. Versions are available for adolescents and adults. The psychometric properties of the BDD-YBOCS were published in a validation study by Phillips et al. (1997). A copy of the instrument and any additional information may be obtained from the author, Katharine A. Phillips, M.D., Butler Hospital, 345 Blackstone Blvd., Providence, RI 02906, USA; (tel) 401-455-6490; (fax) 401-455-6539; (e-mail) Katharine_Phillips@brown. edu; (webpage) www.butler.org/bdd/.

Yale–Brown Obsessive Compulsive Scale–Shopping Version (YBOCS-SV)

The YBOCS-SV is a 10-item clinician-administered interview for assessing the severity of compulsive shopping. It is a modification of the original Y-BOCS. The instrument is reprinted along with its psychometric properties in a paper by the authors (Monahan et al., 1996). Additional information may be obtained from the author, Donald W. Black, M.D., Psychiatry Research–MEB, University of Iowa College of Medicine, Iowa City, IA 52242, USA; (tel) 319-353-4431; (fax) 319-353-3003; (e-mail) donald-black@uiowa.edu.

Yale–Brown Obsessive Compulsive Scale–Trichotillomania Version (YBOCS-TM)

The YBOCS-TM is a 10-item clinician-administered interview for assessing the severity of trichotillomania. It is a modification of the original Y-BOCS. The psychometric properties of this scale are described in the original validation study (Stanley et al., 1993) as well as in a more recent comparison with other instruments (Stanley et al., 1999). Additional information may be obtained from the author, Melinda A. Stanley, Ph.D., University of Texas–Houston Health Sciences Center, 1300 Moursund St., Houston, TX 77030-3497, USA; (tel) 713-500-2600; (fax) 713-500-2530; (e-mail) melinda.a.stanley@uth.tmc.edu.

Yale Global Tic Severity Scale (YGTSS)

The YGTSS is a brief clinician-administered interview for assessing the range and severity of clinical tics. It may be used with children or adults. The scale is reprinted in the original validation paper by Leckman et al. (1989). Psychometric properties are presented in the Leckman et al. (1989) paper as well as in a paper by Walkup, Rosenberg, Brown, and Singer (1992). Additional information may be obtained from the author, James F. Leckman, M.D., Room I-267 SHM, Child Study Center, Yale University, 230 South Frontage Road, P.O. Box 207900, New Haven, CT 06520-7900, USA; (tel) 203-785-7971; (fax) 203-785-7611; (e-mail) james.leckman@yale.edu.

REFERENCES

Amir, N., Foa, E. B., & Coles, M. E. (1997). Factor structure of the Yale–Brown Obsessive Compulsive Scale. *Psychological Assessment, 9*, 312–316.

Baer, L. (2000). *Getting control: Overcoming your obsessions and compulsions, revised edition.* New York: Plume.

Cooper, J. (1970). The Leyton Obsessional Inventory. *Psychological Medicine, 1*, 48–64.

Cottraux, J., Bouvard, M., Defayolle, M., & Messy, P. (1988). Validity and factorial structure study of the Compulsive Activity Checklist. *Behavior Therapy, 19*, 45–53.

Dent, H. R., & Salkovskis, P. M. (1986). Clinical measures of depression, anxiety, and obsessionality in nonclinical populations. *Behaviour Research and Therapy, 24*, 689–691.

Eisen, J. L., Phillips, K. A., Baer, L., Beer, D. A., Atala, K., & Rasmussen, S. A. (1998). The Brown Assessment of Beliefs Scale: Reliability and validity. *American Journal of Psychiatry, 155*, 102–108.

Emmelkamp, P. M. G., Kraaijkamp, H. J. M., & van den Hout, M. A. (1999). Assessment of obsessive-compulsive disorder. *Behavior Modification, 23*, 269–279.

Freeston, M. H., Ladouceur, R., Rheaume, J., Letart, H., Gagnon, F., & Thibodeau, N. (1994). Self-report of obsessions and worry. *Behaviour Research and Therapy, 32*, 29–36.

Frost, R. O., & Gross, R. C. (1993). The hoarding of possessions. *Behaviour Research and Therapy, 31*, 367–381.

Frost, R. O., Steketee, G., & Kyrios, M. *The Saving Inventory.* Northampton, MA: Department of Psychology, Smith College.

Gayton, W. F., Clavin, R. H., Clavin, S. L., & Broida, J. (1994). Further validation of the Indecisiveness Scale. *Psychological Reports, 75*, 1631–1634.

Goodman, W. K., Rasmussen, S. A., & Price, L. H. (1999). *Florida Yale–Brown Obsessive Compulsive Scale (FLY-BOCS).* Gainesville: Department of Psychiatry, University of Florida College of Medicine.

Insel, T. R., Murphy, D. L., Cohen, R. M., Alterman, I., Kilts, C., & Linniola, M. (1983). Obsessive-compulsive disorder: A double-blind trial of clomipramine and clorgyline. *Archives of General Psychiatry, 40*, 605–612.

Kaplan, S. L. (1994). A Self-Rated Scale for Obsessive Compulsive Disorder. *Journal of Clinical Psychology, 50*, 564–574.

Keuthen, N. J., O'Sullivan, R. L., Ricciardi, J. N., Hera, D., Savage, C. R., Borgmann, A. S., Jenike, M. A., & Baer, L. (1995). The Massachusetts General Hospital (MGH) Hairpulling Scale: 1. Development and factor analyses. *Psychotherapy and Psychosomatics, 64*, 141–145.

Kim, S., Dysken, M., & Kuskowski, M. (1990). The Yale–Brown Obsessive Compulsive Scale: A reliability and validity study. *Psychiatry Research, 41*, 37–44.

Klepsch, R., Zaworka, W., Hand, I., Lünenschloss, K., & Jauernig, G. (1991). Derivation and validation of the Hamburg Obsession/Compulsion Inventory–Short Form (HOCI-S): First results. *Psychological Assessment: A Journal of Consulting and Clinical Psychology, 3*, 196–201.

Kyrios, M., Bhar, S., & Wade, D. (1996). The assessment of obsessive-compulsive phenomena: Psychometric and normative data on the Padua Inventory from an Australian non-clinical student sample. *Behaviour Research and Therapy, 34*, 85–95.

Leckman, J. F., Riddle, M. A., Hardin, M. T., Ort, S. I., Swartz, K. L., Stevenson, J., & Cohen, D. J. (1989). The Yale Global Tic Severity Scale: Initial testing of a clinician-rated scale of tic severity. *Journal of the American Academy of Child and Adolescent Psychiatry, 28*, 566–573.

Mancini, F., Gragnani, A., Orazi, F., & Pietrangeli, M. G. (1999). Obsessions and compulsions: Normative data on the Padua Inventory from an Italian non-clinical adolescent sample. *Behaviour Research and Therapy, 37*, 919–925.

Marks, I. M., Stern, R. S., Mawson, D., Cobb, J., & McDonald, R. (1980). Clomipramine and exposure for obsessive-compulsive rituals—I. *British Journal of Psychiatry, 136,* 1–25.

Mawson, D., Marks, I. M., & Ramm, L. (1982). Clomipramine and exposure for chronic obsessive-compulsive rituals: Two year follow-up and further findings. *British Journal of Psychiatry, 140,* 11–18.

McDonald, A. M., & de Silva, P. (1999). The assessment of obsessionality using the Padua Inventory: Its validity in a British non-clinical sample. *Personality and Individual Differences, 27,* 1027–1046.

McKay, D., Danyko, S., Neziroglu, F., & Yaryura-Tobias, J. A. (1995). Factor structure of the Yale–Brown Obsessive-Compulsive Scale: A two dimensional measure. *Behaviour Research and Therapy, 33,* 865–869.

McKay, D., Neziroglu, F., Stevens, K., Yaryura-Tobias, J. A. (1998). The Yale–Brown Obsessive-Compulsive Scale: Confirmatory factor analytic findings. *Journal of Psychopathology and Behavioral Assessment, 20,* 265–274.

Monahan, P., Black, D. W., & Gabel, J. (1996). Reliability and validity of a scale to measure change in persons with compulsive buying. *Psychiatry Research, 64,* 59–67.

Neziroglu, F., Stevens, K. P., Yaryura-Tobias, J. A., & McKay, D. (in press). Predictive validity of the Overvalued Ideas Scale: Outcome in obsessive-compulsive and body dysmorphic disorders. *Behaviour Research and Therapy.*

Obsessive Compulsive Cognitions Working Group. (in press). Development and initial validation of the Obsessive Beliefs Questionnaire and the Interpretation of Intrusions Inventory. *Behaviour Research and Therapy.*

O'Sullivan, R. L., Keuthen, N. J., Hayday, C. F., Ricciardi, J. N., Buttolph, M. L., Jenike, M. A., & Baer, L. (1995). The Massachusetts General Hospital (MGH) Hairpulling Scale: 2. Reliability and validity. *Psychotherapy and Psychosomatics, 64,* 146–148.

Pato, M. T., & Pato, C. N. (1991). Psychometrics in obsessive-compulsive disorder. In J. Zohar, T. Insel, & S. Rasmussen (Eds.), *The psychobiology of obsessive compulsive disorder* (pp. 44–88). Berlin: Springer.

Phillips, K. A., Atala, K. D., & Pope, H. G. (1995). Diagnostic instruments for body dysmorphic disorder [published abstract]. *New research programs and abstracts* [p. 157]. American Psychiatric Association 148th annual meeting. Miami, FL: American Psychiatric Association.

Phillips, K. A., Hollander, E., Rasmussen, S. A., Aronowitz, B. R., de Caria, C., Goodman, W. K. (1997). A severity rating scale for body dysmorphic disorder: Development of reliability and validity of a modified version of the Yale–Brown Obsessive Compulsive Scale. *Psychopharmacology Bulletin, 33,* 17–22.

Philpott, R. (1975). Recent advances in the behavioral measurement of obsessional illness: Difficulties common to these and other instruments. *Scottish Medical Journal, 20,* 33–40.

Rachman, S., & Shafran, R. (1998). Cognitive and behavioral features of obsessive-compulsive disorder. In R. P. Swinson, M. M. Antony, S. Rachman, & M. A. Richter (Eds.), *Obsessive compulsive disorder: Theory, research, and treatment* (pp. 51–78). New York: Guilford.

Radomsky, A S., & Rachman, S. (2000, November). *The Symmetry, Ordering, and Arranging Questionnaire (SOAQ).* Paper presented at the meeting of the Association for Advancement of Behavior Therapy, New Orleans, LA.

Rapoport, J. L., Elkins, R., & Mikkelsen, E. (1980). Clinical controlled trial of clomipramine in adolescents with obsessive-compulsive disorder. *Psychopharmacology Bulletin, 16,* 61–63.

Richter, M. A., Cox, B. J., & Direnfeld, D. M. (1994). A comparison of three assessment instruments for obsessive-compulsive symptoms. *Journal of Behavior Therapy and Experimental Psychiatry, 25,* 143–147.

Rosen, J. C., & Reiter, J. (1996). Development of the Body Dysmorphic Disorder Examination. *Behaviour Research and Therapy, 34,* 755–766.

Rosenfeld, R., Dar, R., Anderson, D., Kobak, K. A., & Greist, J. H. (1992). A computer-administered version of the Yale–Brown Obsessive-Compulsive Scale. *Psychological Assessment, 4,* 329–332.

Salkovskis, P. M. (1985). Obsessional–compulsive problems: A cognitive–behavioural analysis. *Behaviour Research and Therapy, 23,* 571–583.

Salkovskis, P. M. (1998). Psychological approaches to the understanding of obsessional problems. In R. P. Swinson, M. M. Antony, S. Rachman, & M. A. Richter (Eds.), *Obsessive compulsive disorder: Theory, research, and treatment* (pp. 33–50). New York: Guilford.

Sanavio, E. (1988). Obsessions and compulsions: The Padua Inventory. *Behaviour Research and Therapy, 26,* 169–177.

Scahill, L., Riddle, M. A., McSwiggen-Hardin, M., Ort, S. I., King, R. A., Goodman, W. K., Cicchetti, D., & Leckman, J. F. (1997). Children's Yale–Brown Obsessive Compulsive Scale: Reliability and validity. *Journal of the American Academy of Child and Adolescent Psychiatry, 36,* 844–852.

Schutte, N. S., & Malouff, J. M. (1995). *Sourcebook of adult assessment strategies.* New York: Plenum Press.

Shear, M. K., Feske, U., Brown, C., Clark, D. B., Mammen, O., & Scotti, J. (2000). Anxiety disorders measures. In Task Force for the Handbook of Psychiatric Measures (Eds.), *Handbook of psychiatric measures.* Washington, DC: American Psychiatric Association.

Simonds, L. M., Thorpe, S. J., & Elliott, S. A. (2000). The Obsessive Compulsive Inventory: Psychometric properties in a non-clinical student sample. *Behavioural and Cognitive Psychotherapy, 28,* 153–159.

Stanley, M. A., Breckenridge, J. K., Snyder, A. G., & Novy, D. M. (1999). Clinician-rated measures for hair pulling: A preliminary psychometric evaluation. *Journal of Psychopathology and Behavioral Assessment, 21,* 157–170.

Stanley, M. A., Prather, R. C., Wagner, A. L., Davis, M. L., & Swann, A. (1993). Can the Yale–Brown Obsessive-Compulsive Scale be used to assess trichotillomania? A preliminary report. *Behaviour Research and Therapy, 31,* 171–178.

Steketee, G., & Freund, B. (1993). Compulsive Activity Checklist (CAC): Further psychometric analyses and revision. *Behavioural Psychotherapy, 21,* 13–25.

Steketee, G., Frost, R., & Bogart, K. (1996). The Yale–Brown Obsessive Compulsive Scale: Interview versus self-report. *Behaviour Research and Therapy, 34,* 675–684.

Steketee, G., Frost, R. O., & Kyrios, M. (2000). *Assessment of cognition in compulsive hoarding.* Manuscript submitted for publication.

Sternberger, L. G., & Burns, G. L. (1990a). Compulsive Activity Checklist and the Maudsley Obsessional-Compulsive Inventory: Psychometric properties of two measures of obsessive-compulsive disorder. *Behavior Therapy, 21,* 117–127.

Sternberger, L. G., & Burns, G. L. (1990b). Maudsley Obsessional-Compulsive Inventory: Obsessions and compulsions in a nonclinical sample. *Behaviour Research and Therapy, 28,* 337–340.

Sternberger, L. G., & Burns, G. L. (1990c). Obsessions and compulsions: Psychometric properties of the Padua Inventory with an American college population. *Behaviour Research and Therapy, 28,* 341–345.

Summerfeldt, L. J., Richter, M. A., Antony, M. M., & Swinson, R. P. (1999). Symptom structure in obsessive compulsive disorder: A confirmatory factor-analytic study. *Behaviour Research and Therapy, 37,* 297–311.

Swedo, S. E., Leonard, H. L., Rapoport, J. L., Lenane, M. C., Goldberger, E. L., & Cheslow, D. L. (1989). A double-blind comparison of clomipramine and desipramine in the treatment trichotillomania (hair-pulling). *New England Journal of Medicine, 321,* 497–501.

Taylor, S. (1998). Assessment of obsessive-compulsive disorder. In R. P. Swinson, M. M. Antony, S. Rachman, & M. A. Richter (Eds.), *Obsessive compulsive disorder: Theory, research, and treatment* (pp. 229–257). New York: Guilford.

Taylor, S., Kyrios, M., & Thordarson, D. S. (in press). Stage III outcomes for the Obsessive Beliefs Questionnaire and the Interpretation of Intrusions Inventory. In R. O. Frost & G. Steketee (Eds.), *Cognitive approaches to obsessions and compulsions: Theory, assessment, and treatment.* Amsterdam: Elsevier.

Thordarson, D. S., Radomsky, A. S., Rachman, S., Shafran, R., & Sawchuk, C. N. (1997, November). *The Vancouver Obsessional Compulsive Inventory (VOCI).* Paper presented at the meeting of the Association for Advancement of Behavior Therapy, Miami Beach.

van Oppen, P. (1992). Obsessions and compulsions: Dimensional structure, reliability, convergent and divergent validity of the Padua Inventory. *Behaviour Research and Therapy, 30,* 631–637.

van Oppen, P., Emmelkamp, P. M. G., van Balkom, A. J. L. M., & van Dyck, R. (1995). The sensitivity to change of measures for obsessive-compulsive disorder. *Journal of Anxiety Disorders, 9,* 241–248.

van Oppen, P., Hoekstra, R. J., & Emmelkamp, P. M. G. (1995). The structure of obsessive-compulsive symptoms. *Behaviour Research and Therapy, 33,* 15–23.

Walkup, J. T., Rosenberg, L. A., Brown, J., & Singer, H. S. (1992). The validity of instruments measuring tic severity in Tourette's syndrome. *Journal of the American Academy of Child and Adolescent Psychiatry, 31,* 472–477.

Warren, R., Zgourides, G., & Monto, M. (1993). Self-report versions of the Yale–Brown Obsessive-Compulsive Scale: An assessment of a sample of normals. *Psychological Reports, 73,* 574.

Winchel, R. M., Jones, J. S., Molcho, A., Parsons, B., Stanley, B., & Stanley, M. (1992). The Psychiatric Institute Trichotillomania Scale (PITS). *Psychopharmacology Bulletin, 28,* 463–476.

Woody, S. R., Steketee, G., & Chambless, D. L. (1995). Reliability and validity of the Yale–Brown Obsessive-Compulsive Scale. *Behaviour Research and Therapy, 33,* 597–605.

Zaworka, W., Hand, I., Lünenschloss, K., & Jauernig, G. (1983). *Das Hamberger Zwangsinventar* [Hamburg Obsession Compulsion Inventory]. Weinheim, Germany: Beltz.

Chapter 18
Acute Stress Disorder and Posttraumatic Stress Disorder: A Brief Overview and Guide to Assessment

Susan M. Orsillo, Sonja V. Batten, and Charity Hammond

Clinicians working in a wide variety of settings, including inpatient units, outpatient clinics, and primary care centers, will inevitably encounter clients experiencing a range of levels of psychological distress in response to potentially traumatizing events (PTEs). However, whether the trauma history of these clients is identified and included in the clinician's conceptualization of the case is dependent on the nature and scope of the assessment. Post-traumatic stress disorder (PTSD), one of the most significant trauma-related disorders, is frequently overlooked in mental health settings (e.g., Mueser et al., 1998; Zimmerman & Mattia, 1999). Thus, structured assessment of PTEs and related psychopathology is critical for the application of effective treatments.

The purpose of this chapter is to provide a broad overview of issues related to the assessment of both PTEs and possible symptoms associated with these events. The assessment of trauma-related symptomatology will be described as it relates to two of the most common stress-related responses, acute stress disorder (ASD) and PTSD. As a comprehensive review of this topic is beyond the scope of this chapter, readers are referred to in-depth reviews published elsewhere (e.g., Briere, 1997; Foa & Rothbaum, 1998; Litz, Miller, Ruef, & McTeague,

Susan M. Orsillo, Sonja V. Batten, and Charity Hammond • National Center for PTSD–Women's Health Sciences Division, Boston VA Healthcare System, and Boston University School of Medicine, Boston, Massachusetts 02130.

in press; Litz & Weathers, 1994). All instruments mentioned in this chapter are described elsewhere in this book, along with full citations.

POTENTIALLY TRAUMATIZING EVENTS

Definition, Prevalence, and Relationship to Psychopathology

In DSM-IV, a traumatic event, as defined within the diagnostic criteria of ASD and PTSD, is evaluated by both objective and subjective criteria. First, the event must involve some threat to safety and physical integrity. Second, the individual must experience a significant emotional response to the event including fear, helplessness, or horror. This two-part definition of a traumatic event is critical, because responses to events are affected by an individual's context, and not all individuals perceive similar events to be "traumatic." Thus, in this chapter, we will use the term *potentially traumatizing event* to describe events that fit DSM-IV criteria and that may or may not be associated with the development of ASD or PTSD. A list of the specific PTEs that minimally should be assessed was developed following the National Institute of Mental Health–National Center for PTSD Conference on Assessment Standardization (Keane, Weathers, & Foa, 2000; see Table 1).

Epidemiological studies confirm that exposure to PTEs is unfortunately quite common. For instance, in the National Comorbidity Study, 60.7% of men and 51.2% of women reported that they had experienced at least one traumatic event, and the majority of respondents who reported any lifetime trauma were likely to have actually experienced two or more traumatic events (Kessler et al., 1999). However, whereas most individuals demonstrate immediate symptoms of psychological distress immediately following a PTE (e.g., Rothbaum, Foa, Riggs, Murdock, & Walsh, 1992), only a minority will develop chronic psychological distress related to their exposure. A variety of factors contribute to the development of posttrauma psychopathology, including: pretrauma psychological and demographic characteristics, characteristics of the trauma such as type of event, duration, and intensity, immediate psychological reactions to the event, posttrauma social support, additional posttrauma stressful events, and coping efforts directed toward managing posttrauma symptoms (e.g., Boscarino, 1995; Green, Grace, Lindy, Gleser, & Leonard, 1990; Harvey & Bryant, 1998; King, King, Foy, & Gudanowski, 1996).

Table 1. Minimum Categories
of PTEs to be Assessed

War-zone stressors
Sexual assault in childhood and adulthood
Robbery
Accidents
Technological disasters
Natural disasters or hazardous exposures
Sudden death of a loved one
Life-threatening illnesses
Witnessing or experiencing violence

Assessment of PTEs

General Issues. The assessment of PTEs can be a difficult and complex process that requires sensitivity and skill. Given that the assessment process for trauma survivors can be much more distressing and anxiety-provoking than for other clients, it is important that the assessor begin by making an effort to establish rapport with the client. Many trauma survivors, especially those with a history of interpersonal trauma, experience shame or guilt about the nature and extent of their traumatic histories. Clinicians should be sensitive to these possible reactions and should approach their contacts with trauma survivors in a direct but nonjudgmental way that conveys to the client that the therapist is comfortable discussing distressing material, while not insensitive to the personal nature of these experiences. Clinicians also need to be aware of their own emotional response to the client's disclosure and ensure that they do not unintentionally reinforce the client's potential avoidance as a way to manage their own discomfort with the material and with their client's distress.

Finally, as the assessment of trauma may be distressing in and of itself, it is important that the clinician discuss with the client the possibility of symptom exacerbation during the assessment process (Flack, Litz, & Keane, 1998). For example, a female client with PTSD may experience an increase in nightmares after describing her rape during an assessment session. Or, a man with a history of childhood sexual assault may experience significant shame in disclosing this event to a male clinician. Before the assessment process begins, the client's potential use of substances or engagement in self-injurious behaviors as a means of managing symptom intensification should be assessed, as well as the presence of any suicidal or homicidal risk. If necessary, a plan should be developed to help the client identify and manage these behaviors or ask for help if their intensity increases.

The specific questions that are asked to assess the lifetime occurrence of PTEs can significantly impact the accuracy of their assessment. Individuals are more likely to report traumatic experiences when asked directly about specific events than during free recall or unstructured conversation (Lanktree, Briere, & Zaidi, 1991). Further, the exact wording used can affect whether a person reports exposure to a given traumatic event. It is recommended that behaviorally anchored terminology be used to assess PTEs, rather than using more subjective words like "abuse" or "rape" that may be understood differently from individual to individual and may impact on whether an event is reported during an assessment (Keane et al., 2000; Resnick, Falsetti, Kilpatrick, & Freedy, 1996). The skilled clinician should also take a person's cultural context into account and recognize that there are cultural differences with respect to which events are considered traumatic or bear reporting to a clinician (Keane, Kaloupek, & Weathers, 1996). Finally, in addition to simply asking the respondent to indicate whether he or she has experienced a particular event, it is also essential to ask whether the person's response to each event involved intense fear, helplessness, or horror (American Psychiatric Association [APA], 1994). Without this piece of information, a person's response to a PTE cannot be classified as meeting the criteria for ASD or PTSD, and the evaluation may increase the probability of overestimating the presence of psychiatric disorder.

Other considerations involved in the assessment of PTEs include the level of detail gathered during the assessment. Depending on the purpose of the assessment, more or less detail may be required, and clients should not be subjected to a lengthy evaluation process unless there will be a clear clinical or research utility for the assessment. However, especially for clinical purposes, it is often useful to gather comprehensive information about the client's complete trauma history, given the research presented earlier showing that most trauma survivors have experienced more than one PTE (Kessler et al., 1999), and the fact that previous exposure to a PTE often signals a greater risk of developing PTSD in response to a subsequent PTE (Breslau, Chilcoat, Kessler, & Davis, 1999). In addition, it can be of notable clinical relevance to collect details about the PTE to place the event into a more complete context. Such details may include events or situations that preceded the PTE, pretrauma beliefs and functioning, who the perpetrator was, how or why the traumatic situation ended, responses from significant others in the person's life after disclosing the trauma, and coping styles used both before and after the traumatic event occurred. For each event, it can be helpful to obtain information assessing event frequency, duration, perceived life threat, harm, injuries, and age at the time of the event.

Methods of Assessing PTEs. Depending on the purpose of the assessment, a variety of instruments may be utilized to determine exposure to PTEs. Some instruments such as the Stressful Life Events Screening Questionnaire, the Traumatic Events Questionnaire, and the Traumatic Life Events Questionnaire assess a wide variety of PTEs, each with one or two questions. These instruments allow for a breadth of assessment, but they often lack depth. In contrast, some instruments focus on assessing one type of traumatic event, such as exposure to childhood abuse. Measures that assess a wide range of PTEs are reviewed in Chapter 19. Some examples of measures that assess one type of PTE are presented in Table 2.

As the context of the evaluation allows, either interviews, self-report checklists, or a combination of the two may be used,. However, each mode of assessment has potential benefits and limitations. Assessment of PTEs via self-report questionnaires may be helpful, in that individuals may be more likely to disclose personal information in a setting that they feel has less opportunity for social judgment. In addition, such measures are often more efficient to administer. However, the use of semistructured interviews allows for a therapeutic context in which the clinician can provide support and empathy through the assessment process. Further, in an interview, the clinician can better ensure that respondents comprehend the nature and meaning of the assessment questions. Structured interviews for PTEs are sometimes preferable to facilitate the management of potential psychological distress during the evaluation process. Finally, from a clinical standpoint, it would seem that clients might be more likely to disclose their exposure to traumatic events in an interview rather than on a questionnaire. However, the data comparing these formats thus far are equivocal (e.g., Dill, Chu, Grob, & Eisen, 1991; Stinson & Hendrick, 1992).

Table 2. Common Instruments for Assessment of PTEs

Assessment instrument	Type of PTE
Childhood Trauma Questionnaire (Bernstein et al., 1994)	Childhood maltreatment
Psychological and Physical Maltreatment Scale (Briere & Runtz, 1988)	Childhood maltreatment
Assessing Environments III (Berger, Knutson, Mehm, & Perkins, 1988; Knutson & Selner, 1994)	Punitive childhood experiences
Wyatt Sexual History Questionnaire (Wyatt, 1985; Wyatt, Lawrence, Vodounon, & Mickey, 1992)	Childhood sexual abuse
Sexual Experiences Survey (Koss & Gidycz, 1985; Koss & Oros, 1982)	Adolescent and adult sexual assault
Conflict Tactics Scale (Straus, 1979)	Verbal and physical acts of aggression
Psychological Maltreatment of Women (Tolman, 1989)	Psychological aggression
Wartime Stressor Scale (Wolfe, Brown, Furey, & Levin, 1993)	Stressful wartime experiences
Combat Exposure Scale (Keane et al., 1989)	Combat experiences

ASSESSMENT OF POSTTRAUMATIC SYMPTOMATOLOGY

Acute Stress Disorder

Individuals who develop psychological symptoms within 1 month of exposure to a PTE may fulfill the criteria for ASD (APA, 1994). This diagnosis may be given if a person has experienced a PTE during which his or her response involved intense fear, helplessness, or horror. The characteristics of ASD involve symptoms of dissociation or numbing, reexperiencing, avoidance of stimuli related to the trauma, and symptoms of high anxiety or hyperarousal, and the person's level of distress must be enough to cause clinically significant distress or impairment in life functioning. The main feature that distinguishes ASD from PTSD (described below) is the time frame for the development and experience of symptoms. ASD can only be diagnosed if the posttraumatic symptoms develop within 4 weeks of the traumatic event and last between 2 days and 4 weeks. If the symptoms persist for more than 4 weeks, the person's diagnosis must be changed, most often to PTSD or an adjustment disorder. The prevalence of ASD in populations exposed to PTEs depends on the severity and duration of the event (APA, 1994). The Acute Stress Disorder Interview, the Acute Stress Disorder Scale, and the Stanford Acute Stress Reaction Questionnaire are all published measures that were developed for assessing ASD.

Posttraumatic Stress Disorder

As with ASD, PTSD may also be diagnosed when a person has been exposed to a PTE, during which the person experienced fear, helplessness, or horror (APA, 1994). However, PTSD is diagnosed when posttraumatic symptoms last for more than 30 days. There are three main classes of symptoms in PTSD: reexperiencing, avoidance, and arousal. Reexperiencing symptoms may include distressing memories, nightmares, flashbacks, and intense distress or physiological reactivity on exposure to internal or external cues related to the event. Avoidance symptoms may include avoidance of thoughts, feelings, situations, or people associated with the event, problems with memory for the event, anhedonia, and restricted range of affect. Finally, symptoms of increased arousal may consist of trouble sleeping or concentrating, irritability or anger, hypervigilance, and exaggerated startle response.

Estimates of the lifetime prevalence of PTSD in the general population range from 1 to 14%, with 3 to 58% of individuals exposed to a PTE developing PTSD (APA, 1994). A diagnosis of PTSD is often associated with a notably chronic course, and more than one third of individuals diagnosed with PTSD have been found to still meet criteria for the disorder 5 years later (Kessler, Sonnega, Bromet, Hughes, & Nelson, 1995). Special considerations in the assessment of PTSD will be discussed below.

Assessment of PTSD

General Issues.   The general issues related to the assessment of PTSD are quite similar to those discussed in the assessment of PTEs. In addition to the points already raised, part of the assessment can be focused on normalizing the disparate symptoms of PTSD and educating the client as to how these symptoms reflect an attempt to adapt to and cope with the PTE he or she has experienced.

One additional factor to consider when conducting a PTSD assessment is the potential impact of pending compensation for distress related to the traumatic event. For instance, a motor vehicle accident victim may be seeking an insurance settlement at the same time that he or she is seeking an assessment. Or, a veteran may be interested in receiving service-related compensation. Some measures of PTSD such as the Minnesota Multiphasic Personality Inventory PTSD Scale are sensitive to the overendorsement of symptoms that often reflects malingering. However, overendorsement of symptoms can also reflect extreme distress or a cry for help and thus interpretation should be made with caution. There is some suggestion that compensation-seeking malingering may be less common than typically thought (e.g., Blanchard & Hickling, 1997).

Clinical Interview. During the clinical interview, the clinician's main goal is to establish a safe and therapeutic context for the client. In addition to assessing the client's history of PTEs, his or her personal and family psychological history, previous therapy experience, and current functioning should be assessed.

A fear and avoidance hierarchy can be developed, including situations, places, and people that are currently problematic for the client. To our knowledge, there is currently no psychometrically established measure of situational fear and avoidance for PTSD as there is for many other anxiety disorders. The development of such an instrument would greatly facilitate the identification of feared situations. In the absence of such a measure, the clinician should be knowledgeable about the types of situations that are typically problematic for survivors of different types of PTEs (e.g., cologne, alcohol, and sexual activities for a rape victim, forests, helicopters, and people of Asian descent for Vietnam veterans). Further, there may be idiosyncratic stimuli (a particular street, a shirt of a certain color) that are significantly fear inducing and that require careful assessment to identify.

As with other chronic anxiety disorders, it can be difficult for clients to recognize and report on longstanding, chronic avoidance patterns such as driving a particular route to work or preferring quiet evenings at home to interacting with others in a social context. Often a client will see these as personal preferences, and the relationship between these choices and the onset of PTSD can only be demonstrated through a careful, thorough functional analysis.

Semistructured Interviews. A number of semistructured interviews designed to assess PTSD have been developed and psychometrically validated (see Chapter 19). The use of a semistructured interview can greatly increase the probability that the presence of PTSD is identified (e.g., Zimmerman & Mattia, 1999). These interviews differ from one another primarily in the extent of their use and validation across trauma groups, their ability to provide dichotomous and/or continuous measures of severity, and their ease in administration.

Questionnaires. Many different questionnaires have been developed to assess PTSD symptomatology (see Chapter 19). The vast majority of measures consist of 17 questions directly corresponding to the 17 symptoms of PTSD described in DSM-IV criteria B (reexperiencing), C (avoidance and numbing), and D (hyperarousal). Many of the questionnaires allow for estimates of caseness if the requisite number and pattern of symptoms is endorsed. It is important to note that many of the questionnaires have not been validated across a variety of trauma groups, and that the recommended cutoffs may vary for trauma type, gender, and ethnicity. Of the questionnaires reviewed in Chapter 19, only the Posttraumatic Diagnostic Scale includes questions that tap into all of the diagnostic criteria of PTSD (although the Distressing Events Questionnaire includes all criteria with the exception of A-1, the presence of a traumatic event). Most questionnaires also allow continuous estimates of overall symptom severity as well as severity within each symptom cluster.

Very few PTSD questionnaires assess broader clinical features beyond the diagnostic criteria. Some exceptions that include both PTSD symptoms and associated features are the Civilian Mississippi Scale, the Trauma Symptom Inventory, the Los Angeles Symptom Checklist, and the Penn Inventory for PTSD.

Cognitive Factors.   The experience of trauma is thought to significantly impact on an individual's belief system (e.g., Janoff-Bulman, 1992). Thus, assessment of the content of the cognitions of a client with PTSD (e.g., self-blame, meaning of the world) can be helpful in case conceptualization and treatment planning. Several cognitive measures are reviewed in Chapter 19, including the Posttraumatic Cognitions Inventory.

Behavioral Assessment.   Self-monitoring can be an important component of the PTSD assessment. Foa and Rothbaum (1998) suggest that clients self-monitor the occurrence of target behaviors (e.g., nightmares, startle response, outbursts of anger) as they occur over the course of the week. A client can be asked to record the date and time of the symptom, the situation in which it was elicited, thoughts that were present at the time of the symptom, physiological responses, and subjective fear ratings related to the symptom expression.

Little has been written about the use of behavioral assessment tests (BATS) in the assessment of PTSD. However, their utility in the assessment of other anxiety disorders is well established. An example of a BAT for PTSD might include a simulated social interaction with someone of the opposite sex or making small talk with a group of strangers (if applicable to the client's specific avoidance pattern). BATs could also include trips to a crowded mall or a feared parking garage. Self-reported anxiety before and during the BAT could be assessed in addition to behavioral indicators such as eye contact, distance between the client and the confederate, and so on. Psychophysiological response during the BAT can also be continuously assessed. Of course, exposure to feared or avoided situations should only be undertaken when the avoidance is unreasonable and the exposure would not actually constitute a potential threat to the client's well-being.

Psychophysiological Assessment.   Psychophysiological assessment is commonly used in research to examine the response of clients with PTSD to the presentation of trauma cues (e.g., a video of combat-related sights and sounds, the imaginal presentation of a rape script). Several indices have been used including heart rate, skin conductance, and facial EMG. In a recent, large-scale study, Keane et al. (1998) found that a combination of four physiological indices correctly classified two thirds of male Vietnam veterans with current PTSD. Although psychophysiological assessment can be expensive and is often not available to clinicians (but see review in Chapter 19), it can provide additional assessment information that can guide the conceptualization and treatment of PTSD.

Associated Features.   Given that PTSD is associated with high levels of comorbidity (e.g., Orsillo, Weathers, et al., 1996), a full semistructured assessment of additional Axis I and relevant Axis II disorders (e.g., Borderline Personality Disorder, Antisocial Personality Disorder) is recommended (Keane et al., 2000). Also, measures such as the Minnesota Multiphasic Personality Inventory and the Symptom Checklist (SCL-90-R) can both provide an index of PTSD symptomatology and additional psychopathology (see Chapter 19). Certainly the functional relationship between comorbid disorders is critically important to the development of a case conceptualization and treatment plan. For instance, comorbid PTSD and substance abuse often reflects the use of substances as a means of attempting to control the reexperiencing and hyperarousal symptoms that are perceived as unacceptable. A client with comorbid PTSD and panic disorder may need to decrease his or her sensitivity to panic symptoms before exposure therapy is indicated. A client with comorbid PTSD and social phobia may be socially avoidant because of the shame and guilt he or she feels about the traumatic experience or about the social rejection that was endured as a result of the traumatic exposure (Orsillo, Heimberg, Juster, & Garrett, 1996).

Several theorists and researchers have suggested that PTSD does not capture the full range of responses to traumatic events, particularly for traumatized children, rape victims, and battered women (Herman, 1992). Changes in affect regulation, self-identity, and interpersonal functioning seem to be common. The Structured Interview for Disorders of Extreme Stress has been developed to assess the presence of these symptoms. PTSD is also frequently associated with guilt and shame related to the traumatic experience. The Trauma-Related Guilt Inventory can be a useful tool for assessing these emotional responses.

CONCLUSION

In summary, the assessment of posttraumatic symptomatology involves a set of complicated but extremely important methodological issues. Given the fact that virtually all medical professionals and mental health providers will encounter clients who have been exposed to PTEs, it is important that the clinician know how to assess both the stressful event experienced and the possible symptoms related to that event in a manner least likely to lead to either under- or overendorsement of symptoms. The use of a multimethod assessment package, integrating standardized interviews and questionnaires discussed in the current chapter and reviewed in more detail in Chapter 19 is highly recommended.

REFERENCES

American Psychiatric Association. (1994). *Diagnostic and statistical manual of mental disorders* (4th ed.). Washington, DC: Author.

Berger, A. M., Knutson, J. F., Mehm, J. G., & Perkins, K. A. (1988). The self-report of punitive childhood experiences of young adults and adolescents. *Child Abuse and Neglect, 12,* 251–262.

Bernstein, D. P., Fink, L., Handelsman, L., Foote, J., Lovejoy, M., Wenzel, K., Sapareto, E., & Ruggiero, J. (1994). Initial reliability and validity of a new retrospective measure of child abuse and neglect. *American Journal of Psychiatry, 151,* 1132–1136.

Blanchard, E. B., & Hickling, E. J. (1997). *After the crash: Assessment and treatment of motor vehicle accident survivors.* Washington, DC: American Psychological Association.

Boscarino, J. A. (1995). Post-traumatic stress and associated disorders among Vietnam veterans: The significance of combat exposure and social support. *Journal of Traumatic Stress, 8,* 317–336.

Breslau, N., Chilcoat, H. D., Kessler, R. C., & Davis, G. C. (1999). Previous exposure to trauma and PTSD effects of subsequent trauma: Results from the Detroit Area Survey of Trauma. *American Journal of Psychiatry, 156,* 902–907.

Briere, J. (1997). *Psychological assessment of adult posttraumatic states.* Washington, DC: American Psychological Association.

Briere, J., & Runtz, M. (1988). Multivariate correlates of childhood psychological and physical maltreatment among university women. *Child Abuse and Neglect, 12,* 331–341.

Dill, D. L., Chu, J. A., Grob, M. C., & Eisen, S. V. (1991). The reliability of abuse history reports: A comparison of two inquiry formats. *Comprehensive Psychiatry, 32*, 166–169.

Flack, W. F., Litz, B. T., & Keane, T. M. (1998). Cognitive–behavioral treatment of warzone-related posttraumatic stress disorder: A flexible, hierarchical approach. In V. M. Follete, J. I. Ruzek, & F. R. Abueg (Eds.), *Cognitive–behavioral therapies for trauma* (pp. 77–99). New York: Guilford.

Foa, E. B., & Rothbaum, B. O. (1998). *Treating the trauma of rape.* New York: Guilford.

Green, B. L., Grace, M. C., Lindy, J. D., Gleser, G. C., & Leonard, A. (1990). Risk factors for PTSD and other diagnoses in a general sample of Vietnam veterans. *American Journal of Psychiatry, 147*, 729–733.

Harvey, A. G., & Bryant, R. A. (1998). The relationship between acute stress disorder and posttraumatic stress disorder: A prospective evaluation of motor vehicle accident survivors. *Journal of Consulting and Clinical Psychology, 66*, 507–512.

Herman, J. L. (1992). Complex PTSD: A syndrome in survivors of prolonged and repeated trauma. *Journal of Traumatic Stress, 5*, 377–392.

Janoff-Bulman, R. (1992). *Shattered assumptions: Towards a new psychology of trauma.* New York: The Free Press.

Keane, T. M., Fairbank, J. A., Caddell, J. M., Zimering, R. T., Taylor, K. L., & Mora, C. A. (1989). Clinical evaluation of a measure to assess combat exposure. *Psychological Assessment, 1*, 53–55.

Keane, T. M., Kaloupek, D. G., & Weathers, F. W. (1996). Ethnocultural considerations in the assessment of PTSD. In A. J. Marsella & M. J. Friedman (Eds.), *Ethnocultural aspects of posttraumatic stress disorder: Issues, research, and clinical applications* (pp. 183–205). Washington, DC: American Psychological Association.

Keane, T. M., Kolb, L. C., Kaloupek, D. G., Orr, S. P., Blanchard, E. B., Thomas, R. G., Hsieh, F. Y., & Lavori, P. W. (1998). Utility of psychophysiology measurement in the diagnosis of posttraumatic stress disorder: Results from a Department of Veteran's Affairs cooperative study. *Journal of Consulting and Clinical Psychology, 66*, 914–923.

Keane, T. M., Weathers, F. W., & Foa, E. B. (2000). Diagnosis and assessment. In E. B. Foa, T. M. Keane, & M. J. Friedman (Eds.), *Effective treatments for PTSD* (pp. 18–36). New York: Guilford.

Kessler, R. C., Sonnega, A., Bromet, E., Hughes, M., & Nelson, C. B. (1995). Posttraumatic stress disorder in the National Comorbidity Survey. *Archives of General Psychiatry, 52*, 1048–1060.

Kessler, R. C., Sonnega, A., Bromet, E., Hughes, M., Nelson, C. B., & Breslau, N. (1999). Epidemiological risk factors for trauma and PTSD. In R. Yehuda (Ed.), *Risk factors for posttraumatic stress disorder* (pp. 23–59). Washington, DC: American Psychiatric Press.

King, D. W., King, L. A., Foy, D. W., & Gudanowski, D. M. (1996). Prewar factors in combat-related posttraumatic stress disorder: Structural equation modeling with a national sample of female and male Vietnam veterans. *Journal of Consulting and Clinical Psychology, 64*, 520–531.

Knutson, J. F., & Selner, M. B. (1994). Punitive childhood experiences reported by young adults over a 10-year period. *Child Abuse and Neglect, 18*, 155–166.

Koss, M. P., & Gidycz, C. A. (1985). Sexual Experiences Survey: Reliability and validity. *Journal of Consulting and Clinical Psychology, 53*, 422–423.

Koss, M. P., & Oros, C. J. (1982). Sexual Experiences Survey: A research instrument investigating sexual aggression and victimization. *Journal of Consulting and Clinical Psychology, 50*, 455–457.

Lanktree, C., Briere, J., & Zaidi, L. (1991). Incidence and impact of sexual abuse in a child outpatient sample: The role of direct inquiry. *Child Abuse and Neglect, 15*, 447–453.

Litz, B. T., Miller, M. W., Ruef, A. M., & McTeague, L. M. (in press). Assessment of adults exposed to trauma. In M. M. Antony & D. H. Barlow (Eds.), *Handbook of assessment, treatment planning, and outcome evaluation: Empirically supported strategies for psychological disorders.* New York: Guilford.

Litz, B. T., & Weathers, F. W. (1994). The diagnosis and assessment of post-traumatic stress disorder in adults. In M. B. Williams & J. F. Sommer (Eds.), *The handbook of posttraumatic therapy* (pp. 20–37). Westport, CT: Greenwood Press.

Mueser, K. T., Goodman, L. B., Trumbetta, S. L., Rosenberg, S. D., Osher, F. C., Vidaver, R., Auciello, P., & Foy, D. W. (1998). Trauma and posttraumatic stress disorder in severe mental illness. *Journal of Consulting and Clinical Psychology, 66*, 493–499.

Orsillo, S. M., Heimberg, R. G., Juster, H. R., & Garrett, J. (1996). Social phobia in Vietnam veterans. *Journal of Traumatic Stress, 9*, 235–252.

Orsillo, S. M., Weathers, F. W., Litz, B. T., Steinberg, H. R., Huska, J. A., & Keane, T. M. (1996). Current and lifetime psychiatric disorders among veterans with war zone-related posttraumatic stress disorder. *Journal of Nervous and Mental Disease, 184*, 307–313.

Resnick, H. S., Falsetti, S. A., Kilpatrick, D. G., & Freedy, J. R. (1996). Assessment of rape and other civilian trauma-related PTSD: Emphasis on assessment of potentially traumatic events. In T. W. Miller (Ed.), *Theory and assessment of stressful life events* (pp. 235–271). Madison, CT: International Universities Press.

Rothbaum, B. O., Foa, E. B., Riggs, D., Murdock, T., & Walsh, W. (1992). A prospective examination of post-traumatic stress disorder in rape victims. *Journal of Traumatic Stress, 5,* 455–475.

Stinson, M. H., & Hendrick, S. S. (1992). Reported childhood sexual abuse in university counseling center clients. *Journal of Counseling Psychology, 39,* 370–374.

Straus, M. A. (1979). Measuring intrafamily conflict and violence: The Conflict Tactics (CT) Scales. *Journal of Marriage and the Family, 41,* 75–88.

Tolman, R. M. (1989). The development of a measure of psychological maltreatment of women by their male partners. *Violence and Victims, 4,* 159–177.

Wolfe, J., Brown, P. J., Furey, J., & Levin, K. (1993). Development of a war-time stressor scale for women. *Psychological Assessment, 5,* 330–335.

Wyatt, G. E. (1985). The sexual abuse of Afro-American and white American women in childhood. *Child Abuse and Neglect: The International Journal, 9,* 507–519.

Wyatt, G. E., Lawrence, J., Vodounon, A., & Mickey, M. R. (1992). The Wyatt Sex History Questionnaire: A structured interview for female sexual history taking. *Journal of Child Sexual Abuse, 1,* 51–68.

Zimmerman, M., & Mattia, J. I. (1999). Is posttraumatic stress disorder underdiagnosed in routine clinical settings? *Journal of Nervous and Mental Disease, 187,* 420–428.

Chapter 19
Measures for Acute Stress Disorder and Posttraumatic Stress Disorder

Susan M. Orsillo

Note: Throughout this chapter, reference is made to the various DSM-IV criteria for PTSD (American Psychiatric Association, 1994). Criterion A-1 refers to the occurrence of a traumatic event. Criterion A-2 refers to the presence of intense fear, helplessness, and horror at the time of the traumatic event. Criterion B refers to the presence of symptoms involving reexperiencing the traumatic event. Criterion C refers to symptoms of persistent avoidance of stimuli related to the traumatic event and numbing of general responsiveness. Criterion D includes symptoms of increased arousal since experiencing the trauma. Criterion E refers to the duration of the disturbance (at least 1 month for PTSD). Criterion F refers to the presence of clinically significant distress or impairment.

ACCIDENT FEAR QUESTIONNAIRE (AFQ)

Original Citation

Kuch, K., Cox, B. J., & Direnfeld, D. M. (1995). A brief self-rating scale for PTSD after road vehicle accident. *Journal of Anxiety Disorders*, *9*, 503–514.

Susan M. Orsillo • National Center for PTSD–Women's Health Sciences Division, Boston VA Health-care System, and Boston University School of Medicine, Boston, Massachusetts 02130.

Purpose

To measure PTSD-related phobic avoidance following involvement in a motor vehicle accident.

Description

The AFQ is a self-report scale consisting of an MVA profile that includes 10 yes/no questions about the accident and related anxiety, and 10 phobic avoidance items (AFQ-PA) in which the respondent is asked to rate his or her avoidance on a nine-point scale ranging from 0 (would not avoid it) to 8 (would always avoid it). There are also two descriptive questions about the accident and one question that assesses interference from physical illness (e.g., back pain) using the same nine-point scale.

Administration and Scoring

The AFQ can be administered in 5 to 10 minutes. The AFQ-PA subscale can be scored by summing the 10 items. A cutoff score of 15 on the AFQ-PA may be used to detect the presence of PTSD and/or accident phobia (see below).

Psychometric Properties

Sample Scores and Norms.   The mean scores for the AFQ-PA are available from a sample of 54 men and women seeking treatment for pain or some other somatic symptom following a motor vehicle accident (Kuch et al., 1995). Individuals diagnosed with PTSD obtained a mean score of 54.44 (SD = 11.36); those diagnosed with accident phobia had a mean score of 34.00 (SD = 14.77); those with neither disorder had a mean score of 14.66 (SD = 12.46). Lower means were obtained in a sample of 113 accident victims referred to a research study from a rehabilitation center (Asmundson, Cox, Larsen, Frombach, & Norton, 1999). The mean score of individuals diagnosed with PTSD and accident phobia combined was 20.9 (SD = 14.0) and the comparison group obtained a mean of 9.0 (SD = 9.6). The percentages of respondents by diagnosis who endorsed each item in the accident profile are found in Kuch et al. (1995) and Asmundson et al. (1999).

Reliability.   Items making up the MVA profile subscale had fairly low internal consistency (α = .67) likely reflecting the divergent nature of the items (Asmundson et al., 1999). In contrast, good internal consistency was demonstrated for the AFQ-PA subscale (αs .80 to .89; Asmundson et al., 1999; Kuch et al., 1995).

Validity.   The convergent and discriminant validity of the AFQ-PA was evaluated across a number of measures (Asmundson et al., 1999). The AFQ-PA was moderately associated with measures of anxiety sensitivity (.43), alexithymia (.33), and somatization (.28). The measure was not associated with extraversion and perceived self-control.

Individuals diagnosed with PTSD scored significantly higher than those with accident phobia and those with neither disorder in one sample (Kuch et al., 1995). In another sample, the PTSD and phobia groups did not differ, but these groups combined scored significantly higher than individuals with neither disorder (Asmundson et al., 1999).

The diagnostic efficiency of the AFQ-PA was assessed against a structured clinical interview. A cutoff score of 15 on the AFQ-PA appeared to be the optimal score for screening. However, this score yielded a sensitivity of only .67 and specificity of .78 with 55% of those scoring at or above the cutoff meeting diagnostic criteria for PTSD or accident phobia and 85% of those below the cutoff not meeting criteria for either disorder.

Source

The AFQ is reprinted in the original citation and in Appendix B. More information can be obtained by contacting Klaus Kuch, M.D. Forensic Program (4th Floor), Centre for Addiction and Mental Health, Clarke Institute Division, 250 College Street, Toronto, ON M5T 1R8, Canada; (tel) 705-487-2324; (e-mail) klaus.kuch@sympatico.ca.

ACUTE STRESS DISORDER INTERVIEW (ASDI)

Original Citation

Bryant, R. A., Harvey, A. G., Dang, S. T., & Sackville, T. (1998). Assessing acute stress disorder: Psychometric properties of a structured clinical interview. *Psychological Assessment, 10*, 215–220.

Purpose

To diagnose acute stress disorder.

Description

The ASDI is a clinician-rated scale consisting of 19 items that relate to criterion B (*dissociation*, 5 items), criterion C (*reexperiencing*, 4 items), criterion D (*avoidance*, 4 items), and criterion E (*arousal*, 6 items). Each item is scored dichotomously as 0 (symptom absent) or 1 (symptom present). The ASDI also includes items that assess the *objective and subjective experience of the traumatic event* (criterion A, 3 items), the *duration of each symptom* (criterion F), and *impairment* (criterion G, 4 items).

Administration and Scoring

The ASDI can be administered in 10 minutes. Scoring is according to DSM-IV criteria for ASD (see above).

Psychometric Properties

The psychometric properties of the ASDI were evaluated in a multisample, multistudy paper (Bryant et al., 1998).

Sample Scores and Norms. Thirteen patients out of 56 (23%) patients who were admitted to a hospital following a traumatic event met criteria for ASD. Twenty-four patients out of 60 (40%) who were referred to a PTSD unit following a traumatic event were diagnosed with ASD.

Reliability. The internal consistency for the 19 symptom items of the ASDI was found to be excellent ($r = .90$) among a sample of 65 patients admitted to a hospital following a traumatic event. The individual symptom clusters were lower: *dissociation* ($r = .67$), *reexperiencing* ($r = .67$), *avoidance* ($r = .69$), and *arousal* ($r = .76$).

Two- to seven-day test–retest reliability was reported for a sample of 60 adults seeking treatment . Correlations for each of the symptom clusters ranged from .80 to .87. Further, 88% of those who were diagnosed at time 1 were also diagnosed at time 2 and 94% of participants who were not diagnosed at time 1 also did not receive a diagnosis at time 2.

Validity. The items of the ASDI were rated by experts on a five-point scale ranging from 1 (not at all) to 5 (extremely) on their relevance ($M = 4.86$, $SD = 0.93$), specificity ($M = 4.44$, $SD = 0.43$), and clarity ($M = 4.51$, $SD = 0.27$). The content validity of the ASDI was evaluated in a sample of 56 inpatients admitted to a hospital following the occurrence of a traumatic event. The ASDI cluster score for the *dissociation* symptoms was significantly correlated with a measure of dissociation ($r = .35$), the *reexperiencing* cluster correlated with a measure of intrusion ($r = .72$), the *avoidance* cluster correlated with an additional measure of avoidance ($r = .83$), and the *arousal* cluster correlated with a measure of state anxiety ($r = .38$).

Given the lack of a gold standard measure of ASD, the ASDI was validated against the diagnosis of expert clinicians. The sensitivity of the ASDI was 91% and the specificity was 93%. Kappa values were .75 for the overall diagnosis, .79 for the stressor, .65 for *dissociation*, .61 for *reexperiencing*, .73 for *avoidance*, and .41 for *arousal*.

Alternative Forms

A self-report version of the ASDI, the Acute Stress Disorder Scale (ASDS) has also been developed (Bryant, Moulds, & Guthrie, 2000). Patients diagnosed with ASD scored a mean of 65.11 ($SD = 14.74$) on the ASDS and patients without ASD scored a mean of 36.97 ($SD = 19.54$). The internal consistency and test–retest reliability for the ASDS was found to be very good to excellent for the total score and the individual symptom clusters. Convergent validity and predictive validity against the interview version have also been established. The ASDS can be obtained by contacting Dr. Bryant (see source information below) and is reprinted in the original citation (Bryant et al., 2000).

Source

The ASDI can be obtained by contacting Richard A. Bryant, Ph.D., School of Psychology, University of New South Wales, Sydney, NSW 2052, Australia; (e-mail) r.bryant@ unsw.edu.au.

CLINICIAN-ADMINISTERED PTSD SCALE (CAPS)

Original Citations

Blake, D. D., Weathers, F. W., Nagy, L. M., Kaloupek, D. G., Klauminzer, G., Charney, D. S., & Keane, T. M. (1990). A clinician rating scale for assessing current and lifetime PTSD: The CAPS-1. *The Behavior Therapist, 13*, 187–188.

Blake, D. D., Weathers, F. W., Nagy, L. M., Kaloupek, D. G., Gusman, F. D., Charney, D. S., & Keane, T. M. (1995). The development of a clinician-administered PTSD scale. *Journal of Traumatic Stress, 8*, 75–90.

Purpose

To diagnose and assess symptoms of PTSD.

Description

The CAPS is a clinician-rated scale. The most up-to-date version includes a checklist of potentially traumatizing events. After it is administered, up to three events are chosen (based on their severity or recency) and a description of the event and the respondent's emotional response at the time of the event are obtained to establish DSM-IV criterion A. These events are referred to in the subsequent questions. Seventeen items directly assess DSM-IV criteria B, C, and D. Each item is rated on a five-point scale to determine the frequency (for most items 0 = never to 4 = daily or almost every day) and intensity (0 = none to 4 = extreme, with additional specific behavioral descriptions to each item). Raters are also permitted to indicate whether they believe each rating is of questionable validity (e.g., whether the patient is over- or underreporting). Criterion E is established by two questions on onset and duration. Criterion F is established by three questions on distress and impairment in functioning. Three items require the interviewer to make global ratings on the validity of responses, severity of PTSD and, if applicable, improvement since the previous assessment. If criteria are met for PTSD, five items tapping into associated features are administered. This version of the CAPS is able to assess symptoms over the past week, past month, and lifetime.

Administration and Scoring

The CAPS can be administered in 45–60 minutes. A total score is obtained by summing the frequency and intensity scores for each of the 17 symptom items. The CAPS can also be used to obtain a dichotomous rating of the presence or absence of PTSD. The psychometric properties of nine scoring rules (e.g., a symptom is present if the frequency rating is at least 1 and the intensity rating is at least 2; a symptom is present if the severity of a symptom {frequency + intensity} is greater than or equal to 4) have been examined (Weathers, Ruscio, & Keane, 1999). These authors concluded that the appropriate scoring rule should be based on the purpose of the assessment (e.g., screening versus differential diagnosis). Thus, it is highly recommended that users of the CAPS obtain this article.

Psychometric Properties

Sample Scores and Norms. In a sample of motor vehicle accident and sexual assault victims, the mean score on the CAPS was 45.9 ($SD = 29.1$; Blanchard, Jones-Alexander, Buckley, & Forneris, 1996).

Reliability. Internal consistency for intensity of PTSD symptom criteria was examined in a sample of 25 veterans (Blake et al., 1990). Cronbach's alpha ranged from .73 to .85. Similar results were found with a larger sample (Weathers & Litz, 1994). Internal consistency was also high within a sample of older veterans (αs range from .87 to .95; Hyer, Summers, Boyd, Litaker, & Boudewyns, 1996). Interrater reliability on the same interview (with both raters present) was established within a sample of seven veterans for criteria B, C, and D (rs range from .92 to .99 for frequency and intensity; Blake et al., 1990). Diagnostic agreement within the pairs was perfect.

A more conservative test of interrater reliability was conducted in a larger sample of veterans. Three rater pairs independently interviewed veterans on two occasions 2 to 3 days apart (Weathers & Litz, 1994). The correlations for symptom clusters and total scores ranged from .77 to .98. However, the use of questionable validity ratings for each item was not shown to be reliable (Weathers & Litz, 1994).

Validity. A confirmatory factor analysis was conducted on a sample of 524 service-seeking male veterans to examine the relative fit of a number of models hypothesized to reflect the dimensionality of PTSD (King, Leskin, King, & Weathers, 1998). The model of best fit was a four-factor, first order solution containing correlated factors reflecting the reexperiencing, effortful avoidance, emotional numbing, and hyperarousal symptom clusters of PTSD.

Convergent validity of the CAPS was demonstrated for a sample of 25 veterans (Blake et al., 1990). The CAPS was significantly correlated with self-report measures of PTSD (rs range from .70 to .84) and combat exposure ($r = .42$; Blake et al., 1990). In a sample of motor vehicle accident and sexual assault victims, the CAPS was significantly associated with a self-report measure of PTSD ($r = .93$). Within a large service-seeking veteran sample, score on the CAPS was shown to be significantly associated with other self-report measures of PTSD (rs range from .77 to .91), depression (rs range from .69 to .74), and anxiety (rs range from .65 to .76; Weathers & Litz, 1994). In contrast, in the same sample, the CAPS was only weakly associated with a measure of antisocial personality ($r = .14$). Further, when the effects of possible response bias were controlled for, the correlations with measures of PTSD remained strong, whereas the correlations with associated features dropped substantially (Weathers & Litz, 1994). Finally, convergent validity of the symptom subscales of the CAPS was assessed in a large sample of service-seeking veterans (King et al., 1998). A measure of state anxiety was more strongly associated with symptoms of hyperarousal and reexperiencing than the numbing and avoidance clusters. In contrast, numbing and hyperarousal were the symptom clusters most highly associated with depression (King et al., 1998).

The diagnostic utility of nine scoring rules for the CAPS was examined against a diagnosis obtained by structured clinical interview in a sample of service-seeking veterans (Weathers et al., 1999). All nine rules yielded efficiencies ranging from .82 to .87.

Diagnosis based on the CAPS has been shown to be predictive of heart rate reactivity in response to a combat-related priming event (e.g., Litz, Orsillo, Kaloupek, & Weathers, 2000). Treatment sensitivity was demonstrated in a study of trauma management therapy with veterans (Frueh, Turner, Beidel, Mirabella, & Jones, 1996), and in an open trial of exposure therapy with a mixed group of trauma survivors (Thompson, Charlton, Kerry, & Lee, 1995).

Alternative Forms

The CAPS has been translated into several languages including French, Spanish, Japanese, and Russian. A modification of the CAPS for use with Afghan refugees (Pushto and Farsi {Dari} languages) has been demonstrated to have good internal consistency and interrater reliability (Malekzai et al., 1996). The Dutch version has also been psychometrically examined (Hovens, van der Ploeg, Klaarenbeek, Schreuder, & Rivero, 1994a). A computerized version of the CAPS with good validity and reliability has been developed (Neal, Busuttil, Herapath, & Strike, 1994). A child version of the CAPS is available through the National Center for PTSD website. More information on the child version is available by contacting Elana Newman, University of Tulsa, Psychology/Lorton Hall, 600 S. College Ave., Tulsa, OK 74104-3189, USA; (e-mail) newmane@centum.utulsa.edu.

Source

More information about the CAPS, including a request form to obtain a copy of the measure, is available at the National Center for PTSD website (www.ncptsd.org/treatment/assessment/caps.html). In addition, interested readers can contact Carole A. Goguen, Psy.D. at the National Center for PTSD (116D) VA Medical Center & Regional Office Center, 215 North Main St., White River Junction, VT 05009, USA. The CAPS can be obtained through the National Center for PTSD at no cost. In addition, a version of the CAPS is under development with Western Psychological Services. For more information, contact Western Psychological Services, 12031 Wilshire Boulevard, Los Angeles, CA 90025, USA; (tel) 800-648-8857; (fax) 310-478-7838; (e-mail) custsvc@wpspublish.com; (website) www.wpspublish.com.

DAVIDSON TRAUMA SCALE (DTS)

Original Citation

Davidson, J. R. T., Book, S. W., Colket, J. T., Tupler, L. A., Roth, S., David, D., Hertzberg, M., Mellman, T., Beckham, J. C., Smith, R. D., Davison, R. M., Katz, R., & Feldman, M. E. (1997). Assessment of a new self-rating scale for posttraumatic stress disorder. *Psychological Medicine*, 27, 153–160.

Purpose

To assess symptoms of PTSD among individuals with a history of trauma exposure.

Description

The DTS is a self-report scale comprised of 17 items corresponding to each of the DSM-IV symptoms of PTSD. For each item, the respondent rates frequency and severity for the previous week on a five-point scale. The *reexperiencing* symptoms are tied to a specific traumatic event described by the respondent. However, the *numbing*, *withdrawal*, and *hyper-*

arousal events are not specifically linked to the traumatic event (e.g., the respondent is not asked if these symptoms arose as a result of, or at the time of, the trauma). For frequency, the scale ranges from 0 (not at all) to 4 (every day). For severity, the range is from 0 (not at all) to 4 (extremely distressing).

Administration and Scoring

The DTS takes 10 minutes to administer. A total score can be derived by summing all of the items. Subscale scores can be computed separately for frequency and severity. Subscale scores can also be computed separately for each of the symptom clusters: reexperiencing, avoidance, and hyperarousal.

Psychometric Properties

Sample Scores and Norms. Respondents derived from studies on veterans and victims of a natural disaster with PTSD obtained a mean score of 62 ($SD = 38.0$) versus a mean of 15.5 ($SD = 13.8$) for respondents without PTSD (Davidson, et al., 1997).

Reliability. Internal consistency was reported for participants in studies on rape victims, veterans, and victims of a natural disaster (Davidson, Book, et al., 1997). Cronbach's alpha for the combined sample ranged from .97 to .99 for the frequency only, severity only, and total items. Similar internal consistency ratings were found in a sample of survivors of childhood sexual assault (Zlotnick, Davidson, Shea, & Pearlstein, 1996).

Two-week test–retest data were available for 21 participants in a multicenter drug trial for individuals with a variety of trauma histories who were rated with "no change" on an independently derived measure of their symptoms (Davidson, et al., 1997). The test–retest reliability on this subsample was .86.

Factor analysis of a sample of individuals with a history of combat, rape, or natural disaster yielded two factors (Davidson, et al., 1997). The first accounting for 20% of the variance was interpreted as a severity factor. The second accounted for a small amount of the variance and consisted mostly of positive loadings on the *intrusive* items and negative loadings on the *avoidance* and *numbing* items. A factor analysis on only respondents with PTSD yielded six factors, the largest being similar to the severity factor discussed above.

Convergent validity was assessed with the same sample (Davidson, et al., 1997). Individuals diagnosed with PTSD on the basis of a structured clinical interview scored significantly higher than those without PTSD. A score of 40 on the DTS was associated with a sensitivity of 69%, specificity of 95%, and efficiency of 83%. Within the sample of patients treated with an antidepressant, DTS scores were significantly different (in the predicted directions) for five categories of PTSD severity (minimal, subclinical, clinical, severe, and very severe) determined by a physician's rating (Davidson, et al., 1997). Within the rape victim and veteran samples, the DTS was significantly correlated with a self-report ($r = .64$) and an interview ($r = .78$) measure of PTSD. The DTS was also significantly correlated with measures of general psychological distress (rs ranging from .44 to .65), but not with a measure of extroversion ($r = .04$).

In a sample of childhood sexual abuse survivors, DTS scores were significantly correlated with an interview measure of PTSD (rs ranged from .57 to .72 for frequency and severity), a measure of dissociation (rs ranged from .51 to .59), and a measure of affect regulation (rs ranged from .49 to .53; Zlotnick et al., 1996).

Sensitivity to treatment effects was evaluated by comparing the DTS total score in responders versus nonresponders in the antidepressant trial (Davidson, et al., 1997). Responders demonstrated a significant decrease in DTS score, whereas nonresponders did not. Controlling for pretreatment scores, women with a history of childhood sexual assault who received a group treatment demonstrated a nonsignificant trend toward scoring lower on the DTS than individuals in the waitlist control condition (Zlotnick et al., 1996).

Alternative Forms

The DTS is available in French-Canadian and Spanish. A four-item scale called the SPAN (Startle, Physiological arousal, Anger, and Numbness) has been developed as a brief diagnostic screening from the DTS. The psychometric properties of this scale are described in Meltzer-Brody, Churchill, and Davidson (1999). The SPAN is also available from Multi-Health Systems (see below).

Source

The DTS is available through Multi-Health Systems Inc., 908 Niagara Falls Blvd., North Tonawanda, NY 14120-2060, USA; (tel) 800-456-3003 (USA) or 800-268-6011 (Canada); (fax) 416-424-1736; (webpage) www.mhs.com. A kit that contains a manual and 25 scoring forms is available for $47.50 US. More information can also be obtained by contacting Jonathan R. T. Davidson, M.D., Department of Psychiatry, Duke University Medical Center, Box 3812, Durham, NC 27710, USA; (tel) 919-684-2880; (fax) 919-684-8866; (e-mail) tolme@acpub.duke.edu.

DISSOCIATIVE EXPERIENCES SCALE (DES)

Original Citations

Bernstein, E. M., & Putnam, F. W. (1986). Development, reliability and validity of a dissociation scale. *Journal of Nervous and Mental Disease, 174,* 727–735.

Carlson, E. B., & Putnam, F. W. (1993). An update on the Dissociative Experiences Scale. *Dissociation, 6,* 16–27.

Purpose

To measure frequency of dissociative experiences.

Description

The DES has been used in over 400 published studies on a variety of populations. Over 35 studies have been conducted on the psychometric properties of the scale. While the DES appears to be a clinically useful measure of dissociative features, it lacks some clarity because it does not specify a time period for reporting and because it measures experiences that are reflective of both normal and pathological dissociation. The DES consists of 28 items that describe dissociative experiences including experiences of amnesia, depersonalization, derealization, imaginative involvement, and absorption. Respondents are asked to indicate the frequency (not including drug- or alcohol-related experiences) of these experiences using a 100-point scale. The original version of the DES used a visual analogue response scale consisting of a 100 mm line numerically anchored on the end points. A revised version uses a format of numbers from 0 to 100 (by 10s) and asks the respondent to circle the percentage of time that best reflects how much he or she has each experience in their daily life (no specific time window is indicated).

Administration and Scoring

The DES can be administered in 10 to 15 minutes. On the original version, the scale is scored by measuring the mark made by the respondent to the nearest 5 millimeters. On the revised version, the circled numbers are used. A total score is calculated by adding all of the items and dividing by 28. Subscale means based on a factor analysis (Carlson et al., 1991) can also be obtained, although, there is some debate over the validity of these factors (see psychometric review below). *Amnestic dissociation* is measured by taking the mean of items 3–6, 8, 10, 25, and 26. *Absorption and imaginative involvement* is measured by taking the mean of items 2, 14–18, 20, 22, and 23. *Depersonalization and derealization* is the mean of items 7, 11–13, 27, and 28. A score of 30 is used as a cutoff point for defining a respondent as high in dissociation.

Psychometric Properties

Sample Scores and Norms.   Based on a meta-analysis of 85 studies on almost 12,000 respondents, means were derived for individuals with PTSD ($N = 259$, $M = 32.58$), for normal individuals ($N = 1578$, $M = 11.57$), and students ($N = 5676$, $M = 14.27$; van Ijzendoorn & Schuengel, 1996).

Reliability.   The meta-analysis conducted by van Ijzendoorn and Schuengel (1996) included 16 studies that examined internal consistency, and the mean alpha across these studies was .93. The test–retest reliability of the DES has been shown to range from .79 to .96 over 4- to 8-week intervals (e.g., Bernstein & Putnam, 1986; Frischholz et al., 1990; Pitblado & Sanders, 1991).

Validity.   Fischer and Elnitsky (1990) conducted a factor analysis on the DES in a student sample to determine if the three-factor solution (yielding the three subscales discussed earlier) would emerge. However, they found that a one-factor solution best accounted for the data. In contrast, Ross, Joshi, and Currie (1991) conducted a factor analysis on data derived from a large community sample and obtained the three-factor solution that was hypothesized. Carlson et al. (1991) conducted a factor analysis on DES scores derived from a multicenter study including 1574 individuals with and without a variety of psychological disorders (Carlson et al., 1991) and also obtained the three-factor solution. However, Waller (1995) reanalyzed their data set correcting for skewness and confirmed that one general factor best accounted for the variance.

The meta-analysis conducted by van Ijzendoorn and Schuengel (1996) included 26 studies that allowed for an examination of the convergent validity of the DES. The DES showed excellent convergent validity with other self-report and interview measures of dissociation (combined effect size $d = 1.05$, $N = 1705$), PTSD (combined effect size $d = 0.75$, $N = 1099$), and physical or sexual abuse (combined effect size $d = 0.52$, $N = 2108$).

In contrast, the discriminant validity of the DES is somewhat less well established. DES scores do not seem to be strongly associated with gender (combined effect size $d = -0.01$, $N = 4074$) or age ($d = -0.24$, $N = 2474$). However, DES scores have been shown to be significantly related to a number of measures of general psychological distress (rs ranging from .67 to .69; e.g., Walker, Katon, Neraas, Jemelka, & Massoth, 1992; Zlotnick et al., 1995). Although this may indicate that the DES measures general distress, it may also accurately reflect the relationship between general distress level and severity of dissociation.

Alternative Forms

The DES has been translated into at least 17 languages. There is an adolescent DES that is similarly formatted, but that contains different content, and is available through the Sidran Foundation (see below). A brief version of the DES, the DES-T, has been developed to specifically measure pathological dissociation (Waller, Putnam, & Carlson, 1996; Waller & Ross, 1997). A computerized version of the scale is available from Grant Fair, M.S.W., R.S.W., (e-mail) grantf@provcomm.net.

Source

The line version of the DES is reprinted in the Bernstein and Putnam (1986) paper, although the response line is not the correct length and one item is missing. The percentage version of the DES is reprinted in Carlson and Putnam (1993) and in Appendix B. One copy of the instrument (designate the language), a user's manual (the Carlson & Putnam, 1993, article referenced above), and a list of 333 references are available for purchase through the Sidran Foundation, 2328 West Joppa Road, Luterville, MD 21093, USA; (tel) 410-825-8888; (fax) 410-337-0747; (e-mail) sidran@sidran.org; (webpage) www.sidran.org.

DISTRESSING EVENT QUESTIONNAIRE (DEQ)

Original Citation

Kubany, E. S., Leisen, M. B., Kaplan, A. S., & Kelly, M. P. (2000). Validation of a brief measure of posttraumatic stress disorder: The Distressing Event Questionnaire (DEQ). *Psychological Assessment, 12*, 197–209.

Purpose

To assess PTSD and PTSD severity.

Description

The DEQ is a comprehensive measure that has been demonstrated to assess PTSD across a variety of trauma populations. Although the measure does not assess criterion A-1 (the occurrence of a traumatic event), it does assess criterion A-2, with three questions that assess the presence of intense fear, helplessness, and horror at the time of the traumatic event. The DEQ also includes 17 items that assess the diagnostic symptoms of PTSD (criteria B through D). Respondents are asked to indicate the degree to which they experienced each of the symptoms within the last month on a five-point scale ranging from 0 (absent or did not occur) to 4 (present to an extreme or severe degree). Criterion E is assessed by three questions that ask if the respondent had PTSD for more than 30 days, when the symptoms began, and how long they have persisted. Criterion F is assessed by 11 items that measure distress and impairment in various areas of functioning. Additional features associated with PTSD, including trauma-related guilt, anger, and unresolved grief over trauma-related losses, are also assessed.

Administration and Scoring

The DEQ can be administered in 5 to 7 minutes. A PTSD diagnosis can be obtained by following the DSM-IV diagnostic criteria or a symptom severity index can be obtained by summing the appropriate items. Cutoff scores differ for men and women (see below).

Psychometric Properties

Psychometric properties were evaluated in a multisample, multistudy study (Kubany et al., 2000).

Sample Scores and Norms. None are available.

Reliability. Reliability was assessed in a sample of male veterans. The internal consistency of the DEQ was excellent for the total score ($\alpha = .93$) and very good to excellent for each of the B, C, and D symptom clusters (αs .88 to .91). Similar results were found for women with histories of sexual assault, abuse by an intimate partner, prostitution, and substance abuse.

Test–retest reliability for a male veteran sample ($M = 17.5$ days, $SD = 12.3$ days) for the overall scale was .95 with reliability coefficients (rs) for the various symptom clusters ranging from .69 to .72. Similar results were found among battered women (test–retest reliability for total score, $r = .83$; for subscales rs range from .76 to .81). Temporal stability of the DEQ for identifying the presence of a PTSD diagnosis was also demonstrated with the battered women. Utilizing all six DSM-IV criteria to establish a diagnosis resulted in 83% diagnostic agreement.

Validity. Six clinicians who specialize in PTSD rated relevance and representativeness of several aspects of the DEQ (e.g., response format, individual items) for measuring PTSD as defined in DSM-IV . The responses averaged "very well" to "considerably" relevant and representative for all indices.

Convergent validity was assessed in a male veteran sample. A sum of the 20 symptom items of the DEQ was significantly, positively correlated with another measure of PTSD ($r = .83$), a measure of depression ($r =. 76$), and hostility ($r = .55$), and was negatively correlated with a measure of self-esteem ($r = -.67$).

In a mixed sample of veterans and women with histories of sexual assault, abuse by an intimate partner, prostitution, and substance abuse, the DEQ was correlated with two other measures of PTSD (rs range from .82 to .94) and these correlations remained high across a variety of ethnic groups. Further, the sum of the additional items of the DEQ measuring associated features were also found to correlate significantly with three measures of PTSD, a measure of depression and a measure of guilt (rs = .71 to .91 for men and rs = .57 to .78 for women). In contrast, the DEQ was uncorrelated with a measure of social desirability in all samples except for within the group of women with a history of prostitution.

The ability of the DEQ to predict diagnostic status as assessed by another self-report measure of PTSD was examined. The percentage of diagnostic agreement between the two scales was 82%. PTSD designation on the DEQ was based on whether DSM-IV criteria B, C, and D were met using a symptom score of 2 (i.e., present to a moderate degree) or higher. The two measures agreed on positive PTSD cases 75% of the time, and agreement regarding the absence of PTSD occurred in 92% of the cases.

The discriminative validity of the DEQ was evaluated against the CAPS. A cutoff score of 26 for a veteran group correctly classified 86% of the sample. A cutoff score of 18 for a group of treatment-seeking women with histories of rape, incest, partner abuse, prostitution, and substance abuse correctly classified 90% of the sample.

Alternative Forms

There are different initial instruction versions of the DEQ depending on the purpose of the assessment and the setting in which it is conducted. Translations are available in Japanese and Tagalog. A computerized version of the scale (which incorporates this scale and the Traumatic Life Events Questionnaire) is currently being validated in a grant-funded study.

Source

The DEQ is available from Edward S. Kubany, Ph.D., National Center for PTSD, Department of Veterans Affairs, 1132 Bishop Street, Suite 307, Honolulu, HI 96813, USA; (tel) 808-566-1651; (fax) 808-566-1885; (e-mail) kubany@pixi.com. A published version of the DEQ is in development with Western Psychological Services, 12031 Wilshire Boulevard, Los Angeles, CA 90025, USA; (tel) 800-648-8857; (fax) 310-478-7838; (e-mail) custsvc@ wpspublish.com; (website) www.wpspublish.com.

IMPACT OF EVENT SCALE (IES)

Original Citations

Horowitz, M., Wilner, N., & Alvarez, W. (1979). Impact of Event Scale: A measure of subjective stress. *Psychosomatic Medicine, 41,* 209–218.

Weiss, D. S., & Marmar, C. R. (1997). The Impact of Event Scale-Revised. In J. P. Wilson & T. M. Keane (Eds.), *Assessing psychological trauma and PTSD* (pp. 399-411). New York: Guilford.

Purpose

To measure intrusion and avoidance resulting from exposure to traumatic events.

Description

The IES is a 15-item self-report questionnaire based on Horowitz's (1976) conceptualization of the stress response as including alternating phases of intrusions and avoidance. There are two subscales: *intrusion* and *avoidance* (see discussion below). Respondents are asked to indicate a specific life event and to rate the descriptive statements in response to that event. Respondents rate how frequently they have experienced each of the symptoms during the previous 7 days on a four-point scale. Weighted numerical ratings are assigned to the descriptors (not at all = 0, rarely = 1, sometimes = 3, and often = 5). Item values of 2 and 4 are not used. Although the IES can be used to assess responses to any type of stressful event, it has been widely used to measure symptoms of PTSD. However, the IES does not assess criterion D, hyperarousal symptoms (e.g., difficulty concentrating, exaggerated startle response). A revised version of the IES, discussed below, includes six items to assess this symptom cluster.

Administration and Scoring

It takes 10 minutes to administer the IES. The IES is scored by summing all of the items. Subscale scores can also be derived by summing the items that reflect *intrusion* (items 1, 4–6, 10, 11, 14) and *arousal* (items 2, 3, 7–9, 12, 13, 15). Horowitz (1982) identified total score thresholds for clinical concern as low (< 8.5), medium (8.6–19), and high (> 19). However, these cutoff points are not related to diagnostic status and their utility has been questioned (e.g., Joseph, 2000).

Psychometric Properties

Sample Scores and Norms.   There are no published norms on the IES, but some individual studies report mean scores for different groups. For instance, the mean score on the IES in a sample of 130 service seeking veterans was 55.7 (*SD* = 10.6) for the total score and 27.6 (*SD* = 6.8) for the *intrusion* subscale and 28.2 (*SD* = 6.2) for the *avoidance* subscale (McFall, Smith, Roszell, Tarver, & Malas, 1990). Among a sample of survivors of a ferry disaster, the mean score was 35 for total score, 19 for *intrusion*, and 16 for *avoidance* (Joseph, Yule, Williams, & Hodgkinson, 1993). Female bank staff following an armed raid scored an average of 22.57 on the IES total score (Hodgkinson & Joseph, 1995).

Reliability.   Good internal consistency for the total and subscale scores on the IES has been demonstrated in a sample of psychotherapy outpatients who had experienced a serious life event (αs range from .78 to .86; Horowitz et al., 1979) and a sample including outpatients and controls who had experienced parental bereavement (total score IES α = .86; Zilberg, Weiss, & Horowitz, 1982).

Test–retest reliability over 1 week for a small sample of students who had recently dissected a cadaver was .87 for the total score, .89 for *intrusion*, and .79 for *avoidance* (Horowitz et al., 1979). Despite the fact that the IES is widely used, no other studies have reported test–retest reliability data on the scale, raising the concern that these findings might overestimate the true reliability of the scale (Joseph, 2000).

Validity. Psychotherapy outpatients reflecting on significantly distressing life events scored significantly higher on the *intrusion subscale, avoidance subscale*, and the total IES than medical students relating to their first dissection experience, which had occurred during the previous week (Horowitz et al., 1979). Patients seeking therapy for parental bereavement scored significantly higher than individuals recruited from the community who had also lost a parent (Zilberg et al., 1982).

Several factor analyses have confirmed the existence of the two hypothesized factors of the IES (e.g., Hodgkinson & Joseph, 1995; Joseph et al., 1993; Schwarzwald, Solomon, Weisenberg, & Mikulincer, 1987; Zilberg et al., 1982) with minor differences in the item loadings. However, even when the two-factor structure was supported, some of these studies have yielded a weaker, third factor that may in fact reflect the distinction of emotional avoidance or denial from active behavioral avoidance (e.g., Joseph et al., 1993; McDonald, 1997; Schwarzwald et al., 1987). Hodgkinson and Joseph (1995) found a change in the structure of a factor analysis over time. Specifically, they found *intrusion* to be a larger factor immediately posttrauma and *avoidance* to account for more variance at a later follow-up point (Hodgkinson & Joseph, 1995). Finally, other studies with more chronic trauma populations have reported a single factor solution, suggesting that the distinctiveness of intrusion and avoidance lessens over time (Hendrix, Jurich, & Schumm, 1994).

Studies have examined correlations between the subscales of the IES and have, for the most part, supported the notion that they measure separate but related constructs ($rs = .40$ to .78; Hodgkinson & Joseph, 1995; Horowitz et al., 1979, Neal, Busuttil, Rollins, et al., 1994; Zilberg et al., 1982). There is some evidence that the relationship between the two subscales changes over time (e.g., Zilberg et al., 1982).

The IES has been shown to be associated with another self-report measure of PTSD (rs for the total score and subscales ranged from .44 to .67) and a measure of general distress (rs range from .50 to .60) among women receiving inpatient treatment for trauma-related disorders (Allen, Coyne, & Huntoon, 1998). In a mixed sample of veterans seeking treatment and civilians, the IES was significantly associated with a self-report (rs ranged from .73 to .79) and a structured clinical interview measure of PTSD (rs ranged from .75 to .81; Neal, Busuttil, Rollins, et al., 1994). Further, the IES was significantly associated with general distress (rs ranged from .44 to .63) in a sample of women exposed to an armed raid (Hodgkinson & Joseph, 1995).

Neal, Busuttil, Rollins, et al. (1994) found that an optimum cutoff score of 35 for the total IES yielded a sensitivity of 89%, specificity of 88%, and overall diagnostic efficiency of 88%, relative to a structured clinical interview.

Treatment sensitivity has been demonstrated in several studies (Davidson et al., 1993; Foa, Rothbaum, Riggs, & Murdock, 1991; Horowitz et al., 1979).

The predictive validity of the IES has also been demonstrated. Perry, Difede, Musngi, Frances, and Jacobsberg (1992) found that IES *intrusion* scores 2 months posttrauma significantly predicted PTSD at 6 months and that IES *avoidance* scores at 6 months significantly predicted PTSD at 12 months posttrauma. Shalev, Peri, Canetti, and Schreiber (1996) found that IES scores 1 week posttrauma predicted PTSD 6 months later with 92.3% sensitivity, but only 34.2% specificity.

Alternative Forms

The IES has been translated into several languages including Hebrew and Dutch. A revised version of the IES, which includes seven new items presumed to measure hyperarousal and one that measures flashback-type experiences, has been demonstrated to have very good internal consistency and moderate to good test–retest reliability (Weiss & Marmar, 1997). After collecting these psychometric data, the authors made some additional changes to the IES-R with regard to the instructions and the rating scale, which need to be empirically evaluated.

Source

The IES is reprinted in the original citation and in Appendix B. Additional information can be obtained by contacting Mardi Horowitz, M.D., University of California–San Francisco, P.O. Box 0984, Box F-LPP 357, San Francisco, CA 94142, USA. The IES-R is reprinted in Weiss and Marmar (1997). More information can be obtained by contacting Daniel S. Weiss, Ph.D., Director of PTSD Research, SFVAMC, Department of Psychiatry, University of California–San Francisco, San Francisco, CA 94143, USA; (e-mail) dweiss@itsa.ucsf.edu.

LOS ANGELES SYMPTOM CHECKLIST (LASC)

Original Citation

King, L. A., King, D. W., Leskin, G., & Foy, D. W. (1995). The Los Angeles Symptom Checklist: A self-report measure of posttraumatic stress disorder. *Assessment, 2,* 1–17.

Purpose

To measure PTSD symptoms from DSM-IV criteria B, C, and D as well as associated features.

Description

The LASC is a 43-item self-report scale. Seventeen of the items correspond fairly closely with the B, C, and D symptoms of PTSD. Each item is a word or phrase that is rated on a five-point scale ranging from 0 (not a problem) to 4 (extreme problem), reflecting the extent to which the symptom is a problem for the respondent. No time frame is established for rating symptoms.

Administration and Scoring

The LASC can be administered in 10 to 15 minutes. It can be scored in several ways. To be considered a positive PTSD case, a respondent must endorse an appropriate combination of symptoms with a rating of two or higher. Following DSM-IV criteria, the diagnosis of PTSD requires at least one *reexperiencing* (B) symptom (items 5, 23, 28), three *avoidance* (C) symptoms (items 19, 29, 40–43), and two *arousal* (D) symptoms (items 1, 4, 8, 20, 25, 34, 37, 38). A partial PTSD diagnosis may be considered if a respondent endorses two of the three criteria. The LASC may also be scored as a continuous measure of PTSD severity, which requires summing the scores of the 17 items reflecting PTSD symptoms. Finally, the sum of all 43 items provides a global assessment of distress and interference related to traumatic exposure.

Psychometric Properties

Sample Scores and Norms.   Normative information is available for a variety of samples that vary across gender, age, and trauma type derived from 10 studies reported by King, King, Leskin, and Foy (1995). *PTSD severity* scores for male veterans have been found to range from 46.94 to 49.82; in the same samples the *LASC total* score ranged from 94.63 to 107.87 (Leskin & Foy, 1993; Pava, 1993). Mean *PTSD severity* scores for help seeking women with a history of childhood sexual assault ranged from 29.57 to 31.18; in the same samples the *total LASC* scores ranged from 56.83 to 64.62 (Lawrence, 1992; Rowan, Foy, Rodriguez, & Ryan, 1994; Ryan, 1992).

Reliability.   A data set was formed to assess the psychometric characteristics of the LASC by combining data from 10 studies that had used the measure with clinical samples (King et al., 1995). The samples were derived from a diverse set of populations including Vietnam veterans, battered women, adult survivors of childhood sexual abuse, maritally distressed women, psychiatric outpatients, and high-risk adolescents. The total data set included 874 respondents. Coefficient alpha was .94 for the 17 items specifically assessing PTSD symptoms and .95 for the total score. Test–retest reliability over 2 weeks was available for a sample of 19 Vietnam veterans. The 17-item scores yielded a coefficient of .94 and the total scores yielded a coefficient of .90.

Validity.   A factor analysis on the combined data set yielded three factors accounting for a total of 40.8% of the variance in the scale. Factor 1 was represented primarily by items that assessed the specific symptoms of PTSD. Factor 2 included items that tapped into physical manifestations of stress (e.g., severe headaches, abdominal distress, dizziness). Factor 3 included items reflecting issues related to interpersonal functioning (e.g., marked self-consciousness, inability to make and keep same-sex friends).

The LASC PTSD scores have been shown to be moderately but significantly related to measures of combat exposure (rs ranging from .30 to .51; Foy, Sipprelle, Rueger, & Carroll, 1984; Lund, Foy, Sipprelle, & Strachan, 1984; Resnick, Foy, Donahoe, & Miller, 1989) and other self-report measures of PTSD symptomatology (rs ranging from .38 to .48; Astin, Lawrence, & Foy, 1993). Diagnoses based on LASC scores corresponded to diagnosis based on a structured clinical interview with a sensitivity rate of 70% and a specificity rate of 80% (Housekamp & Foy, 1991).

King et al. (1995) also examined the ability of the LASC to predict PTSD diagnosis derived from a structured clinical interview. Although the 17 items were associated with a PTSD diagnosis (a score of 34 on the LASC is associated with approximately a 75% probability of having PTSD), the additional 26 items did not add to the predictive power of the measure. Thus, although these items may be clinically descriptive, their predictive validity is unproven.

Alternate Forms

An adolescent version of the LASC is available (Foy, Wood, King, King, & Resnick, 1997).

Source

The LASC is reprinted in Appendix B. The primary author of the scale is David W. Foy, Ph.D., Graduate School of Education and Psychology, Pepperdine University Plaza, 400 Corporate Pointe, Culver City, CA 90230, USA; (tel) 310-568-5739; (fax) 310-568-5755. More information can also be obtained by contacting Lynda A. King, National Center for PTSD (116B-3), VA Boston Healthcare System, 150 South Huntington Avenue, Boston, MA, 02130, USA; (tel) 617-232-9500, ext. 4938; (fax) 617-566-8508; (e-mail) lking@world. std.com.

MINNESOTA MULTIPHASIC PERSONALITY INVENTORY PTSD SCALE (MMPI-PTSD)

Original Citation

Keane, T. M., Malloy, P. F., & Fairbank, J. A. (1984). Empirical development of an MMPI subscale for the assessment of combat-related posttraumatic stress disorder. *Journal of Consulting and Clinical Psychology, 52*, 888–891.

Purpose

To detect symptoms of posttraumatic stress disorder.

Description

One of the greatest advantages of the MMPI-PTSD scale is that it is widely available to clinicians who regularly administer the MMPI-2 as part of their practice. The original MMPI-PTSD was a 49-item measure derived from the MMPI. When the MMPI was renamed and revised, the MMPI-PTSD scale also underwent some changes including the deletion of three items, the rewording of one item, and a change in item order (thus the current version has 46 items). The items are answered in a true–false format. Although the scale is typically administered as part of the full MMPI-2, it can be useful as a stand-alone scale. The embedded and stand-alone versions have been shown to be highly correlated ($r = .90$; Herman, Weathers, Litz, & Keane, 1996).

Administration and Scoring

It takes 15 minutes to administer the stand-alone version of the MMPI-PTSD scale. A total score is derived by summing the positive answers to the items. The MMPI-2 PTSD is also discussed in the MMPI-2 manual and can be scored by the hand or computer method. A cutoff score of 30 was originally suggested for detecting PTSD among veterans; later studies with the MMPI-2 version suggested a cutoff between 24 and 28. The civilian cutoff is in the range of 15 to 19. Scores greater than 38 or 40 may indicate fabrication of symptoms. Additional information about scoring and interpreting the MMPI-PTSD scale in the context of the MMPI-2 is available in the manual.

Psychometric Properties

Sample Scores and Norms. On the original MMPI-PTSD scale, veterans with PTSD have a mean score between 26 and 37 (Keane et al., 1984; Koretzky & Peck, 1990), whereas psychiatric controls have a mean of 20 (Keane et al., 1984) and non-PTSD patients a mean of 12.30 (Koretzky & Peck, 1990). Veterans with PTSD revealed a mean of 31.5 on the revised stand-alone scale whereas those without PTSD had a mean of 15.5 (Herman et al., 1996). Mean scores for the revised, embedded MMPI-PTSD scale have been shown to range from 30.6 to 36.2 for veterans with PTSD (Herman et al., 1996; Litz et al., 1991), and to be 15.5 for veterans without PTSD (Herman et al., 1996), 22.9 for psychiatric controls, 18.3 for substance abusers, and 5.2 for a comparison group (Litz et al., 1991).

Reliability. The internal consistency of the embedded and stand-alone versions of the MMPI-2 PTSD scale has been shown to be excellent in a veteran sample (αs range from .95 to .96; Herman et al., 1996).

The test–retest reliability of the stand-alone version of the MMPI-2 PTSD scale over 2 to 3 days was also excellent in a veteran sample ($r = .95$; Herman et al., 1996).

Validity. Veterans with PTSD have been shown to score significantly higher than psychiatric controls (Keane et al., 1984) and veterans without PTSD (Herman et al., 1996; Scotti, Sturges, & Lyons, 1996). Further, the MMPI-PTSD scale can differentiate veterans with comorbid PTSD and substance abuse from those with substance abuse alone (Kenderdine, Phillips, & Scurfield, 1992).

A score of 30 correctly classified 82% of veterans with and without PTSD (Keane et al., 1984). A score of 19 correctly classified 88% of patients in a psychotherapy clinic (Koretzky & Peck, 1990).

With regard to convergent validity, the original MMPI-PTSD scale was correlated significantly with other self-report measures of PTSD in a sample of veterans (rs ranged from .79 to .88; Watson et al., 1994) although another study found the associations to be lower (rs ranged from .21 to .71; McFall, Smith, Mackay, & Tarver, 1990). In a sample of battered women, Dutton, Perrin, Chrestman, Halle, and Burghardt (1991) found the MMPI-PTSD scale to be moderately but significantly correlated with other self-report measures of PTSD (rs ranged from .33 to .65). Stronger convergent validity with other measures of PTSD was demonstrated in a mixed trauma sample (Neal, Busuttil, Rollins, et al., 1994; rs ranged from .79 to .85); however, in this sample, the scale was also highly correlated with a measure of general distress ($r = .92$). Further, the MMPI-PTSD scale was significantly correlated with a number of MMPI scales and subscales in a sample of inpatient alcoholics, again suggesting that the measure may assess general psychological distress (Moody & Kish, 1989).

The embedded and stand-alone versions of the MMPI-2 PTSD scale have been shown to be moderately but significantly associated with a measure of combat exposure (rs ranged from .32 to .37), other self-report measures of PTSD (rs ranged from .65 to .85), and a structured clinical interview for PTSD (rs ranged from .77 to .80; Herman et al., 1996).

Cutoffs of 26 and 28 for the embedded MMPI-2 PTSD scale have been shown to correctly classify 76% of veterans with PTSD (Herman et al., 1996; Munley, Bains, Bloem, & Busby, 1995), whereas a cutoff of 24 on the stand-alone version correctly classified 80% of veterans with PTSD (Herman et al., 1996).

Treatment sensitivity for the MMPI-PTSD has been demonstrated in a number of studies (e.g., Brom, Kleber, & Defares, 1989; Thompson et al., 1995).

Source

Additional information about the MMPI-PTSD scale can be obtained by contacting Terence M. Keane, Ph.D., National Center for PTSD (116B-2), VA Boston Healthcare System, 150 South Huntington Avenue, Boston, MA 02130, USA; (tel) 617-232-9500, ext. 4143; (e-mail) terry.keane@med.va.gov.

MISSISSIPPI SCALE FOR PTSD

Original Citations

Keane, T. M., Caddell, J. M., & Taylor, K. L. (1988). Mississippi Scale for Combat-Related Posttraumatic Stress Disorder: Three studies in reliability and validity. *Journal of Consulting and Clinical Psychology, 56,* 85–90.

Purpose

To measure self-reported symptoms of PTSD.

Description

There are several versions of the Mississippi Scale for PTSD. Among the most widely used include the Mississippi Scale for Combat-Related PTSD and the Civilian Mississippi Scale. The original combat scale consists of 35 items that tap into the presence of symptoms reflecting the three main DSM-IV criteria for PTSD: *reexperiencing* (criterion B), *avoidance and numbing* (criterion C), and *hyperarousal* (criterion D) and associated features (e.g., depression, substance abuse). Items are rated on a five-point scale with anchors that vary depending on the item but include phrases such as "not at all true" to "almost always true." Respondents are asked to rate symptoms over the time period occurring "since the event." The original version of the civilian scale used in the civilian/nonveteran component of the National Vietnam Veterans Readjustment Study (NVVRS) also had 35 items. Eleven of the items were rephrased slightly, changing reference to military service to a more general reference to the past. In both the combat and civilian versions, 4 items were added to make the scale consistent with DSM-IV criteria. These items assess symptoms of reexperiencing, psychogenic amnesia, hypervigilance, and increased arousal when confronted with reminders of the event. However, these items have not been found to increase the discriminative validity of the measure, so they are commonly omitted.

ADMINISTRATION AND SCORING

The full Mississippi Scale takes 10 to 15 minutes to administer. After reversing the positively worded items, a total score is derived by summing all of the items. A cutoff score of 107 was originally established for the combat version, although later studies suggested that a cutoff of 121 allows for better differentiation between veterans with and without PTSD. For the version reprinted in Appendix B, there are 9 positively worded items that should be reversed (items 6, 11, 17, 19, 22, 24, 27, 30, 34).

Psychometric Properties

Sample Scores and Norms.   Among a large sample of treatment seeking veterans, the mean score for the 35-item scale was 104.5 ($SD = 26.2$; Keane et al., 1988). Means on the civilian measure for undergraduates ranged from 73.5 to 74.4 on the 35-item scale, and 81.8 to 82.9 on the 39-item scale (Lauterbach, Vrana, King, & King, 1997). The mean score obtained by civilians on the NVVRS was 64.3 ($SD = 13.2$) for the 35-item scale (Vreven, Gudanowski, King, & King, 1995).

Reliability.   In a large sample of veterans seeking treatment, the 35-item Mississippi Scale for Combat-Related PTSD was shown to have excellent internal consistency ($\alpha = .94$; Keane et al., 1988). Test–retest reliability over 1 week in a smaller sample of veterans was .97 (Keane et al., 1988).

Internal consistency for the civilian version has also been demonstrated to be very good for both the 35- and 39-item scales (αs from .86 to .89; Lauterbach et al., 1997; Vreven et al., 1995).

Validity.   Several factor analyses have been conducted on the 35-item Mississippi Scale for Combat-Related PTSD (e.g., Keane et al., 1988; McFall, Smith, Mackay, & Tarver, 1990). King and King (1994) conducted exploratory and higher order confirmatory factor analysis on the Mississippi Scale for Combat-Related PTSD using data from over 2200 veterans who participated in the NVVRS. The results suggest that the latent structure of this scale is best represented as an overarching single PTSD factor with four subsidiary dimensions: (1) reexperiencing and situational avoidance, (2) withdrawal and numbing, (3) arousal and lack of control, and (4) self-persecution.

Factor analyses on the civilian version have yielded mixed results from study to study and for the 35- versus the 39-item scale (Lauterbach et al., 1997; Vreven et al., 1995).

With regard to convergent validity, scores on the Mississippi Scale for Combat-Related PTSD are significantly associated with combat exposure (rs range from .25 to .44; Keane et al., 1988; McFall, Smith, Mackay, & Tarver, 1990; McFall, Smith, Roszell, et al., 1990) and other self-report measures of PTSD (rs range from .44 to .88; McFall, Smith, Mackay, & Tarver, 1990; McFall, Smith, Roszell, et al., 1990; Watson et al., 1994).

The convergent validity of the civilian measure has also been examined. Individuals with symptoms of PTSD score significantly higher than those without any PTSD symptoms, and some relationship has been established between exposure to stressful events and score on the Civilian Mississippi Scale (Lauterbach et al., 1997; Vrenen et al., 1995). Also, civilian scores have been associated with sexual abuse-related posttraumatic symptomatology (Gold & Cardeña, 1998). Further, the scores have been significantly but moderately associated with other measures of PTSD (rs range from .34 to .52; Lauterbach et al., 1997). However, the civilian version has also been found to be strongly associated with general distress ($r = .63$; Vrenen et al., 1995), depression ($r = .71$), and anxiety ($r = .70$; Lauterbach et al., 1997). Overall these findings suggest that the civilian version may be more of a general measure of psychopathology than a specific measure of PTSD (Lauterbach et al., 1997; Vrenen et al., 1995).

Compared with a diagnosis derived by structured interview, the diagnostic accuracy of the Mississippi Scale for Combat-Related PTSD with a cutoff score of 107 was 90%, with a sensitivity of 93% and a specificity of 89% (Keane et al., 1988). McFall, Smith, Mackay, and Tarver (1990) found similar diagnostic efficiency with a lower cutoff score. However, Dalton, Tom, Rosenblum, Garte, and Aubuchon (1989) reported that 77% of nonveterans were able to feign a score on the scale exceeding the 107 cutoff. Lyons, Caddell, Pittman, Rawls, and Perrin (1994) also found that the scale was vulnerable to faking and suggested a cutoff of 121. However, although the sensitivity of this cutoff is good (.95), its specificity is relatively low (.45).

The diagnostic accuracy of the civilian version of the scale was examined in a large sample of individuals recruited from an emergency room (Shalev, Freedman, Peri, Brandes, & Sahar, 1997). With a cutoff of 75, the sensitivity of the scale was .87, and the specificity was .51. No cutoff score was found that could optimize both sensitivity and specificity.

Alternative Forms

The Mississippi Scale for Combat-Related PTSD has been translated into Hebrew and Spanish. A short version of the combat-related version, comprised of 11 items, has been shown to have good internal consistency, high sensitivity and specificity against a cutoff derived from the full scale, and good treatment sensitivity (Fontana & Rosenheck, 1994). Norris and Perilla (1996) developed a 30-item Revised Version of the Civilian Mississippi Scale that has demonstrated internal consistency for both an English and a Spanish translation.

Source

The Mississippi Scale for Combat-Related PTSD can be obtained by contacting Terence M. Keane, Ph.D., National Center for PTSD (116B-2), VA Boston Healthcare System, 150 South Huntington Avenue, Boston, MA 02130, USA; (tel) 617-232-9500, ext. 4143; (e-mail) terry.keane@med.va.gov. The 35-item Civilian Mississippi Scale is reprinted in Appendix B.

PENN INVENTORY FOR PTSD (PENN INVENTORY)

Original Citation

Hammarberg, M. (1992). Penn Inventory for Posttraumatic Stress Disorder: Psychometric properties. *Psychological Assessment, 4,* 67–76.

Purpose

To measure severity of PTSD.

Description

The Penn Inventory is a 26-item self-report measure of the severity of PTSD. Each item comprises four sentences modeled after the Beck Depression Inventory. The meanings of the series of sentences measure the presence or absence of PTSD symptoms over the past week in addition to their degree, frequency, or intensity. The respondent chooses the statement that best describes their experience. Each sentence is rated from 0 to 3 with higher scores representing more symptomatology. Items are not keyed to a specific traumatic event.

Administration and Scoring

The Penn Inventory can be administered in 10 to 15 minutes. A score is derived by summing all of the circled values. A cutoff score of 35 can be used to determine the likely presence of PTSD.

Psychometric Properties

Sample Scores and Norms.   The mean scores for clinical samples of Vietnam veterans range from 51.1 ($SD = 12.3$) to 54.7 ($SD = 8.7$; Hammarberg, 1992). Veterans without PTSD revealed a mean score of 15.6 ($SD = 9.1$) and a nonveteran community sample had a mean of 15.3 ($SD = 8.4$; Hammarberg, 1992).

Reliability.   The Penn Inventory has been demonstrated to have very good to excellent internal consistency (α ranges from .78 to .94) across a variety of clinical and community samples (Hammarberg, 1992). Additionally, test–retest over an average of 5.2 days ranged from .87 to .93 (Hammarberg, 1992).

Validity.   Individuals diagnosed with PTSD on the basis of self-report measures and a clinical interview scored significantly higher than those without PTSD (either confirmed by diagnostic interview or assumed based on nonveteran or community status; Hammarberg, 1992).

The overall diagnostic efficiency of the measure against another self-report measure of PTSD among veterans was 94% (Hammarberg, 1992). In a sample of disaster victims, the hit rate was 95% (Hammarberg, 1992).

Scores on the Penn Inventory have been shown to be moderately but significantly associated with exposure to combat ($r = .39$; Hammarberg, 1992). Further, among a group of veterans diagnosed with PTSD, the Penn Inventory was demonstrated to be associated with measures of anxiety (rs ranged from .74 to .82) and depression ($r = .52$). The Penn Inventory was also significantly associated with additional measures of PTSD (rs from .72 to .85).

Treatment sensitivity was demonstrated in a sample of Vietnam veterans treated for PTSD (Hammarberg & Silver, 1994). Patients changed on average from a score of 55 ($SD = 9.2$) to a score of 45.96 ($SD = 16.0$) over a period of 12 weeks, whereas untreated veterans with PTSD and non-PTSD Vietnam era veterans and nonveterans showed no significant symptom change.

Source

The Penn Inventory may be obtained from Melvyn Hammarberg, Ph.D., Department of Anthropology, 325 Museum, University of Pennsylvania, Philadelphia, PA 19104-6398, USA; (tel) 215-898-0981; (fax) 215-898-7462; (e-mail) mhammarb@ecat.sas.upenn.edu. The cost of the measure is $35.00 US.

POSTTRAUMATIC COGNITIONS INVENTORY (PTCI)

Original Citation

Foa, E. B., Ehlers, A., Clark, D. M., Tolin, D. F., & Orsillo, S. M. (1999). The Posttraumatic Cognitions Inventory (PTCI): Development and validation. *Psychological Assessment*, *11*, 303–314.

Purpose

To measure trauma-related thoughts and beliefs.

Description

The PTCI is a 36-item self-report questionnaire that taps into three constructs related to trauma-related thoughts and beliefs: *negative cognitions about self*, *negative cognitions about the world*, and *self-blame*. Each item presents a statement and is followed by a seven-point response scale representing degree of agreement ranging from 1 (totally disagree) to 7 (totally agree). Items are worded so that higher ratings reflect greater endorsement of pathological cognitions.

Administration and Scoring

The PTCI can be administered in 10 minutes. Scoring consists of summing the items that make up each subscale and dividing the sum by the number of items comprising the subscale. *Negative cognitions about self* is derived from items 2–6, 9, 12, 14, 16, 17, 20, 21, 24–26, 28–30, 33, 35, and 36; *negative cognitions about the world* is derived from items 7, 8, 10, 11, 18, 23, and 27; *self-blame* is derived from items 1, 15, 19, 22, and 31. Items 13, 32, and 34 are experimental and are not included in the subscales. The total score is derived by taking the sum of the items that comprise the three subscales.

Psychometric Properties

The psychometric properties are derived from a sample of 601 volunteers, 392 of whom had experienced a traumatic event, and 170 of whom had reported at least moderate PTSD symptomatology on a self-report measure (Foa et al., 1999). Participants were recruited from clinical, community, and undergraduate settings.

Sample Scores and Norms. The median scores for a sample of individuals with PTSD of at least moderate severity were 133 (*SD* = 44.17) for total score, 3.60 (*SD* = 1.48) for *negative cognitions about self*, 5.00 (*SD* = 1.25) for *negative cognitions about the world*, and 3.20 (*SD* = 1.74) for *self-blame*. Median scores derived from a nontraumatized group were 45.50 (*SD* = 34.76) for total score, 1.08 (*SD* = 0.76) for *negative cognitions about self*, 2.07 (*SD* = 1.43) for *negative cognitions about the world*, and 1.00 (*SD* = 1.45) for *self-blame*.

Reliability. Cronbach's alphas for the three PTCI scales and total scales are good to very good (total score, α = .97; *negative cognitions about self*, α = .97; *negative cognitions about the world*, α = .88; *self-blame*, α = .86). One-week test–retest reliability on a subsample of the respondents was .74 for the total score and ranged from .75 to .89 for the scales. Three-week test–retest reliability in another subsample was .85 for the total score and ranged from .80 to .86 for the scales.

Validity. Factor analysis confirmed the existence of the three-factor structure. The first factor explained 48.5% of the variance, the second factor accounted for an additional 4%, and the third factor accounted for an additional 3.4%. The stability of the structure was validated across three samples.

PTCI scores were found to correlate with PTSD severity (*r* = .79), depression (*r* = .75), and anxiety (*r* = .75). The scales of the PTCI were significantly associated with similar scales assessing trauma-related cognitions. Traumatized individuals with PTSD scored significantly higher than traumatized individuals without PTSD and nontraumatized individuals on all of the PTCI scales. Further, the PTCI compared favorably with other measures of trauma-related cognitions for predicting PTSD. Scores on the PTCI scales classified 86% of the traumatized individuals correctly into those with and without PTSD with a sensitivity of .78 and a specificity of .93.

Source

The PTCI is reprinted in the original citation and in Appendix B. Additional information about the measure can be obtained by contacting Edna B. Foa, Ph.D., Center for the Study and Treatment of Anxiety, University of Pennsylvania, School of Medicine, 3535 Market Street, 6th floor, Philadelphia, PA 19104, USA; (tel) 215-746-3327; (fax) 215-746-3311; (e-mail) foa@mail.med.upenn.edu.

POSTTRAUMATIC DIAGNOSTIC SCALE (PDS)

Original Citation

Foa, E. B., Cashman, L. A., Jaycox, L., & Perry, K. (1997). The validation of a self-report measure of posttraumatic stress disorder: The Posttraumatic Diagnostic Scale. *Psychological Assessment, 4,* 445–451.

Purpose

To assess the DSM-IV diagnostic criteria and symptom severity of PTSD.

Description

The PDS is a revised version of an earlier self-report scale entitled the PTSD Symptom Scale (Foa, Riggs, Dancu, & Rothbaum, 1993). The PDS consists of 49 items arranged into four sections. Part I includes a checklist of 12 traumatic events one could experience or witness. In Part 2, the event causing the most distress in the past month is chosen, described in more detail and referred to in subsequent questions. Criterion A is established via four questions that assess physical threat and feelings of helplessness related to the event. Part 3 includes 17 items corresponding to PTSD criteria B, C, and D that assess the frequency of each symptom in the past month on a four-point scale. Part 4 assesses criterion F with 9 items that determine impairment in major life areas (e.g., work, leisure) using a yes/no format.

Administration and Scoring

The PDS can be administered in 10 to 15 minutes. It may be scored by hand or by computer program. A number of scoring indices can be derived including PDS diagnosis, symptom severity score, number of symptoms endorsed, symptom severity rating, and level of impairment in functioning. Following DSM-IV criteria, the diagnosis of PTSD requires the presence of physical injury or perception of life threat; a sense of helplessness or terror during the event; endorsement of at least one reexperiencing (criterion B) symptom, three avoidance (criterion C) symptoms, and two arousal (criterion D) symptoms; duration of at least 1 month; and impairment in at least one area of life functioning. An index of PTSD severity is obtained by summing the 17 symptom items.

Psychometric Properties

The psychometric properties are derived from a sample of 248 volunteers recruited from several PTSD treatment centers as well as from non-treatment seeking populations who may be at high risk for trauma (e.g., staff at police stations, individuals at women's shelters; Foa et al., 1997).

Sample Scores and Norms.   The mean scores for a sample of 128 individuals with PTSD were 33.59 (*SD* = 9.96) for total symptom severity, 8.95 (*SD* = 3.68) for reexperiencing, 13.63 (*SD* = 4.76) for avoidance, and 11.02 (*SD* = 3.53) for arousal. The non-PTSD group (*N* = 120) obtained a mean score of 12.54 (*SD* = 10.54) on the total scale, 3.64 (*SD* = 3.18) on the reexperiencing scale, 4.54 (*SD* = 4.83) on the avoidance scale, and 4.36 (*SD* = 3.97) on the arousal scale.

Reliability.   The PDS has been shown to have excellent internal consistency overall (α = .92) and very good internal consistency for the symptom subscales (αs ranging from .78 to .84). Additionally, repeated administration over 2 to 3 weeks yielded an 87% agreement rate (kappa = .74) between diagnoses and adequate stability in symptom severity (all *rs* = .77 to .85).

Validity.   Satisfactory agreement was found between the diagnoses derived from the PDS and those obtained from a structured clinical interview (kappa of .65, 82% agreement). Sensitivity of the PDS was .89 and specificity was .75. Scores reflecting symptom severity on the PDS correlated with another measure of PTSD ($r = .78$), a measure of anxiety (rs range from .73 to .74), and a measure of depression ($r = .79$). These correlations raise the issue of whether the PDS is a specific measure of PTSD or a more general measure of psychological distress. However, given the high comorbidity of PTSD with anxiety and mood disorders, and the symptom overlap between disorders, this pattern of findings is not surprising.

Alternative Forms

The PTSD Symptom Scale Interview (PSS-I) is an interview version of the PTSD Symptom Scale Self-Report Scale that was the predecessor of the PDS. Psychometric properties of this scale are available in Foa et al. (1993).

Source

The PDS is available from National Computer Systems, P.O. Box 1416, Minneapolis, MN 55440, USA; (tel) 800-627-7271; (webpage) www.ncs.com. The PDS on-line version requires the purchase of Microtest Q Assessment Systems Software with an annual licensing fee of $89.00 US. Each assessment profile costs $4.25 US for the first 50 reports. The pencil-and-paper starter kit (including 1 manual, 10 answer sheets, and 1 scoring sheet) is $44.00 US. The reorder kit (50 answer sheets, 50 work sheets, and 1 scoring sheet) is $117.00 US. Additional information about the measure can be obtained by contacting Edna B. Foa, Ph.D., Center for the Study and Treatment of Anxiety, University of Pennsylvania, School of Medicine, 3535 Market Street, 6th floor, Philadelphia, PA 19104, USA; (tel) 215-746-3327; (fax) 215-746-3311; (e-mail) foa@mail.med.upenn.edu.

PTSD CHECKLIST (PCL)

Original Citations

Weathers, F. W., Litz, B. T., Herman, D. S., Huska, J. A., & Keane, T. M. (1993, October). *The PTSD checklist: Reliability, validity and diagnostic utility.* Paper presented at the Annual Meeting of the International Society for Traumatic Stress Studies, San Antonio, TX.

Blanchard, E. B., Jones-Alexander, J., Buckley, T. C., & Forneris, C. A. (1996). Psychometric properties of the PTSD Checklist (PCL). *Behaviour Research and Therapy, 34,* 669–673.

Purpose

To assess PTSD symptom severity.

Description

The PCL is a 17-item inventory that assesses the specific symptoms of PTSD. The respondent is asked to rate how much the problem described in each statement has bothered him or her over the past month on a five-point scale ranging from 1 (not at all) to 5 (extremely). The authors have also suggested that the time frame (e.g., last week) can be changed to accommodate the goals of the assessment.

Administration and Scoring

The PCL takes 5 to 10 minutes to administer. A total score is an indicator of PTSD symptom severity. Cutoff scores of 50 for military samples and 44 for nonmilitary samples have been proposed (see below). Although the authors originally suggested that a PTSD diagnosis could be derived by considering a score of 3 or higher as reflecting the presence of a particular symptom, and by following the DSM-IV diagnostic rules to determine the appropriate number and pattern of symptoms, Blanchard et al. (1996) caution against this approach (see below).

Psychometric Properties

Sample Scores and Norms.   In a sample of combat veterans, those with a diagnosis of PTSD obtained a mean of 63.58 (SD = 14.14) and those without a diagnosis of PTSD obtained a mean of 34.40 (SD = 14.09; Weathers et al., 1993). Individuals with MVA-related PTSD scored 60.0 (SD = 9.4) and those without PTSD scored 26.6 (SD = 4.6). Sexual assault victims diagnosed with PTSD scored 55 (SD = 16.7) versus 22.8 (SD = 11.8) for the no-PTSD assault group (Blanchard et al., 1996). Additional sample means are available for mothers of cancer survivors (Manne, Du Hamel, Gallelli, Sorgen, & Redd, 1998) and for breast cancer survivors (Andrykowski, Cordova, Studts, & Miller, 1998).

Reliability.   The PCL has been shown to have excellent internal consistency in Vietnam and Persian Gulf veterans, victims of motor vehicle accidents, and sexual assault survivors (rs ranging from .94 to .97; Blanchard et al., 1996; Weathers et al., 1993). Test–retest reliability over 2 to 3 days was .96 for the Vietnam veterans (Weathers et al., 1993).

Validity.   A factor analysis on data derived from the Persian Gulf war veterans suggested that the items are best accounted for by a single factor (Weathers et al., 1993). In a Vietnam veteran sample, the PCL-M was significantly correlated with other measures of PTSD (rs range from .77 to .93) and a measure of combat exposure (r = .46; Weathers et al., 1993). Among Persian Gulf veterans, the PCL-M was significantly associated with another measure of PTSD (.85; Weathers et al., 1993).

Several studies have examined the diagnostic efficiency of the PCL. Weathers et al. (1993) found that at a cutoff of 50, the PCL-M predicted PTSD diagnosis derived from a structured clinical interview with a sensitivity of .82 and a specificity of .84. Blanchard et al. (1996) found the same cutoff yielded a sensitivity of .78 and a specificity of .86, and that a cutoff of 44 improved the sensitivity to .94 and specificity to .86 with an overall diagnostic efficiency of 90%. However, they also found variability in the most efficient cutoff score for each item (3 versus 4), thus they caution against the use of a score of 3 on a sufficient number of criterion B, C, and D symptoms to derive a diagnosis.

Additional diagnostic efficiency for cancer groups is found in Manne et al. (1998) and Andrykowski et al. (1998).

Alternative Forms

There are several versions of the PCL: the PCL-Military, the PCL-S (which is tied to a specified stressor), and the PCL-C (which is not tied to a specific stressful event, but instead asks about "response to stressful life events"). A parent report on child symptoms is also available (PCL-PR).

Source

The PCL-C is reprinted in Appendix B. More information about the scale can be obtained from Frank Weathers, Ph.D., Department of Psychology, 226 Thach Hall, Auburn University, AL 36849, USA, (tel) 334-844-6495; (e-mail) weathfw@mail.auburn.edu.

PURDUE PTSD SCALE-REVISED (PPTS-R)

Original Citation

Lauterbach, D., & Vrana, S. (1996). Three studies on the reliability and validity of a self report measure of posttraumatic stress disorder. *Assessment*, *3*, 17–25.

Purpose

To assess the frequency of each PTSD symptom.

Description

The PPTSD-R is a self-report measure comprised of 17 items corresponding to the symptoms found within PTSD criteria B, C, and D. Respondents rate the frequency of occurrence within the previous month of each item on a five-point scale ranging from 1 (not at all) to 5 (often).

Administration and Scoring

The PPTSD-R can be administered in 10 minutes. The scale can be scored to yield a dichotomous index reflecting the presence or absence of PTSD or to yield a continuous measure of severity. Continuous scores are obtained by summing the 17 items. The diagnosis of PTSD requires the endorsement of at least one *reexperiencing* (criterion B) symptom (items 1–4, 8), three *avoidance* (criterion C) symptoms (items 5–7, 9–12) and two *arousal* (criterion D) symptoms (items 13–17).

Psychometric Properties

The psychometric properties reported below are published in a multisample, multistudy paper (Lauterbach & Vrana, 1996).

Sample Scores and Norms. Mean scores for a sample of 440 undergraduate students are 31.5 (*SD* = 12.9) for the total score, 8.5 (*SD* = 4.1) for *reexperiencing*, 12.6 (*SD* = 5.5) for *avoidance*, and 10.4 (*SD* = 4.9) for *arousal*. Within a sample of 35 students receiving psychotherapy at a university-based counseling center the means were 38.7 (*SD* = 15.9) for the total score, 9.5 (*SD* = 4.6) for *reexperiencing*, 15.6 (*SD* = 6.7) for *avoidance* and 13.6 (*SD* = 6.3) for *arousal*.

Reliability. The PPTSD-R has excellent internal consistency overall (α = .91) and very good internal consistency for the symptom subscales (αs ranging from .79 to .84). Test–retest reliability for 51 undergraduate students over 2 weeks reflected adequate stability in symptom severity for the total score (*r* = .72); however, stability was somewhat lower for the *avoidance* (*r* = .67), *arousal* (*r* = .71), and *reexperiencing* subscales (*r* = .48).

Validity. The PPTSD-R has been shown to be more strongly correlated with other measures of PTSD symptomatology (*r*s range from .50 to .66) than measures of anxiety (*r* = .37) and depression (*r* = .39). Further, students who experienced at least one traumatic event scored significantly higher on the PPTSD-R than those who did not report any traumatic events on the total score, *reexperiencing* and *arousal* subscales. Although the traumatized group scored higher on the *avoidance* scale as well, this difference did not reach conventional levels of significance.

Alternative Forms

There is a military and a civilian version of the measure.

Source

The PPTSD-R is reprinted in Appendix B. More information is available from Dean Lauterbach, Ph.D., 350 Sam Sibley Drive, Room 313, Bienvenu Hall, Department of Psychology, Northwestern State University, Natchitoches, LA 71497, USA; (tel) 318-357-5453; (fax) 318-357-6802.

SHORT SCREENING SCALE FOR PTSD

Original Citation

Breslau, N., Peterson, E. L., Kessler, R. C., & Schultz, L. R. (1999). Short screening scale for DSM-IV posttraumatic stress disorder. *American Journal of Psychiatry*, *156*, 908–911.

Purpose

To screen for PTSD in persons exposed to a DSM-IV qualifying traumatic event.

Description

The Short Screening Scale for PTSD is a seven-item (yes/no format) clinician-administered interview measure derived from the modified National Institute of Mental Health Diagnostic Interview Schedule and the World Health Organization Composite International Diagnostic Interview developed and used in the Detroit Area Survey of Trauma (Breslau, Kessler, & Peterson, 1998). The majority of PTSD symptom measures ask about symptoms in connection with only one event. Often, respondents have experienced multiple events, but they are asked to choose the worst or most distressing event to complete the measure. The Short Screening Scale for PTSD was developed to enable interviewers to quickly and efficiently assess PTSD in response to a number of traumas.

Administration and Scoring

The Short Screening Scale for PTSD can be administered in less than 3 minutes. Scoring consists of counting the number of positive answers to the seven items. A score of 4 or more seems to be the best cutoff for predicting PTSD diagnosis.

Psychometric Properties

Sample Scores and Norms.   None are available.

Reliability.   The reliability of the seven-item screening scale has not been directly examined. However, the reliability of the PTSD module from which it was derived has been assessed. A random sample of 32 baseline PTSD cases and 23 noncases was selected to be reassessed 12 to 18 months after the baseline interview (Breslau et al., 1998). There was agreement on 83% of the cases.

Validity.   The predictive validity of the Short Screening Scale for PTSD relative to the full diagnostic interview was examined in a representative sample of 1830 men and women who were interviewed as part of the 1996 Detroit Area Survey of Trauma (Breslau et al., 1999). With 4 as a cutoff, the sensitivity was 80.3% and the specificity was 97.3%.

Although this measure appears to be a promising screening tool, particularly for researchers, it is important to note that the validity of the scale has not been examined in a study in which the seven items were administered as a freestanding scale.

Source

The Short Screening Scale for PTSD is reprinted in Appendix B. More information about the scale can be obtained by contacting Naomi Breslau, Ph.D., Henry Ford Health Systems, Psychiatry Service, 3A, Detroit, MI 48202-3450, USA; (tel) 313-876-2516; (fax) 313-874-6221; (e-mail) nbresla1@hfhs.org.

STANFORD ACUTE STRESS REACTION QUESTIONNAIRE (SASRQ)

Original Citation

Cardeña, E., Koopman, C., Classen, C., Waelde, L. C., & Spiegel, D. (2000). Psycho-metric properties of the Stanford Acute Stress Reaction Questionnaire: A valid and reliable measure of acute stress. *Journal of Traumatic Stress, 13,* 719–734.

Purpose

To assess the psychological symptoms experienced in the aftermath of a traumatic event.

Description

The SASRQ is a 30-item self-report measure of ASD. The instructions allow the administrator to specify the time period during which the respondent's symptoms should be rated. The respondent is asked to describe the stressful event and rate how much disturbance it caused. Then, the respondent rates 30 items on a six-point scale ranging from 0 (not experi-enced) to 5 (very often experienced). Items tap into dissociation (10 items), reexperiencing (6 items), avoidance (6 items), anxiety and hyperarousal (6 items), and impairment in functioning (2 items). A final question asks the respondent how many days he or she experienced the worst symptoms of distress.

Administration and Scoring

The SASRQ can be administered in 15 minutes. It can be scored continuously by summing all of the items or dichotomously (ratings between 0 and 2 = 0, ratings between 3 and 5 = 1) for the presence of a symptom. To meet criterion B, a respondent must endorse three or more of the symptom criteria for dissociation: numbing (items 20, 28), reduction in awareness of surroundings (items 4, 24), derealization (items 3, 18), depersonalization (items 10, 13), dissociative amnesia (items 16, 25). A respondent must endorse a symptom within each of the remaining criterion symptom clusters to obtain an ASD diagnosis: criterion C (items 6, 7, 15, 19, 23, 29), criterion D (items 5, 11, 14, 17, 22, 30), criterion E (items 1, 2, 8, 12, 21, 27), and criterion F (items 9, 26).

Psychometric Properties

The psychometric properties of an earlier version and of the final version of the SASRQ were evaluated together in a multisample, multistudy paper (Cardeña et al., 2000).

Sample Scores and Norms. In a sample of 43 adult emergency rescue workers the mean score was 26.37 (*SD* = 25.52). In contrast, within a group of 97 nonexposed rescue workers the mean was 4.91 (*SD* = 8.34).

Reliability. The internal consistency for the 30 symptom items of the SASRQ was found to be very good to excellent for the total score (*r*s range from .80 to .95) and acceptable to excellent for the subscales (*r*s range from .64 to .91).

Test–retest reliability over 3 to 4 weeks with a sample of students who had not experienced a severe stressor in the interim was .69.

Validity. In several samples, hypothesized group differences on the SASRQ were confirmed. For instance, participants exposed to a rescue operation scored significantly higher on the SASRQ than their nonexposed colleagues. Gulf War veterans with PTSD scored significantly higher than controls.

Convergent and discriminant validity have been demonstrated with the SASRQ. Scores on the dissociation and anxiety subscales of the SASRQ were significantly correlated with a measure of intrusion and avoidance (*r*s ranging from .55 to .75). The association of these subscales with a measure of schizophrenic symptoms was weaker (*r*s ranging from .22 to .47). In another sample, score on the SASRQ was significantly associated with a measure of peritraumatic dissociation ($r = .72$).

Some preliminary support exists for the predictive validity of the SASRQ. Among workers in a building where a mass shooting occurred, all participants who met criteria for ASD had significant PTSD symptoms 7 months later. Individuals diagnosed with ASD on the SASRQ had significantly greater odds of being considered a PTSD case, based on a self-report measure, at 6-month follow-up.

Source

The SASRQ is reprinted in Appendix B. Additional information can be obtained by contacting Etzel Cardeña, Ph.D., Department of Psychology and Anthropology, University of Texas-Pan American, 1201 West University Drive, Edinburg, TX 78639, USA; (tel) 956-381-3329, ext. 3323; (fax) 956-381-3333; (e-mail) ecardena@panam.edu.

STRESSFUL LIFE EVENTS SCREENING QUESTIONNAIRE (SLESQ)

Original Citation

Goodman, L. S., Corcoran, C., Turner, K., Yuan, N., & Green, B. L. (1998). Assessing traumatic event exposure: General issues and preliminary findings for the Stressful Life Events Screening Questionnaire. *Journal of Traumatic Stress, 11*, 521–542.

Purpose

To assess lifetime exposure to a variety of traumatic events.

Description

The SLESQ is a 15-item self-report measure of lifetime exposure to traumatic events. Respondents are asked whether they have experienced an event (e.g., life-threatening illness, physically forced sexual relations), and if they endorse the item, they are asked a series of questions about the nature of their exposure that vary from item to item (e.g., the age at the time of the event, injuries they may have received, the nature of the relationship with the perpetrator). In addition to answering the questions, the respondents are also asked to describe each event. Finally, respondents indicate whether multiple items refer to the same event, and if an event happened more than once, they are asked to describe the nature of the additional episodes of the event. Criterion A-2 is not assessed with this measure. Although the majority of psychometric data derive from a college sample, the SLESQ was developed for use with community samples, and the psychometric properties are currently being evaluated in samples of low-income and ethnic minority women (L. A. Goodman, personal communication, August 16, 2000).

Administration and Scoring

The SLESQ takes 10 minutes to administer for most respondents; those with multiple traumas may need up to 20 minutes. The authors suggest that some level of screening of the description of each endorsed event be conducted to ensure that the responses are appropriate and that they truly reflect criterion A events (rather than stressful, but not traumatic, events). Depending on the question of interest, users can score the scale in a number of ways (for instance, count the total number of endorsed events, or the number of events in a specific category such as interpersonal versus noninterpersonal events).

Psychometric Properties

Sample Means and Norms.   In a large sample of college students, 72% of respondents reported exposure to at least one traumatic event (Goodman et al., 1998). The mean number of events endorsed by this sample was 1.83 ($SD = 1.96$). The prevalence of each event was reported by Goodman et al. (1998). In a sample of 2507 women recruited from six college campuses, 65% of the sample reported at least one event (ruling out other events that were coded as nontraumatic; Green et al., 2000).

Reliability.   Two-week test–retest reliability in college students for the number of events endorsed at each time point was .89 (Goodman et al., 1998). Kappas for specific events ranged from .31 for attempted sexual assault to 1.0 for robbery or mugging. Four items fell below a kappa of .40: attempted rape, witness to a traumatic event, other serious injury or life-threatening situation such as military combat or living in a war zone, other frightening or horrifying event (Goodman et al., 1998).

Validity.   Overall prevalence rates for many of the traumatic events reported in the Goodman et al. (1998) sample were consistent with rates found in other large samples (e.g., sexual assault rates consistent with Koss, Gidycz, & Wisniewski, 1987). Rates of traumatic events were consistent with expected gender differences; women were more likely to have experienced molestation and attempted sexual assault whereas men were more likely to have experienced adult physical assault, and other serious injury or life threat (Goodman et al., 1998).

In a large multisite study, scores on a measure assessing posttraumatic functioning were significantly higher for women with interpersonal traumas than those who had experienced noninterpersonal traumas or no reported events (Green et al., 2000). Women with multiple interpersonal trauma events had significantly higher means than women with a single event (Green et al., 2000).

The convergent validity of the SLESQ against a clinical interview was assessed in a sample of students (Goodman et al., 1998). The correlation between the total number of events endorsed was .77. Kappas for the specific events ranged from .26 for witnessed death/assault to .90 for life threatening illness. Six items fell below a kappa of .60 with increased reporting in the interview condition (Goodman et al., 1998).

To assess the ability of the SLESQ to detect criterion A events, Goodman et al. (1998) reviewed the responses to a randomly selected subsample of questionnaires and rated the descriptions against a conservative definition of criterion A. The first three authors made decisions about whether an event surpassed the threshold. Eighty-five percent of the events described in the SLESQ met the authors' severity threshold for a traumatic event (Goodman et al., 1998).

Source

The SLESQ is reprinted in the original article. More information about the measure can be obtained by contacting Lisa Goodman, Ph.D., Counseling Psychology Program, School of Education, Boston College, Chestnut Hill, MA 02467, USA; (tel) 617-552-1725; (e-mail) goodmalc@bc.edu.

STRUCTURED INTERVIEW FOR DISORDERS OF EXTREME STRESS (SIDES)

Original Citation

Pelcovitz, D., van der Kolk, B., Roth, S., Mandel, F., Kaplan, S., & Resick, P. (1997). Development of a criteria set and a structured interview for disorders of extreme stress (SIDES). *Journal of Traumatic Stress*, *10*, 3–16.

Purpose

To measure alterations that may accompany exposure to extremely traumatic events.

Description

Several theorists and researchers have suggested that PTSD does not capture the full range of responses to traumatic events, particularly for traumatized children, rape victims, and battered women. Changes in affect regulation, self-identity, and interpersonal functioning seem to be common. The SIDES was developed to assess these proposed symptoms as part of the DSM-IV field trials. The SIDES consists of 48 items that tap into seven areas: (1) regulation of affect and impulses, (2) attention or consciousness, (3) self-perception, (4) perception of the perpetrator, (5) relations with others, (6) somatization, and (7) systems of meaning. There are also 27 subscales. Items have been described as being scored dichotomously

(Pelcovitz et al., 1997) and rated on a four-point scale ranging from "none or no problem with symptom" to "extremely problematic" (Zlotnick & Pearlstein, 1997).

Administration and Scoring

The original article developed criteria for determining the number of items in each subscale and scale necessary to meet a diagnostic cutoff (Pelcovitz et al., 1997).

Psychometric Properties

Reliability. In a sample of 520 community participants and treatment seekers who were part of the DSM-IV field trials, internal consistency for the scales ranged from .53 to .90 and was .96 for the total scale (Pelcovitz et al., 1997). Interrater reliability was established within a subsample of the community sample. The kappa coefficient rating for lifetime disorders was .81 (Pelcovitz et al., 1997).

Cronbach's alpha in a sample of survivors of childhood sexual assault was .90 for current (last 6 months) diagnosis and ranged from .42 to .84 for the individual scales (Zlotnick & Pearlstein, 1997).

Validity. The validity of the SIDES was examined in a sample of childhood sexual assault survivors. The *affect regulation* scale was correlated with a measure of borderline personality ($r = .45$), avoidance ($r = .71$), hypervigiliance ($r = .50$), impulsivity ($r = .50$), hostility ($r = .55$), and somatization ($r = .51$). *Alterations in attention and consciousness* was correlated with dissociation ($r = .60$) and avoidance ($r = .57$). *Alterations in self-perception* was correlated with avoidance ($r = .56$), disconnection ($r = .51$), and borderline personality ($r = .46$). *Somatization* was correlated with another measure of somatization ($r = .68$), avoidance ($r = .63$), and hypervigilance ($r = .57$). None of these scales were significantly correlated with a measure of narcissism (Zlotnick & Pearlstein, 1997).

Source

The SIDES can be obtained by contacting David Pelcovitz, Ph.D., Department of Psychiatry, North Shore University Hospital–Cornell University Medical College, Manhassett, NY, 11030, USA.

STRUCTURED INTERVIEW FOR PTSD (SIP)

Original Citations

Davidson, J., Smith, R., & Kudler, H. (1989). Validity and reliability of the DSM-III criteria for posttraumatic stress disorder: Experience with a structured interview. *Journal of Nervous and Mental Disease, 177,* 336–341.

Davidson, J. R. T., Malik, M. A., & Travers, J. (1997). Structured Interview for PTSD (SIP): Psychometric validation for DSM-IV criteria. *Depression and Anxiety, 5,* 127–129.

Purpose

To assess diagnostic status and symptom severity of PTSD.

Description

The SIP was originally developed to capture DSM-III symptoms or PTSD, but it has been revised and updated for DSM-IV. The SIP consists of 17 items representing the DSM-IV criteria for PTSD along with two measures of survivor and behavior guilt. Each item is rated on a five-point scale ranging from 0 (not at all) to 4 (extremely severe, daily or produces so much distress that patient cannot work or function socially).

Administration and Scoring

The SIP takes 10 to 30 minutes to administer depending on the complexity and severity of the individual's symptoms. The SIP can be scored using DSM-IV diagnostic criteria to yield a dichotomous score reflecting the presence or absence of the diagnosis, or the items can be summed to obtain a measure of symptom severity.

Psychometric Properties

Sample Scores and Norms.   Among a sample of patients diagnosed with PTSD and enrolled in a clinical trial, the mean pretreatment SIP score was 36 ($SD = 9.7$; Davidson et al., 1997).

Reliability.   Cronbach's alpha was .94 for a veteran sample (Davidson et al., 1989) and .80 for the clinical trial sample described above (Davidson et al., 1997). Interrater reliability on a subsample from the clinical trial ranged from .97 to .99 for total SIP score, for symptoms over the past 4 weeks and during the worst ever period (Davidson et al., 1997).

Test–retest reliability for a subsample of patients in the clinical trial who showed no clinical change on an independent measure of functioning between weeks 2 and 4 of the trial was .71 (Davidson et al., 1997). Test–retest reliability in a subsample of the veterans who demonstrated no change between weeks 4 and 8 of a clinical trial was .89 (Davidson et al., 1989).

Validity.   A factor analysis conducted on an earlier version of the SIP revealed three factors representing arousal and intrusiveness (which accounted for the majority of the variance), guilt and avoidance, and problems with sleep, concentration, and numbing (Davidson et al., 1989). A factor analysis on the revised scale, conducted with a mostly female, chronic PTSD sample, yielded seven factors, with one strong factor accounting for most of the variance, and six weaker factors, some comprised of only a single item (Davidson et al., 1997).

The SIP has been shown to be significantly correlated with other measures of PTSD (rs range from .49 to .67, Davidson et al., 1989, 1997), but not with measures of combat exposure ($r = .08$) or intensity of combat ($r = .27$; Davidson et al., 1989). The SIP is also associated with interview measures of anxiety (rs range from .48 to .51) and depression (rs range from .42 to .57; Davidson et al., 1989, 1997). A small but significant relationship was found between several measures of disability and the SIP (*r*s range from .25 to .33), but not social support (*r* = .14; Davidson et al., 1997).

The diagnostic sensitivity of the SIP as relative to the Structured Clinical Interview for DSM was 96% and the specificity was 80% (Davidson et al., 1989). At a score of 25, the SIP showed an efficiency of 94% relative to a structured interview diagnosis (Davidson et al., 1997).

The SIP showed treatment sensitivity in that those with PTSD following treatment in a clinical trial had higher scores than patients who no longer met diagnostic criteria (Davidson et al., 1997).

Alternative Forms

Carlier, Lamberts, Van Uchelen, and Gersons (1998) describe the development and validation of the Self-Rating Scale for PTSD, an abridged self-report version of the SIP. The scale is reprinted in the Carlier et al. (1998) article. The TOP-8, a scale derived from the SIP, includes the items that occurred most frequently and that demonstrated the most change in response to treatment (Davidson & Colket, 1997). The TOP-8 can be administered in 5 to 10 minutes and has been shown to have very good to excellent internal consistency, test–retest reliability, interrater reliability, convergent validity, and treatment sensitivity. More information about the TOP-8 can be obtained by contacting Jonathan Davidson, M.D. (see contact information below).

Source

The SIP can be obtained by contacting Jonathan R. T. Davidson, M.D., Department of Psychiatry, Duke University Medical Center, Box 3812, Durham, NC 27710, USA; (tel) 919-684-2880; (fax) 919-684-8866; (e-mail) tolme@acpub.duke.edu.

TRAUMA-RELATED GUILT INVENTORY (TRGI)

Original Citation

Kubany, E. S., Haynes, S. N., Aubueg, F. R., Manke, F. P., Brennan, J. M., & Stahura, C. (1996). Development and validation of the Trauma-Related Guilt Inventory. *Psychological Assessment, 8,* 428–444.

Purpose

To assess cognitive and emotional aspects of guilt associated with exposure to a traumatic event.

Description

The TRGI is a 32-item self-report questionnaire designed to measure guilt associated with the experience of a traumatic event. It includes three scales—*global guilt, distress,* and *guilt cognitions*—and three subscales (all part of guilt cognitions)—*hindsight-bias/responsibility, wrongdoing,* and *lack of justification.*

Psychometric Properties

Psychometric data are all derived from a multistudy, multisample report by Kubany et al. (1996).

Sample Scores and Norms. Means for each of the three scales and subscales are available for the TRGI on a sample of 325 college students, 168 battered women, and 74 veterans (Kubany et al., 1996).

Reliability. Internal consistency in a sample of 100 women receiving services from a battered women's shelter was .86 to .90 for the scales and .67 to .82 for the subscales. Similar results were found for combat veterans.

In a sample of 32 students, 1-week test–retest reliability ranged from .73 to .86 for the scales and from .74 to .83 for the subscales. Similar results were found for veterans over an average of 8.4 days ($SD = 6.01$).

Validity. Three factor-analytic studies were conducted (on students with a history of traumatic events and battered women) to refine the TRGI and determine its factor structure. The final factor structure that best accounts for the data seems to be a four-factor solution that consists of a distress factor and three cognitive factors termed hindsight-bias/responsibility, wrongdoing, and lack of justification.

Convergent validity was demonstrated with a traumatized student sample in that the *global guilt* scale correlated with a measure of PTSD ($r = .48$) and depression ($r = .60$). The *guilt cognitions* subscale was correlated moderately with PTSD ($r = .32$) and depression ($r = .32$) and the *distress* scale was correlated .77 with PTSD and .59 with depression. Correlations for the subscales were smaller, and no relationship was found between lack of justification and depression or PTSD.

Convergent validity was also demonstrated for the veteran and battered women groups with scores on each of the TRGI measures correlated highly with other measures of guilt, PTSD, depression, self-esteem, shame, and social anxiety. Some discriminant validity was demonstrated for both the battered women and veteran groups in that the TRGI was only weakly associated with a measure assessing guilt over commonplace events.

Alternative Forms

The TRGI was validated and cross-validated with an ethnically diverse sample. A translation into Tagalog is available.

Source

The TRGI can be obtained by contacting Edward S. Kubany, Ph.D., National Center for PTSD, Department of Veterans Affairs, 1132 Bishop Street, Suite 307, Honolulu, HI 96813, USA; (tel) 808-566-1651; (fax) 808-566-1885; (e-mail) kubany@pixi.com. A published version of the TRGI is in development with Western Psychological Services, 12031 Wilshire Boulevard, Los Angeles, CA 90025, USA; (tel) 800-648-8857; (fax) 310-478-7838; (e-mail) custsvc@wpspublish.com; (website) www.wpspublish.com.

TRAUMA SYMPTOM INVENTORY (TSI)

Original Citation

Briere, J. (1995). *Trauma Symptom Inventory professional manual*. Odessa, FL: Psychological Assessment Resources.

Briere, J., Elliot, D. M., Harris, K., & Cotman, A. (1995). Trauma Symptom Inventory: Psychometrics and association with childhood and adult victimization in clinical samples. *Journal of Interpersonal Violence, 10*, 387–401.

Purpose

To evaluate acute and chronic posttraumatic symptomatology.

Description

The TSI is unique from many other measures of posttraumatic symptomatology in that it includes symptoms beyond those typically associated with PTSD and ASD such as other intra- and interpersonal problems that often arise in individuals with a history of chronic psychological trauma. The TSI is a 100-item self-report scale that is comprised of 3 validity scales and 10 clinical scales. The validity scales assess underendorsement, overendorsement, and random or inconsistent response style. The clinical scales include *anxious arousal, depression, anger/ irritability, intrusive experiences, defensive avoidance, dissociation, sexual concerns, dysfunctional sexual behavior, impaired self-reference*, and *tension reduction behavior*. Respondents are asked to indicate how often each symptom has occurred within the past 6 months on a four-point scale ranging from 0 (never) to 3 (often).

Administration and Scoring

The TSI can be administered in 20 minutes, except in the case of significantly clinically impaired patients. Raw scores are derived by summing the items that comprise each scale. Directions are included in the manual for the handling of responses that are left blank. Raw scores are converted to T scores using the appropriate profile for the respondent based on age and gender. Interpretation of the respondent's profile is described in the professional manual using each elevated scale and common two-point profiles.

Psychometric Properties

Sample Scores and Norms. A normative sample is described in the professional manual including norms for male and female Navy recruits (Briere, 1995). Means and standard deviations are also available for males and females with and without a victimization history from a sample of 370 patients recruited from inpatient and outpatient treatment facilities (Briere et al., 1995).

Reliability. The TSI has been demonstrated to have very good to excellent internal consistency for the individual scales (αs ranging from .74 to .90) in a sample of 370 patients (Briere et al., 1995), and similar reliability was demonstrated in a university sample, the standardization sample, and a Navy recruit sample of 3569 (Briere, 1995). No test–retest reliability data are available.

Validity. Exploratory factor analysis in the standardization sample yielded two independent factors labeled "Generalized Trauma and Distress" and "Self-Dysfunction" (Briere, 1995). Similar results were obtained with the clinical sample (Briere et al., 1995). Confirmatory factor analysis supported a three-factor model theoretically developed by the author with the dimensions of posttraumatic stress, self-dysfunction, and dysphoric mood.

Individuals with a history of physical or sexual abuse scored significantly higher than those who did not report such a history on all 10 clinical scales of the TSI (Briere et al., 1995). In discriminant function analyses on the normative sample, the experience of adult and childhood interpersonal violence and disaster was associated with elevated TSI scores (Briere, 1995). Data bearing on the convergent and discriminant validity of the clinical scales are published in the manual, along with data supporting the incremental and criterion validity of the scale (Briere, 1995). For instance, in a subsample of the standardization sample ($N = 449$), an optimally weighted combination of TSI scales correctly predicted 92% of the true positive and 91% of the true negative cases of a self-report derived diagnosis of PTSD.

Alternative Forms

The TSC-40 is a similar scale that predates the TSI and is designed only for use in research (Briere & Runtz, 1989). The TSI-A is an 86-item alternate version of the TSI that contains very few sexual items (items from the *sexual concerns* or *dysfunctional sexual behavior* scales are dropped). There is a Trauma Symptom Checklist for Children that is somewhat comparable. The TSI has been translated into other languages for research purposes only.

Source

The TSI is available from Psychological Assessment Resources, Inc., P.O. Box 998, Odessa, FL 33556, USA; (tel) 800-331-TEST or 813-968-3003; (webpage) www.parinc.com. A TSI introductory kit that includes the manual, 10 item booklets, 25 hand-scorable answer sheets, and 25 each of the male and female profile forms is priced at $89.00 US. A computerized scoring program of the TSI is available that provides raw scores, T scores, and a profile of the scales for a one time cost of $199.00 US. Interpretation of the profile is not included. Information about the scale is also available from John Briere, Ph.D., Department of Psychiatry, USC School of Medicine, 1934 Hospital Place, Los Angeles, CA 90033, USA; (tel) 323-226-5697; (fax) 323-226-5502; (e-mail) jbriere@hsc.usc.edu.

TRAUMATIC EVENTS QUESTIONNAIRE (TEQ)

Original Citation

Vrana, S., & Lauterbach, D. (1994). Prevalence of traumatic events and post-traumatic psychological symptoms in a non-clinical sample of college students. *Journal of Traumatic Stress, 7,* 289–302.

Purpose

To assess the frequency, type, and severity of trauma experienced.

Description

The TEQ is a self-report instrument that assesses experiences with 11 specific types of trauma selected from DSM-III-R and the relevant literature as potentially eliciting posttraumatic symptoms. Two residual categories are also included, in which respondents can record additional events that are not included in the list, and events that the individual feels are so traumatic that they cannot be discussed. For each event endorsed, respondents are asked the number of times the event occurred, their age at the time of the event, and on a seven-point scale ranging from 1 (not at all) to 7 (extremely), whether they were injured at the time of the event, whether their life was threatened, how traumatic the event was for them at the time, and how traumatic it is presently. Finally, respondents who endorsed more than one item are asked to indicate which event was the worst for them. Those who do not endorse any of the items in the scale are asked to describe the worst, stressful experience that they have encountered.

Administration and Scoring

The TEQ can be administered in 10 minutes. Several indices of traumatic exposure can be obtained including the total number of experiences (sum all "yes" responses to item A; continuous events such as sexual abuse are counted as one event) and severity of experiences (sum all responses to items C through F).

Psychometric Properties

The psychometric properties described below were derived from a sample of 440 college students (Vrana & Lauterbach, 1994).

Sample Scores and Norms.   Eighty-four percent of the sample reported at least one traumatic event, and approximately one-third of the sample reported exposure to four or more individual events. Males experienced significantly more events than females.

Reliability.   No published data are available.

Validity.   Respondents with at least one traumatic event reported significantly more depression, anxiety, and PTSD symptomatology than those who did not report exposure to any traumatic events. Further, the number of traumatic events was a significant predictor of depression, anxiety, and PTSD symptom severity.

Alternative Forms

There is a military and a civilian version of the TEQ.

Source

The TEQ (civilian version) is reprinted in Appendix B. More information is available from Dean Lauterbach, Ph.D., 350 Sam Sibley Drive, Room 313, Bienvenu Hall, Department of Psychology, Northwestern State University, Natchitoches, LA 71497, USA; (tel) 318-357-5453; (fax) 318-357-6802.

TRAUMATIC LIFE EVENTS QUESTIONNAIRE (TLEQ)

Original Citation

Kubany, E. S., Haynes, S. N., Leisen, M. B., Owens, J. A., Kaplan, A. S., Watson, S. B., & Burns, K. (2000). Development and preliminary validation of a brief broad-spectrum measure of trauma exposure: The Traumatic Life Events Questionnaire. *Psychological Assessment, 12,* 210–224.

Purpose

To assess exposure to a broad range of potentially traumatic events.

Description

The TLEQ is a self-report scale that assesses exposure to 21 types of potentially traumatic events. An open-ended question that assesses exposure to some other life threatening or highly disturbing events is also included. The events are described in behaviorally descriptive terms, and emotionally charged terms such as *rape* or *abuse* are avoided. For each event, respondents are asked to indicate the number of times the event occurred on a seven-point scale ranging from never to five times or more. Respondents are asked whether each event evoked fear, helplessness, or horror. Additional questions ask about physical injury and immediate emotional response to the event. Finally, in the case of exposure to multiple events, respondents are asked to indicate which event they perceive as the worst.

Administration and Scoring

The TLEQ can be administered in 10 to 15 minutes.

Psychometric Properties

Psychometric properties were evaluated in a multisample, multistudy report (Kubany et al., 2000).

Sample Scores and Norms.   Reports of occurrences of traumatic events across five samples are presented by Kubany et al. (2000).

Reliability.   The temporal stability of the TLEQ was evaluated in a sample of 42 battered women. Kappa coefficients assessing agreement over 2 weeks were above .40 for 20 of the 21 items and .60 or above for 12 items. The overall mean percentage of test–retest agreement was 86%. Correlations of frequency of occurrence reports for each event (with the exception of combat) averaged .77 and ranged from .50 to .93. The test–retest reliability of the occurrence or nonoccurrence of criterion A-2 (intense fear, helplessness, and horror) yielded kappa coefficients of .40 or higher for 19 of the 21 items and .60 or higher for 16 items. The overall percentage of agreement for criteria A-2 was 89%.

Validity.   Seven experts in the area of PTSD rated relevance and representativeness of several aspects of the TLEQ (e.g., response format, individual items) for measuring PTSD as defined in DSM-IV. Overall item wording was rated very positively, as was adequacy of coverage for traumatic events.

Convergent validity was assessed in a sample of 62 undergraduate students. Agreement was evaluated between a self-report and interview version of a slightly modified version of the TLEQ. Kappa coefficients were .40 for 15 of the 16 items and above .60 for 13 items. The overall mean percentage of agreement was 92%. Convergent validity was also assessed for the two formats administered 1 week apart with similar, but slightly lower, agreement.

All but one Vietnam veteran with documented service records endorsed exposure to combat on the TLEQ. Among the battered women, 98% of those who met the cutoff for PTSD, indicated that they had experienced partner abuse with fear, helplessness, and horror at the time of the event on the TLEQ.

Discriminative validity was assessed in a sample of battered women. Women who met the cutoff for PTSD on a self-report measure reported significantly more types of traumatic events, more total events, and more events that evoked intense fear, helplessness, and horror on the TLEQ than women who did not meet the PTSD cutoff.

Alternative Forms

A computerized version is currently being validated in a grant-funded project.

Source

The TLEQ is available from Edward S. Kubany, Ph.D., National Center for PTSD, Department of Veterans Affairs, 1132 Bishop Street, Suite 307, Honolulu, HI 96813, USA; (tel)

808-566-1651; (fax) 808-566-1885; (e-mail) kubany@pixi.com. A published version of the TLEQ is in development with Western Psychological Services, 12031 Wilshire Boulevard, Los Angeles, CA 90025, USA; (tel) 800-648-8857; (fax) 310-478-7838; (e-mail) custsvc@wpspublish.com; (website) www.wpspublish.com.

BRIEF DESCRIPTIONS OF ADDITIONAL MEASURES

Evaluation of Life-time Stressors (ELS)

The ELS is a comprehensive questionnaire and interview protocol designed to assess exposure to potentially traumatic events across the life span. The ELS-Q is a 53-item screening questionnaire that addresses exposure to traumatic events in addition to behavioral correlates of a wide range of potentially traumatic events. For each event, respondents indicate "yes," "no," "I'm not sure," or "It happened to someone I knew." All nonnegative responses on the questionnaire are followed up on the ELS-I (interview). Initial psychometrics on the protocol are quite promising. The ELS-Q is not used as a stand-alone questionnaire. The ELS can be obtained from Karen E. Krinsley, Ph.D., PTSD 116B-2, VA Boston Healthcare System, 150 South Huntington Avenue, Boston, MA 02130, USA; (e-mail) krinsley.karen@boston.va.gov.

Harvard Trauma Questionnaire (HTQ)

The HTQ is a self-report scale designed to measure trauma and torture events and to assess symptoms of PTSD and current functioning among individuals affected by torture, trauma and war-related violence. It is available in over 30 languages including Cambodian, Vietnamese, Laotian, Bosnian, Croatian, Ethiopian, Spanish, and Japanese. Cultural validity, reliability, and the instrument's psychometric properties have been established in a number of culturally diverse settings. The measure and more information can be obtained from Richard F. Mollica, M.D., M.A.R., Harvard Program in Refugee Trauma, 8 Story Street, 3rd floor, Cambridge, MA 02138, USA; (tel) 617-496-5550; (fax) 617-496-5530; (e-mail) rmollica@hprt.harvard.edu.

Life Stressor Checklist-Revised (LSCL-R)

The LSCL-R is a measure of lifetime exposure to stressful and traumatic events. It is still under development and the authors request that those who wish to use it consult with them first. The scale is reprinted in a paper by Wolfe and Kimerling (1997). For more information about the scale, contact Rachel Kimerling, Ph.D., Assistant Adjunct Professor, Department of Psychiatry, UCSF School of Medicine, San Francisco General Hospital, 1001 Potrero Ave., Suite 2100, San Francisco, CA 94110, USA; (tel) 415-206-6447; (fax) 415-206-3855; (e-mail) rachelk@itsa.ucsf.edu.

Modified PTSD Symptom Scale (MPSS-SR)

The MPSS-SR is a 17-item self-report measure designed to assess the frequency and severity of PTSD symptoms corresponding to DSM-III-R criteria. It was developed from the

Foa et al. (1993) PTSD Symptom Scale. Updates to the scale were made to be consistent with DSM-IV criteria, but this updated version is not published. The measure was validated against the Structured Clinical Interview for DSM in the DSM-IV field trials and some promising psychometric data are discussed in the original reference by Falsetti, Resnick, Resick, and Kilpatrick (1993). More information about the scale is available from Sherri Falsetti, Ph.D., National Crime Victims Center, Medical University of South Carolina, 171 Ashley Avenue, Charleston, SC 29425, USA; (tel) 843-792-2945; (fax) 843-792-3388; (e-mail) falsetsa@musc.edu.

Peri-Traumatic Dissociative Experiences Questionnaire (PDEQ)

The PDEQ is a 10-item self-report measure of dissociation at the time of a traumatic event. A recently completed meta-analysis of PTSD predictors found that greater dissociation at the time of trauma, as assessed with the PDEQ, was the most robust predictor of current PTSD (Ozer, Best, Lipsey, & Weiss, manuscript under review). A rater version of the scale is also available. Both versions are available in Marmar, Weiss, and Metzler (1997). For more information about the scale, contact Charles R. Marmar, M.D., Langley Porter Institute, 401 Parnassus Avenue, Box F 0984, San Francisco, CA 94122, USA; (tel) 415-750-2126; (fax) 415-221-6347; (e-mail) marmar@itsa.ucsf.edu.

Personal Beliefs and Reactions Scale (PBRS)

The PBRS is a self-report scale that was developed to assess cognitive schemas that are often disrupted in the aftermath of sexual trauma. It consists of 40 items and eight scales: esteem, trust, self-blame, safety, intimacy, control, negative rape beliefs, and undoing. Preliminary psychometrics on the scale appear promising. The scale can be obtained by contacting Mindy B. Mechanic, Ph.D., Department of Psychology, University of Missouri-St. Louis, 8001 Natural Bridge Road, St. Louis, MO 63121, USA; (e-mail) mbmechanic@umsl.edu.

Posttraumatic Dissociation Scale (PTDS)

The PTDS is a 24-item self-report measure that assesses the frequency of occurrences of derealization, depersonalization, gaps in awareness, amnesia, and gaps in awareness accompanied by reexperiencing over the previous week. The measure is currently under development and has not yet been published. More information about the scale can be obtained from Eve Carlson, Ph.D., National Center for PTSD (352-117 MP), VA Palo Alto Health Care System, 795 Willow Road, Menlo Park, CA 94025, USA; (tel) 650-493-5000, ext. 24058; (fax) 650-617-2684; (e-mail) carlson@icon.palo-alto.med.va.gov.

PTSD Interview

The PTSD Interview is based on DSM-III-R criteria of PTSD. To date, it has been used primarily with veterans. A description of the measure and some psychometric data are available in a paper by Watson, Juba, Manifold, Kucala, and Anderson (1991). More information about the scale can be obtained from Dr. Charles Watson, VA Medical Center, Research Service, 4801 8th Street North, St. Cloud, MN 56303, USA.

PTSD Inventory

The PTSD Inventory is a 17-item self-report diagnostic questionnaire that assesses war-related PTSD. The measure has been demonstrated to have very good validity relative to a structured interview. A revised version of the scale, consistent with DSM-IV criteria, is described and reprinted in Solomon et al. (1993). A Hebrew version of the scale is available from the author. More information about the scale can be obtained from Zahava Solomon, Ph.D., Bob Shapell School of Social Work, Tel Aviv University, Ramat Aviv, Tel Aviv, Israel.

SCL-90-R PTSD Scale

A 28-item scale derived from the SCL-90-R has been developed and validated to detect crime-related PTSD (Saunders, Arata, & Kilpatrick, 1990). This scale was not designed to be administered independent of the SCL-90, instead it is interpreted in the context of the entire measure. Similarly, a 25-item war-zone-related PTSD scale with strong psychometric properties has been derived from the SCL-90-R (Weathers et al., 1996). The item numbers that make up these measures and the psychometric properties are available in the respective papers. More information about the crime-related PTSD scale is available from Benjamin Saunders, Ph.D., National Crime Victims Center, Medical University of South Carolina, 171 Ashley Avenue, Charleston, SC 29425, USA; (tel) 843-792-2945; (fax) 843-792-3388; (e-mail) saunders@musc.edu. More information about the war-zone-related PTSD scale can be obtained from Frank Weathers, Ph.D., Department of Psychology, 226 Thach Hall, Auburn University, Auburn, AL 36849, USA; (tel) 334-844-6495; (e-mail) weathfw@mail.auburn.edu.

Self-Rating Inventory for Posttraumatic Stress Disorder (SIP)

The SIP is a 47-item Dutch language self-rating questionnaire that assesses PTSD symptoms and associated features. Psychometric data on the scale are found in Hovens, van der Ploeg, Klaarenbeek, Schreuder, and Rivero (1994b). More information is available from J. E. Hovens, Ph.D., Centre '45, National Center for the Treatment of WWII Victims, Hermanstraat 6, NL-2315 KS, Leiden, the Netherlands.

Stress Response Rating Scale (SRRS)

The SRRS is a clinician rating scale that assesses response to serious life-events. It consists of 40 items that reflect signs and symptoms of intrusion, avoidance, and distress. Symptoms are rated over the previous 7 days. More information about this measure and its psychometric properties are available in Weiss, Horowitz, and Wilner (1984). The scale is available from Daniel S. Weiss, Ph.D., Department of Psychiatry, University of California–San Francisco, Box F-0984, San Francisco, CA 94143, USA; (tel) 415-476-7557; (fax) 415-502-7296; (e-mail) dweiss@itsa.ucsf.edu.

Trauma Assessment for Adults (TAA)

There is a self-report and an interview version of the TAA, a brief screen for exposure to traumatic events. It is adapted from the Potential Stressful Events Interview (Falsetti, Resnick,

Kilpatrick, & Freedy, 1994) and the National Women's Study Event History and PTSD Module. More information about the scale can be obtained by contacting Heidi Resnick, Ph.D., National Crime Victims Research and Treatment Center, Department of Psychiatry and Behavioral Sciences, 171 Ashley Avenue, Charleston, SC 29425, USA. The Brief Trauma Interview, designed to briefly assess lifetime trauma exposure according to DSM-IV criteria in a clinically sensitive format, is also based on this measure. More information can be obtained by contacting Paula P. Schnurr, Ph.D., National Center for PTSD (116D), VA Medical and Regional Office Center, White River Junction, VT 05009, USA; (tel) 802-296-5132; (fax) 802-296-5135; (e-mail) paula.p.schnurr@dartmouth.edu.

Trauma History Questionnaire (THQ)

The THQ is a 24-item measure that assesses history of exposure to traumatic events. It is based on the High Magnitude Stressor Questionnaire from the DSM-IV field trials. It is currently considered an experimental instrument and thus the authors require a data sharing agreement. Preliminary psychometrics are available in a paper by Green (1996). The scale is available from Bonnie L. Green, Ph.D., Department of Psychiatry, Georgetown University, 611 Kober Cogan Hall, Washington, DC 20007, USA; (tel) 202-687-4812; (fax) 202-687-6658.

Traumatic Experiences Inventory (TEI)

The TEI is a 38-item self-report measure of the existence, intensity, and duration of symptoms that develop in response to a crime or natural disaster in which lives were lost. The factors include avoidance, reexperiencing, increased arousal, and victimization. More information on the scale is available in Sprang (1997).

Traumatic Stress Institute Belief Scale (TSI)

The TSI is designed to measure disrupted cognitive schemas that reflect trauma-sensitive needs. It was developed by Laurie Anne Pearlman, Ph.D., at the Traumatic Stress Institute/ Center for Adult & Adolescent Psychotherapy LLC, 22 Morgan Farms Drive, South Windsor, CT 06074, USA; (tel) 860-644-2541; (fax) 860-644-6891; (e-mail) laurie.pearlman@snet.net. A published version of the TSI is in development with Western Psychological Services, 12031 Wilshire Boulevard, Los Angeles, CA 90025, USA; (tel) 800-648-8857; (fax) 310-478-7838; (e-mail) custsvc@wpspublish.com; (website) www.wpspublish.com.

Traumatic Stress Schedule (TSS)

The TSS is a measure designed to detect the occurrence and impact of exposure to traumatic events. Respondents are asked about the occurrence of six types of events, as well as any additional events, and they are queried about the impact of these events on their life. The scale is reprinted in a paper by Norris (1990). More information is available from Fran Norris, Ph.D., Department of Psychology, Georgia State University, University Plaza, Atlanta, GA 30303, USA; (tel) 404-651-1607; (fax) 404-651-1391; (e-mail) fnorris@gsu.edu.

World Assumption Scale (WAS)

The WAS is a 32-item self-report measure of assumptions that are presumed to be impacted by exposure to traumatic events. The WAS taps into assumptions about the benevolence of the world, the meaning of the world, and self-worth. The measure is reprinted in a paper by Janoff-Bulman (1996) and some psychometric data are also available. More information about the scale is available from Ronnie Janoff-Bulman, Ph.D., Department of Psychology, University of Massachusetts, Amherst, MA 01003, USA; (tel) 413-545-0264; (fax) 413-545-0996; (e-mail) janbul@psych.umass.edu.

REFERENCES

Allen, J. G., Coyne, L., & Huntoon, J. (1998). Trauma pervasively elevates Brief Symptom Inventory profiles in inpatient women. *Psychological Reports, 83*, 499–513.

Andrykowski, M. A., Cordova, M. J., Studts, J. L., & Miller, T. W. (1998). Posttraumatic stress disorder after treatment for breast cancer: Prevalence of diagnosis and use of the PTSD Checklist–Civilian Version (PCL-C) as a screening instrument. *Journal of Consulting and Clinical Psychology, 66*, 586–590.

Asmundson, G. J. G., Cox, B. J., Larsen, D. K., Frombach, I. K., & Norton, G. R. (1999). Psychometric properties of the Accident Fear Questionnaire: An analysis based on motor vehicle accident survivors in a rehabilitation setting. *Rehabilitation Psychology, 44*, 373–387.

Astin, M. C., Lawrence, K. J., & Foy, D. W. (1993). Posttraumatic stress disorder among battered women: Risk and resiliency factors. *Violence and Victims, 8*, 17–29.

Blake, D. D., Weathers, F. W., Nagy, L. M., Kaloupek, D. G., Klauminzer, G., Charney, D. .., & Keane, T. M. (1990). A clinician rating scale for assessing current and lifetime PTSD: The CAPS-1. *The Behavior Therapist, 13*, 187–188.

Blanchard, E. B., Jones-Alexander, J., Buckley, T. C., & Forneris, C. A. (1996). Psychometric properties of the PTSD Checklist (PCL). *Behaviour Research and Therapy, 34*, 669–673.

Breslau, N., Kessler, R. C., & Peterson, E. L. (1998). PTSD assessment with a structured interview: Reliability and concordance with a standardized clinical interview. *International Journal of Methods in Psychiatric Research, 7*, 121–127.

Briere, J., & Runtz, M. (1989). The Trauma Symptom Checklist (TSC-33): Early data on a new scale. *Journal of Interpersonal Violence, 4*, 151–163.

Brom, D., Kleber, R. J., & Defares, P. B. (1989). Brief psychotherapy for posttraumatic stress disorders. *Journal of Consulting and Clinical Psychology, 57*, 607–612.

Bryant, R. A., Harvey, A. G., Dang, S. T., & Sackville, T. (1998). Assessing acute stress disorder: Psychometric properties of a structured clinical interview. *Psychological Assessment, 10*, 215–220.

Bryant, R. A., Moulds, M. L., & Guthrie, R. M. (2000). Acute Stress Disorder Scale: A self-report measure of acute stress disorder. *Psychological Assessment, 12*, 61–68.

Cardeña, E., Koopman, C., Classen, C., Waelde, L. C., & Spiegel, D. (2000). Psychometric properties of the Stanford Acute Stress Reaction Questionnaire: A valid and reliable measure of acute stress. *Journal of Traumatic Stress, 13*, 719–734.

Carlier, I. V. E., Lamberts, R. D., Van Uchelen, A. J., & Gersons, B. P. R. (1998). Clinical utility of a brief diagnostic test for posttraumatic stress disorder. *Psychosomatic Medicine, 60*, 42–47.

Carlson, E. B., Putnam, F. W., Ross, C. A., Anderson, G., Clark, P., Torem, M., Coons, P., Bowman, E., Chu, J. A., Dill, D., Loewenstein, R. J., & Braun, B. G. (1991). Factor analysis of the Dissociative Experiences Scale: A multicenter study. In B. G. Braun & E. B. Carlson (Eds.), *Proceedings of the Eighth International Conference on Multiple Personality and Dissociative States.* Chicago: Rush.

Dalton, J. E., Tom, A., Rosenblum, M. L., Garte, S. H., & Aubuchon, I. N. (1989). Faking on the Mississippi Scale for Combat-Related Posttraumatic Stress Disorder. *Psychological Assessment, 1*, 56–57.

Davidson, J. R. T., & Colket, J. T. (1997). The eight-item Treatment-Outcome Post-Traumatic Stress Disorder Scale: A brief measure to assess treatment outcome in post-traumatic stress disorder. *International Clinical Psychopharmacology, 12*, 41–45.

Davidson, J. R., Kudler, H. S., Saunders, W. B., Erickson, L., Smith, R. D., Stein, R. M., Lipper, S., Hammett, E. B., Mahorney, S. L., & Cavenar, J. O. (1993). Predicting response to amitriptyline in posttraumatic stress disorder. *American Journal of Psychiatry, 150*, 1024–1029.

Dutton, M. A., Perrin, S., Chrestman, K., Halle, P., & Burghardt, K. (1991, August). *Posttraumatic stress disorder in battered women: Concurrent validity.* Paper presented at the 99th Annual Convention of the American Psychological Association, San Francisco.

Falsetti, S., Resnick, H., Kilpatrick, D., & Freedy, J. (1994). A review of the Potential Stressful Events Interview. *The Behavior Therapist, 17,* 66–67.

Falsetti, S. A., Resnick, H. S., Resick, P. A., & Kilpatrick, D. G. (1993). The Modified PTSD Symptom Scale: A brief self-report measure of posttraumatic stress disorder. *Behavioral Assessment Review, 16,* 161–162.

Fischer, D., & Elnitsky, S. (1990). A factor analytic study of two scales measuring dissociation. *American Journal of Clinical Hypnosis, 32,* 201–207.

Foa, E. B., Riggs, D. S., Dancu, C. V., & Rothbaum, B. O. (1993). Reliability and validity of a brief instrument for assessing posttraumatic stress disorder. *Journal of Traumatic Stress, 6,* 459–473.

Foa, E. B., Rothbaum, B. O., Riggs, D. S., & Murdock, T. B. (1991). Treatment of posttraumatic stress disorder in rape victims: A comparison between cognitive-behavioral procedures and counseling. *Journal of Consulting and Clinical Psychology, 59,* 715–723.

Fontana, A., & Rosenheck, R. (1994). A short form of the Mississippi Scale for measuring change in combat-related PTSD. *Journal of Traumatic Stress, 7,* 407–414.

Foy, D. W., Sipprelle, R. C., Rueger, D. B., & Carroll, E. M. (1984). Etiology of posttraumatic stress disorder in Vietnam veterans: Analysis of premilitary, military, and combat exposure influences. *Journal of Consulting and Clinical Psychology, 52,* 79–87.

Foy, D. W., Wood, J. L., King, D. W., King, L. A., & Resnick, H. S. (1997). Los Angeles Symptom Checklist: Psychometric evidence with an adolescent sample. *Assessment, 4,* 377–384.

Frischholz, E. J., Braun, B. G., Sachs, R. G., Hopkins, L., Shaeffer, D. M., Lewis, J., Leavitt, F., Pasquotto, M. A., & Schwartz, D. R. (1990). The Dissociative Experiences Scale: Further replication and validation. *Dissociation, 3,* 151–153.

Frueh, B. C., Turner, S. M., Beidel, D. C., Mirabella, R. F., & Jones, W. J. (1996). Trauma Management Therapy: A preliminary evaluation of a multicomponent behavioral treatment for chronic combat-related PTSD. *Behaviour Research and Therapy, 34,* 533–543.

Gold, J. W., & Cardeña, E. (1998). Convergent validity of three posttraumatic symptoms inventories among adult sexual abuse survivors. *Journal of Traumatic Stress, 11,* 173–180.

Green, B. L. (1996). Psychometric review of Trauma History Questionnaire (Self-Report). In B. H. Stamm (Ed.), *Measurement of stress, trauma and adaptation* (pp. 366–388). Lutherville, MD: Sidran Press.

Green, B. L., Goodman, L. A., Krupnick, J. L., Corcoran, C. B., Petty, R. M., Stockton, P., & Stern, N. M. (2000). Outcomes of single versus multiple trauma exposure in a screening sample. *Journal of Traumatic Stress, 13,* 271–286.

Hammarberg, M. (1992). Penn Inventory for Posttraumatic Stress Disorder: Psychometric properties. *Psychological Assessment, 4,* 67–76.

Hammarberg, M., & Silver, S. M. (1994). Outcome of treatment for post-traumatic stress disorder in a primary care unit serving Vietnam veterans. *Journal of Traumatic Stress, 7,* 195–216.

Hendrix, C. C., Jurich, A. P., & Schumm, W. R. (1994). Validation of the Impact of Event Scale on a sample of American Vietnam veterans. *Psychological Reports, 75,* 321–322.

Herman, D. S., Weathers, F. W., Litz, B. T., & Keane, T. M. (1996). Psychometric properties of the embedded and stand-alone versions of the MMPI-2 Keane PTSD scale. *Assessment, 3,* 437–442.

Hodgkinson, P., & Joseph, S. (1995). Factor analysis of the Impact of Event Scale with female bank staff following an armed raid. *Personality and Individual Differences, 19,* 773–775.

Horowitz, M. (1976). *Stress response syndromes.* New York: Jason Aronson.

Horowitz, M. (1982). Stress response symptoms and their treatment. In L. Goldberger & S. Breznitz (Eds.), *Handbook of stress: Theoretical and clinical aspects* (pp. 711–732). New York: Free Press.

Housekamp, B. M., & Foy, D. W. (1991). The assessment of posttraumatic stress disorder in battered women. *Journal of Interpersonal Violence, 6,* 368–376.

Hovens, J. E., van der Ploeg, H. M., Klaarenbeek, M. T. A., Schreuder, J. N., & Rivero, V. V. (1994a). The assessment of posttraumatic stress disorder with the Clinician Administered PTSD Scale: Dutch results. *Journal of Clinical Psychology, 50,* 325–340.

Hovens, J. E., van der Ploeg, H. M., Klaarenbeek, M. T. A., Schreuder, J. N., & Rivero, V. V. (1994b). The development of the Self-Rating Inventory for Posttraumatic Stress Disorder. *Acta Psychiatrica Scandinavica, 90,* 172–183.

Hyer, L., Summers, M. N., Boyd, S., Litaker, M., & Boudewyns, P. (1996). Assessment of older combat veterans with the Clinician-Administered PTSD Scale. *Journal of Traumatic Stress, 9,* 587–593.

Janoff-Bulman, R. (1996). Psychometric review of World Assumption Scale. In B. H. Stamm (Ed.), *Measurement of stress, trauma and adaptation* (pp. 440–442). Lutherville, MD: Sidran Press.

Joseph, S. (2000). Psychometric evaluation of Horowitz's Impact of Event Scale: A review. *Journal of Traumatic Stress, 13*, 101–113.

Joseph, S., Yule, W., Williams, R., & Hodgkinson, P. (1993). The Herald of Free Enterprise disaster: Measuring post-traumatic symptoms 30 months on. *British Journal of Clinical Psychology, 32*, 327–331.

Kenderdine, S. K., Phillips, E. J., & Scurfield, R. M. (1992). Comparison of the MMPI-PTSD subscale with PTSD and substance abuse patient populations. *Journal of Clinical Psychology, 48*, 136–139.

King, D. W., Leskin, G. A., King, L. A., & Weathers, F. W. (1998). Confirmatory factor analysis of the Clinician-Administered PTSD Scale: Evidence for the dimensionality of posttraumatic stress disorder. *Psychological Assessment, 10*, 90–96.

King, L. A., & King, D. W. (1994). Latent structure of the Mississippi Scale for Combat-Related Post-Traumatic Stress Disorder: Exploratory and higher-order confirmatory factor analyses. *Assessment, 1*, 275–291.

Koretzky, M. B., & Peck, A. H. (1990). Validation and cross-validation of the PTSD subscale of the MMPI with civilian trauma victims. *Journal of Clinical Psychology, 46*, 296–300.

Koss, M. P., Gidycz, C. A., & Wisniewski, N. (1987). The scope of rape: Incidence and prevalence of sexual aggression and victimization in a national sample of higher education students. *Journal of Consulting and Clinical Psychology, 55*, 162–170.

Lauterbach, D., Vrana, S., King, D. W., & King, L. A. (1997). Psychometric properties of the civilian version of the Mississippi PTSD Scale. *Journal of Traumatic Stress, 10*, 499–513.

Lawrence, K. J. (1992). *Assessment of posttraumatic stress disorder among survivors of ritual abuse.* Unpublished doctoral dissertation, Fuller Theological Seminary, Pasadena, CA.

Leskin, G., & Foy, D. W. (1993, October). Development and psychometric validation of the LA Symptom Checklist. In L. A. King (Chair), *Assessment of PTSD by self-report measure: Implications for construct validity.* Symposium presented at the annual meeting of the International Society for Traumatic Stress Studies, San Antonio, TX.

Litz, B. T., Orsillo, S. M., Kaloupek, D., & Weathers, F. (2000). Emotional-processing in posttraumatic stress disorder. *Journal of Abnormal Psychology, 109*, 26–39.

Litz, B. T., Penk, W. E., Walsh, S., Hyer, L., Blake, D. D., Marx, B., Keane, T. M., & Bitman, D. (1991). Similarities and differences between MMPI and MMPI-2 applications to the assessment of posttraumatic stress disorder. *Journal of Personality Assessment, 57*, 238–253.

Lund, M., Foy, D. W., Sipprelle, R. C., & Strachan, A. M. (1984). The Combat Exposure Scale: A systematic assessment of trauma in the Vietnam war. *Journal of Clinical Psychology, 40*, 1323–1328.

Lyons, J. A., Caddell, J. M., Pittman, R. L., Rawls, R., & Perrin, S. (1994). The potential for faking on the Mississippi Scale for Combat-Related PTSD. *Journal of Traumatic Stress, 7*, 441–445.

Malekzai, A. S. B., Niazi, J. M., Paige, S. R., Hendricks, S. E., Fitzpatrick, D., Leuschen, M. P., & Millimet, C. R. (1996). Modification of CAPS-1 for diagnosis of PTSD in Afghan refugees. *Journal of Traumatic Stress, 9*, 891–898.

Manne, S. L., Du Hamel, K., Gallelli, K., Sorgen, K., & Redd, W. H. (1998). Posttraumatic stress disorder among mothers of pediatric cancer survivors: Diagnosis, comorbidity, and utility of the PTSD Checklist as a screening instrument. *Journal of Pediatric Psychology, 23*, 357–366.

Marmar, C. R., Weiss, D. S., & Metzler, T. (1997). The Peritraumatic Dissociative Experiences Questionnaire. In J. P. Wilson & T. M. Keane (Eds.), *Assessing psychological trauma and PTSD* (pp. 412–428). New York: Guilford.

McDonald, A. S. (1997). Factor structure of the Impact of Event Scale in a non-clinical sample. *Personality and Individual Differences, 23*, 419–424.

McFall, M. E., Smith, D. E., Mackay, P. W., & Tarver, D. J. (1990). Reliability and validity of Mississippi Scale for Combat-Related Posttraumatic Stress Disorder. *Psychological Assessment, 2*, 114–121.

McFall, M. E., Smith, D. E., Roszell, D. K., Tarver, D. J., & Malas, K. L. (1990). Convergent validity of measures of PTSD in Vietnam combat veterans. *American Journal of Psychiatry, 147*, 645–648.

Meltzer-Brody, S., Churchill, E., & Davidson, J. R. T. (1999). Derivation of the SPAN, a brief diagnostic screening test for post-traumatic stress disorder. *Psychiatry Research, 88*, 63–70.

Moody, D. R., & Kish, G. B. (1989). Clinical meaning of the Keane PTSD scale. *Journal of Clinical Psychology, 45*, 542–546.

Munley, P. H., Bains, D. S., Bloem, W. D., & Busby, R. M. (1995). Post-traumatic stress disorder and the MMPI-2. *Journal of Traumatic Stress, 8*, 171–178.

Neal, L. A., Busuttil, W., Herapath, R., & Strike, P. W. (1994). Development and validation of the computerized Clinician Administered Posttraumatic Stress Disorder Scale-1-Revised. *Psychological Medicine, 24*, 701–706.

Neal, L. A., Busuttil, W., Rollins, J., Herepath, R., Strike, P., & Turnbull, G. (1994). Convergent validity of measures of post-traumatic stress disorder in a mixed military and civilian population. *Journal of Traumatic Stress, 7*, 447–455.

Norris, F. H. (1990). Screening for traumatic stress: A scale for use in the general population. *Journal of Applied Social Psychology, 20*, 1704–1718.

Norris, F. H., & Perilla, J. L. (1996). The Revised Civilian Mississippi Scale for PTSD: Reliability, validity, and cross-language stability. *Journal of Traumatic Stress, 9*, 285–298.

Pava, W. (1993). {Administration of LASC}. Unpublished data.

Perry, S., Difede, J., Musngi, G., Frances, A. J., & Jacobsberg, L. (1992). Predictors of posttraumatic stress disorder after burn injury. *American Journal of Psychiatry, 149*, 931–935.

Pitblado, C. B., & Sanders, B. (1991). Reliability and short-term stability of scores on the Dissociative Experiences Scale. In B. G. Braun & E. B. Carlson (Eds.), *Proceedings of the Eighth International Conference on Multiple Personality and Dissociative States*. Chicago: Rush.

Resnick, H. S., Foy, D. W., Donahoe, C. P., & Miller, E. N. (1989). Antisocial behavior and posttraumatic stress disorder in Vietnam veterans. *Journal of Clinical Psychology, 45*, 860–866.

Ross, C. A., Joshi, S., & Currie, R. (1991). Dissociative experiences in the general population: A factor analysis. *Hospital and Community Psychiatry, 42*, 297–301.

Rowan, A. B., Foy, D. W., Rodriguez, N., & Ryan, S. (1994). Posttraumatic stress disorder in adults sexually abused as children. *International Journal of Child Abuse and Neglect, 18*, 51–61.

Ryan, S. (1992). *Psychometric analysis of the Sexual Abuse Exposure Questionnaire*. Unpublished doctoral dissertation, Fuller Theological Seminary, Pasadena, CA.

Saunders, B. E., Arata, C. M., & Kilpatrick, D. G. (1990). Development of a crime-related post-traumatic stress disorder scale for women within the Symptom Checklist-90-Revised. *Journal of Traumatic Stress, 3*, 439–448.

Schwarzwald, J., Solomon, Z., Weisenberg, M., & Mikulincer, M. (1987). Validation of the Impact of Event Scale for psychological sequelae of combat. *Journal of Consulting and Clinical Psychology, 55*, 251–256.

Scotti, J. R., Sturges, L. V., & Lyons, J. A. (1996). The Keane PTSD Scale extracted from the MMPI: Sensitivity and specificity with Vietnam veterans. *Journal of Traumatic Stress, 9*, 643–650.

Shalev, A. Y., Freedman, S., Peri, T., Brandes, D., & Sahar, T. (1997). Predicting PTSD in trauma survivors: Prospective evaluation of self-report and clinician-administered instruments. *British Journal of Psychiatry, 170*, 558–564.

Shalev, A. Y., Peri, T., Canetti, L., & Schreiber, S. (1996). Predictors of PTSD in injured trauma survivors: A prospective study. *American Journal of Psychiatry, 153*, 219–225.

Solomon, Z., Benbenishty, R., Neria, Y., Abramowitz, M., Ginzburg, K., & Ohry, A. (1993). Assessment of PTSD: Validation of the revised PTSD Inventory. *Israel Journal of Psychiatry and Related Sciences, 30*, 110–115.

Sprang, G. (1997). The Traumatic Experiences Inventory (TEI): A test of psychometric properties. *Journal of Psychopathology and Behavioral Assessment, 19*, 257–271.

Thompson, J. A., Charlton, P. F. C., Kerry, R., & Lee, D. (1995). An open trial of exposure therapy based on deconditioning for post-traumatic stress disorder. British *Journal of Clinical Psychology, 34*, 407–416.

van Ijzendoorn, M. H., & Schuengel, C. (1996). The measurement of dissociation in normal and clinical populations: Meta-analytic validation of the Dissociative Experiences Scale (DES). *Clinical Psychology Review, 16*, 365–382.

Vrenen, D. L., Gudanowski, D. M., King, L. A., & King, D. W. (1995). The civilian version of the Mississippi PTSD Scale: A psychometric evaluation. *Journal of Traumatic Stress, 8*, 91–109.

Walker, E. A., Katon, W. J., Neraas, K., Jemelka, R. P., & Massoth, D. (1992). Dissociation in women with chronic pelvic pain. *American Journal of Psychiatry, 149*, 534–537.

Waller, N. G. (1995). The Dissociative Experiences Scale. In J. C. Conoley & J. C. Impara (Eds.), *Twelfth mental measurements yearbook* (pp. 317–318). Lincoln, NE: Buros Institute of Mental Measurement.

Waller, N. G., Putnam, F. W., & Carlson, E. B. (1996). Types of dissociation and dissociative types: A taxometric analysis of dissociative experiences. *Psychological Methods, 1*, 300–321.

Waller, N. G., & Ross, C. A. (1997). The prevalence and biometric structure of pathological dissociation in the general population: Taxometric and behavior genetic findings. *Journal of Abnormal Psychology, 106*, 499–510.

Watson, C. G., Juba, M. P., Manifold, V., Kucala, T., & Anderson, P. E. D. (1991). The PTSD Interview: Rationale, description, reliability, and concurrent validity of a DSM-III-based technique. *Journal of Clinical Psychology, 47*, 179–188.

Watson, C. G., Plemel, D., DeMotts, J., Howard, M. T., Tuorila, J., Moog, R., Thomas, D., & Anderson, D. (1994). A comparison of four PTSD measures' convergent validities in Vietnam veterans. *Journal of Traumatic Stress, 7*, 75–82.

Weathers, F. W., & Litz, B. T. (1994). Psychometric properties of the Clinician Administered PTSD Scale, CAPS-1. PTSD *Research Quarterly, 5*, 2–6.

Weathers, F. W., Litz, B. T., Keane, T. M., Herman, D. S., Steinberg, H. R., Huska, J. A., & Kraemer, H. C. (1996). The utility of the SCL-90-R for the diagnosis of war-zone related posttraumatic stress disorder. *International Society for Traumatic Stress Studies, 9*, 111–128.

Weathers, F. W., Ruscio, A. M., & Keane, T. M. (1999). Psychometric properties of nine scoring rules for the Clinician Administered Posttraumatic Stress Disorder Scale. *Psychological Assessment, 11*, 124–133.

Weiss, D. S., Horowitz, M. J., & Wilner, N. (1984). The Stress Response Rating Scale: A clinician's measure for rating the response to serious life-events. *British Journal of Clinical Psychology, 23,* 202–215.

Weiss, D. S., & Marmar, C. R. (1997). The Impact of Event Scale-Revised. In J. P. Wilson & T. M. Keane (Eds.), *Assessing psychological trauma and PTSD* (pp. 98–135). New York: Guilford.

Wolfe, J., & Kimerling, R. (1997). Gender issues in the assessment of posttraumatic stress disorder. In J. P. Wilson & T. M. Keane (Eds.), *Assessing psychological trauma and PTSD* (pp. 192–238). New York: Guilford.

Zilberg, N. J., Weiss, D. S., & Horowitz, M. J. (1982). Impact of Event Scale: A cross-validation study and some empirical evidence supporting a conceptual model of stress response syndromes. *Journal of Consulting and Clinical Psychology, 50,* 407–414.

Zlotnick, C., Davidson, J., Shea, M. T., & Pearlstein, T. (1996). Validation of the Davidson Trauma Scale in a sample of survivors of childhood sexual abuse. *Journal of Nervous and Mental Disease, 184,* 255–257.

Zlotnick, C., & Pearlstein, T. (1997). Validation of the Structured Interview for Disorders of Extreme Stress. *Comprehensive Psychiatry, 38,* 243–247.

Zlotnick, C., Shea, M., Zakriski, A., Costello, E., Begin, A., Pearlstein, T., & Simpson, E. (1995). Stressors and close relationships during childhood and dissociative experiences in survivors of sexual abuse among inpatient psychiatric women. *Comprehensive Psychiatry, 36,* 207–212.

Appendix A
Quick-View Guides

Compiled by Jennifer S. Mills

Table I. Measures for Anxiety and Related Constructs (Chapter 7)

Name of instrument	Type of measure	Measurement focus	Time to complete (minutes)	Fee involved?	Alternate forms
Anxiety Control Questionnaire	Self-report	Perceived control over emotional reactions and external threats	5–10	No	
Beck Anxiety Inventory	Self-report	Symptoms of anxiety minimally shared with depression	5–10	Yes	Computerized version; Spanish, French, Turkish
Depression Anxiety Stress Scales	Self-report	Core symptoms of depression, anxiety, and stress	5–10	Yes (manual)	Brief version
Fear Questionnaire	Self-report	Severity of phobias, also anxiety and depression	<10	No	Catalan, Chinese, Dutch, French, German, Italian, Spanish
Frost Multidimensional Perfectionism Scale	Self-report	Dimensions of perfectionism	10	No	Chinese, French, Egyptian, German, Hebrew, Japanese, Portuguese, Spanish
Hamilton Anxiety Rating Scale and Clinical Anxiety Scale	Clinician-administered	Generalized anxiety	15–30	No	Computerized version; structured interview
Hospital Anxiety and Depression Scale	Self-report	Levels of depression and anxiety in nonpsychiatric medical patients	5	No	11 languages
Meta-Cognitions Questionnaire	Self-report	Beliefs about worry and intrusive thoughts	15–20	No	
Positive and Negative Affect Schedule	Self-report	Positive and negative affect	<5	No	Child version; expanded version; French, German, Norwegian, Polish, Russian, Spanish
Self-Rating Anxiety Scale	Self-report	Symptoms of anxiety	5	No	Interview format; Chinese, Italian, Portuguese, Spanish
State–Trait Anxiety Inventory (Form Y)	Self-report	State and trait levels of anxiety	10	Yes	Child version; Brief version; 30 languages
Thought Control Questionnaire	Self-report	Strategies for controlling unpleasant and unwanted thoughts	5–10	No	
Trimodal Anxiety Questionnaire	Self-report	Somatic, behavioral, and cognitive aspects of anxiety	5–10	No	Dutch

Table II. Measures for Panic Disorder and Agoraphobia (Chapter 9)

Name of instrument	Type of measure	Measurement focus	Time to complete (minutes)	Fee involved?	Alternate forms
Agoraphobic Cognitions Questionnaire	Self-report	Panic-related cognitions	5–10	No	Dutch, German, French, Greek, Spanish, Swedish, Portuguese, Mandarin
Agoraphobic Cognitions Scale	Self-report	Fearful cognitions	3	No	Norwegian
Agoraphobic Self-Statements Questionnaire	Self-report	Agoraphobic positive/negative self-statements	5	No	Dutch
Albany Panic and Phobia Questionnaire	Self-report	Situational and interoceptive fear	5	No	Spanish
Anxiety Sensitivity Index	Self-report	Fear of anxiety symptoms	3–5	Yes	Child version; brief version; Spanish, Italian, Chinese, Dutch, German, Hebrew
Anxiety Sensitivity Index-Revised 36	Self-report	Fear of anxiety symptoms	5	No	Dutch, Spanish
Anxiety Sensitivity Profile	Self-report	Cognitive aspects of anxiety sensitivity	10	No	Dutch, Spanish
Body Sensations Interpretation Questionnaire	Self-report	Anxious misinterpretations	10–15	No	Brief version; Swedish
Body Sensations Questionnaire	Self-report	Fear of arousal	5–10	No	Dutch, German, French, Greek, Spanish, Swedish, Portuguese, Mandarin
Body Vigilance Scale	Self-report	Body vigilance	3–5	No	
Mobility Inventory for Agoraphobia	Self-report	Severity of agoraphobic avoidance and panic	5–10	No	Dutch, German, French, Greek, Spanish, Swedish, Portuguese; version available for ratings "with and without medication"
Panic and Agoraphobia Scale	Clinician-administered	Severity of panic disorder with or without agoraphobia	5–10	Yes	17 languages
Panic Attack Questionnaire-Revised	Self-report	Detailed information on panic attacks	20–30	No	Version available for individuals not already diagnosed with panic disorder; self-report version in development
Panic Disorder Severity Scale	Clinician-administered	Severity of panic disorder in individuals already diagnosed	10–15	No	
Phobic Avoidance Rating Scale	Clinician-administered	Severity of agoraphobic avoidance	10–15	No	Norwegian
Texas Safety Maneuver Scale	Self-report	Safety behaviors	5–10	No	

Table III. Measures for Specific Phobia (Chapter 11)

Name of instrument	Type of measure	Measurement focus	Time to complete (minutes)	Fee involved?	Alternate forms
Acrophobia Questionnaire	Self-report	Anxiety and avoidance of heights	5	No	
Blood–Injection Symptom Scale	Self-report	Anxiety, tension, and faintness to blood and injections	1–2	No	State version
Claustrophobia General Cognitions Questionnaire	Self-report	Cognitions related to claustrophobic situations	5	No	
Claustrophobia Questionnaire	Self-report	Fears of suffocation and restriction	5–10	No	
Claustrophobia Situations Questionnaire	Self-report	Anxiety in and avoidance of claustrophobic situations	5–10	No	
Dental Anxiety Inventory	Self-report	Severity of dental anxiety	5–10	No	Brief version; Dutch, French, German, Italian, Norwegian, Spanish
Dental Cognitions Questionnaire	Self-report	Negative cognitions related to dental treatment	5–7	No	Dutch, German, Norwegian
Dental Fear Survey	Self-report	Dental avoidance of fear of dental stimuli	2–5	No	Spanish, Korean, Portuguese, Chinese, Swedish, Dutch, Japanese, Hebrew
Fear of Spiders Questionnaire	Self-report	Severity of spider phobia	5	No	
Fear Survey Schedule	Self-report	Identification of specific fears of objects/ situations	10–15	Yes	Child version; revised and extended version; various languages
Medical Fear Survey	Self-report	Severity of medical fears	5	No	Translations in development
Mutilation Questionnaire	Self-report	Verbal–cognitive component of mutilation and blood/injury fears	5	No	Various languages
Snake Questionnaire	Self-report	Verbal–cognitive component of snake fear	5	No	Various languages
Spider Phobia Beliefs Questionnaire	Self-report	Fearful beliefs about spiders	10–15	No	Dutch
Spider Questionnaire Self-report	Self-report	Verbal–cognitive component of spider fear	5	No	Child version; several languages

Table IV. Measures for Social Phobia (Chapter 13)

Name of instrument	Type of measure	Measurement focus	Time to complete (minutes)	Fee involved?	Alternate forms
Brief Social Phobia Scale	Clinician-administered	Social fear, avoidance, and physiological arousal	5–15	No	Computerized version
Fear of Negative Evaluation	Self-report	Fear of negative evaluation by others	10–15	No	Brief version; Japanese
Liebowitz Social Anxiety Scale	Clinician-administered	Social fear and avoidance	20–30	No	Computerized version; French, Spanish
Self-Statements during Public Speaking Scale	Self-report	Self-statements during public speaking	5	No	Spanish, German
Social Avoidance and Distress Scale	Self-report	Social distress and avoidance	10–15	No	Hindi, Japanese
Social Interaction Anxiety Scale	Self-report	Fear of social interaction	5	No	
Social Interaction Self-Statement Test	Self-report	Positive and negative thoughts associated with social interaction	5–10	No	French, Spanish
Social Phobia and Anxiety Inventory	Self-report	Severity of social anxiety and social phobia	20–30	Yes	Child version; South American Portuguese, Icelandic, Canadian French, U.S. Spanish, Swedish, Dutch
Social Phobia Inventory	Self-report	Symptoms of social phobia	10	No	
Social Phobia Scale	Self-report	Fear of being observed during routine activities	5	No	

APPENDIX

Table V. Measures for Generalized Anxiety Disorder (Chapter 15)

Name of instrument	Type of measure	Measurement focus	Time to complete (minutes)	Fee involved?	Alternate forms
Consequences of Worrying Scale	Self-report	Beliefs about the consequences of worry	5–10	No	
Generalized Anxiety Disorder Questionnaire	Self-report	Diagnostic criteria of GAD	3–4	No	
Intolerance of Uncertainty Scale	Self-report	Difficulty tolerating uncertainty	3–4	No	
Penn State Worry Questionnaire	Self-report	Trait worry	3	No	Child and adolescent versions; Chinese, Dutch, French, German, Greek, Italian, Spanish, Thai; weekly assessment version
Why Worry Scale (I & II)	Self-report	Reasons that people worry	3–4	No	French; WWII available as structured interview
Worry Domains Questionnaire	Self-report	Nonpathological worry	5	No	French; revised version with health worry domain
Worry Scale for Older Adults	Self-report	Extent of worry among older adults	5–10	No	French, Spanish, Hebrew

Table VI. Measures for Obsessive Compulsive Disorder (Chapter 17)

Name of instrument	Type of measure	Measurement focus	Time to complete (minutes)	Fee involved?	Alternate forms
Compulsive Activity Checklist	Self-report	Impairment due to obsessive compulsive symptoms	5	No	Numerous versions of various titles and lengths; French
Frost Indecisiveness Scale	Self-report	Indecisiveness	3–5	No	
Maudsley Obsessional Compulsive Inventory	Self-report	Obsessional-compulsive complaints	5	No	Portuguese
Obsessive Compulsive Inventory	Self-report	Severity of obsessive-compulsive symptoms	10–15	No	
Overvalued Ideas Scale	Clinician-administered	Strength of belief in obsessive compulsive and related disorders	5–10	No	Portuguese, Spanish, French, Italian
Padua Inventory–Washington State University Revision	Self-report	Obsessions and compulsions	10	No	Spanish, German; original PI in various languages; PI-Revised
Responsibility Attitude Scale	Self-report	Responsibility beliefs as they relate to OCD	5–10	No	
Responsibility Interpretations Questionnaire	Self-report	Responsibility beliefs as they relate to OCD	5–10	No	
Thought–Action Fusion Scale	Self-report	Cognitive distortions associated with OCD	5–10	No	
Yale–Brown Obsessive Compulsive Scale	Clinician-administered or self-report	Severity and types of symptoms in OCD	30+	No	Computerized version; child version; versions for related disorders

Table VII. Measures for Posttraumatic Stress Disorder (Chapter 19)

Name of instrument	Type of measure	Measurement focus	Time to complete (minutes)	Fee involved?	Alternate forms
Accident Fear Questionnaire	Self-report	Phobic avoidance following involvement in a motor vehicle accident	5–10	No	
Acute Stress Disorder Interview	Clinician-administered	Acute stress disorder	10	No	Self-report version
Clinician-Administered PTSD Scale	Clinician-administered	PTSD symptom severity and diagnosis	45–60	No	Child version; computerized version; several languages
Davidson Trauma Scale	Self-report	PTSD symptom severity and diagnosis	10	Yes	Brief diagnostic screening version; French-Canadian, Spanish
Dissociative Experiences Scale	Self-report	Frequency of dissociative experiences	10–15	No	Adolescent version; brief version; computerized version; 17 languages
Distressing Events Questionnaire	Self-report	PTSD symptom severity and diagnosis	5–7		Computerized version; Japanese, Tagalog
Impact of Event Scale	Self-report	Intrusion and avoidance following trauma exposure	10	No	Revised version; several languages
Los Angeles Symptom Checklist	Self-report	PTSD symptom severity	10–15	No	Adolescent version
Minnesota Multiphasic Personality Inventory–PTSD Scale	Self-report	PTSD symptom severity	15	Yes	
Mississippi Scale for PTSD	Self-report	PTSD symptom severity	10–15	Yes (some versions)	Combat-related (Spanish, Hebrew, brief); revised civilian (Spanish)

Measure	Format	Construct	Time (min)	Standardized	Notes
Penn Inventory for PTSD	Self-report	PTSD symptom severity	10–15	Yes	
Posttraumatic Cognitions Inventory	Self-report	Trauma-related thoughts and beliefs	10	Yes	
Posttraumatic Diagnostic Scale	Self-report	PTSD symptom severity	10–15	Yes	Interview version
PTSD Checklist	Self-report	PTSD symptom severity	5–10	No	Military version; specific or general stressors; parent report for a child
Purdue PTSD Scale-Revised	Self-report	PTSD symptom severity	10	No	Military and civilian versions
Short Screening Scale for PTSD	Clinician-administered	Screen for PTSD among those with known trauma exposure	<3	No	
Stanford Acute Stress Reaction Questionnaire	Self-report	Acute Stress Disorder	15	No	
Stressful Life Events Screening Questionnaire	Self-report	Lifetime exposure to various traumatic events	10	No	
Structured Interview for Disorders of Extreme Stress	Interview	Alterations resulting from extreme stress	45	No	
Structured Interview for PTSD	Interview	PTSD symptom severity and diagnosis	10–30	No	Self-report; brief version
Trauma-Related Guilt Inventory	Self-report	Guilt associated with exposure to a traumatic event	15	Yes	Tagalog
Trauma Symptom Inventory	Self-report	Acute and chronic posttraumatic stress symptoms	20	Yes	Excluding sexual items; child version; research version
Traumatic Events Questionnaire	Self-report	Frequency, type, and severity of trauma	10	Yes	Military, civilian
Traumatic Life Events Questionnaire	Self-report	Exposure to potentially traumatic events	5–10	Yes	Computerized version

Appendix B
Reprinted Measures

Measures for Anxiety and Related Constructs

Anxiety Control Questionnaire (ACQ)

Listed below are a number of statements describing a set of beliefs. Please read each statement carefully and, on the 0–5 scale below, indicate how much you think <u>each</u> statement is typical of <u>you</u>.

0	1	2	3	4	5
Strongly Disagree	Moderately Disagree	Slightly Disagree	Slightly Agree	Moderately Agree	Strongly Agree

_____ 1. I am usually able to avoid threat quite easily.

_____ 2. How well I cope with difficult situations depends on whether I have outside help.

_____ 3. When I am put under stress, I am likely to lose control.

_____ 4. I can usually stop my anxiety from showing.

_____ 5. When I am frightened by something, there is generally nothing I can do.

_____ 6. My emotions seem to have a life of their own.

_____ 7. There is little I can do to influence people's judgments of me.

_____ 8. Whether I can successfully escape a frightening situation is always a matter of chance with me.

_____ 9. I often shake uncontrollably.

_____ 10. I can usually put worrisome thoughts out of my mind easily.

_____ 11. When I am in a stressful situation, I am able to stop myself from breathing too hard.

_____ 12. I can usually influence the degree to which a situation is potentially threatening to me.

_____ 13. I am able to control my level of anxiety.

_____ 14. There is little I can do to change frightening events.

_____ 15. The extent to which a difficult situation resolves itself has nothing to do with my actions.

_____ 16. If something is going to hurt me, it will happen no matter what I do.

_____ 17. I can usually relax when I want.

_____ 18. When I am under stress, I am not always sure how I will react.

_____ 19. I can usually make sure people like me if I work at it.

_____ 20. Most events that make me anxious are outside my control.

_____ 21. I always know exactly how I will react to difficult situations.

_____ 22. I am unconcerned if I become anxious in a difficult situation, because I am confident in my ability to cope with my symptoms.

_____ 23. What people think of me is largely outside of my control.

_____ 24. I usually find it hard to deal with difficult problems.

_____ 25. When I hear someone has a serious illness, I worry that I am next.

_____ 26. When I am anxious, I find it hard to focus on anything other than my anxiety.

_____ 27. I am able to cope as effectively with unexpected anxiety as I am with anxiety that I expect to occur.

0	1	2	3	4	5
Strongly Disagree	Moderately Disagree	Slightly Disagree	Slightly Agree	Moderately Agree	Strongly Agree

_____ 28. I sometimes think, "Why even bother to try coping with my anxiety when nothing I do seems to affect how frequently or intensely I experience it?"

_____ 29. I often have the ability to get along with "difficult" people.

_____ 30. I will avoid conflict due to my inability to successfully resolve it.

APPENDIX

Clinical Anxiety Scale (CAS)

Instructions: The Scale is an instrument for the assessment of the present state of anxiety; therefore the emphasis on eliciting information for the ratings should be on how the patient feels at the present time. However, the interview itself may raise, or lower, the severity of anxiety and the interviewer should inform the patient that he should describe how he has felt during the period of the past two days.

Psychic tension (care should be taken to distinguish tension from muscular tension—see next item).

Score 4: Very marked and distressing feeling of being 'on edge', 'keyed up', 'wound up' or 'nervous' which persists with little change throughout the waking hours.
Score 3: As above, but with some fluctuation of severity during the course of the day.
Score 2: A definite experience of being tense which is sufficient to cause some, although not severe, distress.
Score 1: A slight feeling of being tense which does not cause distress.
Score 0: No feeling of being tense apart from the normal degree of tension experienced in response to stress and which is acceptable as normal for the population.

Ability to relax (muscular tension)

Score 4: The experience of severe tension throughout much of the bodily musculature which may be accompanied by such symptoms as pain, stiffness, spasmodic contractions, and lack of control over movements. The experience is present throughout most of the waking day and there is no ability to produce relaxation at will.
Score 3: As above, but the muscular tension may only be experienced in certain groups of muscles and may fluctuate in severity throughout the day.
Score 2: A definite experience of muscular tension in some part of the musculature sufficient to cause some, but not severe, distress.
Score 1: Slight recurrent muscular tension of which the patient is aware but which does not cause distress. Very mild degrees of tension headache or pain in other groups of muscles should be scored here.
Score 0: No subjective muscular tension or of such degree which, when it occurs, can easily be controlled at will.

Startle response (hyperarousability)

Score 4: Unexpected noise causes severe distress so that the patient may complain in some such phrase as "I jump out of my skin". Distress is experienced in psychic *and* somatic modalities so that, in addition to the experience of fright, there is muscular activity and autonomic symptoms such as sweating or palpitation.
Score 3: Unexpected noise causes severe distress in psychic or somatic, but not in both modalities.
Score 2: Unexpected noise causes definite but not severe distress.
Score 1: Patient agrees that he is slightly 'jumpy' but is not distressed by this.
Score 0: The degree of startle response is entirely acceptable as normal for the population.

Worrying (The assessment must take into account the degree to which worry is out of proportion to actual stress).

Score 4: The patient experiences almost continuous preoccupation with painful thoughts which cannot be stopped voluntarily and the distress is quite out of proportion to the subject matter of the thoughts.

Score 3: As above, but there is some fluctuation in intensity throughout the waking hours and the distressing thoughts may cease for an hour or two, especially if the patient is distracted by activity requiring his attention.

Score 2: Painful thoughts out of proportion to the patient's situation keep intruding into consciousness but he is able to dispel or dismiss them.

Score 1: The patient agrees that he tends to worry a little more than necessary about minor matters but this does not cause much distress.

Score 0: The tendency to worry is accepted as being normal for the population; for instance even marked worrying over a severe financial crisis or unexpected illness in a relative should be scored as 0 if it is judged to be entirely in keeping with the degree of stress.

Apprehension

Score 4: The experience is that of being on the brink of some disaster which cannot be explained. The experience need not be continuous and may occur in short bursts several times a day.

Score 3: As above, but the experience does not occur more than once a day.

Score 2: The sensation of groundless apprehension of disaster which is not severe although it causes definite distress. The patient may not use strong terms such as "disaster" or "catastrophe" but may express his experience in some such phrase as "I feel as if something bad is about to happen."

Score 1: A slight degree of apprehensiveness of which the patient is aware but which does not cause distress.

Score 0: No experience of groundless anticipation of disaster.

Restlessness

Score 4: The patient is unable to keep still for more than a few minutes and engages in restless pacing or other purposeless activity.

Score 3: Same as above, but he is able to keep still for an hour or so at a time.

Score 2: There is a feeling of "needing to be on the move" which causes some, but not severe, distress.

Score 1: Slight experience of restlessness which causes no distress.

Score 0: Absence of restlessness.

The following item may be rated if required, but should not be added to the CAS Score

Panic attacks

Score 4: Episodes, occurring several times a day, of the sudden experience of groundless terror accompanied by marked autonomic symptoms, feelings of imminent collapse or loss of control over reason and self-integrity.

Score 3: As above, but the episodes do not occur more than once a day.

Score 2: The episodes may occur only once or twice a week; they are generally less severe than described above but still cause distress.

Score 1:   Episodic slight increases in the level of anxiety which are only precipitated by definite events or activities. For instance, the experience of a patient who is recovering from agoraphobia and who experiences a perceptible rise of anxiety on leaving the house would be scored here.

Score 0:   No episodic sudden increase in the level of anxiety.

Depression Anxiety Stress Scales (DASS)

INSTRUCTIONS: Please read each statement and choose the number which indicates how much the statement applied to you over the past week. There are no right or wrong answers. Do not spend too much time on any statement. The rating scale is as follows:

0 = Did not apply to me at all
1 = Applied to me to some degree, or some of the time
2 = Applied to me to a considerable degree, or a good part of the time
3 = Applied to me very much, or most of the time

_____ 1. I found myself getting upset by quite trivial things.

_____ 2. I was aware of dryness of my mouth.

_____ 3. I couldn't seem to experience any positive feeling at all.

_____ 4. I experienced breathing difficulty (e.g., excessively rapid breathing, breathlessness in the absence of physical exertion).

_____ 5. I just couldn't seem to get going.

_____ 6. I tended to over-react to situations.

_____ 7. I had a feeling of shakiness (e.g., legs going to give way).

_____ 8. I found it difficult to relax.

_____ 9. I found myself in situations that made me so anxious I was most relieved when they ended.

_____ 10. I felt that I had nothing to look forward to.

_____ 11. I found myself getting upset rather easily.

_____ 12. I felt that I was using a lot of nervous energy.

_____ 13. I felt sad and depressed.

_____ 14. I found myself getting impatient when I was delayed in any way (e.g., elevators, traffic lights, being kept waiting).

_____ 15. I had a feeling of faintness.

_____ 16. I felt that I had lost interest in just about everything.

_____ 17. I felt I wasn't worth much as a person.

_____ 18. I felt that I was rather touchy.

_____ 19. I perspired noticeably (e.g., hands sweaty) in the absence of high temperatures or physical exertion.

_____ 20. I felt scared without any good reason.

_____ 21. I felt that life wasn't worthwhile.

Reminder of Rating Scale:

0 = Did not apply to me at all
1 = Applied to me to some degree, or some of the time
2 = Applied to me to a considerable degree, or a good part of the time
3 = Applied to me very much, or most of the time

_____ 22. I found it hard to wind down.

_____ 23. I had difficulty in swallowing.

_____ 24. I couldn't seem to get any enjoyment out of the things I did.

_____ 25. I was aware of the action of my heart in the absence of physical exertion (e.g., sense of heart rate increase, heart missing a beat).

_____ 26. I felt down-hearted and blue.

_____ 27. I found that I was very irritable.

_____ 28. I felt I was close to panic.

_____ 29. I found it hard to calm down after something upset me.

_____ 30. I feared that I would be "thrown" by some trivial but unfamiliar task.

_____ 31. I was unable to become enthusiastic about anything.

_____ 32. I found it difficult to tolerate interruptions to what I was doing.

_____ 33. I was in a state of nervous tension.

_____ 34. I felt I was pretty worthless.

_____ 35. I was intolerant of anything that kept me from getting on with what I was doing.

_____ 36. I felt terrified.

_____ 37. I could see nothing in the future to be hopeful about.

_____ 38. I felt that life was meaningless.

_____ 39. I found myself getting agitated.

_____ 40. I was worried about situations in which I might panic and make a fool of myself.

_____ 41. I experienced trembling (e.g., in the hands).

_____ 42. I found it difficult to work up the initiative to do things.

Fear Questionnaire (FQ)

Choose a number from the scale below to show how much you would avoid each of the situations listed below because of fear or other unpleasant feelings. Then write the number you chose on the line beside each situation.

```
0————1————2————3————4————5————6————7————8
Would not      Slightly      Definitely      Markedly      Always
 avoid it      avoid it       avoid it       avoid it     avoid it
```

1. Main phobia you want treated (describe in your own words):
   _____   _____

2. Injections or minor surgery ....   _____
3. Eating or drinking with other people ....   _____
4. Hospitals ....   _____
5. Traveling alone by bus or coach ....   _____
6. Walking alone in busy streets ....   _____
7. Being watched or stared at ....   _____
8. Going into crowded shops ....   _____
9. Talking to people in authority ....   _____
10. Sight of blood ....   _____
11. Being criticized ....   _____
12. Going alone far from home ....   _____
13. Thought of injury or illness ....   _____
14. Speaking or acting to an audience ....   _____
15. Large open spaces ....   _____
16. Going to the dentist ....   _____
17. Other situations (describe) _____   _____

AG + BL + SOC = TOTAL

_____   _____   _____   _____

Now choose a number from the scale below to show how much you are troubled by each problem listed and write the number on the line opposite.

```
0————1————2————3————4————5————6————7————8
 Hardly        Slightly      Definitely      Markedly     Very severely
 at all       troublesome   troublesome    troublesome    troublesome
```

18. Feeling miserable or depressed ....   _____
19. Feeling irritable or angry ....   _____
20. Feeling tense of panicky ....   _____
21. Upsetting thoughts coming into your mind ....   _____
22. Feeling you or your surrounding are strange or unreal ....   _____
23. Other feelings (describe) _____   _____

24. How would you rate the present state of your phobic symptoms on the scale below?

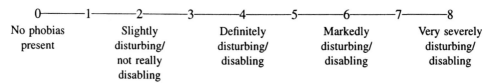

0————1————2————3————4————5————6————7————8				
No phobias present	Slightly disturbing/ not really disabling	Definitely disturbing/ disabling	Markedly disturbing/ disabling	Very severely disturbing/ disabling

Circle one number between 0 and 8

Frost Multidimensional Perfectionism Scale (FMPS)

Please write in the space provided beside each item the number that best corresponds to your agreement with each statement below. Use the scale provided.

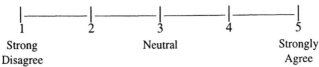

| | | | | |
|1|2|3|4|5|

Strong   Neutral   Strongly
Disagree   Agree

_____ 1. My parents set very high standards for me.

_____ 2. Organization is very important to me.

_____ 3. As a child, I was punished for doing things less than perfectly.

_____ 4. If I do not set the highest standards for myself, I am likely to end up a second rate person.

_____ 5. My parents never tried to understand my mistakes.

_____ 6. It is important to me that I be thoroughly competent in everything that I do.

_____ 7. I am a neat person.

_____ 8. I try to be an organized person.

_____ 9. If I fail at work/school, I am a failure as a person.

_____ 10. I should be upset if I make a mistake.

_____ 11. My parents wanted me to be the best at everything.

_____ 12. I set higher goals than most people.

_____ 13. If someone does a task at work/school better than I, then I feel like I failed the whole task.

_____ 14. If I fail partly, it is as bad as being a complete failure.

_____ 15. Only outstanding performance is good enough for my family.

_____ 16. I am very good at focusing my efforts on attaining a goal.

_____ 17. Even when I do something very carefully, I often feel that it is not quite right.

_____ 18. I hate being less than the best at things.

_____ 19. I have extremely high goals.

_____ 20. My parents have expected excellence from me.

_____ 21. People will probably think less of me if I make a mistake.

_____ 22. I never felt like I could meet my parents' expectations.

_____ 23. If I do not do as well as other people, it means that I am an inferior human being.

_____ 24. Other people seem to accept lower standards from themselves than I do.

_____ 25. If I do not do well all the time, people will not respect me.

_____ 26. My parents have always had higher expectations for my future than I have.

_____ 27. I try to be a neat person.

_____ 28. I usually have doubts about the simple everyday things I do.

_____ 29. Neatness is very important to me.

_____ 30. I expect higher performance in my daily tasks than most people.

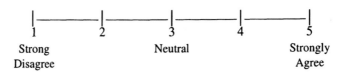

Strong
Disagree
Neutral
Strongly
Agree

_____ 31. I am an organized person.

_____ 32. I tend to get behind in my work because I repeat things over and over.

_____ 33. It takes me a long time to do something "right."

_____ 34. The fewer mistakes I make, the more people will like me.

_____ 35. I never felt like I could meet my parents' standards.

Hamilton Anxiety Rating Scale (HARS)

0 = none; 1 = mild; 2 = moderate; 3 = severe; 4 = very severe, grossly disabling

1. ANXIOUS MOOD	Worries, anticipation of the worst, apprehension (fearful anticipation) irritability	0 1 2 3 4
2. TENSION	Feelings of tension, fatiguability, inability to relax, startle response, moved to tears easily, trembling, feelings of restlessness	0 1 2 3 4
3. FEARS	Of dark, strangers, being left alone, large animals, traffic, crowds	0 1 2 3 4
4. INSOMNIA	Difficulty in falling asleep, broken sleep, unsatisfying sleep and fatigue on waking, dreams, nightmares, night terrors	0 1 2 3 4
5. INTELLECTUAL (COGNITIVE)	Difficulty in concentration, poor memory	0 1 2 3 4
6. DEPRESSED MOOD	Loss of interest, lack of pleasure in hobbies, depression, early waking, diurnal swing	0 1 2 3 4
7. GENERAL SOMATIC (MUSCULAR)	Muscular pains and aches, muscular stiffness, muscular twitchings, clonic jerks, grinding of teeth, unsteady voice	0 1 2 3 4
8. GENERAL SOMATIC (SENSORY)	Tinnitus, blurring of vision, hot and cold flushes, feelings of weakness, pricking sensations	0 1 2 3 4
9. CARDIOVASCULAR SYMPTOMS	Tachycardia, palpitations, pain in chest, throbbing of vessels, fainting feelings, missing beat	0 1 2 3 4
10. RESPIRATORY SYMPTOMS	Pressure or constriction in chest, choking feelings, sighings, dyspnoea	0 1 2 3 4
11. GASTROINTESTINAL SYMPTOMS	Difficulty in swallowing, wind, dyspepsia, pain before and after meals, burning sensations, fullness, waterbrash, nausea, vomiting, sinking feelings; 'working' in the abdomen, borborygmi, looseness of bowels, loss of weight, constipation	0 1 2 3 4
12. GENITO-URINARY	Frequency of micturition, urgency of micturition, amenorrhea, menorrhagia, development of frigidity, premature ejaculation, loss of erection, impotence	0 1 2 3 4
13. AUTONOMIC SYMPTOMS	Dry mouth, flushing, pallor, tendency to sweat, giddiness, tension headache, raising of hair	0 1 2 3 4

0 = none; 1 = mild; 2 = moderate; 3 = severe; 4 = very severe, grossly disabling

| 14. BEHAVIOR AT INTERVIEW | GENERAL: tense, not relaxed, fidgeting (hands, picking fingers, clenching, tics, handkerchief), restlessness (pacing) tremor of hands, furrowed brow, strained face, increased muscular tone, sighing respirations, facial pallor; PHYSIOLOGICAL: swallowing, belching, high resting pulse rate, respiration rate over 20/min, brisk tendon jerks, tremor, dilated pupils, exophthalmos, sweating, eye-lid twitching | 0 1 2 3 4 |

GENERAL COMMENTS:

Meta-Cognitions Questionnaire (MCQ)

This questionnaire is concerned with beliefs people have about their thinking. Listed below are a number of beliefs that people have expressed. Please read each item and say how much you generally agree with it by circling the appropriate number. Please respond to all the items. There are no right or wrong answers.

	Do not agree	Agree slightly	Agree moderately	Agree very much
1. Worrying helps me to avoid problems in the future.	1	2	3	4
2. My worrying is dangerous for me.	1	2	3	4
3. I have difficulty knowing if I have actually done something, or just imagined it.	1	2	3	4
4. I think a lot about my thoughts.	1	2	3	4
5. I could make myself sick with worrying.	1	2	3	4
6. I am aware of the way my mind works when I am thinking through a problem.	1	2	3	4
7. If I did not control a worrying thought, and then it happened, it would be my fault.	1	2	3	4
8. If I let my worrying thoughts get out of control, they will end up controlling me.	1	2	3	4
9. I need to worry in order to remain organized.	1	2	3	4
10. I have little confidence in my memory for words and names.	1	2	3	4
11. My worrying thoughts persist, no matter how I try to stop them.	1	2	3	4
12. Worrying helps me to get things sorted out in my mind.	1	2	3	4
13. I cannot ignore my worrying thoughts.	1	2	3	4
14. I monitor my thoughts.	1	2	3	4
15. I should be in control of my thoughts all of the time.	1	2	3	4
16. My memory can mislead me at times.	1	2	3	4
17. I could be punished for not having certain thoughts.	1	2	3	4
18. My worrying could make me go mad.	1	2	3	4
19. If I do not stop my worrying thoughts, they could come true	.1	2	3	4
20. I rarely question my thoughts.	1	2	3	4
21. Worrying puts my body under a lot of stress.	1	2	3	4
22. Worrying helps me to avoid disastrous situations.	1	2	3	4

	Do not agree	Agree slightly	Agree moderately	Agree very much
23. I am constantly aware of my thinking.	1	2	3	4
24. I have a poor memory.	1	2	3	4
25. I pay close attention to the way my mind works.	1	2	3	4
26. People who do not worry have no depth.	1	2	3	4
27. Worrying helps me cope.	1	2	3	4
28. I imagine having not done things and then doubt my memory for doing them.	1	2	3	4
29. Not being able to control my thoughts is a sign of weakness.	1	2	3	4
30. If I did not worry, I would make more mistakes.	1	2	3	4
31. I find it difficult to control my thoughts.	1	2	3	4
32. Worrying is a sign of a good person.	1	2	3	4
33. Worrying thoughts enter my head against my will.	1	2	3	4
34. If I could not control my thoughts I would go crazy.	1	2	3	4
35. I will lose out in life if I do not worry.	1	2	3	4
36. When I start worrying, I cannot stop.	1	2	3	4
37. Some thoughts will always need to be controlled.	1	2	3	4
38. I need to worry in order to get things done.	1	2	3	4
39. I will be punished for not controlling certain thoughts.	1	2	3	4
40. My thoughts interfere with my concentration.	1	2	3	4
41. It is alright to let my thoughts roam free.	1	2	3	4
42. I worry about my thoughts.	1	2	3	4
43. I am easily distracted.	1	2	3	4
44. My worrying thoughts are not productive.	1	2	3	4
45. Worry can stop me from seeing a situation clearly.	1	2	3	4
46. Worrying helps me to solve problems.	1	2	3	4
47. I have little confidence in my memory for places.	1	2	3	4
48. My worrying thoughts are uncontrollable.	1	2	3	4
49. It is bad to think certain thoughts.	1	2	3	4
50. If I do not control my thoughts, I may end upembarrassing myself.	1	2	3	4

APPENDIX

	Do not agree	Agree slightly	Agree moderately	Agree very much
51. I do not trust my memory.	1	2	3	4
52. I do my clearest thinking when I am worrying.	1	2	3	4
53. My worrying thoughts appear automatically.	1	2	3	4
54. I would be selfish if I never worried.	1	2	3	4
55. If I could not control my thoughts, I would not be able to function.	1	2	3	4
56. I need to worry, in order to work well.	1	2	3	4
57. I have little confidence in my memory for actions.	1	2	3	4
58. I have difficulty keeping my mind focused on one thing for a long time.	1	2	3	4
59. If a bad thing happens which I have not worried about, I feel responsible.	1	2	3	4
60. It would not be normal if I did not worry.	1	2	3	4
61. I constantly examine my thoughts.	1	2	3	4
62. If I stopped worrying, I would become glib, arrogant and offensive.	1	2	3	4
63. Worrying helps me plan the future more effectively.	1	2	3	4
64. I would be a stronger person if I could worry less.	1	2	3	4
65. I would be stupid and complacent not to worry.	1	2	3	4

Items reprinted from Cartwright-Hatton, S., & Wells, A. (1997). Beliefs about worry and intrusions: The Meta-Cognitions Questionnaire and its correlates. *Journal of Anxiety Disorders, 11*, 279–296. Full measure reprinted in Wells A. (1997). *Cognitive therapy of anxiety disorder: A practise manual and conceptual guide.* Chichester, UK: Wiley (pp. 286–290). © 1997 John Wiley & Sons Limited. Reproduced with permission from Elsevier Science, John Wiley & Sons Limited and Adrian Wells, Ph.D.

The Positive and Negative Affect Scales (PANAS)

This scale consists of a number of words that describe different feelings and emotions. Read each item and then mark the appropriate answer in the space next to that word. Indicate to what extent [INSERT APPROPRIATE TIME INSTRUCTIONS HERE]. Use the following scale to record your answers.

1	2	3	4	5
very slightly or not at all	a little	moderately	quite a bit	extremely

_____ interested   _____ irritable

_____ distressed   _____ alert

_____ excited   _____ ashamed

_____ upset   _____ inspired

_____ strong   _____ nervous

_____ guilty   _____ determined

_____ scared   _____ attentive

_____ hostile   _____ jittery

_____ enthusiastic   _____ active

_____ proud   _____ afraid

Time instructions that have been used:

Moment	(you feel this way right now, that is, at the present moment)
Today	(you have felt this way today)
Past few days	(you have felt this way during the past few days)
Week	(you have felt this way during the past week)
Past few weeks	(you have felt this way during the past few weeks)
Year	(you have felt this way during the past year)
General	(you generally feel this way, that is, how you feel on the average)

Self-Rating Anxiety Scale (SAS)

	None OR A little of the time	Some of the time	Good part of the time	Most OR All of the time
1. I feel more nervous and anxious than usual	1	2	3	4
2. I feel afraid for no reason at all	1	2	3	4
3. I get upset easily or feel panicky	1	2	3	4
4. I feel like I'm falling apart and going to pieces	1	2	3	4
5. I feel that everything is all right and nothing bad will happen	1	2	3	4
6. My arms and legs shake and tremble	1	2	3	4
7. I am bothered by headaches, neck and back pains	1	2	3	4
8. I feel weak and get tired easily	1	2	3	4
9. I feel calm and can sit still easily	1	2	3	4
10. I can feel my heart beating fast	1	2	3	4
11. I am bothered by dizzy spells	1	2	3	4
12. I have fainting spells or feel like it	1	2	3	4
13. I can breathe in and out easily	1	2	3	4
14. I get feelings of numbness and tingling in my fingers, toes	1	2	3	4
15. I am bothered by stomachaches or indigestion	1	2	3	4
16. I have to empty my bladder often	1	2	3	4
17. My hands are usually dry and warm	1	2	3	4
18. My face gets hot and blushes	1	2	3	4
19. I fall asleep easily and get a good night's rest	1	2	3	4
20. I have nightmares	1	2	3	4

Adapted from Zung, W. W. K. (1971). A rating instrument for anxiety disorders. *Psychosomatics*, *12*, 371–379. Reprinted with permission from the American Psychiatric Press on behalf of the Academy of Psychosomatic Medicine.

Thought Control Questionnaire (TCQ)

Most people experience unpleasant, and/or unwanted thoughts (in verbal and/or picture form) which can be difficult to control. We are interested in the techniques that you **generally** use to control such thoughts.

Below are a number of things that people do to control these thoughts. Please read each statement carefully, and indicate how often you use each technique by **circling** the appropriate number. There are no right or wrong answers. Do not spend too much time thinking about each one.

When I experience an unpleasant/unwanted thought:

	Never	Sometimes	Often	Almost Always
1. I call to mind positive images instead.	1	2	3	4
2. I tell myself not to be so stupid.	1	2	3	4
3. I focus on the thought.	1	2	3	4
4. I replace the thought with a more trivial bad thought.	1	2	3	4
5. I don't talk about the thought to anyone.	1	2	3	4
6. I punish myself for thinking the thought.	1	2	3	4
7. I dwell on other worries.	1	2	3	4
8. I keep the thought to myself.	1	2	3	4
9. I occupy myself with work instead.	1	2	3	4
10. I challenge the thought's validity.	1	2	3	4
11. I get angry at myself for having the thought.	1	2	3	4
12. I avoid discussing the thought.	1	2	3	4
13. I shout at myself for having the thought.	1	2	3	4
14. I analyse the thought rationally.	1	2	3	4
15. I slap or pinch myself to stop the thought.	1	2	3	4
16. I think pleasant thoughts instead.	1	2	3	4
17. I find out how my friends deal with these thoughts.	1	2	3	4
18. I worry about more minor things instead.	1	2	3	4
19. I do something that I enjoy.	1	2	3	4
20. I try to reinterpret the thought.	1	2	3	4
21. I think about something else.	1	2	3	4
22. I think more about the more minor problems I have.	1	2	3	4
23. I try a different way of thinking about it.	1	2	3	4
24. I think about past worries instead.	1	2	3	4
25. I ask my friends if they have similar thoughts.	1	2	3	4
26. I focus on different negative thoughts.	1	2	3	4

APPENDIX

	Never	Sometimes	Often	Almost Always
27. I question the reasons for having the thought.	1	2	3	4
28. I tell myself that something bad will happen if I think the thought.	1	2	3	4
29. I talk to a friend about the thought.	1	2	3	4
30. I keep myself busy.	1	2	3	4

Items reprinted from Wells, A., & Davies, M. (1994). The Thought Control Questionnaire—A measure of individual differences in the control of unwanted thoughts. *Behaviour Research and Therapy, 32,* 871–878. Full measure reprinted in Wells A. (2001). *Emotional disorders and metacognition: Innovative cognitive therapy.* Chichester, UK: Wiley. © 2001 John Wiley & Sons Limited. Reproduced with permission from Elsevier Science, John Wiley & Sons Limited, and Adrian Wells, Ph.D.

Trimodal Anxiety Questionnaire (TAQ)

Please circle the number that indicates how you feel for each item. <u>For example</u>, if you feel happy often, but not all of the time, put ...

I feel happy

0	1	2	3	4	5	⑥	7	8
Never								Extremely Often

---

1. My throat gets dry.

0	1	2	3	4	5	6	7	8
Never								Extremely Often

2. I have difficulty in swallowing.

0	1	2	3	4	5	6	7	8
Never								Extremely Often

3. I try to avoid starting conversations.

0	1	2	3	4	5	6	7	8
Never								Extremely Often

4. My heart pounds.

0	1	2	3	4	5	6	7	8
Never								Extremely Often

5. I picture some future misfortune.

0	1	2	3	4	5	6	7	8
Never								Extremely Often

6. I avoid talking to people in authority (my boss, policemen).

0	1	2	3	4	5	6	7	8
Never								Extremely Often

7. My limbs tremble.

0	1	2	3	4	5	6	7	8
Never								Extremely Often

8. I can't get some thoughts out of my mind.

0	1	2	3	4	5	6	7	8
Never								Extremely Often

9. I avoid going into a room by myself where people are already gathered and talking.

0	1	2	3	4	5	6	7	8
Never								Extremely Often

APPENDIX

10. My stomach hurts.

0	1	2	3	4	5	6	7	8
Never								Extremely Often

11. I dwell on mistakes that I have made.

0	1	2	3	4	5	6	7	8
Never								Extremely Often

12. I avoid new or unfamiliar situations.

0	1	2	3	4	5	6	7	8
Never								Extremely Often

13. My neck feels tight.

0	1	2	3	4	5	6	7	8
Never								Extremely Often

14. I feel dizzy.

0	1	2	3	4	5	6	7	8
Never								Extremely Often

15. I think about possible misfortunes to my loved ones.

0	1	2	3	4	5	6	7	8
Never								Extremely Often

16. I cannot concentrate at a task or job without irrelevant thoughts intruding.

0	1	2	3	4	5	6	7	8
Never								Extremely Often

17. I pass by school friends, or people I know but have not seen for a long time, unless they speak to me first.

0	1	2	3	4	5	6	7	8
Never								Extremely Often

18. I breathe rapidly.

0	1	2	3	4	5	6	7	8
Never								Extremely Often

19. I keep busy to avoid uncomfortable thoughts.

0	1	2	3	4	5	6	7	8
Never								Extremely Often

20. I can't catch my breath.

0	1	2	3	4	5	6	7	8
Never								Extremely Often

21. I can't get some pictures or images out of my mind.

0	1	2	3	4	5	6	7	8
Never								Extremely Often

22. I try to avoid social gatherings.

0	1	2	3	4	5	6	7	8
Never								Extremely Often

23. My arms or legs feel stiff.

0	1	2	3	4	5	6	7	8
Never								Extremely Often

24. I imagine myself appearing foolish with a person whose opinion of me is important.

0	1	2	3	4	5	6	7	8
Never								Extremely Often

25. I find myself staying home rather than involving myself in activities outside.

0	1	2	3	4	5	6	7	8
Never								Extremely Often

26. I prefer to avoid making specific plans for self-improvement.

0	1	2	3	4	5	6	7	8
Never								Extremely Often

27. I am concerned that others might not think well of me.

0	1	2	3	4	5	6	7	8
Never								Extremely Often

28. I try to avoid challenging jobs.

0	1	2	3	4	5	6	7	8
Never								Extremely Often

29. My muscles twitch or jump.

0	1	2	3	4	5	6	7	8
Never								Extremely Often

30. I experience a tingling sensation somewhere in my body.

0	1	2	3	4	5	6	7	8
Never								Extremely Often

31. My arms or legs feel weak.

0	1	2	3	4	5	6	7	8
Never								Extremely Often

32. I have to be careful not to let my real feelings show.

0	1	2	3	4	5	6	7	8
Never								Extremely Often

33. I experience muscular aches and pains.

0	1	2	3	4	5	6	7	8
Never								Extremely Often

34. I feel numbness in my face, limbs or tongue.

0	1	2	3	4	5	6	7	8
Never								Extremely Often

35. I experience chest pains.

0	1	2	3	4	5	6	7	8
Never								Extremely Often

36. I have an uneasy feeling.

0	1	2	3	4	5	6	7	8
Never								Extremely Often

Measures for Panic Disorder and Agoraphobia

Agoraphobic Cognitions Questionnaire (ACQ)

Below are some thoughts or ideas that may pass through your mind when you are nervous or frightened. Please indicate how often each thought occurs when you are nervous. Rate from 1–5 using the scale below:

1	2	3	4	5
thought **never** occurs	thought **rarely** occurs	thought occurs **during half of the times**	thought **usually** occurs	thought **always** occurs

...... when I am nervous

Please rate all items.

1. I am going to throw up	1	2	3	4	5
2. I am going to pass out	1	2	3	4	5
3. I must have a brain tumor	1	2	3	4	5
4. I will have a heart attack	1	2	3	4	5
5. I will choke to death	1	2	3	4	5
6. I am going to act foolish	1	2	3	4	5
7. I am going blind	1	2	3	4	5
8. I will not be able to control myself	1	2	3	4	5
9. I will hurt someone	1	2	3	4	5
10. I am going to have a stroke	1	2	3	4	5
11. I am going crazy	1	2	3	4	5
12. I am going to scream	1	2	3	4	5
13. I am going to babble or talk funny	1	2	3	4	5
14. I am going to be paralyzed by fear	1	2	3	4	5
15. other ideas not listed (please describe and rate them)					
....	1	2	3	4	5
....	1	2	3	4	5
....	1	2	3	4	5

Agoraphobic Cognitions Scale (ACS)

To what extent do you fear the following:

	Not at all	A little	Moderate	Much	Very much
1. Fear of fainting	0	1	2	3	4
2. Fear of having a heart attack	0	1	2	3	4
3. Fear of another illness	0	1	2	3	4
4. Fear of dying	0	1	2	3	4
5. Fear of becoming helpless	0	1	2	3	4
6. Fear of going crazy	0	1	2	3	4
7. Fear of losing control	0	1	2	3	4
8. Fear that anxiety will be visible	0	1	2	3	4
9. Fear of making a scene	0	1	2	3	4
10. Fear of fear	0	1	2	3	4

Agoraphobic Self-Statements Questionnaire (ASQ)

<u>Instructions</u>

Listed below are a number of thoughts, all of which can go through your mind when you are in a situation in which you feel/become anxious or tense. Read each statement and put a circle around the most appropriate number to indicate how often you have these thoughts.

	Never				Continuously
1. I will become panicky	0	1	2	3	4
2. Tension is easing	0	1	2	3	4
3. I am not normal	0	1	2	3	4
4. I can not leave as fast as I want to	0	1	2	3	4
5. I will just try and see how things go	0	1	2	3	4
6. I am pleased with myself	0	1	2	3	4
7. I feel alone and abandoned	0	1	2	3	4
8. I am going to faint	0	1	2	3	4
9. I feel confused	0	1	2	3	4
10. If only there was someone to help me	0	1	2	3	4
11. It is pleasant to be able to enter this situation	0	1	2	3	4
12. I am doing fine	0	1	2	3	4
13. I can't make it	0	1	2	3	4
14. I feel unreal	0	1	2	3	4
15. I will lose control over myself	0	1	2	3	4
16. Others manage, why shouldn't I?	0	1	2	3	4
17. I feel safe and at ease	0	1	2	3	4
18. I will go on, I will pull myself through this	0	1	2	3	4
19. I am really anxious and tense	0	1	2	3	4
20. I can handle this situation	0	1	2	3	4
21. What I feel is not dangerous, but a reaction to tension	0	1	2	3	4
22. I will make a scene	0	1	2	3	4
23. Nothing will happen	0	1	2	3	4
24. I feel relaxed	0	1	2	3	4
25. I can't stay any longer, I have to go	0	1	2	3	4

Albany Panic and Phobia Questionnaire (APPQ)

Please rate, on the following scale, the *amount of fear* that you think you would experience in each of the situations listed below if they were to occur *in the next week*. Try to imagine yourself actually doing each activity and how you would feel.

Fear Scale

```
0 -------1 -------2 -------3 -------4 -------5 -------6 -------7 -------8
No Fear        Slight        Moderate        Marked        Extreme
                Fear           Fear            Fear           Fear
```

_____ 1. Talking to people
_____ 2. Going through a car wash
_____ 3. Playing a vigorous sport on a hot day
_____ 4. Blowing up an airbed quickly
_____ 5. Eating in front of others
_____ 6. Hiking on a hot day
_____ 7. Getting gas at a dentist
_____ 8. Interrupting a meeting
_____ 9. Giving a speech
_____ 10. Exercising vigorously alone
_____ 11. Going long distances from home alone
_____ 12. Introducing yourself to groups
_____ 13. Walking alone in isolated areas
_____ 14. Driving on highways
_____ 15. Wearing striking clothes
_____ 16. Possibility of getting lost
_____ 17. Drinking a strong cup of coffee
_____ 18. Sitting in the center of a cinema
_____ 19. Running up stairs
_____ 20. Riding on a subway
_____ 21. Speaking on the telephone
_____ 22. Meeting strangers
_____ 23. Writing in front of others
_____ 24. Entering a room full of people
_____ 25. Staying overnight away from home
_____ 26. Feeling the effects of alcohol
_____ 27. Going over a long, low bridge

Anxiety Sensitivity Index (ASI)

Circle the one number that best represents the extent to which you agree with the item. If any of the items concern something that is not part of your experience (e.g., "It scares me when I feel shaky" for someone who has never trembled or had the "shakes"), answer on the basis of how you might feel *if you had* such an experience. Otherwise, answer all the items on the basis of your own experience.

	Very Little	A Little	Moderate	Much	Very Much
1. It is important to me not to appear nervous.	0	1	2	3	4
2. When I cannot keep my mind on a task, I worry that I might be going crazy.	0	1	2	3	4
3. It scares me when I feel "shaky" (trembling).	0	1	2	3	4
4. It scares me when I feel faint.	0	1	2	3	4
5. It is important to me to stay in control of my emotions.	0	1	2	3	4
6. It scares me when my heart beats rapidly.	0	1	2	3	4
7. It embarrasses me when my stomach growls.	0	1	2	3	4
8. It scares me when I am nauseous.	0	1	2	3	4
9. When I notice my heart is beating rapidly, I worry that I might have a heart attack.	0	1	2	3	4
10. It scares me when I become short of breath.	0	1	2	3	4
11. When my stomach is upset, I worry that I might be seriously ill.	0	1	2	3	4
12. It scares me when I am unable to keep my mind on a task.	0	1	2	3	4
13. Other people notice when I feel shaky.	0	1	2	3	4
14. Unusual body sensations scare me.	0	1	2	3	4
15. When I am nervous, I worry that I might be mentally ill.	0	1	2	3	4
16. It scares me when I am nervous.	0	1	2	3	4

Anxiety Sensitivity Index-Revised 36 (ASI-R-36)

Please circle the number that best corresponds to how much you agree with each item. If any of the items concern something that is not part of your experience (for example, "It scares me when I feel shaky" for someone who has never trembled or felt shaky) answer on the basis of how you expect you might feel if you had such an experience. Otherwise, answer all items on the basis of your own experience. Be careful to circle only one number for each item and please answer all items.

	Very Little	A Little	Moderate	Much	Very Much
1. It is important to me not to appear nervous.	0	1	2	3	4
2. When I cannot keep my mind on a task, I worry that I might be going crazy.	0	1	2	3	4
3. It scares me when I feel "shaky" (trembling).	0	1	2	3	4
4. It scares me when I feel faint.	0	1	2	3	4
5. It scares me when my heart beats rapidly.	0	1	2	3	4
6. It scares me when I am nauseous.	0	1	2	3	4
7. When I notice my heart is beating rapidly, I worry that I might have a heart attack.	0	1	2	3	4
8. It scares me when I become short of breath.	0	1	2	3	4
9. When my stomach is upset, I worry that I might be seriously ill.	0	1	2	3	4
10. It scares me when I am unable to keep my mind on a task.	0	1	2	3	4
11. When my head is pounding, I worry I could have a stroke.	0	1	2	3	4
12. When I tremble in the presence of others, I fear what people might think of me.	0	1	2	3	4
13. When I feel like I'm not getting enough air, I get scared that I might suffocate.	0	1	2	3	4
14. When I get diarrhea, I worry that I might have something wrong with me.	0	1	2	3	4
15. When my chest feels tight, I get scared that I won't be able to breathe properly.	0	1	2	3	4
16. When my breathing becomes irregular, I fear that something bad will happen.	0	1	2	3	4

	Very Little	A Little	Moderate	Much	Very Much
17. It frightens me when my surroundings seem strange or unreal.	0	1	2	3	4
18. Smothering sensations scare me.	0	1	2	3	4
19. When I feel pain in my chest, I worry that I'm having a heart attack.	0	1	2	3	4
20. I believe it would be awful to vomit in public.	0	1	2	3	4
21. It scares me when my body feels strange or different in some way.	0	1	2	3	4
22. I worry that other people will notice my anxiety.	0	1	2	3	4
23. When I feel "spacey" or spaced out, I worry that I may be mentally ill.	0	1	2	3	4
24. It scares me when I blush in front of people.	0	1	2	3	4
25. When I feel a strong pain in my stomach, I worry that it could be cancer.	0	1	2	3	4
26. When I have trouble swallowing, I worry that I could choke.	0	1	2	3	4
27. When I notice my heart skipping a beat, I worry that there is something seriously wrong with me.	0	1	2	3	4
28. It scares me when I feel tingling or pricking sensations in my hands.	0	1	2	3	4
29. When I feel dizzy, I worry there is something wrong with me.	0	1	2	3	4
30. When I begin to sweat in social situations, I fear people will think negatively of me.	0	1	2	3	4
31. When my thoughts seem to speed up, I worry that I might be going crazy.	0	1	2	3	4
32. When my throat feels tight, I worry that I could choke to death.	0	1	2	3	4
33. When my face feels numb, I worry that I might be having a stroke.	0	1	2	3	4
34. When I have trouble thinking clearly, I worry that there is something wrong with me.	0	1	2	3	4
35. I think it would be horrible for me to faint in public.	0	1	2	3	4

	Very Little	A Little	Moderate	Much	Very Much
36. When my mind goes blank, I worry that there is something terribly wrong with me.	0	1	2	3	4

APPENDIX

Anxiety Sensitivity Profile (ASP)

INSTRUCTIONS. It is very important that you read these instructions carefully so that you will be able to answer the questions that follow. The purpose of this questionnaire is to measure your level of **fear of anxiety-related sensations.** There are many anxiety-related sensations, including the following: palpitations (pounding heart or accelerated heart rate), sweating, trembling, shortness of breath, chest pain or discomfort, nausea, dizziness, feelings of unreality, chills, and hot flashes. People differ in their fears of these sensations; some people have little or no fear, others have mild or moderately severe fears, while others have very strong fears.

Anxiety sensations are feared if a person believes that these sensations have bad consequences. For example, people are frightened of palpitations if they believe these sensations could lead to a heart attack. People are frightened of dizziness if they believe that this sensation could mean that they are going crazy. People are frightened of publicly observable anxiety reactions (e.g., blushing or trembling) if they believe these reactions could cause others to ridicule or reject them.

We would like you to do two things for each of the items on the following pages:

1. Imagine that you are experiencing the sensation. Try to imagine this as vividly as possible.
2. Using the scale provided, rate the likelihood that if YOU experienced the sensation, **it would lead to something bad happening to you,** such as dying, going crazy, losing control, or being ridiculed or rejected by others. There are no right or wrong answers, and all responses will remain anonymous. Please note: We are not assessing whether or not you experience these sensations as a result of being anxious. We want to assess whether you believe that anxiety-related sensations would **lead to** something **bad** to happen to **you.**

Practice item:

Imagine that you're experiencing the following sensation. **What is the likelihood that this sensation would LEAD to something BAD happening to YOU?** Circle the number that best indicates your choice:

	Not at all likely	Somewhat likely	Extremely likely
0. Your legs feel unsteady	1 . . . . . 2 . . . . . 3 . . . . . 4 . . . . . 5 . . . . . 6 7

Before you answer the following questions, please place a checkmark here if you fully understand the instructions you have read: _____

If you don't understand the instructions, please ask for clarification.

What is the likelihood that this sensation would LEAD to something BAD happening to YOU?

	Not at all likely	Somewhat likely	Extremely likely
1. Your heart is pounding	1 . . . . . 2 . . . . . 3 . . . . . 4 . . . . . 5 . . . . . 6 7
2. Your thoughts seem slower than usual	1 . . . . . 2 . . . . . 3 . . . . . 4 . . . . . 5 . . . . . 6 7
3. You feel like you can't take a deep breath	1 . . . . . 2 . . . . . 3 . . . . . 4 . . . . . 5 . . . . . 6 7

What is the likelihood that this sensation would LEAD to something BAD happening to YOU?

	Not at all likely	Somewhat likely	Extremely likely

4. Your stomach is making loud noises .... 1 ..... 2 ..... 3 ..... 4 ..... 5 ..... 6 7

5. You have tingling sensations in your hands .... 1 ..... 2 ..... 3 ..... 4 ..... 5 ..... 6 7

6. You have pain in your chest .... 1 ..... 2 ..... 3 ..... 4 ..... 5 ..... 6 7

7. Your thoughts seem jumbled ... 1 ..... 2 ..... 3 ..... 4 ..... 5 ..... 6 7

8. Your heart is beating so loud that you can hear it .... 1 ..... 2 ..... 3 ..... 4 ..... 5 .... 6 7

9. You feel like you're in a fog ... 1 ..... 2 ..... 3 ..... 4 ..... 5 ..... 6 7

10. Hot flushes sweep over you .... 1 ..... 2 ..... 3 ..... 4 ..... 5 ..... 6 7

11. You have diarrhea .... 1 ..... 2 ..... 3 ..... 4 ..... 5 ..... 6 7

12. You are "jumpy" or easily startled .... 1 ..... 2 ..... 3 ..... 4 ..... 5 ..... 6 7

13. You keeping getting distracted by unwanted thoughts .... 1 ..... 2 ..... 3 ..... 4 ..... 5 ..... 6 7

14. Your heart beats rapidly .... 1 ..... 2 ..... 3 ..... 4 ..... 5 ..... 6 7

15. You feel like you're suffocating .... 1 ..... 2 ..... 3 ..... 4 ..... 5 ..... 6 7

16. You have a knot in your stomach .... 1 ..... 2 ..... 3 ..... 4 ..... 5 ..... 6 7

17. You feel numb all over .... 1 ..... 2 ..... 3 ..... 4 ..... 5 ..... 6 7

18. Thoughts seem to race through your mind .... 1 ..... 2 ..... 3 ..... 4 ..... 5 ..... 6 7

19. You feel out of breath even though you haven't been exerting yourself .... 1 ..... 2 ..... 3 ..... 4 ..... 5 ..... 6 7

20. Your heart pounds in your ears .... 1 ..... 2 ..... 3 ..... 4 ..... 5 ..... 6 7

21. You feel like something is stuck in your throat .... 1 ..... 2 ..... 3 ..... 4 ..... 5 ..... 6 7

22. Your body feels strange or different in some way .... 1 ..... 2 ..... 3 ..... 4 ..... 5 ..... 6 7

23. Your face sweats even though you're not hot .... 1 ..... 2 ..... 3 ..... 4 ..... 5 ..... 6 7

24. Your voice quavers (trembles or sounds shaky) .... 1 ..... 2 ..... 3 ..... 4 ..... 5 ..... 6 7

25. You can't keep your mind on a task .... 1 ..... 2 ..... 3 ..... 4 ..... 5 ..... 6 7

What is the likelihood that this sensation would LEAD to something BAD happening to YOU?

	Not at all likely	Somewhat likely	Extremely likely
26. You have difficulty swallowing	1 .... 2 3	.... 4 5	.... 6 7
27. Your stomach aches	1 .... 2 3	.... 4 5	.... 6 7
28. You have burning sensations in your chest (heartburn)	1 .... 2 3	.... 4 5	.... 6 7
29. Familiar surroundings seem strange or unreal to you	1 .... 2 3	.... 4 5	.... 6 7
30. You feel like you're choking	1 .... 2 3	.... 4 5	.... 6 7
31. You feel your heartbeat pulsing in your neck	1 .... 2 3	.... 4 5	.... 6 7
32. You are constipated	1 .... 2 3	.... 4 5	.... 6 7
33. You feel faint or lightheaded	1 .... 2 3	.... 4 5	.... 6 7
34. Your heart starts beating slower	1 .... 2 3	.... 4 5	.... 6 7
35. You shiver even though you're not cold	1 .... 2 3	.... 4 5	.... 6 7
36. You have trouble thinking clearly	1 .... 2 3	.... 4 5	.... 6 7
37. You feel that there's a lump in your throat	1 .... 2 3	.... 4 5	.... 6 7
38. You feel like you're about to vomit	1 .... 2 3	.... 4 5	.... 6 7
39. You're awake but feel like you're in a daze	1 .... 2 3	.... 4 5	.... 6 7
40. Your stomach is upset	1 .... 2 3	.... 4 5	.... 6 7
41. You have trouble remembering things	1 .... 2 3	.... 4 5	.... 6 7
42. Your heart beats erratically	1 .... 2 3	.... 4 5	.... 6 7
43. You have tingling sensations in your lips	1 .... 2 3	.... 4 5	.... 6 7
44. Your mind goes blank	1 .... 2 3	.... 4 5	.... 6 7
45. Your throat feels tight	1 .... 2 3	.... 4 5	.... 6 7
46. You feel "spacey" or spaced out	1 .... 2 3	.... 4 5	.... 6 7
47. You feel like you're not getting enough air	1 .... 2 3	.... 4 5	.... 6 7
48. Your face blushes red	1 .... 2 3	.... 4 5	.... 6 7
49. You feel bloated (gassy)	1 .... 2 3	.... 4 5	.... 6 7

What is the likelihood that this sensation would LEAD to something BAD happening to YOU?

	Not at all likely	Somewhat likely	Extremely likely
50. You feel sick in your stomach (nausea)	1 ..... 2 ..... 3 ..... 4 ..... 5 ..... 6 7		
51. Your heart skips a beat	1 ..... 2 ..... 3 ..... 4 ..... 5 ..... 6 7		
52. Your face feels numb	1 ..... 2 ..... 3 ..... 4 ..... 5 ..... 6 7		
53. The muscles in your face twitch	1 ..... 2 ..... 3 ..... 4 ..... 5 ..... 6 7		
54. You are easily distracted	1 ..... 2 ..... 3 ..... 4 ..... 5 ..... 6 7		
55. Your chest feels tight	1 ..... 2 ..... 3 ..... 4 ..... 5 ..... 6 7		
56. You have difficulty concentrating	1 ..... 2 ..... 3 ..... 4 ..... 5 ..... 6 7		
57. You have to urinate more frequently than usual	1 ..... 2 ..... 3 ..... 4 ..... 5 ..... 6 7		
58. Your hands are trembling	1 ..... 2 ..... 3 ..... 4 ..... 5 ..... 6 7		
59. You feel like you can't breathe properly	1 ..... 2 ..... 3 ..... 4 ..... 5 ..... 6 7		
60. You feel like things are spinning around you (vertigo)	1 ..... 2 ..... 3 ..... 4 ..... 5 ..... 6 7		

Body Sensations Interpretation Questionnaire (BSIQ)

NOTE: The BSIQ is administered in a booklet form. On the following pages, the BSIQ instructions and items are reprinted. However, the instrument is not meant to be completed in this format. For a full description of the BSIQ, see Chapter 9 of this book.

Instructions for Part 1

Here are some outline descriptions of situations in which it is not quite clear what is happening. Read each one, and then answer the question below it very briefly. Write down the first thing that comes into your mind without thinking too long about it. Please write down what you think is happening before you continue. Be as specific as possible.

When you have done that, turn over the page and you will see three possible explanations for the situation. Arrange these in the order in which they would be most likely to come to your mind if you found yourself in a similar situation. So the one that you would consider most likely to be true should come first, and the one that you would consider least likely to be true should come third. Do not think too long before deciding. We want your first impressions, and do not worry if none of them fits with what you actually did think.

Instructions for Part 2

Now that you have answered the preceding questions, we would be grateful if you would answer one more question about each of the ambiguous situations. Please return to the start of the booklet and then rate the extent to which you think each of the three explanations for a situation would likely to be true if you found yourself in that situation.

Use the scale below for your ratings. Put a number between 0 and 8 next to each of the three explanations in the text. Do not worry if your ratings appear to be different from your previous answers, and please do not change any of your original answers.

0 -------1 -------2 -------3 -------4 -------5 -------6 -------7 -------8

| No Fear | Slight Fear | Moderate Fear | Marked Fear | Extreme Fear |

BSIQ Items

1. You notice that your heart is beating quickly and pounding. Why?

   a) Because you have been physically active.
   b) Because there is something wrong with your heart.
   c) Because you are feeling excited.

2. A member of your family is late arriving home. Why?

   a) Because they have had a serious accident on the way home.
   b) They met a friend and are talking with them.
   c) It took longer than usual to get home.

3. You go into a shop and the assistant ignores you. Why?

   a) They are bored with their job, and this makes them rude.
   b) They are concentrating very hard on something else.
   c) They find you irritating and resent your presence.

4. You have developed a small spot on the back of your hand. Why?

   a) You have been eating the wrong things, or have a mild allergy.
   b) You are developing skin cancer.
   c) You have been bitten by an insect.

5. You are talking to an acquaintance who briefly looks out of the window. Why?

   a) Something outside has caught their attention.
   b) They are bored with you.
   c) They are tired and can't concentrate.

6. You feel lightheaded and weak. Why?

   a) You are about to faint.
   b) You need to get something to eat.
   c) You didn't get enough sleep last night.

7. You wake with a start in the middle of the night, thinking you heard a noise, but all is quiet. What woke you up?

   a) You were woken by a dream.
   b) A burglar broke into your house.
   c) A door or window rattled in the wind.

8. Your chest feels uncomfortable and tight. Why?

   a) You have indigestion.
   b) You have a sore muscle.
   c) Something is wrong with your heart.

9. You notice a frowning stranger approaching you in the street. Why?

   a) You have done something wrong and are about to be told.
   b) He's lost and wants directions.
   c) You dropped something and he's returning it.

10. You have a sudden pain in your stomach. Why?

    a) You have appendicitis or an ulcer.
    b) You have indigestion.
    c) You are hungry.

11. A crisis comes up at work and you can't immediately think of what to do. Why?

    a) It's an unusual situation, which you haven't encountered before.
    b) You need a moment to think about a solution.
    c) You are inadequate to deal with the problem.

12. You are introduced to someone at a party who fails to reply to a question you ask. Why?

    a) They did not hear the question.
    b) They think you are uninteresting and boring.
    c) They were preoccupied with something else at the time.

13. You have a pain in the small of your back. Why?

    a) You have pulled a muscle while bending and stretching.
    b) You are sitting awkwardly.
    c) There is something wrong with your spine.

14. You suddenly feel confused and are having difficulty thinking straight. Why?

    a) You are going out of your mind.
    b) You are coming down with a cold.
    c) You've been working too hard and need a rest.

15. You have visitors round for a meal and they leave sooner than you expected. Why?

    a) They did not wish to outstay their welcome.
    b) They had another pressing engagement to go to.
    c) They did not enjoy the visit and were bored with your company.

16. You are under a great deal of pressure and finding it difficult to manage everything you have to do. Why?

    a) You are tired and will be better after a rest.
    b) You re getting to the point where you will just stop coping.
    c) There are just too many things to do in the time available.

17. You find a lump under the skin of your neck. Why?

    a) You have a mild cold virus and your glands are slightly swollen.
    b) The lump is normally there, but you have just noticed it.
    c) You are developing cancer.

18. You notice that some people you know are looking in your direction. Why?

    a) They are criticizing you.
    b) They are being friendly and want you to join them.
    c) They just happen to be looking your way.

19. You feel short of breath. Why?

    a) You are developing flu.
    b) You are about to suffocate or stop breathing.
    c) You are physically "out of shape".

20. A letter marked "URGENT" arrives. What is in the letter?

    a) It is a circular designed to attract your attention.
    b) You forgot to pay a bill.
    c) News that someone you know has died or is seriously ill.

21. A friend suggests that you change the way that you're doing a job in your own house. Why?

    a) They are trying to be helpful.
    b) They think you're incompetent.
    c) They have done the job more often and know an easier way.

22. You notice that your heart is pounding, you feel breathless, dizzy and unreal. Why?

    a) You have been overdoing it and are overtired.
    b) Something you ate disagreed with you.
    c) You are dangerously ill or going mad.

23. You have been eating normally but have recently lost some weight. Why?

    a) You have cancer.
    b) It's a normal fluctuation.
    c) You have been rushing about more than usual.

24. You smell smoke. What's burning?

    a) Your house is on fire.
    b) Some food is burning.
    c) Someone is smoking a cigarette.

25. Your vision has become slightly blurred. Why?

    a) You have strained your eyes slightly.
    b) You need to get glasses or change your existing glasses.
    c) This is the sign of a serious illness.

26. An old acquaintance passes you in the street without acknowledging you. Why?

    a) They recognized you but think you're not worth talking to.
    b) Your appearance has changed since they last saw you and so they did not recognize you.
    c) They had other things on their mind.

27. You doctor tells you your headaches are caused by tension, but he wants you to see a specialist. Why?

    a) He wants to confirm his diagnosis.
    b) He actually thinks you've got a serious illness.
    c) The specialist knows more about how to treat tension headaches.

Body Sensations Questionnaire (BSQ)

Below is a list of specific body sensations that may occur when you are nervous or in a feared situation. Please mark down how afraid you are of these feelings. Use the following five point scale:

1	2	3	4	5
not at all	somewhat	moderately	very	extremely

...... frightened by this sensation.

1. heart palpitations	1	2	3	4	5
2. pressure or a heavy feeling in chest	1	2	3	4	5
3. numbness in arms or legs	1	2	3	4	5
4. tingling in the fingertips	1	2	3	4	5
5. numbness in another part of your body	1	2	3	4	5
6. feeling short of breath	1	2	3	4	5
7. dizziness	1	2	3	4	5
8. blurred or distorted vision	1	2	3	4	5
9. nausea	1	2	3	4	5
10. having "butterflies" in your stomach	1	2	3	4	5
11. feeling a knot in your stomach	1	2	3	4	5
12. having a lump in your throat	1	2	3	4	5
13. wobbly or rubber legs	1	2	3	4	5
14. sweating	1	2	3	4	5
15. a dry throat	1	2	3	4	5
16. feeling disoriented and confused	1	2	3	4	5
17. feeling disconnected from your body: only partly present	1	2	3	4	5
18. other (please describe)	1	2	3	4	5
....	1	2	3	4	5
....	1	2	3	4	5

Body Vigilance Scale (BVS)

Instructions: This measure is designed to index how sensitive you are to internal bodily sensations such as heart palpitations or dizziness. Fill it out according to how you have felt for the **past week**.

1. I am the kind of person who pays close attention to internal bodily sensations.

0	1	2	3	4	5	6	7	8	9	10
Not at all Like Me				Moderately Like Me					Extremely Like Me	

2. I am very sensitive to changes in my internal bodily sensations.

0	1	2	3	4	5	6	7	8	9	10
Not at all Like Me				Moderately Like Me					Extremely Like Me	

3. On average, **how much time** do you spend each day "scanning" your body for sensations (e.g., sweating, heart palpitations, dizziness)?

0	10	20	30	40	50	60	70	80	90	100
No Time				Half of the Time					All of the Time	

4. Rate how much attention you pay to each of the following sensations using this scale:

0	1	2	3	4	5	6	7	8	9	10
None		Slight			Moderate			Substantial		Extreme

1. Heart palpitations   _____
2. Chest pain/discomfort   _____
3. Numbness   _____
4. Tingling   _____
5. Short of breath/smothering _____
6. Faintness   _____
7. Vision changes   _____
8. Feelings of unreality   _____
9. Feeling detached from self _____
10. Dizziness   _____
11. Hot flash   _____
12. Sweating/clammy hands _____
13. Stomach upset   _____
14. Nausea   _____
15. Choking/throat closing _____

Mobility Inventory for Agoraphobia (MI)

1. Please indicate the degree to which you avoid the following places or situations because of discomfort or anxiety. Rate your amount of avoidance when you are with a trusted companion and when you are alone. Do this by using the following scale:

1	2	3	4	5
never avoid	rarely avoid	avoid about half of the time	avoid most of the time	always avoid

Circle the number for each situation or place under both conditions: when accompanied and when alone. Leave blank situations that do not apply to you.

Places	When **accompanied**	When **alone**
Theaters	1 2 3 4 5	1 2 3 4 5
Supermarkets	1 2 3 4 5	1 2 3 4 5
Shopping malls	1 2 3 4 5	1 2 3 4 5
Classrooms	1 2 3 4 5	1 2 3 4 5
Department stores	1 2 3 4 5	1 2 3 4 5
Restaurants	1 2 3 4 5	1 2 3 4 5
Museums	1 2 3 4 5	1 2 3 4 5
Elevators	1 2 3 4 5	1 2 3 4 5
Auditoriums or stadiums	1 2 3 4 5	1 2 3 4 5
Garages	1 2 3 4 5	1 2 3 4 5
High places	1 2 3 4 5	1 2 3 4 5
Please tell how high	_____	_____
Enclosed places	1 2 3 4 5	1 2 3 4 5

Open spaces	When **accompanied**	When **alone**
Outside (for example: fields, wide streets, courtyards)	1 2 3 4 5	1 2 3 4 5
Inside (for example: large rooms, lobbies)	1 2 3 4 5	1 2 3 4 5

Riding	When **accompanied**	When **alone**
Buses	1 2 3 4 5	1 2 3 4 5
Trains	1 2 3 4 5	1 2 3 4 5
Subways	1 2 3 4 5	1 2 3 4 5
Airplanes	1 2 3 4 5	1 2 3 4 5
Boats	1 2 3 4 5	1 2 3 4 5

Driving or riding in car	When **accompanied**	When **alone**
A. at anytime	1 2 3 4 5	1 2 3 4 5
B. on expressways	1 2 3 4 5	1 2 3 4 5

Situations	When **accompanied**					When **alone**				
Standing in lines	1	2	3	4	5	1	2	3	4	5
Crossing bridges	1	2	3	4	5	1	2	3	4	5
Parties or social gatherings	1	2	3	4	5	1	2	3	4	5
Walking on the street	1	2	3	4	5	1	2	3	4	5
Staying at home alone						1	2	3	4	5
Being far away from home	1	2	3	4	5	1	2	3	4	5
Other (specify):										
	1	2	3	4	5	1	2	3	4	5

2. After completing the first step, circle the five items with which you are most concerned. Of the items listed, these are the five situations or places where avoidance/anxiety most affects your life in a negative way.

Panic Attacks

3. We define a panic attack as:

   A high level of anxiety accompanied by …

   1. strong body reactions (heart palpitations, sweating, muscle tremors, dizziness, nausea) with …
   2. the temporary loss of the ability to plan, think, or reason and …
   3. the intense desire to escape or flee the situation. (Note: This is different from high anxiety or fear alone).

Please indicate the total number of panic attacks you have had in the last 7 days:

In the last 3 weeks:

How severe or intense have the panic attacks been? (Place an X on the line below):

very mild	mild	moderately severe	very severe	extremely severe
1	2	3	4	5

Safety Zone

4. Many people are able to travel alone freely in an area (usually around their home) called their safety zone. Do you have such a zone? If yes, please describe:

a. its location:

b. its size (e.g., radius from home):

Panic and Agoraphobia Scale (PAS)–Patient Questionnaire

This questionnaire is designed for people suffering from panic attacks and agoraphobia.
Rate the severity of your symptoms in the **past week**.

Panic attacks are defined as the sudden outburst of anxiety, accompanied by some of the following symptoms:

- ◯ palpitating or pounding heart, or accelerated heart rate
- ◯ sweating
- ◯ trembling or shaking
- ◯ dry mouth
- ◯ difficulty in breathing
- ◯ feeling of choking
- ◯ chest pain or discomfort
- ◯ nausea or abdominal distress (e.g. churning in stomach)
- ◯ feeling dizzy, unsteady, faint, or light headed
- ◯ feelings that objects are unreal (like in a dream), or that the self is distant or "not really here
- ◯ fear of losing control, "going crazy," or passing out
- ◯ fear of dying
- ◯ hot flushes or cold chills
- ◯ numbness or tingling sensations

Panic attacks develop suddenly and increase in intensity within about ten minutes.

A.1. How frequently did you have panic attacks?

- ☐ 0 no panic attack in the past week
- ☐ 1 1 panic attack in the past week
- ☐ 2 2 or 3 panic attacks in the past week
- ☐ 3 4–6 panic attacks in the past week
- ☐ 4 more than 6 panic attacks in the past week

A.2. How severe were the panic attacks in the past week?

- ☐ 0 no panic attacks
- ☐ 1 attacks were usually mild
- ☐ 2 attacks were usually moderate
- ☐ 3 attacks were usually severe
- ☐ 4 attacks were usually extremely severe

A.3. How long did the panic attacks usually last?

- ☐ 0 no panic attacks
- ☐ 1 1 to 10 minutes
- ☐ 2 over 10 to 60 minutes
- ☐ 3 over 1 to 2 hours
- ☐ 4 over 2 hours and more

U. *Were most of the attacks expected (occurring in feared situations) or unexpected (spontaneous)?*

- ☐ 9   no panic attacks
- ☐ 0   mostly unexpected
- ☐ 1   more unexpected than expected
- ☐ 2   some unexpected, some expected
- ☐ 3   more expected than unexpected
- ☐ 4   mostly expected

B.1. In the past week, did you avoid certain situations because you feared having a panic attack or a feeling of discomfort?

- ☐ 0   no avoidance (or: my attacks don't occur in certain situations)
- ☐ 1   infrequent avoidance of feared situations
- ☐ 2   occasional avoidance of feared situations
- ☐ 3   frequent avoidance of feared situations
- ☐ 4   very frequent avoidance of feared situations

B.2. Please tick the situations you avoided or in which you developed panic attacks or a feeling of discomfort when you are not accompanied:

- ☐ 1   Aeroplanes
- ☐ 2   Subways (underground)
- ☐ 3   Buses, trains
- ☐ 4   Ships
- ☐ 5   Theatres, cinemas
- ☐ 6   Supermarkets
- ☐ 7   Standing in queues (lines)
- ☐ 8   Auditoriums, stadiums
- ☐ 9   Parties or social gatherings
- ☐ 10   Crowds
- ☐ 11   Restaurants
- ☐ 12   Museums
- ☐ 13   Lifts
- ☐ 14   Enclosed spaces (e.g. tunnels)
- ☐ 15   Classrooms, lecture theatres

- ☐ 16   Driving or riding in a car (e.g., in a traffic jam)
- ☐ 17   Large rooms (lobbies)
- ☐ 18   Walking on the street
- ☐ 19   Fields, wide streets, courtyards_
- ☐ 20   High places
- ☐ 21   Crossing bridges
- ☐ 22   Traveling away from home
- ☐ 23   Staying at home alone

other situations:

- ☐ 24   _____
- ☐ 25   _____
- ☐ 26   _____

B.3. How important were the avoided situations?

- ☐ 0   unimportant (or no agoraphobia)
- ☐ 1   not very important
- ☐ 2   moderately important
- ☐ 3   very important
- ☐ 4   extremely important

C.1. In the past week, did you suffer from the fear of having a panic attack (anticipatory anxiety or "fear of being afraid")?

☐ 0   no anticipatory anxiety
☐ 1   infrequent fear of having a panic attack
☐ 2   sometimes fear of having a panic attack
☐ 3   frequent fear of having a panic attack
☐ 4   fear of having a panic attack all the time

C.2. How strong was this "fear of fear?"

☐ 0   no
☐ 1   mild
☐ 2   moderate
☐ 3   marked
☐ 4   extreme

D.1. In the past week, did your panic attacks or agoraphobia lead to restrictions (impairment) in your family relationships (partnership, children, etc.)?

☐ 0   no impairment
☐ 1   mild impairment
☐ 2   moderate impairment
☐ 3   marked impairment
☐ 4   extreme impairment

D.2. In the past week, did your panic attacks or agoraphobia lead to restrictions (impairment) in your social life and leisure activities (e.g., weren't you able to go to a cinema or to parties)?

☐ 0   no impairment
☐ 1   mild impairment
☐ 2   moderate impairment
☐ 3   marked impairment
☐ 4   extreme impairment

D.3. In the past week, did your panic attacks or agoraphobia lead to restrictions (impairment) in your work (or household) responsibilities?

☐ 0   no impairment
☐ 1   mild impairment
☐ 2   moderate impairment
☐ 3   marked impairment
☐ 4   extreme impairment

E.1. In the past week, did you worry about suffering harm from your anxiety symptoms (e.g., having a heart attack, or collapsing and being injured)?

☐ 0   not true
☐ 1   hardly true
☐ 2   partly true
☐ 3   mostly true
☐ 4   definitely true

E.2. Did you sometimes think that your doctor was wrong, when he told you that your symptoms like pounding heart, dizziness, tingling sensations, shortness of breath have a psychological cause? Did you believe that, in reality, a somatic (physical, bodily) cause lies behind these symptoms that hasn't been found yet?

☐ 0   not at all true (rather psychic disease)
☐ 1   hardly true
☐ 2   partly true
☐ 3   mostly true
☐ 4   definitely true (rather organic disease)

Panic Disorder Severity Scale (PDSS)

TIME PERIOD OF RATING   (Circle one):   one month
                                              other (specify) _____

General Instructions for Raters

The goal is to obtain a measure of overall severity of DSM IV symptoms of panic disorder, with or without agoraphobia. Ratings are generally made for the past month, to allow for a stable estimation of panic frequency and severity. Users may choose a different time frame, but time frame should be consistent for all items.

Each item is rated from 0–4, where 0 = none or not present; 1 = mild, occasional symptoms, slight interference; 2 = moderate, frequent symptoms, some interference with functioning, but still manageable; 3 = severe, preoccupying symptoms, substantial interference in functioning, and 4 = extreme, pervasive near constant symptoms, disabling/incapacitating.

A suggested script is provided as a guide to questioning, but is not essential. Probes should be used freely to clarify ratings. As an overall caution, please note that this is not an observer administered self-rating scale. The patient is not asked to rate a symptom as "mild, moderate or severe". Rather the symptom is explored and rated by the interviewer. However, to clarify a boundary between two severity levels, it is appropriate to utilize the descriptors above. For example, the interviewer might ask the patient whether it is more accurate to describe a given symptom as occurring "frequently, with definite interference but still manageable", or if it is "preoccupying, with substantial interference". Similarly, it may be appropriate to ask whether a symptom is "preoccupying, with substantial interference", or "pervasive, near constant, and incapacitating".

In rating items 6 and 7, the interviewer should be alert to inconsistencies. For example, sometimes a subject will describe a symptom from items 1–5 as causing substantial impairment in functioning, but then will report that overall panic disorder symptoms cause only mild or moderate work and social impairment. This should be pointed out and clarified.

There are some types of anxiety, common in panic disorder patients, but not rated by this instrument. Anticipatory anxiety about situations feared for reasons other than panic (e.g. related to a specific phobia or social phobia) is not considered panic-related anticipatory anxiety and is not rated by this instrument. Similarly, generalized anxiety is not rated by this instrument. The concerns of someone experiencing generalized anxiety are focused on the probability of adverse events in the future. Such worries often include serious health problems in oneself or a loved one, financial ruin, job loss, or other possible calamitous outcomes of daily life problems.

1. PANIC ATTACK FREQUENCY, INCLUDING LIMITED SYMPTOM EPISODES

Begin by explaining to the patient that we define a *Panic Attack* as a feeling of fear or apprehension that begins suddenly and builds rapidly in intensity, usually reaching a peak in less than 10 minutes. This feeling is associated with uncomfortable physical sensations like racing or pounding heart, shortness of breath, choking, dizziness, sweating, trembling. Often there are distressing, catastrophic thoughts such as fear of losing control, having a heart attack or dying. A full panic episode has at least four such symptoms. A *Limited Symptom Episode (LSE)* is similar to a full panic attack, but has fewer than 4 symptoms. Given these definitions, please tell me

Q: In the past month, how many full panic attacks did you experience, the kind with 4 or more symptoms? How about limited symptom episodes, the kind with less than 4 symptoms? On average, did you have more than one limited symptom episodes/day? *(Calculate weekly frequencies by dividing the total number of full panic attacks over the rating interval by the number of weeks in the rating interval.)*

0 = No panic or limited symptom episodes

1 = Mild, less than an average of one full panic a week, and no more than 1 limited symptom episode/day

2 = Moderate, one or two full panic attacks a week, and/or multiple limited symptom episodes/day

3 = Severe, more than 2 full attacks/week, but not more than 1/day on average

4 = Extreme, full panic attacks occur more than once a day, more days than not

2. DISTRESS DURING PANIC ATTACKS, INCLUDE LIMITED SYMPTOM EPISODES

Q: Over the past month, when you had panic or limited symptom attacks, how much distress did they cause you? I am asking you now about the distress you felt during the attack itself.

(This item rates the average degree of distress and discomfort the patient experienced during panic attacks experienced over the rating interval. Limited symptom episodes should be rated only if they caused more distress than full panic. Be sure to distinguish between distress DURING panic and anticipatory fear that an attack will occur.)

Possible further probes: How upset or fearful did you feel during the attacks? Were you able to continue doing what you were doing when panic occurred? Did you lose your concentration? If you had to stop what you were doing, were you able to stay in the situation where the attack occurred or did you have to leave?

0 = No panic attacks or limited symptoms episodes, or no distress during episodes

1 = Mild distress but able to continue activity with little or no interference

2 = Moderate distress, but still manageable, able to continue activity and/or maintain concentration, but does so with difficulty

3 = Severe, marked distress and interference, loses concentration and/or must stop activity, but able to remain in the room or situation

4 = Extreme, severe and disabling distress, must stop activity, will leave the room or situation if possible, otherwise remains, unable to concentrate, with extreme distress

3. SEVERITY OF ANTICIPATORY ANXIETY (panic-related fear, apprehension or worry)

Q: Over the past month, on average, how much did you worry, feel fearful or apprehensive about when your next panic would occur or about what panic attacks might mean about your physical or mental health? I am asking about times when you were not actually having a panic attack.

(Anticipatory anxiety can be related to the meaning of the attacks rather than to having an attack, so there can be considerable anxiety about having an attack even if the distress during the attacks was low. Remember that sometimes a patient does not worry about when the next attack will occur, but instead worries about the meaning of the attacks for his or her physical or mental health.)

Possible further probes: How intense was your anxiety? How often did you have these worries or fears? Did the anxiety get to the point where it interfered with your life? IF SO, How much did it interfere?

0 = No concern about panic

1 = Mild, there is occasional fear, worry or apprehension about panic

2 = Moderate, often worried, fearful or apprehensive, but has periods without anxiety. There is a noticeable modification of lifestyle, but anxiety is still manageable and overall functioning is not impaired

3 = Severe, preoccupied with fear, worry or apprehension about panic, substantial interference with concentration and/or ability to function effectively

4 = Extreme, near constant and disabling anxiety, unable to carry out important tasks because of fear, worry or apprehension about panic

4. AGORAPHOBIC FEAR/AVOIDANCE

Q: Over the past month, were there places where you felt afraid, or that you avoided, because you thought if you had a panic attack, it could be difficult to get help or to easily leave?

Possible further probes: Situations like using public transportation, driving in a car, being in a tunnel or on a bridge, going to the movies, to a mall or supermarket, or being in other crowded places? anywhere else? Were you afraid of being at home alone or completely alone in other places? How often did you experience fear of these situations? How intense was the fear? Did you avoid any of these situations? Did having a trusted companion with you make a difference? Were there things you would do with a companion that you would not do alone? How much did the fear and/or avoidance affect your life? Did you need to change your lifestyle to accommodate your fears?

0 = None, no fear or avoidance

1 = Mild, occasional fear and/or avoidance, but will usually confront or endure the situation. There is little or no modification of lifestyle

2 = Moderate, noticeable fear and/or avoidance, but still manageable, avoids feared situations but can confront with a companion. There is some modification of lifestyle, but overall functioning is not impaired

3 = Severe, extensive avoidance; substantial modification of lifestyle is required to accommodate phobia, making it difficult to manage usual activities

4 = Extreme pervasive disabling fear and/or avoidance. Extensive modification in lifestyle is required such that important tasks are not performed

5. PANIC-RELATED SENSATION FEAR/ AVOIDANCE

Q: Sometimes people with panic disorder experience physical sensations that may be reminiscent of panic and cause them to feel frightened or uncomfortable. Over the past month, did you avoid doing anything because you thought you it might cause this kind of uncomfortable physical sensations?

Possible further probes: For example, things that made your heart beat rapidly, such as strenuous exercise or walking? playing sports? working in the garden? What about exciting sports events, frightening movies or having an argument? Sexual activity or orgasm? Did you fear or avoid sensations on your skin such as heat or tingling? Sensations of feeling dizzy or out of breath? Did you avoid any food, drink or other substance because it might bring on physical sensations, such as coffee or alcohol or medications like cold medication? How much did the avoidance of situations or activities like these affect your life? Did you need to change your lifestyle to accommodate your fears?

0 = No fear or avoidance of situations or activities that provoke distressing physical sensations

1 = Mild, occasional fear and/or avoidance, but usually will confront or endure with little distress activities and situations which provoke physical sensations. There is little modification of lifestyle

2 = Moderate, noticeable avoidance, but still manageable; there is definite, but limited modification of lifestyle, such that overall functioning not impaired

3 = Severe, extensive avoidance, causes substantial modification of lifestyle or interference in functioning

4 = Extreme pervasive and disabling avoidance. Extensive modification in lifestyle is required such that important tasks or activities are not performed

6. IMPAIRMENT/INTERFERENCE IN WORK FUNCTIONING DUE TO PANIC DISORDER

(Note to raters: This item focuses on work. If the person is not working, ask about school, and if not in school full time, ask about household responsibilities.)

Q: Over the past month, considering all the symptoms, the panic attacks, limited symptom episodes, anticipatory anxiety and phobic symptoms, how much did your panic disorder interfere with your ability to do your job, (or your schoolwork, or carry out responsibilities at home?)

Possible further probes: Did the symptoms affect the quality of your work? Were you able to get things done as quickly and effectively as usual? Did you notice things you were not doing because of your anxiety, or things you couldn't do as well? Did you take short cuts or request assistance to get things done? Did anyone else notice a change in your performance? Was there a formal performance review or warning about work performance? Any comments from co-workers or from family members about your work?

0 = No impairment from panic disorder symptoms

1 = Mild, slight interference, feels job is harder to do but performance is still good

2 = Moderate, symptoms cause regular, definite interference but still manageable. Job performance has suffered but others would say work is still adequate

3 = Severe, causes substantial impairment in occupational performance, such that others have noticed, may be missing work or unable to perform at all on some days

4 = Extreme, incapacitating symptoms, unable to work (or go to school or carry out household responsibilities)

7. IMPAIRMENT/INTERFERENCE IN SOCIAL FUNCTIONING DUE TO PANIC DISORDER

Q: Over the past month, considering all the panic disorder symptoms together, how much did they interfere with your social life?

Possible further probes: Did you spend less time with family or other relatives than you used to? Did you spend less time with friends? Did you turn down opportunities to socialize because of panic disorder? Did you have restrictions about where or how long you would socialize because of panic disorder? Did the panic disorder symptoms affect your relationships with family members or friends?

0 = No impairment

1 = Mild, slight interference, feels quality of social behavior is somewhat impaired but social functioning is still adequate

2 = Moderate, definite, interference with social life but still manageable. There is some decrease in frequency of social activities and/or quality of interpersonal interactions but still able to engage in most usual social activities

3 = Severe, causes substantial impairment in social performance. There is marked decrease in social activities, and/or marked difficulty interacting with others; can still force self to interact with others, but does not enjoy or function well in most social or interpersonal situations

4 = Extreme, disabling symptoms, rarely goes out or interacts with others, may have ended a relationship because of panic disorder

TOTAL SCORE (sum of items 1–7): _____

Phobic Avoidance Rating Scale (PARS)

The rating is based on a semi-structured clinical interview. The purpose is to evaluate degree of anxiety-motivated avoidance of each of 13 situations under otherwise usual motivational conditions. When variations within a situation make a difference, e.g., "I am able to go to parties with people I know well, but not to parties with strangers," the interviewer should choose the variant that the subject seems to fear the most. The interviewer should consider whether the subject diminishes or exaggerates his/her avoidance. The more biases are suspected, the more the interviewer has to ask for concrete details with respect to avoidance.

Avoidance is rated by the examiner according to the following criteria:

0—No avoidance;
1—Does not avoid the situation, but has avoidant tendencies within it;
2—Sometimes avoid and sometimes not, depending on how one feels at that specific time;
3—Avoids the situation regularly, but is able to expose oneself to it in the presence of safeguarding conditions;
4—Avoids the situation regularly, safeguarding conditions make no difference.

Firstly, the subject is asked to specify degree of avoidance when safeguarding conditions are not present. Examples of safeguarding conditions should be given (intake of drugs before exposure, bringing drugs with him/her, being assured that a hospital is within reach, having an appointment with a trusted person after exposure, etc.). If the subject apparently does not avoid the situation, he/she is asked whether he/she has avoidant tendencies within the situation (to decide between scale step 0 and 1). Examples of avoidant tendencies should be given (hurrying through the situation, sitting near the exit at the cinema, etc.). If the subject apparently avoids the situation regularly, he/she is asked whether he/she nevertheless is able to enter the situation when safeguarding conditions are present (to decide between scale step 3 and 4). Examples of such conditions may be repeated.

Item List

_____ 1. Walk away from home alone.
_____ 2. Walking on the street alone.
_____ 3. Walking across open spaces alone.
_____ 4. Traveling by bus or train alone.
_____ 5. Going to a theatre, cinema unaccompanied.
_____ 6. Shopping, standing in lines unaccompanied.
_____ 7. Going to meetings.
_____ 8. Going to parties.
_____ 9. Receiving guests at home.
_____10. Riding lifts.
_____11. Being in high places.
_____12. Walking over bridges.
_____13. Being in enclosed spaces.

Texas Safety Maneuver Scale (TSMS)

INSTRUCTIONS: Listed below are behaviors that people sometimes use to manage or avoid panic or anxiety. Read each item carefully and rate how often you use each behavior to manage panic or anxiety. For example, if you use a car phone for business but *never* use it to manage or avoid panic or anxiety, place a ✓ in the first column "YES, BUT NOT TO MANAGE ANXIETY". However, if you *usually* use your car phone to manage or avoid panic or anxiety, place a ✓ in the column labeled "USUALLY TO MANAGE ANXIETY OR PANIC".

		YES, BUT NOT to manage anxiety or panic	NEVER to manage anxiety or panic	RARELY to manage anxiety or panic	SOMETIMES to manage anxiety or panic	USUALLY to manage anxiety or panic	ALWAYS to manage anxiety or panic
1	Carrying food in car or on your person						
2	Carrying water in car or on your person						
3	Carrying alcohol or medication in car or on your person						
4	Carrying vital telephone nos in car or on your person						
5	Having a phone or CB radio in your car						
6	Relying on a companion for travel						
7	Relying on a companion for shopping						
8	Relying on a companion for attending social gatherings						
9	Relying on a companion to eat in restaurants						
10	Listening to music						
11	Reading						

		YES, BUT NOT to manage anxiety or panic	NEVER to manage anxiety or panic	RARELY to manage anxiety or panic	SOMETIMES to manage anxiety or panic	USUALLY to manage anxiety or panic	ALWAYS to manage anxiety or panic
12	Watching television						
13	Using mental distractions (e.g., using thoughts or images)						
14	Staying busy						
15	Conversing with others						
16	Using relaxation, meditation, yoga, or breathing techniques						
17	Checking the presence/location of phones						
18	Checking the presence/location of bathrooms						
19	Checking the presence/location of exits						
20	Checking the presence/location of hospitals or clinics						
21	Checking pulse, breathing, blood pressure						
22	Avoiding stressful encounters						
23	Avoiding anger-provoking situations						
24	Avoiding emotionally-arousing events (e.g., concerts, sporting events)						
25	Avoiding emotionally-arousing films						
26	Avoiding stress at work or school						

	YES, BUT NOT to manage anxiety or panic	NEVER to manage anxiety or panic	RARELY to manage anxiety or panic	SOMETIMES to manage anxiety or panic	USUALLY to manage anxiety or panic	ALWAYS to manage anxiety or panic
27	Avoiding saunas, Jacuzzis or hot showers					
28	Avoiding drinks containing caffeine					
29	Avoiding vigorous exercise					
30	Avoiding tight-fitting clothes					
31	Avoiding specific foods or getting too full					
32	Avoiding merry-go-rounds or other amusement park rides that might make you dizzy					
33	Avoiding alcohol					
34	Avoiding marijuana or other drugs					
35	Avoiding crowded stores					
36	Avoiding driving on busy freeways					
37	Avoiding using public transportation (e.g. buses, trains or planes)					
38	Avoiding parties or other social activities					
39	Avoiding long lines (e.g. bank, post-office)					
40	Avoiding sit-down meals at formal restaurants					

APPENDIX

		YES, BUT NOT to manage anxiety or panic	NEVER to manage anxiety or panic	RARELY to manage anxiety or panic	SOMETIMES to manage anxiety or panic	USUALLY to manage anxiety or panic	ALWAYS to manage anxiety or panic
41	Avoiding staying home alone						
42	Avoiding being far from home						
43	Having to sit close to an exit						
44	Taking one's own car to avoid traveling with another person						
45	Having to drive in the right-hand lane on the freeway						
46	Thinking of excuses that you can use to leave a social situation early						
47	Using muscle relaxation exercises						
48	Using meditation or yoga						
49	Deep breathing exercises						
50	Listening to stress/anxiety reduction tapes						
51	Other (list):						
52	Other (list):						
53	Other (list):						
54	Other (list):						

Measures for Specific Phobia

Acrophobia Questionnaire (AQ)–Part 1: Anxiety Scale

Below we have compiled a list of situations involving height. We are interested to know how anxious (tense, uncomfortable) you would feel in each situation <u>nowadays</u>. Please indicate how you would feel by putting one of the following numbers (0, 1, $\overline{2, 3, 4, 5}$, or 6) in the space to the left of each item:

0 Not at all anxious; calm and relaxed
1
2 Slightly anxious
3
4 Moderately anxious
5
6 Extremely anxious

_____ 1. Diving off the low board at a swimming pool.
_____ 2. Stepping over rocks crossing a stream.
_____ 3. Looking down a circular stairway form several flights up.
_____ 4. Standing on a ladder leaning against a house, second story.
_____ 5. Sitting in the front of a second balcony of a theater.
_____ 6. Riding a Ferris wheel.
_____ 7. Walking up a steep incline in country hiking.
_____ 8. Airplane trip (to San Francisco).
_____ 9. Standing next to an open window on the third floor.
_____ 10. Walking on a footbridge over a highway.
_____ 11. Driving over a large bridge (Golden Gate, George Washington).
_____ 12. Being away from window in an office on the 15th floor of a building.
_____ 13. Seeing window washers ten flights up on a scaffold.
_____ 14. Walking over a sidewalk grating.
_____ 15. Standing on the edge of a subway platform.
_____ 16. Climbing up a fire escape to the 3rd floor landing.
_____ 17. On the roof of a ten story apartment building.
_____ 18. Riding an elevator to the 50th floor.
_____ 19. Standing on a chair to get something off a shelf.
_____ 20. Walking up the gangplank of an ocean liner.

Acrophobia Questionnaire (AQ)—Part 2: Avoidance Scale

Now that you have rated each item according to anxiety, we would like you to rate them as to avoidance. Indicate in the space to the left of the items below how much you would <u>now</u> avoid the situation, if it arose.

0 Would not avoid doing it
1 Would try to avoid doing it
2 Would not do it under any circumstances

_____ 1. Diving off the low board at a swimming pool.

_____ 2. Stepping over rocks crossing a stream.

_____ 3. Looking down a circular stairway form several flights up.

_____ 4. Standing on a ladder leaning against a house, second story.

_____ 5. Sitting in the front of a second balcony of a theater.

_____ 6. Riding a Ferris wheel.

_____ 7. Walking up a steep incline in country hiking.

_____ 8. Airplane trip (to San Francisco).

_____ 9. Standing next to an open window on the third floor.

_____ 10. Walking on a footbridge over a highway.

_____ 11. Driving over a large bridge (Golden Gate, George Washington).

_____ 12. Being away from window in an office on the 15th floor of a building.

_____ 13. Seeing window washers ten flights up on a scaffold.

_____ 14. Walking over a sidewalk grating.

_____ 15. Standing on the edge of a subway platform.

_____ 16. Climbing up a fire escape to the 3rd floor landing.

_____ 17. On the roof of a ten story apartment building.

_____ 18. Riding an elevator to the 50th floor.

_____ 19. Standing on a chair to get something off a shelf.

_____ 20. Walking up the gangplank of an ocean liner.

Blood–Injection Symptom Scale (BISS)

These questions ask about sensations that you may experience in situations involving blood or injections. For each sensation, circle 'yes' if you noticed the sensation during one of your worst experiences involving blood or injections and circle 'no' if you did not notice the sensation during one of your worst experiences involving blood or injections.

1. Did you have tightness, pain or discomfort in your chest?	No	Yes
2. Were you anxious?	No	Yes
3. Did you have blurred vision?	No	Yes
4. Did you have cold or clammy hands?	No	Yes
5. Were you dizzy or lightheaded?	No	Yes
6. Did you feel faint?	No	Yes
7. Were you fatigued?	No	Yes
8. Did you faint?	No	Yes
9. Did you feel unreal?	No	Yes
10. Did your heart pound?	No	Yes
11. Were you particularly irritable?	No	Yes
12. Did you feel nauseous?	No	Yes
13. Did the room spin?	No	Yes
14. Did you sweat?	No	Yes
15. Did your muscles feel tense, sore, or ache?	No	Yes
16. Did you tremble?	No	Yes
17. Did you have trouble walking?	No	Yes

Claustrophobia General Cognitions Questionnaire (CGCQ)

Listed below are some thoughts that people might have when they are in a claustrophobic situation(s). What are situations in which you would feel claustrophobic? Please list some:

If you were to enter these situations, how likely would you be to have each of the thoughts below? Rate the likelihood of having each thought by using the following scale:

____ 1 _____ 2 _____ 3 _____ 4 _____ 5 ____
Not likely   **Somewhat likely**   **Very likely**

Likelihood Rating

1. I might not be able to leave. _____
2. I might lose control. _____
3. I might scream. _____
4. I might die. _____
5. I might suffocate. _____
6. I might not be able to escape if I had to. _____
7. I might run out of air. _____
8. I might get dizzy. _____
9. I might be paralyzed by fear. _____
10. I might not be able to get enough air. _____
11. I might start to choke. _____
12. I might lose control of my senses. _____
13. I might panic. _____
14. Something might be hiding in there. _____
15. I won't be able to see what's in there. _____
16. I might pass out. _____
17. People will think I'm crazy. _____
18. I might not be able to move. _____
19. I might be trapped. _____
20. People will wonder what's wrong with me. _____
21. I might act foolishly. _____
22. People will think I'm strange. _____
23. I might have difficulty breathing. _____
24. I might not be able to get out. _____
25. I might hurt myself. _____
26. I might go crazy. _____

What other thoughts might you have when in that situation(s)?

Claustrophobia Questionnaire (CLQ)

How <u>anxious</u> would you feel in the following places or situations? *Circle* the most appropriate number:

0 = Not at all anxious   3 = Very anxious
1 = Slightly anxious   4 = Extremely anxious
2 = Moderately anxious

SS

1. Swimming while wearing a nose plug   0   1   2   3   4

2. Working under a sink for 15 minutes   0   1   2   3   4

3. Standing in an elevator on the ground floor with the doors closed   0   1   2   3   4

4. Trying to catch your breath during vigorous exercise   0   1   2   3   4

5. Having a bad cold and finding it difficult to breathe through your nose   0   1   2   3   4

6. Snorkeling in a safe practice tank for 15 minutes   0   1   2   3   4

7. Using an oxygen mask   0   1   2   3   4

8. Lying on a bottom bunk bed   0   1   2   3   4

9. Standing in the middle of the 3rd row at a packed concert realizing that you will be unable to leave until the end   0   1   2   3   4

10. In the center of a full row at a cinema   0   1   2   3   4

11. Working under a car for 15 minutes   0   1   2   3   4

12. At the furthest point from an exit on a tour of an underground mine shaft   0   1   2   3   4

13. Lying in a sauna for 15 minutes   0   1   2   3   4

14. Waiting for 15 minutes in a plane on the ground with the door closed   0   1   2   3   4

RS

1. Locked in a small DARK room without windows for 15 minutes   0   1   2   3   4

2. Locked in a small WELL LIT room without windows for 15 minutes   0   1   2   3   4

3. Handcuffed for 15 minutes   0   1   2   3   4

4. Tied up with hands behind back for 15 minutes   0   1   2   3   4

5. Caught in tight clothing and unable to remove it   0   1   2   3   4

6. Standing for 15 minutes in a straitjacket   0   1   2   3   4

7. Lying in a tight sleeping bag enclosing legs and arms, tied at the neck, unable to get out for 15 minutes   0   1   2   3   4

8. Head first into a zipped up sleeping bag, able to leave whenever you wish   0   1   2   3   4

9. Lying in the trunk of a car with air flowing through freely for 15 minutes   0   1   2   3   4

10. Having your legs tied to an immovable chair   0   1   2   3   4

11.	In a public washroom and the lock jams	0	1	2	3	4
12.	In a crowded train which stops between stations	0	1	2	3	4

Claustrophobia Situations Questionnaire (CSQ)

Please indicate the degree to which you would feel **anxious** in and **avoid** being in the situations below. Use the following scale:

1 = not anxious/never avoid
2 = slightly anxious/rarely avoid
3 = moderately anxious/avoid about half the time
4 = very anxious/avoid most of the time
5 = extremely anxious/always avoid

	Anxiety Rating	Avoidance Rating
1. Being in a cave.	____	____
2. Being held down by several people.	____	____
3. Trying on clothes in a small fitting room with the door closed.	____	____
4. Being in a closet.	____	____
5. Being in a tunnel.	____	____
6. Being in handcuffs.	____	____
7. Being in a crowd where you cannot move.	____	____
8. Being covered in sand up to your neck.	____	____
9. Being in the middle of a crowded church.	____	____
10. Being in a dark, windowless chamber with the door closed.	____	____
11. Being in a crowded restaurant.	____	____
12. Being under a car.	____	____
13. Being in the middle of a crowded bar.	____	____
14. Being in the middle of a crowded subway.	____	____
15. Being on a crowded train.	____	____
16. Being in the middle section at a crowded concert.	____	____
17. Being in a small, locked room.	____	____
18. Being in a crowded bus that stops at a traffic light.	____	____
19. Being in a well-lit, windowless room with the door closed.	____	____
20. Wearing a tight jacket.	____	____
21. Being in a body cast.	____	____
22. Being in a small, windowless attic.	____	____
23. Being in a small, tight shower with the curtain closed.	____	____
24. Being in a small, underground cellar.	____	____
25. Lying in bed under covers.	____	____
26. Being on a crowded elevator.	____	____
27. Being in a windowless bathroom with the lock jammed.	____	____

	Anxiety Rating	Avoidance Rating
28. Being on a small elevator alone.	——	——
29. Being in a tunnel with cars on both sides.	——	——
30. Being in a crowded shopping mall.	——	——
31. Being in the middle of a line at a supermarket.	——	——
32. Going through a narrow passage.	——	——
33. Being in the back of a crowded bus.	——	——
34. Being in a barber's/hairdresser's chair.	——	——
35. Being in a dentist's chair.	——	——
36. Sitting by the window in the middle of an airplane.	——	——
37. Trying on clothes with a tight neck.	——	——
38. Being in a neck brace.	——	——
39. Putting you head underwater.	——	——
40. Being in a dark, windowless room with the door closed.	——	——
41. Being in a small, compact car alone.	——	——
42. Being in the back of a small two-door car with a person on either side of you.	——	——

What other situations would you feel anxious in?

_____

_____

Dental Anxiety Inventory (DAI)

INSTRUCTIONS

This questionnaire consists of 36 statements about going to the dentist. Each statement represents a reaction to a particular situation. Read through all the statements carefully.

For each statement, you are asked to indicate to what extent it applies to you personally. It is possible that you may not have been in the given situation before. In that case, try to imagine the situation as clearly as you can and indicate what your reaction would be.

Please circle the number that belongs to the statement which matches your feelings best. For example, consider the item: "I would like the dentist to explain the treatment to me."

If you think the above statement applies to you, (in other words, if you agree that the dentist should explain the treatment to you before he actually does anything), then you would circle the number 4 ("quite true"). If you would like to change your answer, for example if you would like it very much if the dentist explained the treatment to you, then please cross out the wrong number (in this example number 4) and circle the correct answer, which here would be the number 5 ("completely true").

Although some statements may be similar, they are not the same. Please answer all the questions as best as you can, even if you find it difficult to choose. Please do not skip any questions either. Also, try to answer quickly: your first response is the most important.

1	2	3	4	5
totally untrue	hardly true	partly true	quite true	completely true

1. I become nervous when the dentist invites me to sit down in the chair.   1 2 3 4 5

2. I need to go to the toilet more often when I sit in the waiting room thinking that the dentist will say my teeth look bad.   1 2 3 4 5

3. When I'm on my way to the dentist and thinking about the anaesthetic, I would rather go back.   1 2 3 4 5

4. I sleep badly when I think about having to make an appointment with the dentist.   1 2 3 4 5

5. When I lie back in the dentist's chair I think about never coming back again.   1 2 3 4 5

6. When I know the dentist is going to extract a tooth I am already afraid in the waiting room.   1 2 3 4 5

7. When I think of the sound of the drilling machine on my way to the dentist, I would rather go back.   1 2 3 4 5

8. I already feel uncomfortable at home when I think that the dentist will make a remark about my teeth.   1 2 3 4 5

9. When the dentist is about to give me an anaesthetic I cling onto the arms of the chair.   1 2 3 4 5

10. I become afraid in the waiting room when I hear sounds coming from the dentist's surgery.   1 2 3 4 5

11. On my way to the dentist, I sweat or freeze at the thought that the dentist will say I brush my teeth badly.   1 2 3 4 5

1	2	3	4	5
totally untrue	hardly true	partly true	quite true	completely true

12. When I think of the moment when the dentist blows air into a cavity, I would like to cancel the appointment.   1 2 3 4 5

13. When the dentist looks into my mouth, my breathing becomes faster.   1 2 3 4 5

14. I want to walk out of the waiting room the moment I think the dentist will not explain what s/he is going to do in my mouth.   1 2 3 4 5

15. On my way to the dentist, I feel nervous when I know my teeth will be scaled.   1 2 3 4 5

16. I like to postpone making an appointment with the dentist as long as I can.   1 2 3 4 5

17. I feel uncertain when discussing the treatment of my teeth with the dentist.   1 2 3 4 5

18. When I am in the waiting room knowing the dentist is going to scale my teeth, I am unable to concentrate on a magazine.   1 2 3 4 5

19. When I am on my way to the dentist and think of the smell of the practice I feel uncomfortable.   1 2 3 4 5

20. Before going to the dentist, I get palpitations when I think of how the dentist will be displeased at my teeth.   1 2 3 4 5

21. As soon as the dentist gets his/her needle ready for the anaesthetic, I shut my eyes tight.   1 2 3 4 5

22. In the waiting room, I sweat or freeze when I think of sitting down in the dentist's chair.   1 2 3 4 5

23. When I am on my way to the dentist and think that s/he will say my teeth look bad, then I want to go home again.   1 2 3 4 5

24. I already feel nervous at home when I know the dentist is going to give me an anaesthetic.   1 2 3 4 5

25. When the dentist's chair reclines backwards, I tell myself that the treatment will not take long.   1 2 3 4 5

26. In the waiting room, I feel nervous at the thought that the dentist will say my teeth are badly brushed.   1 2 3 4 5

27. On my way to the dentist, I get anxious at the thought that s/he will have to drill.   1 2 3 4 5

28. I already feel uncertain at home thinking of the moment when the dentist will look into my mouth.   1 2 3 4 5

29. When I am sitting in the dentist's chair not knowing what is going on in my mouth, I break in a cold sweat.   1 2 3 4 5

30. When I am sitting in the waiting room and thinking about the check-up, I would prefer to go home.   1 2 3 4 5

31. When I am on my way to the dentist and I imagine his/her instruments, my hands become clammy.   1 2 3 4 5

1	2	3	4	5
totally untrue	hardly true	partly true	quite true	completely true

32. I think about cancelling the appointment if I suspect the dentist will be displeased at my teeth.   1   2   3   4   5

33. I become nervous when the dentist is about to start checking my teeth.   1   2   3   4   5

34. When I'm waiting for the dentist's assistant to call me in, I try to think of something else.   1   2   3   4   5

35. On my way to the dentist, the idea of being in the chair already makes me nervous.   1   2   3   4   5

36. I sleep badly the night before I have to have a tooth extracted.   1   2   3   4   5

Dental Cognitions Questionnaire (DCQ)

This questionnaire refers to your thoughts about dental treatment

Part 1—Instructions:

Below you will find a number of thoughts people may have <u>about dentistry in general or about oneself as a person</u>. Would you please indicate for each of these thoughts:

1. <u>the degree to which you believe that this statement (thought) is true.</u> In other words: "How true does it feel to you now?" Indicate a percentage between 0 ("I don't believe this at all"; "I believe this for 0%") and 100 ("I am absolutely convinced that this is true"; "I believe this for 100%"). You may use any percentage between 0% and 100%.

2. <u>whether or not this thought comes up</u> when you know that you will soon have to undergo dental treatment (tick: 'Yes' or 'No').

I believe this thought for _____ %	When knowing that I will soon have to undergo dental treatment, I think		
_____% Dentists do as they please	☐ Yes	☐ No	1
_____% Dentists are often impatient	☐ Yes	☐ No	2
_____% The dentist does not care if it hurts	☐ Yes	☐ No	3
_____% Dentists do not understand you	☐ Yes	☐ No	4
_____% Dentist are often incapable	☐ Yes	☐ No	5
_____% Dentists think you act childish	☐ Yes	☐ No	6
_____% Treatments often fail	☐ Yes	☐ No	7
_____% My teeth can't be saved	☐ Yes	☐ No	8
_____% I should be ashamed about my teeth	☐ Yes	☐ No	9
_____% My teeth might break	☐ Yes	☐ No	10
_____% I can't stand pain	☐ Yes	☐ No	11
_____% I am a tense person	☐ Yes	☐ No	12
_____% I am a difficult patient	☐ Yes	☐ No	13
_____% I am someone with very long roots	☐ Yes	☐ No	14

Part 2—Instructions:

Below you will find again a number of examples of thoughts. This time, these are thoughts people may have <u>during dental treatment</u>. Would you please indicate for each example:

1. <u>the degree to which you believe that this statement (thought) is true.</u> In other words: "How true does it feel to you now?" Indicate a percentage between 0 ("I don't believe this at all"; "I believe this for 0%") and 100 ("I am absolutely convinced that this is true"; "I believe this for 100%"). You may use any percentage between 0% and 100%.

2. <u>whether or not this thought comes up</u> during a dental treatment (tick: 'Yes' or 'No').

I believe this thought for ____ %	While being treated I think ......

____% Everything goes wrong	☐ Yes ☐ No	15
____% This treatment will hurt	☐ Yes ☐ No	16
____% My teeth will break	☐ Yes ☐ No	17
____% Something surely will go wrong	☐ Yes ☐ No	18
____% It never runs smoothly	☐ Yes ☐ No	19
____% I am helpless	☐ Yes ☐ No	20
____% I can't control myself	☐ Yes ☐ No	21
____% I can't escape, I'm locked in	☐ Yes ☐ No	22
____% Anesthetics often do not work	☐ Yes ☐ No	23
____% The sound of the drill frightens me	☐ Yes ☐ No	24
____% The dentist will drill my tongue, gums or cheek	☐ Yes ☐ No	25
____% The nerve will be touched	☐ Yes ☐ No	26
____% I have no control over what happens	☐ Yes ☐ No	27
____% I will die during treatment	☐ Yes ☐ No	28
____% I will panic during treatment	☐ Yes ☐ No	29
____% I will faint during treatment	☐ Yes ☐ No	30
____% I will suffocate during treatment	☐ Yes ☐ No	31
____% I can't stand this treatment for long	☐ Yes ☐ No	32
____% I will certainly have pain afterwards	☐ Yes ☐ No	33
____% This filling will certainly fall out and has to be made again	☐ Yes ☐ No	34
____% This treatment fails	☐ Yes ☐ No	35
____% I become sick	☐ Yes ☐ No	36
____% The dentist will lose control over his drill	☐ Yes ☐ No	37
____% The dentist believes that I am a difficult patient and act childish	☐ Yes ☐ No	38

Dental Fear Survey (DFS)

The items in this questionnaire refer to various situations, feelings, and reactions related to dental work. Please rate your feeling or reaction on these items by circling the number (1, 2, 3, 4, or 5) or the category which most closely corresponds to your reaction.

1. Has fear of dental work ever caused you to put off making an appointment?

1	2	3	4	5
never	once or twice	a few times	often	nearly every time

2. Has fear of dental work ever caused you to cancel or not appear for an appointment?

1	2	3	4	5
never	once or twice	a few times	often	nearly every time

When having dental work done:

3. My muscles become tense ...

1	2	3	4	5
never	once or twice	a few times	often	nearly every time

4. My breathing rate increases ...

1	2	3	4	5
never	once or twice	a few times	often	nearly every time

5. I perspire ...

1	2	3	4	5
never	once or twice	a few times	often	nearly every time

6. I feel nauseated and sick to my stomach ...

1	2	3	4	5
never	once or twice	a few times	often	nearly every time

7. My heart beats faster ...

1	2	3	4	5
never	once or twice	a few times	often	nearly every time

Part 2: Following is a list of things and situations that many people mention as being somewhat anxiety or fear producing. Please rate how much fear, anxiety or unpleasantness each of them causes you. Use the numbers 1–5, from the following scale (1 = no fear; 5 = extreme fear). Make a check in the appropriate space. (If it helps, try to imagine yourself in each of these situations and describe what your common reaction is.)

	1	2	3	4	5
8. Making an appointment for dentistry ...	___	___	___	___	___
9. Approaching the dentist's office ...	___	___	___	___	___
10. Sitting in the waiting room ...	___	___	___	___	___

	1	2	3	4	5
11. Being seated in the dental chair ...	——	——	——	——	——
12. The smell of the dentist's office ...	——	——	——	——	——
13. Seeing the dentist walk in ...	——	——	——	——	——
14. Seeing the anesthetic needle ...	——	——	——	——	——
15. Feeling the needle injected ...	——	——	——	——	——
16. Seeing the drill ...	——	——	——	——	——
17. Hearing the drill ...	——	——	——	——	——
18. Feeling the vibrations of the drill ...	——	——	——	——	——
19. Having your teeth cleaned ...	——	——	——	——	——
20. All things considered, how fearful are you of having dental work done?	——	——	——	——	——

Fear of Spiders Questionnaire (FSQ)

For each item, please record a number to indicate how much you agree with the statement. Ratings can include any number between 0 (totally disagree) and 7 (totally agree).

Totally Disagree   Totally Agree

0 ——— 1 ——— 2 ——— 3 ——— 4 ——— 5 ——— 6 ——— 7

_____ 1. If I came across a spider now, I would get help from someone else to remove it

_____ 2. Currently, I am sometimes on the look out for spiders.

_____ 3. If I saw a spider now, I would think it will harm me.

_____ 4. I now think a lot about spiders.

_____ 5. I would be somewhat afraid to enter a room now, where I have seen a spider before.

_____ 6. I now would do anything to try to avoid a spider.

_____ 7. Currently, I sometimes think about getting bit by a spider.

_____ 8. If I encountered a spider now, I wouldn't be able to deal effectively with it.

_____ 9. If I encountered a spider now, it would take a long time to get it out of my mind.

_____ 10. If I came across a spider now, I would leave the room.

_____ 11. If I saw a spider now, I would think it will try to jump on me.

_____ 12. If I saw a spider now, I would ask someone else to kill it.

_____ 13. If I encountered a spider now, I would have images of it trying to get me.

_____ 14. If I saw a spider now, I would be afraid of it.

_____ 15. If I saw a spider now, I would feel very panicky.

_____ 16. Spiders are one of my worst fears.

_____ 17. I would feel very nervous if I saw a spider now.

_____ 18. If I saw a spider now, I would probably break out in a sweat and my heart would beat faster.

Fear Survey Schedule II (FSS-II)

Below are 51 different stimuli that can cause fear in people. Please rate how much fear you feel using the following rating scale and record your answer in the space provided.

0 = None   3 = Some fear   6 = Terror
1 = Very little fear   4 = Much fear
2 = A little fear   5 = Very much fear

_____ 1. Sharp objects

_____ 2. Being a passenger in a car

_____ 3. Dead bodies

_____ 4. Suffocating

_____ 5. Failing a test

_____ 6. Looking foolish

_____ 7. Being a passenger in an airplane

_____ 8. Worms

_____ 9. Arguing with parents

_____ 10. Rats and mice

_____ 11. Life after death

_____ 12. Hypodermic needles

_____ 13. Being criticized

_____ 14. Meeting someone for the first time

_____ 15. Roller coasters

_____ 16. Being alone

_____ 17. Making mistakes

_____ 18. Being misunderstood

_____ 19. Death

_____ 20. Being in a fight

_____ 21. Crowded places

_____ 22. Blood

_____ 23. Heights

_____ 24. Being a leader

_____ 25. Swimming alone

_____ 26. Illness

_____ 27. Being with drunks

_____ 28. Illness or injury to loved ones

_____ 29. Being self-conscious

_____ 30. Driving a car

_____ 31. Meeting authority

_____ 32. Mental illness

_____ 33. Closed places

_____ 34. Boating

_____ 35. Spiders

_____ 36. Thunderstorms

_____ 37. Not being a success

_____ 38. God

_____ 39. Snakes

_____ 40. Cemeteries

_____ 41. Speaking before a group

_____ 42. Seeing a fight

_____ 43. Death of a loved one

_____ 44. Dark places

_____ 45.]Strange dogs

_____ 46. Deep water

_____ 47. Being with a member of the opposite sex

_____ 48. Stinging insects

_____ 49. Untimely or early death

_____ 50. Losing a job

_____ 51. Automobile accident

Medical Fear Survey (MFS)

The following situations are known to cause some people to experience fear and apprehension. Please rate for each situation listed, how much **fear** or **tension** you would experience if you were exposed to that situation at this time.

Use the following scale to evaluate each situation and place a mark (X) in the space corresponding to how much **fear** or **tension** you would experience in the listed situation.

0 = no fear or concern at all   **3** = intense fear
1 = mild fear   **4** = terror
2 = considerable fear

HOW MUCH FEAR OR DISCOMFORT WOULD YOU EXPERIENCE FROM:

	0	1	2	3	4
1. handling a hypodermic needle	___	___	___	___	___
2. cutting with a hunting knife	___	___	___	___	___
3. operating a power saw	___	___	___	___	___
4. seeing a nurse for an illness	___	___	___	___	___
5. seeing a small vial of your own blood	___	___	___	___	___
6. receiving an anesthetic injection in the mouth	___	___	___	___	___
7. observing someone chop with an ax	___	___	___	___	___
8. feeling like you will faint	___	___	___	___	___
9. seeing a small test tube of animal blood	___	___	___	___	___
10. seeing a large beaker of animal blood	___	___	___	___	___
11. seeing a preserved brain in a jar	___	___	___	___	___
12. seeing a bleeding wound to a person's arm	___	___	___	___	___
13. feeling pains in your chest	___	___	___	___	___
14. observing a surgical amputation	___	___	___	___	___
15. observing someone cut with a butcher knife	___	___	___	___	___
16. receiving a hypodermic injection in the arm	___	___	___	___	___
17. having a severe headache	___	___	___	___	___
18. seeing a mutilated body on TV	___	___	___	___	___
19. seeing a small bottle of human blood on TV	___	___	___	___	___
20. having blood drawn from your arm	___	___	___	___	___
21. observing someone operate a power saw	___	___	___	___	___
22. feeling dizzy	___	___	___	___	___
23. seeing a photo of a large blood vein	___	___	___	___	___
24. observing someone getting their finger stitched	___	___	___	___	___
25. seeing a large bottle of your own blood	___	___	___	___	___
26. handling a butcher knife	___	___	___	___	___

	0	1	2	3	4
27. having a blood sample drawn from your finger tip	——	——	——	——	——
28. going to a doctor for an illness	——	——	——	——	——
29. observing someone operate a meat cutter	——	——	——	——	——
30. seeing a dead person, unknown to you	——	——	——	——	——
31. seeing blood being drawn from someone's arm	——	——	——	——	——
32. handling an open pocket knife	——	——	——	——	——
33. observing blood pulse through a vein	——	——	——	——	——
34. seeing someone receiving an injection in the arm	——	——	——	——	——
35. seeing a large bottle of human blood on TV	——	——	——	——	——
36. seeing a bleeding wound to a person's eye	——	——	——	——	——
37. feeling your heart race for no obvious reason	——	——	——	——	——
38. seeing the mutilated body of a dog that had been run over by a car	——	——	——	——	——
39. receiving a diagnosis from a doctor	——	——	——	——	——
40. seeing a large bottle of human blood	——	——	——	——	——
41. observing an open heart surgery operation	——	——	——	——	——
42. chopping wood with an ax	——	——	——	——	——
43. feeling odd tingling in your arm	——	——	——	——	——
44. operating a meat slicer	——	——	——	——	——
45. seeing someone receiving an injection in the mouth	——	——	——	——	——
46. seeing photos of wounded soldiers from war	——	——	——	——	——
47. seeing someone handling a hypodermic needle	——	——	——	——	——
48. feeling nauseated	——	——	——	——	——
49. seeing a small vial of human blood	——	——	——	——	——
50. seeing the remains of bodies following an airline crash	——	——	——	——	——

Mutilation Questionnaire (MQ)

Answer each of the following statements either True or False as you feel they generally apply to you. If the statement is true most of the time or mostly true for you, you should answer **true**. If it is mostly false or false most of the time, mark it **false**. Indicate your answer by placing a mark (**X**) in the appropriate column.

TRUE   FALSE

_____ _____ 1. I could not remove the hook from a fish that was caught.

_____ _____ 2. I would feel some revulsion looking at a preserved brain in a bottle.

_____ _____ 3. If a badly injured person appears on TV, I turn my head away.

_____ _____ 4. I dislike looking at pictures of accidents or injuries in magazines.

_____ _____ 5. I do not mind visiting a hospital and seeing ill or injured persons.

_____ _____ 6. Medical odors make me tense and uncomfortable.

_____ _____ 7. I would not go hunting because I could not stand the sight of a dead animal.

_____ _____ 8. Watching a butcher at work would make me anxious.

_____ _____ 9. A career as a doctor or nurse is very attractive to me.

_____ _____ 10. I would feel faint if I saw someone with a wound in the eye.

_____ _____ 11. Watching people use sharp power tools makes me nervous.

_____ _____ 12. The prospect of getting an injection or seeing someone else get one bothers me quite a bit.

_____ _____ 13. I feel sick at the sight of blood.

_____ _____ 14. I enjoy reading articles about modern medical techniques.

_____ _____ 15. Injuries, accidents, blood, etc. bother me more than anything else.

_____ _____ 16. Under no circumstance would I accept an invitation to watch a surgical operation.

_____ _____ 17. When I see an accident I feel tense.

_____ _____ 18. It would not bother me to see a bad cut as long as it had been cleaned and stitched.

_____ _____ 19. Using very sharp knives makes me nervous.

_____ _____ 20. Not only do cuts and wounds upset me, but the sight of people with amputated limbs, large scars, or plastic surgery also bothers me.

_____ _____ 21. If instruments were available, it would be interesting to see the action of the internal organs in a living body.

_____ _____ 22. I am frightened at the idea of someone drawing a blood sample from me.

_____ _____ 23. I don't believe anyone could help a person with a bloody wound without feeling at least a little upset.

_____ _____ 24. I am terrified by the idea of having surgery.

_____ _____ 25. I am frightened by the thought that I might some day have to help a person badly hurt in a car wreck.

TRUE	FALSE	
_____	_____	26. I shudder to think of accidentally cutting myself.
_____	_____	27. The sight of dried blood is repulsive.
_____	_____	28. Blood and gore upset me no more than the average person.
_____	_____	29. The sight of an open wound nauseates me.
_____	_____	30. I could never swab out a wound.

© 1974 Rafael Klorman, James E. Hastings, Theodore C. Weerts, Barbara G. Melamed, & Peter J. Lang. The authors acknowledge support from NIMH Grant MH10993 (P.J. Lang, Principal Investigator). Reprinted with permission.

Snake Questionnaire (SNAQ)

Answer each of the following statements either True or False as you feel they generally apply to you. If the statement is true most of the time or mostly true for you, you should answer **true**. If it is mostly false or false most of the time, mark it **false**. Indicate your answer by placing a mark (**X**) in the appropriate column.

TRUE   FALSE

1. I avoid going to parks or on camping trips because there may be snakes about.
2. I would feel some anxiety holding a toy snake in my hand.
3. If a picture of a snake appears on the screen during a motion picture, I turn my head away.
4. I dislike looking at pictures of snakes in a magazine.
5. Although it may not be so, I think of snakes as slimy.
6. I enjoy watching snakes at the zoo.
7. I am terrified by the thought of touching a harmless snake.
8. If someone says that there are snakes anywhere about, I become alert and on edge.
9. I would not go swimming at the beach if snakes had ever been reported in the area.
10. I would feel uncomfortable wearing a snakeskin belt.
11. When I see a snake, I feel tense and restless.
12. I enjoy reading articles about snakes and other reptiles.
13. I feel sick when I see a snake.
14. Snakes are sometimes useful.
15. I shudder when I think of snakes.
16. I don't mind being near a non-poisonous snake if there is someone there in whom I have confidence.
17. Some snakes are very attractive to look at.
18. I don't believe anyone could hold a snake without some fear.
19. The way snakes move is repulsive.
20. It wouldn't bother me to touch a dead snake with a long stick.
21. If I came upon a snake in the woods I would probably run.
22. I'm more afraid of snakes than any other animal.
23. I would not want to travel "down south" or in tropical countries because of the greater prevalence of snakes.
24. I wouldn't take a course like biology if I thought I might have to dissect a snake.
25. I have no fear of non-poisonous snakes.
26. Not only am I afraid of snakes, but worms and most reptiles make me feel anxious.
27. Snakes are very graceful animals.

TRUE   FALSE

_____ _____ 28. I think that I'm no more afraid of snakes than the average person.

_____ _____ 29. I would prefer not to finish a story if something about snakes was introduced into the plot.

_____ _____ 30. Even if I was late for a very important appointment, the thought of snakes would stop me from taking a shortcut through an open field.

© 1974 Rafael Klorman, James E. Hastings, Theodore C. Weerts, Barbara G. Melamed, & Peter J. Lang. The authors acknowledge support from NIMH Grant MH10993 (P.J. Lang, Principal Investigator). Reprinted with permission.

Spider Phobia Beliefs Questionnaire (SBQ)

This questionnaire is concerned with thoughts that might run through your mind at the moment that you encounter a spider. The questionnaire presents many thoughts which people might have when there is a spider in their vicinity. Fill in after each thought the degree that you believe in it (that is, the extent that you believe at that moment that it might happen). Do not indicate the strength of your belief at this moment, but the strength of your belief in the thought at the moment that you encounter a spider and you are possibly anxious. Rate the strength of your belief of each thought by writing down a number between 0 and 100 [0 = I do not believe it at all (0%); 100 = I absolutely believe it (100%)]. You can express your belief in percentages. Thus, you can write down any number from 0 to 100 as long as it expresses the strength of your belief in the thought right at the moment you encounter a spider.

When there is a spider in my vicinity, I believe that the spider …

_____ 1. will come towards me.

_____ 2. will jump onto me.

_____ 3. will crawl into my clothes.

_____ 4. will bite me.

_____ 5. will attack me.

_____ 6. will crawl towards my private parts.

_____ 7. senses that I'm anxious.

_____ 8. knows that I'm anxious and that I cannot stand it.

_____ 9. does things on purpose to tease me.

_____ 10. is mean.

_____ 11. is poisonous.

_____ 12. is deadly.

_____ 13. is dangerous.

_____ 14. is horrible.

_____ 15. is dirty.

_____ 16. is unpredictable.

_____ 17. is vicious.

_____ 18. is incalculable.

_____ 19. is very quick.

_____ 20. is uncontrollable.

_____ 21. runs in an elusive way.

_____ 22. usually travels in pairs.

_____ 23. will become larger.

_____ 24. hides itself.

_____ 25. runs very fast.

_____ 26. will chase me.

_____ 27. is staring at me.

_____ 28. will settle in spots I do not want, like my bed.

_____ 29. will pop up unexpectedly.

_____ 30. will control me.

_____ 31. will walk all over me during the night.

_____ 32. will hide itself and pop up unexpectedly 10 times as big, or with other spiders.

_____ 33. will drive me to the wall.

_____ 34. cannot be shaken off once it is on me.

_____ 35. especially selects me because of my fear.

_____ 36. hides itself in order to pop up unexpectedly.

_____ 37. wants to come upon me on parts of me I cannot reach.

_____ 38. becomes (in my imagination) very large and holds me with its legs.

_____ 39. will settle on my face.

_____ 40. is never alone, there are always more of them.

_____ 41. will drop from the ceiling on me.

_____ 42. is spying on me.

Part 2: The following section presents thoughts that you might have about yourself at the moment that you encounter a spider and are possibly anxious.

If the spider does not go away and crawls on me, I will …

_____ 43. become crazy because of anxiety.

_____ 44. not be able to stand it.

_____ 45. panic completely and not know what I'm doing.

_____ 46. die of fear.

_____ 47. lose control.

_____ 48. have to be transported to a hospital or psychiatric ward.

_____ 49. become so anxious that other people will think I'm an idiot.

_____ 50. endanger myself or others.

_____ 51. lash out fiercely.

_____ 52. become sick with anxiety.

_____ 53. jump out of a window or out of a moving car.

_____ 54. get a heart attack.

_____ 55. scream or yell uncontrollably.

_____ 56. get creepy dreams.

_____ 57. think of myself as a hysterical or as an idiot.

_____ 58. become even more anxious about spiders.

_____ 59. faint.

_____ 60. come to see spiders everywhere.

_____ 61. cause an accident.

_____ 62. damage my heart.

_____ 63. vomit.

_____ 64. be unable to function normally anymore.

_____ 65. beat up someone.

_____ 66. dare nothing anymore and be overwhelmed with fear.

_____ 67. cry uncontrollably.

_____ 68. become paralyzed.

_____ 69. be unable to sleep for days.

_____ 70. become aggressive (beat, kick, throw).

_____ 71. become hysterical.

_____ 72. stiffen completely from anxiety.

_____ 73. be unable to get the animal out of my mind.

_____ 74. want to be dead.

_____ 75. run away blindly.

_____ 76. be unable to think rationally.

_____ 77. get nightmares of creepy spiders.

_____ 78. be unable to do anything.

DID YOU FILL IN ALL THE QUESTIONS ?

Spider Questionnaire (SPQ)

Answer each of the following statements either True or False as you feel they generally apply to you. If the statement is true most of the time or mostly true for you, you should answer **true**. If it is mostly false or false most of the time, mark it **false**. Indicate your answer by placing a mark (**X**) in the appropriate column.

TRUE   FALSE

_____   _____   1. I avoid going to parks or on camping trips because there may be spiders about.

_____   _____   2. I would feel some anxiety holding a toy spider in my hand.

_____   _____   3. If a picture of spider crawling on a person appears on the screen during a motion picture, I turn my head away.

_____   _____   4. I dislike looking at pictures of spiders in a magazine.

_____   _____   5. If there is a spider on the ceiling over my bed, I cannot go to sleep unless someone kills it for me.

_____   _____   6. I enjoy watching spiders build webs.

_____   _____   7. I am terrified by the thought of touching a harmless spider.

_____   _____   8. If someone says that there are spiders anywhere about, I become alert and on edge.

_____   _____   9. I would not go down to the basement to get something if I thought there might be spiders down there.

_____   _____   10. I would feel uncomfortable if a spider crawled out of my shoe as I took it out of the closet to put it on.

_____   _____   11. When I see a spider, I feel tense and restless.

_____   _____   12. I enjoy reading articles about spiders.

_____   _____   13. I feel sick when I see a spider.

_____   _____   14. Spiders are sometimes useful.

_____   _____   15. I shudder when I think of spiders.

_____   _____   16. I don't mind being near a harmless spider if there is someone there in whom I have confidence.

_____   _____   17. Some spiders are very attractive to look at.

_____   _____   18. I don't believe anyone could hold a spider without some fear.

_____   _____   19. The way spiders move is repulsive.

_____   _____   20. It wouldn't bother me to touch a dead spider with a long stick.

_____   _____   21. If I came upon a spider while cleaning the attic I would probably run.

_____   _____   22. I'm more afraid of spiders than any other animal.

_____   _____   23. I would not want to travel to Mexico or Central America because of the greater prevalence of tarantulas.

_____   _____   24. I am cautious when buying fruit because bananas may attract spiders.

_____   _____   25. I have no fear of non-poisonous spiders.

TRUE   FALSE

_____ _____   26. I wouldn't take a course in biology if I thought I might have to handle live spiders.

_____ _____   27. Spider webs are very artistic.

_____ _____   28. I think that I'm no more afraid of spiders than the average person.

_____ _____   29. I would prefer not to finish a story if something about spiders was introduced into the plot.

_____ _____   30. Even if I was late for a very important appointment, the thought of spiders would stop me from taking a shortcut through an underpass.

_____ _____   31. Not only am I afraid of spiders, but millipedes and caterpillars make me feel anxious.

© 1974 Rafael Klorman, James E. Hastings, Theodore C. Weerts, Barbara G. Melamed, & Peter J. Lang. The authors acknowledge support from NIMH Grant MH10993 (P.J. Lang, Principal Investigator). Reprinted with permission.

Measures for
Social Phobia

Brief Social Phobia Scale (BSPS)

Instructions: The time period will cover the previous week, unless otherwise specified (e.g., at the initial evaluation interview, when it could be the previous month).

Part I. (Fear/Avoidance)

How much do you fear and avoid the following situations? Please give separate ratings for fear and avoidance.

	Fear Rating	Avoidance Rating
	0 = None	0 = Never
	1 = Mild	1 = Rare
	2 = Moderate	2 = Sometimes
	3 = Severe	3 = Frequent
	4 = Extreme	4 = Always
	Fear (F)	Avoidance (A)
1. Speaking in public or in front of others	_____	_____
2. Talking to people in authority	_____	_____
3. Talking to strangers	_____	_____
4. Being embarrassed or humiliated	_____	_____
5. Being criticized	_____	_____
6. Social gathering	_____	_____
7. Doing something while being watched (this does not include speaking)	_____	_____

Part II. Physiologic (P)

When you are in a situation that involves contact with other people, or when you are thinking about such a situation, do you experience the following symptoms?

	0 = None
	1 = Mild
	2 = Moderate
	3 = Severe
	4 = Extreme
8. Blushing	_____
9. Palpitations	_____
10. Trembling	_____
11. Sweating	_____

Total scores: F = _____   A = _____   P = _____   Total = _____

Fear of Negative Evaluation Scale (FNE)

For the following statements, please answer each in terms of whether it is true or false for you. Circle T for true or F for false.

T F 1. I rarely worry about seeming foolish to others.

T F 2. I worry about what people will think of me even when I know it doesn't make any difference.

T F 3. I become tense and jittery if I know someone is sizing me up.

T F 4. I am unconcerned even if I know people are forming an unfavorable impression of me.

T F 5. I feel very upset when I commit some social error.

T F 6. The opinions that important people have of me cause me little concern.

T F 7. I am often afraid that I may look ridiculous or make a fool of myself.

T F 8. I react very little when other people disapprove of me.

T F 9. I am frequently afraid of other people noticing my shortcomings.

T F 10. The disapproval of others would have little effect on me.

T F 11. If someone is evaluating me I tend to expect the worst.

T F 12. I rarely worry about what kind of impression I am making on someone.

T F 13. I am afraid that others will not approve of me.

T F 14. I am afraid that people will find fault with me.

T F 15. Other people's opinions of me do not bother me.

T F 16. I am not necessarily upset if I do not please someone.

T F 17. When I am talking to someone, I worry about what they may be thinking about me.

T F 18. I feel that you can't help making social errors sometimes, so why worry about it.

T F 19. I am usually worried about what kind of impression I make.

T F 20. I worry a lot about what my superiors think of me.

T F 21. If I know someone is judging me, it has little effect on me.

T F 22. I worry that others will think I am not worthwhile.

T F 23. I worry very little about what others may think of me.

T F 24. Sometimes I think I am too concerned with what other people think of me.

T F 25. I often worry that I will say or do the wrong things.

T F 26. I am often indifferent to the opinions others have of me.

T F 27. I am usually confident that others will have a favorable impression of me.

T F 28. I often worry that people who are important to me won't think very much of me.

T F 29. I brood about the opinions my friends have about me.

T F 30. I become tense and jittery if I know I am being judged by my superiors.

Liebowitz Social Anxiety Scale (LSAS)

INSTRUCTIONS

The clinician should rate each item with 0 (none), 1 (mild), 2 (moderate) or 3 (severe) based upon the patient's actual experience of the past week. Each item should be given only one score for Fear and one score for Avoidance. If the patient did not enter the feared situation in the past week, rate the item according to what would have been the patient's level of fear if the feared situation was encountered and would the patient have avoided it.

	Fear or Anxiety 0 = None 1 = Mild 2 = Moderate 3 = Severe	Avoidance 0 = Never (0%) 1 = Occasionally (1–33%) 2 = Often (33–67%) 3 = Usually (67–100%)
1. Telephoning in public (P)		
2. Participating in small groups (P)		
3. Eating in public places (P)		
4. Drinking with others in public places (P)		
5. Talking to people in authority (S)		
6. Acting, performing or giving a talk in front of audience (P)		
7. Going to a party (S)		
8. Working while being observed (P)		
9. Writing while being observed (P)		
10. Calling someone you don't know very well (S)		
11. Talking with people you don't know very well (S)		
12. Meeting strangers (S)		
13. Urinating in a public bathroom (P)		
14. Entering a room when others are already seated (P)		
15. Being the centre of attention (S)		
16. Speaking up at a meeting (P)		
17. Taking a test (P)		
18. Expressing a disagreement or disapproval to people you don't know very well (S)		

APPENDIX

	Fear or Anxiety	Avoidance
	0 = None 1 = Mild 2 = Moderate 3 = Severe	0 = Never (0%) 1 = Occasionally (1–33%) 2 = Often (33–67%) 3 = Usually (67–100%)
19. Looking at people you don't know very well in the eyes (S)		
20. Giving a report to a group (P)		
21. Trying to pick up someone (P)		
22. Returning goods to a store (S)		
23. Giving a party (S)		
24. Resisting a high pressure salesperson (S)		

Performance (P) Anxiety   (Add all (P) scores):   _____   Avoidance (Ps) _____
    Subscore:

Social (S) Anxiety   (Add all (S) scores):   _____   Avoidance (Ss) _____
    Subscore:

Total Anxiety (P + S): _____   Total Avoidance (P + S) _____

From Liebowitz, M.R. (1987). Social phobia. *Modern Problems in Pharmacopsychiatry, 22*, 141–173. Published by S. Karger AG, Basel, Switzerland. Reprinted with permission from S. Karger AG and Michael R. Liebowitz, M.D.

Self-Statements during Public Speaking Scale (SSPS)

Please imagine what you have typically felt and thought to yourself during any kind of public speaking situations. Imagining these situations, how much do you agree with the statements given below. Please rate the degree of your agreement on a scale between 0 (if you do not agree at all) to 5 (if you agree extremely with the statement).

1. What do I have to lose it's worth a try ------------------------------ 0 1 2 3 4 5
2. I'm a loser -- 0 1 2 3 4 5
3. This is an awkward situation but I can handle it -------------------- 0 1 2 3 4 5
4. A failure in this situation would be more proof of my incapacity 0 1 2 3 4 5
5. Even if things don't go well, it's no catastrophe -------------------- 0 1 2 3 4 5
6. I can handle everything --- 0 1 2 3 4 5
7. What I say will probably sound stupid ------------------------------ 0 1 2 3 4 5
8. I'll probably "bomb out" anyway ----------------------------------- 0 1 2 3 4 5
9. Instead of worrying I could concentrate on what I want to say -- 0 1 2 3 4 5
10. I feel awkward and dumb; they're bound to notice ----------------- 0 1 2 3 4 5

Social Avoidance and Distress Scale (SADS)

For the following statements, please answer each in terms of whether it is true or false for you. Circle T for true or F for false.

T F   1. I feel relaxed even in unfamiliar social situations.

T F   2. I try to avoid situations which force me to be very sociable.

T F   3. It is easy for me to relax when I am with strangers.

T F   4. I have no particular desire to avoid people.

T F   5. I often find social occasions upsetting.

T F   6. I usually feel calm and comfortable at social occasions.

T F   7. I am usually at ease when talking to someone of the opposite sex.

T F   8. I try to avoid talking to people unless I know them well.

T F   9. If the chance comes to meet new people, I often take it.

T F 10. I often feel nervous or tense in casual get-togethers in which both sexes are present.

T F 11. I am usually nervous with people unless I know them well.

T F 12. I usually feel relaxed when I am with a group of people.

T F 13. I often want to get away from people.

T F 14. I usually feel uncomfortable when I am in a group of people I don't know.

T F 15. I usually feel relaxed when I meet someone for the first time.

T F 16. Being introduced to people makes me tense and nervous.

T F 17. Even though a room is full of strangers, I may enter it anyway.

T F 18. I would avoid walking up and joining a large group of people.

T F 19. When my superiors want to talk with me, I talk willingly.

T F 20. I often feel on edge when I am with a group of people.

T F 21. I tend to withdraw from people.

T F 22. I don't mind talking to people at parties or social gatherings.

T F 23. I am seldom at ease in a large group of people.

T F 24. I often think up excuses in order to avoid social engagements.

T F 25. I sometimes take the responsibility for introducing people to each other.

T F 26. I try to avoid formal social occasions.

T F 27. I usually go to whatever social engagement I have.

T F 28. I find it easy to relax with other people.

Social Interaction Anxiety Scale (SIAS)

For each question, please circle a number to indicate the degree to which you feel the statement is characteristic or true of you. The rating scale is as follows:

0 = Not at all characteristic or true of me
1 = Slightly characteristic or true of me
2 = Moderately characteristic or true of me

3 = Very characteristic or true of me
4 = Extremely characteristic or true of me

	Not at all	Slightly	Moderately	Very	Extremely
1. I get nervous if I have to speak with someone in authority (teacher, boss, etc.).	0	1	2	3	4
2. I have difficulty making eye-contact with others.	0	1	2	3	4
3. I become tense if I have to talk about myself or my feelings.	0	1	2	3	4
4. I find difficulty mixing comfortably with the people I work with.	0	1	2	3	4
5. I find it easy to make friends of my own age.	0	1	2	3	4
6. I tense-up if I meet an acquaintance on the street.	0	1	2	3	4
7. When mixing socially, I am uncomfortable.	0	1	2	3	4
8. I feel tense if I am alone with just one person.	0	1	2	3	4
9. I am at ease meeting people at parties, etc.	0	1	2	3	4
10. I have difficulty talking with other people.	0	1	2	3	4
11. I find it easy to think of things to talk about.	0	1	2	3	4
12. I worry about expressing myself in case I appear awkward.	0	1	2	3	4
13. I find it difficult to disagree with another's point of view.	0	1	2	3	4
14. I have difficulty talking to an attractive person of the opposite sex.	0	1	2	3	4
15. I find myself worrying that I won't know what to say in social situations.	0	1	2	3	4

	Not at all	Slightly	Moderately	Very	Extremely
16. I am nervous mixing with people I don't know well.	0	1	2	3	4
17. I feel I'll say something embarrassing when talking.	0	1	2	3	4
18. When mixing in a group, I find myself worrying I will be ignored.	0	1	2	3	4
19. I am tense mixing in a group.	0	1	2	3	4
20. I am unsure whether to greet someone I know only slightly.	0	1	2	3	4

Items reprinted from Mattick, R.P., & Clarke, J.C. (1998). Development and validation of measures of social phobia scrutiny fear and social interaction anxiety. *Behaviour Research and Therapy, 36*, 455-470, with permission from Elsevier Science and Richard P. Mattick, M.D.

Social Interaction Self-Statement Test (SISST)

It is obvious that people think a variety of things when they are involved in different social situations. Below is a list of things that you may have thought to yourself at some time before, during, or after the interaction in which you were engaged. Read each item and decide how frequently you were thinking a similar thought before, during, and after the interaction. Circle the number from 1 to 5 for each item. The scale is interpreted as follows:

1 = hardly ever had the thought   4 = often had the thought
2 = rarely had the thought   5 = very often had the thought
3 = sometimes had the thought

Please answer as honestly as possible.

1. When I can't think of anything to say I can feel myself getting very anxious.

1	2	3	4	5
Hardly ever	Rarely	Sometimes	Often	Very often

2. I can usually talk to women pretty well.

1	2	3	4	5
Hardly ever	Rarely	Sometimes	Often	Very often

3. I hope I don't make a fool of myself.

1	2	3	4	5
Hardly ever	Rarely	Sometimes	Often	Very often

4. I'm beginning to feel more at ease.

1	2	3	4	5
Hardly ever	Rarely	Sometimes	Often	Very often

5. I'm really afraid of what she'll think of me.

1	2	3	4	5
Hardly ever	Rarely	Sometimes	Often	Very often

6. No worries, no fears, no anxieties.

1	2	3	4	5
Hardly ever	Rarely	Sometimes	Often	Very often

7. I'm scared to death.

1	2	3	4	5
Hardly ever	Rarely	Sometimes	Often	Very often

8. She probably won't be interested in me.

1	2	3	4	5
Hardly ever	Rarely	Sometimes	Often	Very often

9. Maybe I can put her at ease by starting things going.

1	2	3	4	5
Hardly ever	Rarely	Sometimes	Often	Very often

10. Instead of worrying I can figure out how best to get to know her.

1	2	3	4	5
Hardly ever	Rarely	Sometimes	Often	Very often

11. I'm not too comfortable meeting women, so things are bound to go wrong.

1	2	3	4	5
Hardly ever	Rarely	Sometimes	Often	Very often

12. What the heck—the worst that can happen is that she won't go for me.

1	2	3	4	5
Hardly ever	Rarely	Sometimes	Often	Very often

13. She may want to talk to me as much as I want to talk to her.

1	2	3	4	5
Hardly ever	Rarely	Sometimes	Often	Very often

14. This will be a good opportunity.

1	2	3	4	5
Hardly ever	Rarely	Sometimes	Often	Very often

15. If I blow this conversation, I'll really lose my confidence.

1	2	3	4	5
Hardly ever	Rarely	Sometimes	Often	Very often

16. What I say will probably sound stupid.

1	2	3	4	5
Hardly ever	Rarely	Sometimes	Often	Very often

17. What do I have to lose? It's worth a try.

1	2	3	4	5
Hardly ever	Rarely	Sometimes	Often	Very often

18. This is an awkward situation, but I can handle it.

1	2	3	4	5
Hardly ever	Rarely	Sometimes	Often	Very often

19. Wow—I don't want to do this.

1	2	3	4	5
Hardly ever	Rarely	Sometimes	Often	Very often

20. It would crush me if she didn't respond to me.

1	2	3	4	5
Hardly ever	Rarely	Sometimes	Often	Very often

21. I've just got to make a good impression on her or I'll feel terrible.

1	2	3	4	5
Hardly ever	Rarely	Sometimes	Often	Very often

22. You're such an inhibited idiot.

1	2	3	4	5
Hardly ever	Rarely	Sometimes	Often	Very often

23. I'll probably "bomb out" anyway.

1	2	3	4	5
Hardly ever	Rarely	Sometimes	Often	Very often

24. I can handle anything.

1	2	3	4	5
Hardly ever	Rarely	Sometimes	Often	Very often

25. Even if things don't go well it's no catastrophe.

1	2	3	4	5
Hardly ever	Rarely	Sometimes	Often	Very often

26. I feel awkward and dumb; she's bound to notice.

1	2	3	4	5
Hardly ever	Rarely	Sometimes	Often	Very often

27. We probably have a lot in common.

1	2	3	4	5
Hardly ever	Rarely	Sometimes	Often	Very often

28. Maybe we'll hit it off real well.

1	2	3	4	5
Hardly ever	Rarely	Sometimes	Often	Very often

29. I wish I could leave and avoid the whole situation.

1	2	3	4	5
Hardly ever	Rarely	Sometimes	Often	Very often

30. Ah! Throw caution to the wind.

1	2	3	4	5
Hardly ever	Rarely	Sometimes	Often	Very often

Glass, C.R., Merluzzi, T.V., Biever, J.L., & Larsen, K.H. (1982). Cognitive assessment of social anxiety: Development and validation of a self-statement questionnaire. *Cognitive Therapy and Research*, 6, 37–55. Reprinted with permission from Dr. Carol Glass and Kluwer Academic/Plenum Publishers.

Social Phobia Scale (SPS)

For each question, please circle a number to indicate the degree to which you feel the statement is characteristic or true of you. The rating scale is as follows:

0 = Not at all characteristic or true of me
1 = Slightly characteristic or true of me
2 = Moderately characteristic or true of me

3 = Very characteristic or true of me
4 = Extremely characteristic or true of me

	Not at all	Slightly	Moderately	Very	Extremely
1. I become anxious if I have to write in front of other people.	0	1	2	3	4
2. I become self-conscious when using public toilets.	0	1	2	3	4
3. I can suddenly become aware of my own voice and of others listening to me.	0	1	2	3	4
4. I get nervous that people are staring at me as I walk down the street.	0	1	2	3	4
5. I fear I may blush when I am with others.	0	1	2	3	4
6. I feel self-conscious if I have to enter a room where others are already seated.	0	1	2	3	4
7. I worry about shaking or trembling when I'm watched by other people.	0	1	2	3	4
8. I would get tense if I had to sit facing other people on a bus or a train.	0	1	2	3	4
9. I get panicky that others might see me faint or be sick or ill.	0	1	2	3	4
10. I would find it difficult to drink something if in a group of people.	0	1	2	3	4
11. It would make me feel self-conscious to eat in front of a stranger in a restaurant.	0	1	2	3	4
12. I am worried people will think my behavior odd.	0	1	2	3	4
13. I would get tense if I had to carry a tray across a crowded cafeteria.	0	1	2	3	4

	Not at all	Slightly	Moderately	Very	Extremely
14. I worry I'll lose control of myself in front of other people.	0	1	2	3	4
15. I worry I might do something to attract the attention of other people.	0	1	2	3	4
16. When in an elevator, I am tense if people look at me	0	1	2	3	4
17. I can feel conspicuous standing in a line	0	1	2	3	4
18. I can get tense when I speak in front of other people.	0	1	2	3	4
19. I worry my head will shake or nod in front of others.	0	1	2	3	4
20. I feel awkward and tense if I know people are watching me.	0	1	2	3	4

Items reprinted from Mattick, R.P., & Clarke, J.C. (1998). Development and validation of measures of social phobia scrutiny fear and social interaction anxiety. *Behaviour Research and Therapy*, *36*, 455–470, with permission from Elsevier Science and Richard P. Mattick, M.D.

Measures for Generalized Anxiety Disorder

Consequences of Worry (COWS)

Please indicate, by circling the appropriate number, how much you think each of the following statements describes YOU when you worry.

1 = Not at all
2 = A little
3 = Moderately
4 = Quite a bit
5 = A lot

1. Worrying distorts the problem I have and so I am unable to solve it.
   1   2   3   4   5

2. By worrying, I reorganize and plan my time better—if I stick to it, it makes me feel better.
   1   2   3   4   5

3. Worrying starts off as a process of preparing me to meet new situations.
   1   2   3   4   5

4. Worrying makes me depressed and therefore makes it harder to concentrate and get on with things.
   1   2   3   4   5

5. When I worry, it stops me from taking decisive action.
   1   2   3   4   5

6. Worrying weakens me by affecting my levels of energy in response to those events that worry me.
   1   2   3   4   5

7. Worrying makes me tense and irritable.
   1   2   3   4   5

8. Worrying clarifies my thoughts and concentration.
   1   2   3   4   5

9. Worrying acts as a stimulant.
   1   2   3   4   5

10. Worrying causes me stress.
    1   2   3   4   5

11. Worrying stops me dealing with certain situations.
    1   2   3   4   5

12. Worrying makes me irrational.
    1   2   3   4   5

13. Worrying challenges and motivates me, without them I would not achieve much in life.
    1   2   3   4   5

14. Worrying gets me worked up.
    1   2   3   4   5

15. Deep down I know I do not need to worry that much, but I can't help it.
    1   2   3   4   5

16. Worrying increases my anxiety and so decreases my performance.
    1   2   3   4   5

1 = Not at all
2 = A little
3 = Moderately
4 = Quite a bit
5 = A lot

17. Worrying gives me the opportunity to analyze situations and work out the pros and cons.
    1   2   3   4   5

18. Problems are magnified when I dwell on them.
    1   2   3   4   5

19. Worrying increases my anxiety.
    1   2   3   4   5

20. Worrying stops me from thinking straight.
    1   2   3   4   5

21. Worrying allows me to work through the worst that can happen, so when it doesn't happen, things are better.
    1   2   3   4   5

22. Worrying makes me do things by increasing my adrenalin levels.
    1   2   3   4   5

23. Worry makes me focus on the wrong things.
    1   2   3   4   5

24. In order to get something done, I have to worry about it.
    1   2   3   4   5

25. Worrying makes me reflect on life by asking questions I might not usually ask when happy.
    1   2   3   4   5

26. I become paranoid when I worry.
    1   2   3   4   5

27. Worrying gives me a pessimistic and fatalistic outlook.
    1   2   3   4   5

28. Worrying adds concern to the problem and as such leads me to explore different possibilities.
    1   2   3   4   5

29. Worrying increases my awareness, thus increasing my performance.
    1   2   3   4   5

© 1996 Plenum Publishing Corporation. Items reprinted in Davey, G.C.L., Tallis, F., & Capuzzo, N. (1996). Beliefs about the Consequences of Worrying. *Cognitive Therapy and Research*, *20*, 499–520. Reprinted with permission from Kluwer Academic/Plenum Publishers Corporation and Graham C. L. Davey, Ph.D.

Generalized Anxiety Disorder Questionnaire—IV (GADQ-IV)

1. Do you experience excessive worry? Yes _____ No _____

2. Is your worry excessive in intensity, frequency, or amount of distress it causes?
   Yes _____ No _____

3. Do you find it difficult to control your worry (or stop worrying) once it starts?
   Yes _____ No _____

4. Do you worry excessively or uncontrollably about <u>minor things</u> such as being late for an appointment, minor repairs, homework, etc.? Yes _____ No _____

5. Please list the most frequent topics about which you worry excessively or uncontrollably:

   a. _____   d. _____
   b. _____   e. _____
   c. _____   f. _____

6. During the <u>last six months</u>, have you been bothered by excessive worries more days than not? Yes _____ No _____

7. During the past six months, have you often been bothered by any of the following symptoms? Place a check next to each symptom that you have had more days than not:

   _____ restlessness or feeling keyed up or on edge   _____ irritability
   _____ difficulty falling/staying asleep or restless/   _____ being easily fatigued
         unsatisfying sleep   _____ muscle tension
   _____ difficulty concentrating or mind going blank

8. How much do worry and physical symptoms interfere with your life, work, social activities, family, etc.? Circle one <u>number</u>:

0	1	2	3	4	5	6	7	8
None		Mild		Moderate		Severe		Very Severe

9. How much are you bothered by worry and physical symptoms (how much distress does it cause you)? Circle one <u>number</u>:

0	1	2	3	4	5	6	7	8
No Distress		Mild Distress		Moderate Distress		Severe Distress		Very Severe Distress

Reprinted with permission from Michelle G. Newman, Ph.D.

Intolerance of Uncertainty Scale (IUS)

You will find below a series of statements which describe how people may react to the uncertainties of life. Please use the scale below to describe to what extent each item is characteristic of you (please write the number that describes you best in the space before each item).

1	2	3	4	5
not at all characteristic of me	a little characteristic of me	somewhat characteristic of me	very characteristic of me	entirely characteristic of me

_____ 1. Uncertainty stops me from having a firm opinion.

_____ 2. Being uncertain means that a person is disorganized.

_____ 3. Uncertainty makes life intolerable.

_____ 4. It's not fair that there are no guarantees in life.

_____ 5. My mind can't be relaxed if I don't know what will happen tomorrow.

_____ 6. Uncertainty makes me uneasy, anxious, or stressed.

_____ 7. Unforeseen events upset me greatly.

_____ 8. It frustrates me not having all the information I need.

_____ 9. Being uncertain allows me to foresee the consequences beforehand and to prepare for them.

_____ 10. One should always look ahead so as to avoid surprises.

_____ 11. A small unforeseen event can spoil everything, even with the best of planning.

_____ 12. When it's time to act uncertainty paralyses me.

_____ 13. Being uncertain means that I am not first rate.

_____ 14. When I am uncertain I can't go forward.

_____ 15. When I am uncertain I can't function very well.

_____ 16. Unlike me, others always seem to know where they are going with their lives.

_____ 17. Uncertainty makes me vulnerable, unhappy, or sad.

_____ 18. I always want to know what the future has in store for me.

_____ 19. I hate being taken by surprise.

_____ 20. The smallest doubt stops me from acting.

_____ 21. I should be able to organize everything in advance.

_____ 22. Being uncertain means that I lack confidence.

_____ 23. I think it's unfair that other people seem sure about their future.

_____ 24. Uncertainty stops me from sleeping well.

_____ 25. I must get away from uncertain situations.

_____ 26. The ambiguities in life stress me.

_____ 27. I can't stand being undecided about my future.

Penn State Worry Questionnaire (PSWQ)

Enter the number that best describes how typical or characteristic each item is of you, putting the number next to the item.

1	2	3	4	5
Not at all typical		Somewhat typical		Very typical

_____ 1. If I don't have enough time to do everything, I don't worry about it.

_____ 2. My worries overwhelm me.

_____ 3. I do not tend to worry about things.

_____ 4. Many situations make me worry.

_____ 5. I know I shouldn't worry about things, but I just cannot help it.

_____ 6. When I am under pressure I worry a lot.

_____ 7. I am always worrying about something.

_____ 8. I find it easy to dismiss worrisome thoughts.

_____ 9. As soon as I finish one task, I start to worry about everything else I have to do.

_____ 10. I never worry about anything.

_____ 11. When there is nothing more I can do about a concern, I don't worry about it anymore.

_____ 12. I've been a worrier all my life.

_____ 13. I notice that I have been worrying about things.

_____ 14. Once I start worrying, I can't stop.

_____ 15. I worry all the time.

_____ 16. I worry about projects until they are done.

©1990 Elsevier Science. Items reprinted in Meyer, T.J., Miller, M.L., Metzger, R.L., & Borkovec, T.D. (1990). Development and validation of the Penn State Worry Questionnaire. *Behaviour Research and Therapy, 28,* 487–495. Reprinted with permission from Elsevier Science and T.D. Borkovec, Ph.D.

Why Worry Scale II (WW-II)

Below are a series of statements that can be related to worry. Please think back to times when you are worried, and indicate by circling a number (1 to 5), to what extent these statements are true for you.

	Not at all True	Slightly True	Somewhat True	Very True	Absolutely True
1. If I did not worry, I would be careless and irresponsible.	1	2	3	4	5
2. If I worry, I will be less disturbed when unforeseen events occur.	1	2	3	4	5
3. I worry in order to know what to do.	1	2	3	4	5
4. If I worry in advance, I will be less disappointed if something serious occurs.	1	2	3	4	5
5. The fact that I worry helps me plan my actions to solve a problem.	1	2	3	4	5
6. The act of worrying itself can prevent mishaps from occurring.	1	2	3	4	5
7. If I did not worry, it would make me a negligent person.	1	2	3	4	5
8. It is by worrying that I finally undertake the work that I must do.	1	2	3	4	5
9. I worry because I think it can help me find a solution to my problem.	1	2	3	4	5
10. The fact that I worry shows that I am a person who takes care of their affairs.	1	2	3	4	5
11. Thinking too much about positive things can prevent them from occurring.	1	2	3	4	5
12. The fact that I worry confirms that I am a prudent person.	1	2	3	4	5

	Not at all True	Slightly True	Somewhat True	Very True	Absolutely True
13. If misfortune comes, I will feel less responsible if I have been worrying about it beforehand.	1	2	3	4	5
14. By worrying, I can find a better way to do things.	1	2	3	4	5
15. Worrying stimulates me and makes me more effective.	1	2	3	4	5
16. The fact that I worry incites me to act.	1	2	3	4	5
17. The act of worrying itself reduces the risk that something serious will occur.	1	2	3	4	5
18. By worrying, I do certain things which I would not decide to do otherwise.	1	2	3	4	5
19. The fact that I worry motives me to do the things I must do.	1	2	3	4	5
20. My worries can, by themselves, reduce the risks of danger.	1	2	3	4	5
21. If I worry less, I decrease my chances of finding the best solution.	1	2	3	4	5
22. The fact that I worry will allow me to feel less guilty if something serious occurs.	1	2	3	4	5
23. If I worry, I will be less unhappy when a negative event occurs.	1	2	3	4	5
24. By not worrying, one can attract misfortune.	1	2	3	4	5
25. The fact that I worry shows that I am a good person.	1	2	3	4	5

Reprinted with permission from Michel Dugas, Ph.D., Laboratoire de thérapies behaviorales, École de psychologie, Université Laval, Québec, 1998.

Worry Domains Questionnaire (WDQ)

Please tick an appropriate box to show how much you **WORRY** *about the following:*

I worry ...	*Not at all*	*A little*	*Moderately*	*Quite a bit*	*Extremely*
1. that my money will run out	☐	☐	☐	☐	☐
2. that I cannot be assertive or express my opinions	☐	☐	☐	☐	☐
3. that my future job prospects are not good	☐	☐	☐	☐	☐
4. that my family will be angry with me or disapprove of something that I do	☐	☐	☐	☐	☐
5. that I'll never achieve my ambitions	☐	☐	☐	☐	☐
6. that I will not keep my workload up to date	☐	☐	☐	☐	☐
7. that financial problems will restrict holidays and travel	☐	☐	☐	☐	☐
8. that I have no concentration	☐	☐	☐	☐	☐
9. that I am not able to afford things	☐	☐	☐	☐	☐
10. that I feel insecure	☐	☐	☐	☐	☐
11. that I can't afford to pay bills	☐	☐	☐	☐	☐
12. that my living conditions are inadequate	☐	☐	☐	☐	☐
13. that life may have no purpose	☐	☐	☐	☐	☐
14. that I don't work hard enough	☐	☐	☐	☐	☐
15. that others will not approve of me	☐	☐	☐	☐	☐
16. that I find it difficult to maintain a stable relationship	☐	☐	☐	☐	☐
17. that I leave work unfinished	☐	☐	☐	☐	☐
18. that I lack confidence	☐	☐	☐	☐	☐

I worry ...	*Not at all*	*A little*	*Moderately*	*Quite a bit*	*Extremely*
19. that I am unattractive	☐	☐	☐	☐	☐
20. that I might make myself look stupid	☐	☐	☐	☐	☐
21. that I will lose close friends	☐	☐	☐	☐	☐
22. that I haven't achieved much	☐	☐	☐	☐	☐
23. that I am not loved	☐	☐	☐	☐	☐
24. that I will be late for an appointment	☐	☐	☐	☐	☐
25. that I make mistakes at work	☐	☐	☐	☐	☐

Items reprinted in Tallis, F., Eysenck, M., & Mathews, A. (1992). A questionnaire for the measurement of nonpathological worry. *Personality and Individual Differences, 13,* 161–168. © Elsevier Science. Full measure reprinted in Tallis, F., Davey, G.C.L., & Bond, A. (1994). The Worry Domains Questionnaire. In G.C.L. Davey & F. Tallis (Eds.), *Worrying: Perspectives on theory, assessment, and treatment* (pp. 287–292). New York: Wiley. © John Wiley & Sons Limited. Reprinted with permission of Elsevier Science, John Wiley & Sons Limited, and Frank Tallis, Ph.D.

Worry Scale for Older Adults (WS)

Instructions: Below is a list of problems that often concern many Americans. Please read each one carefully. After you have done so, please fill in one of the spaces to the right with a check that describes how much that problem worries you. Make only one check mark for each item.

THINGS THAT WORRY ME ……	Never	Rarely 1–2 times per month	Sometimes 1–2 times per week	Often 1–2 times per day	Much of the time More than 2 times a day
Finances					
1	that I'll lose my home				
2	that I won't be able to pay for the necessities of life (such as food, clothing, or medicine)				
3	that I won't be able to support myself independently				
4	that I won't be able to enjoy the "good things" in life (such as travel, recreation, entertainment)				
5	that I won't be able to help my children financially				
Health					
6	that my eyesight or hearing will get worse				
7	that I'll lose control of my bladder or kidneys				

	Never	Rarely 1–2 times per month	Sometimes 1–2 times per week	Often 1–2 times per day	Much of the time More than 2 times a day
8	that I won't be able to remember important things				
9	that I won't be able to get around by myself				
10	that I won't be able to enjoy my food				
11	that I'll have to be taken care of by my family				
12	that I'll have to be taken care of by strangers				
13	that I won't be able to take care of my spouse				
14	that I'll have to go to a nursing home or hospital				
15	that I won't be able to sleep at night				
16	that I may have a serious illness or accident				
17	that my spouse or close family member may have a serious illness or accident				
18	that I won't be able to enjoy sex				
19	that my reflexes will slow down				
20	that I won't be able to make decisions				

	Never	Rarely 1–2 times per month	Sometimes 1–2 times per week	Often 1–2 times per day	Much of the time More than 2 times a day
21	that I won't be able to drive a car				
22	that I'll have to use a mechanical aid (such as a hearing aid, bifocals, a cane)				

Social Conditions

	Never	Rarely 1–2 times per month	Sometimes 1–2 times per week	Often 1–2 times per day	Much of the time More than 2 times a day
23	that I'll look "old"				
24	that people will think me unattractive				
25	that no one will want to be around me				
26	that no one will love me anymore				
27	that I'll be a burden to my loved ones				
28	that I won't be able to visit my family and friends				
29	that I may be attacked by muggers or robbers on the street				
30	that my home may be broken into and vandalized				
31	that no one will come to my aid if I need it				
32	that my friends and family won't visit me				

		Never	Rarely 1–2 times per month	Sometimes 1–2 times per week	Often 1–2 times per day	Much of the time More than 2 times a day
33	that my friends and family will die					
34	that I'll get depressed					
35	that I'll have serious psychological problems					

Other Worries

		Never	Rarely 1–2 times per month	Sometimes 1–2 times per week	Often 1–2 times per day	Much of the time More than 2 times a day
36						
37						
38						
39						
40						

© 1986 Patricia A. Wisocki, Ph.D. Items reprinted in Wisocki, P.A. (1988). Worry as a phenomenon relevant to the elderly. *Behavior Therapy, 19*, 369–379. Reprinted with permission from the Association for Advancement of Behavior Therapy and Patricia A. Wisocki, Ph.D.

Measures for Obsessive-Compulsive Disorder

Compulsive Activity Checklist (CAC)

Instructions: Rate each activity on the scale below according to how much impairment is present due to obsessive and compulsive symptoms.

0 No problem with activity—Takes about same time as average person. Does not need to repeat it or avoid it.

1 Activity takes about *twice* as long as most people, or has to repeat it *twice*, or *tends* to avoid it.

2 Activity takes about *three* times as long as most people, or has to repeat it *three* or more times, or usually avoids it.

3 Is unable to complete or attempt activity.

_____ 1. Retracting steps
_____ 2. Having a bath or shower
_____ 3. Washing hands and face
_____ 4. Care of hair (e.g., washing, combing, brushing)
_____ 5. Brushing teeth
_____ 6. Dressing and undressing
_____ 7. Using toilet to urinate
_____ 8. Using toilet to defecate
_____ 9. Touching people or being touched
_____ 10. Handling garbage or waste basket
_____ 11. Washing clothing
_____ 12. Washing dishes
_____ 13. Handling or cooking food
_____ 14. Cleaning house
_____ 15. Keeping things neat and orderly
_____ 16. Bed making
_____ 17. Cleaning shoes
_____ 18. Touching door handles
_____ 19. Touching your genitals, petting or sexual intercourse
_____ 20. Visiting a hospital
_____ 21. Switching lights and spigots on or off
_____ 22. Locking or closing doors or windows
_____ 23. Checking electrical appliances
_____ 24. Doing arithmetic or accounts
_____ 25. Getting ready for work
_____ 26. Doing your work
_____ 27. Writing
_____ 28. Form filling
_____ 29. Mailing letters
_____ 30. Reading
_____ 31. Walking down the street
_____ 32. Traveling by bus, train, or car
_____ 33. Touching the floor
_____ 34. Eating in restaurants
_____ 35. Going to cinemas or theatres
_____ 36. Using public bathrooms
_____ 37. Keeping appointments
_____ 38. Throwing things away

APPENDIX

Frost Indecisiveness Scale (FIS)

	Strongly Disagree				Strongly Agree
1. I try to put off making decisions.	1	2	3	4	5
2. I always know exactly what I want.	1	2	3	4	5
3. I find it easy to make decisions.	1	2	3	4	5
4. I have a hard time planning my free time.	1	2	3	4	5
5. I like to be in a position to make decisions.	1	2	3	4	5
6. Once I make a decision, I feel fairly confident that it is a good one.	1	2	3	4	5
7. When ordering from a menu, I usually find it difficult to decide what to get.	1	2	3	4	5
8. I usually make decisions quickly.	1	2	3	4	5
9. Once I make a decision, I stop worrying about it.	1	2	3	4	5
10. I become anxious when making a decision.	1	2	3	4	5
11. I often worry about making the wrong choice.	1	2	3	4	5
12. After I have chosen or decided something, I often believe I've made the wrong choice or decision.	1	2	3	4	5
13. I do not get assignments done on time because I cannot decide what to do first.	1	2	3	4	5
14. I have trouble completing assignments because I can't prioritize what is more important.	1	2	3	4	5
15. It seems that deciding on the most trivial thing takes me a long time.	1	2	3	4	5

Maudsley Obsessional Compulsive Inventory (MOCI)

Instructions: Please answer each question by putting a circle around the 'TRUE' or the 'FALSE' following the question. There are no right or wrong answers, and no trick questions. Work quickly and do not think too long about the exact meaning of the question.

1.	I avoid using public telephones because of possible contamination.	TRUE	FALSE
2.	I frequently get nasty thoughts and have difficulty in getting rid of them.	TRUE	FALSE
3.	I am more concerned than most people about honesty.	TRUE	FALSE
4.	I am often late because I can't seem to get through everything on time.	TRUE	FALSE
5.	I don't worry unduly about contamination if I touch an animal.	TRUE	FALSE
6.	I frequently have to check things (e.g., gas or water taps, doors, etc.) several times.	TRUE	FALSE
7.	I have a very strict conscience.	TRUE	FALSE
8.	I find that almost everyday I am upset by unpleasant thoughts that come into my mind against my will.	TRUE	FALSE
9.	I do not worry unduly if I accidentally bump into somebody.	TRUE	FALSE
10.	I usually have serious doubts about the simple everyday things I do.	TRUE	FALSE
11.	Neither of my parents was very strict during my childhood.	TRUE	FALSE
12.	I tend to get behind in my work because I repeat things over and over again.	TRUE	FALSE
13.	I use only an average amount of soap.	TRUE	FALSE
14.	Some numbers are extremely unlucky.	TRUE	FALSE
15.	I do not check letters over and over again before posting them.	TRUE	FALSE
16.	I do not take a long time to dress in the morning.	TRUE	FALSE
17.	I am not excessively concerned about cleanliness.	TRUE	FALSE
18.	One of my major problems is that I pay too much attention to detail.	TRUE	FALSE
19.	I can use well-kept toilets without any hesitation.	TRUE	FALSE
20.	My major problem is repeated checking.	TRUE	FALSE
21.	I am not unduly concerned about germs and disease.	TRUE	FALSE
22.	I do not tend to check things more than once.	TRUE	FALSE
23.	I do not stick to a very strict routine when doing ordinary things.	TRUE	FALSE
24.	My hands do not feel dirty after touching money.	TRUE	FALSE
25.	I do not usually count when doing a routine task.	TRUE	FALSE
26.	I take rather a long time to complete my washing in the morning.	TRUE	FALSE
27.	I do not use a great deal of antiseptics.	TRUE	FALSE
28.	I spend a lot of time everyday checking things over and over again.	TRUE	FALSE

29. Hanging and folding my clothes at night does not take up a lot of time.   TRUE   FALSE

30. Even when I do something very carefully I often feel that it is not quite right.   TRUE   FALSE

Obsessive Compulsive Inventory (OCI)

The following statements refer to experiences that many people have in their everyday lives. Under the column labeled FREQUENCY, **CIRCLE** the number next to each statement that best describes how **FREQUENTLY YOU HAVE HAD THE EXPERIENCE IN THE PAST MONTH**. The numbers in this column refer to the following verbal labels:

0 = Never   2 = Sometimes   4 = Almost always
1 = Almost never   3 = Often

Then, in the column labeled DISTRESS, **CIRCLE** the number that best describes HOW MUCH that experience has **DISTRESSED or BOTHERED YOU DURING THE PAST MONTH**. The numbers in the column refer to the following verbal labels:

0 = Not at all   2 = Moderately   4 = Extremely
1 = A little   3 = A lot

	FREQUENCY	DISTRESS
1. Unpleasant thoughts come into my mind against my will and I cannot get rid of them.	0 1 2 3 4	0 1 2 3 4
2. I think contact with bodily secretions (perspiration, saliva, blood, urine, etc.) may contaminate my clothes or somehow harm me.	0 1 2 3 4	0 1 2 3 4
3. I ask people to repeat things to me several times, even though I understood them the first time.	0 1 2 3 4	0 1 2 3 4
4. I wash and clean obsessively.	0 1 2 3 4	0 1 2 3 4
5. I have to review mentally past events, conversations, and actions to make sure that I didn't do something wrong.	0 1 2 3 4	0 1 2 3 4
6. I have saved up so many things that they get in the way.	0 1 2 3 4	0 1 2 3 4
7. I check things more often than necessary.	0 1 2 3 4	0 1 2 3 4
8. I avoid using public toilets because I am afraid of disease or contamination.	0 1 2 3 4	0 1 2 3 4
9. I repeatedly check doors, windows, drawers, etc.	0 1 2 3 4	0 1 2 3 4
10. I repeatedly check gas and water taps and light switches after turning them off.	0 1 2 3 4	0 1 2 3 4
11. I collect things I don't need.	0 1 2 3 4	0 1 2 3 4
12. I have thoughts of hurting someone and not knowing it.	0 1 2 3 4	0 1 2 3 4
13. I have thoughts that I might want to harm myself or others.	0 1 2 3 4	0 1 2 3 4
14. I get upset if objects are not arranged properly.	0 1 2 3 4	0 1 2 3 4
15. I feel obliged to follow a particular order in dressing, undressing, and washing myself.	0 1 2 3 4	0 1 2 3 4
16. I feel compelled to count while I am doing things.	0 1 2 3 4	0 1 2 3 4

	FREQUENCY	DISTRESS
17. I am afraid of impulsively doing embarrassing or harmful things.	0 1 2 3 4	0 1 2 3 4
18. I need to pray to cancel bad thoughts or feelings.	0 1 2 3 4	0 1 2 3 4
19. I keep on checking forms or other things I have written.	0 1 2 3 4	0 1 2 3 4
20. I get upset at the sight of knives, scissors, and other sharp objects in case I lose control with them.	0 1 2 3 4	0 1 2 3 4
21. I am excessively concerned with cleanliness.	0 1 2 3 4	0 1 2 3 4
22. I find it difficult to touch an object when I know it has been touched by strangers or certain people.	0 1 2 3 4	0 1 2 3 4
23. I need things to be arranged in a particular order.	0 1 2 3 4	0 1 2 3 4
24. I get behind in my work because I repeat things over and over again.	0 1 2 3 4	0 1 2 3 4
25. I feel I have to repeat certain numbers.	0 1 2 3 4	0 1 2 3 4
26. After doing something carefully, I still have the impression that I have not finished it.	0 1 2 3 4	0 1 2 3 4
27. I find it difficult to touch garbage or dirty things.	0 1 2 3 4	0 1 2 3 4
28. I find it difficult to control my own thoughts.	0 1 2 3 4	0 1 2 3 4
29. I have to do things over and over again until it feels right.	0 1 2 3 4	0 1 2 3 4
30. I am upset by unpleasant thoughts that come into my mind against my will.	0 1 2 3 4	0 1 2 3 4
31. Before going to sleep I have to do certain things in a certain way.	0 1 2 3 4	0 1 2 3 4
32. I go back to places to make sure that I have not harmed anyone.	0 1 2 3 4	0 1 2 3 4
33. I frequently get nasty thoughts and have difficulty in getting rid of them.	0 1 2 3 4	0 1 2 3 4
34. I avoid throwing things away because I am afraid I might need them later.	0 1 2 3 4	0 1 2 3 4
35. I get upset if others change the way I have arranged things.	0 1 2 3 4	0 1 2 3 4
36. I feel that I must repeat certain words or phrases in my mind in order to wipe out bad thoughts, feelings, or actions.	0 1 2 3 4	0 1 2 3 4
37. After I have done things, I have persistent doubts about whether I really did them.	0 1 2 3 4	0 1 2 3 4
38. I sometimes have to wash or clean myself simply because I feel contaminated.	0 1 2 3 4	0 1 2 3 4
39. I feel that there are good and bad numbers.	0 1 2 3 4	0 1 2 3 4

	FREQUENCY	DISTRESS
40. I repeatedly check anything which might cause a fire.	0 1 2 3 4	0 1 2 3 4
41. Even when I do something very carefully I feel that it is not quite right.	0 1 2 3 4	0 1 2 3 4
42. I wash my hands more often and longer than necessary.	0 1 2 3 4	0 1 2 3 4

Overvalued Ideas Scale (OVIS)

Complete the following questions about obsessions and/ or compulsions which the patient reports as being applicable on the average in the **PAST WEEK INCLUDING TODAY.**

List the <u>main</u> belief which the patient has had in the last week. It should be the one that is associated with the greatest distress or impairment in social and occupational functioning to the patient as assessed by the rater (e.g., I will get AIDS if I do not wash properly after visiting the hospital, my house may burn down if I do not check the stove before leaving the house, I may lose important information if I throw out items that I collect, I am unattractive, my nose is misshapen, my complexion is full of pimples, etc.). The ratings should reflect the patient's beliefs (e.g., how reasonable does the patient perceive the belief, how effective does the patient believe the compulsions are in preventing the feared consequences, etc.). **Only list a belief related to obsessive-compulsive disorder. Rate all items according to your evaluation of the patient=s belief. You may use the three questions provided below each category to assess various aspects of the belief, e.g. strength, reasonableness.**

Describe the main belief below:

_____

_____

_____

As you rate the patient on each of the items, incorporate the patient's specific belief, e.g., How strong is your belief that you will get AIDS if you visit the hospital?

1) STRENGTH OF BELIEF

In the past week, including today;

How strongly do you believe that _____ is true?
How certain/convinced are you this belief is true?
Can your belief be 'shaken' if it is challenged by you or someone else?

1	2	3	4	5	6	7	8	9	10
Belief is Very Weak		Belief is Somewhat Weak		Belief is Weaker Than Stronger	Belief is Stronger Than Weaker		Belief is Somewhat Strong		Belief is Very Strong

(Very weak to very strong refer to the possibility of the belief being true, i.e., very weak–minimally possible; very strong–extremely possible.)

Rating Item 1: _____

2) REASONABLENESS OF BELIEF

In the past week, including today;

How reasonable is your belief?
Is your belief justified or rational?
Is the belief logical or seem reasonable?

1	2	3	4	5	6	7	8	9	10
Totally Unreasonable		Almost Unreasonable		More Low Than High Reasonableness	More High Than Low Reasonableness		Almost Reasonable		Completely Reasonable

Rating Item 2: _____

3) LOWEST STRENGTH OF BELIEF IN PAST WEEK

In the last week, what would you say was the lowest rating of strength for your belief?
How weak did your belief become in the last weak?
Were there times in the past week that you doubted your belief, even for a fleeting
moment, whether _____ was true? If so, tell me more about it?

```
1        2        3        4        5        6        7        8        9        10
| -------- | -------- | -------- |-------- | -------- |-------- | -------- |-------- | --------- |
```
Belief is   Belief is   Belief is Weaker Belief is Stronger   Belief is   Belief is
Very Weak   Somewhat Weak   Than Stronger   Than Weaker   Somewhat Strong   Very Strong

Rating Item 1: _____

4) HIGHEST STRENGTH OF BELIEF IN PAST WEEK

In the last week, what was your highest rating of strength for your belief?
How strong did your belief become in the last week?
How certain/convinced were you about your belief in the past week?

```
1        2        3        4        5        6        7        8        9        10
| -------- | -------- | -------- |-------- | -------- |-------- | -------- |-------- | --------- |
```
Belief is   Belief is   Belief is Weaker Belief is Stronger   Belief is   Belief is
Very Weak   Somewhat Weak   Than Stronger   Than Weaker   Somewhat Strong   Very Strong

Rating Item 4: _____

5) ACCURACY OF BELIEF
In the past week, including today;

How accurate is your belief?
How correct is your belief?
To what degree is your belief erroneous?

```
1        2        3        4        5        6        7        8        9        10
| -------- | -------- | -------- |-------- | -------- |-------- | -------- |-------- | --------- |
```
Totally   Almost   More Low Than   More High Than   Almost   Completely
Inaccurate   Inaccurate   High Agreement   Low Agreement   Agree   Agree

Rating Item 5: _____

6) EXTENT OF ADHERENCE BY OTHERS

How likely is it that others in the general population (in the community, state, country, etc.)
have the same beliefs?
How strongly do these others agree with your belief?
To what extent do these others share your belief?

```
1        2        3        4        5        6        7        8        9        10
| -------- |-------- | -------- |--------- | -------- | -------- |-------- | -------- | --------- |
```
Totally   Almost   More Low Than   More High Than   Almost   Completely
Disagree   Disagree   High Agreement   Low Agreement   Agree   Agree

Rating Item 6: _____

7) ATTRIBUTION OF DIFFERING VIEWS BY OTHERS

Do others share the same belief as you? Yes _____ No _____
b3If the patient answers Yes go to 7a, if the patient answers No go to 7b.

7a) VIEWS OTHERS AS POSSESSING SAME BELIEF

Since you think others agree with your belief, do you think they are as knowledgeable as you about this belief?

To what extent do you believe others are as knowledgeable about the belief as you are?

Do you believe others have as much information as you about this belief?

```
 1        2        3        4        5        6        7        8        9        10
| -------- | -------- | -------- | -------- | -------- | -------- | -------- | -------- | --------- |
```

Lacking	Somewhat Lacking	Less		More	Almost As	Equally as
Total	Knowledge	Knowledgeable		Knowledgeable	Knowledgeable	Knowledgeable
Knowledge		Than More		Than Less		

Rating Item 7a: _____

7b) VIEWS OTHERS AS HOLDING DIFFERING BELIEF

Since you think others disagree with you, do you think they are less knowledgeable than you about this belief?

To what extent do you believe others are less knowledgeable about the belief than you are?

Do you believe others have less information than you about this belief?

```
 1        2        3        4        5        6        7        8        9        10
| -------- | -------- | -------- | -------- | -------- | -------- | -------- | -------- | --------- |
```

Equally as	Almost as	More	Less	Somewhat Lacking	Lacking
Knowledgeable	Knowledgeable	Knowledgeable	Knowledgeable	Knowledge	Total
		Than Less	Than More		Knowledge

Rating Item 7b: _____

8) EFFECTIVENESS OF COMPULSIONS

In the past week, including today;

How effective are the compulsions/ritualistic behaviors in preventing negative consequences other than anxiety?

Are your compulsions of any value in stopping the feared outcome?

Is it possible that your compulsions may not help prevent the negative outcomes?

```
 1        2        3        4        5        6        7        8        9        10
| -------- | -------- | -------- | -------- | -------- | -------- | -------- | -------- | --------- |
```

| Totally | Almost | More Low Than | More High Than | Almost | Completely |
| Ineffective | Ineffective | High Effect | Low Effect | Effective | Effective |

Rating Item 8: _____

9) INSIGHT

To what extent do you think that your disorder has caused you to have this belief?

How probable is it that your beliefs are due to psychological or psychiatric reasons?

Do you think that your belief is due to a disorder?

```
 1        2        3        4        5        6        7        8        9        10
| -------- | -------- | -------- | -------- | -------- | -------- | -------- | -------- | --------- |
```

| Totally | Somewhat | More Probable | More Improbable | Somewhat | Totally |
| Probable | Probable | Than Improbable | Than Probable | Improbable | Improbable |

Rating Item 9: _____

10) STRENGTH OF RESISTANCE

How much energy do you put into rejecting your belief?

How strongly do you try to change your belief?

Do you attempt to resist your belief?

1	2	3	4	5	6	7	8	9	10
|--------	|--------	|--------	|--------	|--------	|--------	|--------	|--------	|--------	|

Total Resistance	Much Resistance	More Resistance Than Less	Less Resistance Than More	Little Resistance	No Resistance

Rating Item 10: _____

11) DURATION OF BELIEF

a) During the time that you have had this belief did it ever fluctuate?

If so, within what period of time?

Check one of the following:

_____   _____   _____   _____

Day   Week   Month   Year

b) In retrospect, how long have you held this particular belief?

Check one of the following:

_____   _____   _____   _____

Day   Week   Month   Year

Padua Inventory–Washington State University Revision (PI-WSUR)

INSTRUCTIONS: The following statements refer to thoughts and behaviors which may occur to everyone in everyday life. For each statement, choose the reply which best seems to fit you and the degree of disturbance which such thoughts or behaviors may create. Rate your replies as follows:

0 = not at all
1 = a little
2 = quite a lot
3 = a lot
4 = very much

_____ 1. I feel my hands are dirty when I touch money.

_____ 2. I think even the slightest contact with bodily secretions (perspiration, saliva, urine, etc.) may contaminate my clothes or somehow harm me.

_____ 3. I find it difficult to touch an object when I know it has been touched by strangers or by certain people.

_____ 4. I find it difficult to touch garbage or dirty things.

_____ 5. I avoid using public toilets because I am afraid of disease and contamination.

_____ 6. I avoid using public telephones because I am afraid of contagion and disease.

_____ 7. I wash my hands more often and longer than necessary.

_____ 8. I sometimes have to wash or clean myself simply because I think I may be dirty or "contaminated."

_____ 9. If I touch something I think is "contaminated," I immediately have to wash or clean myself.

_____ 10. If an animal touches me, I feel dirty and immediately have to wash myself or change clothing.

_____ 11. I feel obliged to follow a particular order in dressing, undressing, and washing myself.

_____ 12. Before going to sleep, I have to do certain things in a certain order.

_____ 13. Before going to bed, I have to hang up or fold my clothes in a special way.

_____ 14. I have to do things several times before I think they are properly done.

_____ 15. I tend to keep on checking things more often than necessary.

_____ 16. I check and recheck gas and water taps and light switches after turning them off.

_____ 17. I return home to check doors, windows, drawers, etc., to make sure they are properly shut.

_____ 18. I keep checking forms, documents, checks, etc., in detail to make sure I have filled them in correctly.

_____ 19. I keep on going back to see that matches, cigarettes, etc., are properly extinguished.

_____ 20. When I handle money, I count and recount it several times.

_____ 21. I check letters carefully many times before posting them.

_____ 22. Sometimes I am not sure I have done things, which in fact I know I have done.

_____ 23. When I read, I have the impression I have missed something important and must go back and reread the passage at least two or three times.

0 = not at all
1 = a little
2 = quite a lot
3 = a lot
4 = very much

_____ 24. I imagine catastrophic consequences as a result of absent-mindedness or minor errors, which I make.

_____ 25. I think or worry at length about having hurt someone without knowing it.

_____ 26. When I hear about a disaster, I think it is somehow my fault.

_____ 27. I sometimes worry at length for no reason that I have hurt myself or have some disease.

_____ 28. I get upset and worried at the sight of knives, daggers, and other pointed objects.

_____ 29. When I hear about suicide or crime, I am upset for a long time and find it difficult to stop thinking about it.

_____ 30. I invent useless worries about germs and disease.

_____ 31. When I look down from a bridge or a very high window, I feel an impulse to throw myself into space.

_____ 32. When I see a train approaching, I sometimes think I could throw myself under its wheels.

_____ 33. At certain moments, I am tempted to tear off my clothes in public.

_____ 34. While driving, I sometimes feel an impulse to drive the car into someone or something.

_____ 35. Seeing weapons excites me and makes me think violent thoughts.

_____ 36. I sometimes feel the need to break or damage things for no reason.

_____ 37. I sometimes have an impulse to steal other people's belongings, even if they are of no use to me.

_____ 38. I am sometimes almost irresistibly tempted to steal something from the supermarket.

_____ 39. I sometimes have an impulse to hurt defenseless children or animals.

Responsibility Attitude Scale (RAS)

This questionnaire lists different attitudes or beliefs which people sometimes hold. Read each statement carefully and decide how much you agree or disagree with it.

For each of the attitudes, show your answer by putting a circle round the words which best describe how you think. Be sure to choose only one answer for each attitude. Because people are different, there is no right answer or wrong answer to these statements.

To decide whether a given attitude is typical of your way of looking at things, simply keep in mind what you are like most of the time.

1. I often feel responsible for things which go wrong.

TOTALLY AGREE	AGREE VERY MUCH	AGREE SLIGHTLY	NEUTRAL	DISAGREE SLIGHTLY	DISAGREE VERY MUCH	TOTALLY DISAGREE

2. If I don't act when I can foresee danger, then I am to blame for any consequences if it happens.

TOTALLY AGREE	AGREE VERY MUCH	AGREE SLIGHTLY	NEUTRAL	DISAGREE SLIGHTLY	DISAGREE VERY MUCH	TOTALLY DISAGREE

3. I am too sensitive to feeling responsible for things going wrong.

TOTALLY AGREE	AGREE VERY MUCH	AGREE SLIGHTLY	NEUTRAL	DISAGREE SLIGHTLY	DISAGREE VERY MUCH	TOTALLY DISAGREE

4. If I think bad things, this is as bad as <u>doing</u> bad things.

TOTALLY AGREE	AGREE VERY MUCH	AGREE SLIGHTLY	NEUTRAL	DISAGREE SLIGHTLY	DISAGREE VERY MUCH	TOTALLY DISAGREE

5. I worry a great deal about the effects of things which I do or don't do.

TOTALLY AGREE	AGREE VERY MUCH	AGREE SLIGHTLY	NEUTRAL	DISAGREE SLIGHTLY	DISAGREE VERY MUCH	TOTALLY DISAGREE

6. To me, not acting to prevent disaster is as bad as making disaster happen.

TOTALLY AGREE	AGREE VERY MUCH	AGREE SLIGHTLY	NEUTRAL	DISAGREE SLIGHTLY	DISAGREE VERY MUCH	TOTALLY DISAGREE

7. If I know that harm is possible, I should always try to prevent it, however unlikely it seems.

TOTALLY AGREE	AGREE VERY MUCH	AGREE SLIGHTLY	NEUTRAL	DISAGREE SLIGHTLY	DISAGREE VERY MUCH	TOTALLY DISAGREE

8. I must always think through the consequences of even the smallest actions.

TOTALLY AGREE	AGREE VERY MUCH	AGREE SLIGHTLY	NEUTRAL	DISAGREE SLIGHTLY	DISAGREE VERY MUCH	TOTALLY DISAGREE

9. I often take responsibility for things which other people don't think are my fault.

TOTALLY AGREE   AGREE   NEUTRAL   DISAGREE   DISAGREE   TOTALLY
AGREE   VERY   SLIGHTLY   SLIGHTLY   VERY   DISAGREE
     MUCH   MUCH

10. Everything I do can cause serious problems.

TOTALLY AGREE   AGREE   NEUTRAL   DISAGREE   DISAGREE   TOTALLY
AGREE   VERY   SLIGHTLY   SLIGHTLY   VERY   DISAGREE
     MUCH   MUCH

11. I am often close to causing harm.

TOTALLY AGREE   AGREE   NEUTRAL   DISAGREE   DISAGREE   TOTALLY
AGREE   VERY   SLIGHTLY   SLIGHTLY   VERY   DISAGREE
     MUCH   MUCH

12. I must protect others from harm.

TOTALLY AGREE   AGREE   NEUTRAL   DISAGREE   DISAGREE   TOTALLY
AGREE   VERY   SLIGHTLY   SLIGHTLY   VERY   DISAGREE
     MUCH   MUCH

13. I should never cause even the slightest harm to others.

TOTALLY AGREE   AGREE   NEUTRAL   DISAGREE   DISAGREE   TOTALLY
AGREE   VERY   SLIGHTLY   SLIGHTLY   VERY   DISAGREE
     MUCH   MUCH

14. I will be condemned for my actions.

TOTALLY AGREE   AGREE   NEUTRAL   DISAGREE   DISAGREE   TOTALLY
AGREE   VERY   SLIGHTLY   SLIGHTLY   VERY   DISAGREE
     MUCH   MUCH

15. If I can have even a slight influence on things going wrong, then I must act to prevent it.

TOTALLY AGREE   AGREE   NEUTRAL   DISAGREE   DISAGREE   TOTALLY
AGREE   VERY   SLIGHTLY   SLIGHTLY   VERY   DISAGREE
     MUCH   MUCH

16. To me, not acting where disaster is a slight possibility is as bad as making that disaster happen.

TOTALLY AGREE   AGREE   NEUTRAL   DISAGREE   DISAGREE   TOTALLY
AGREE   VERY   SLIGHTLY   SLIGHTLY   VERY   DISAGREE
     MUCH   MUCH

17. For me, even slight carelessness is inexcusable when it might affect other people.

TOTALLY AGREE   AGREE   NEUTRAL   DISAGREE   DISAGREE   TOTALLY
AGREE   VERY   SLIGHTLY   SLIGHTLY   VERY   DISAGREE
     MUCH   MUCH

18. In all kinds of daily situations, my inactivity can cause as much harm as deliberate bad intentions.

TOTALLY AGREE   AGREE   NEUTRAL   DISAGREE   DISAGREE   TOTALLY
AGREE   VERY   SLIGHTLY   SLIGHTLY   VERY   DISAGREE
     MUCH   MUCH

19. Even if harm is a very unlikely possibility, I should always try to prevent it at any cost.

| TOTALLY AGREE | AGREE VERY MUCH | AGREE SLIGHTLY | NEUTRAL | DISAGREE SLIGHTLY | DISAGREE VERY MUCH | TOTALLY DISAGREE |

20. Once I think it is possible that I have caused harm, I can't forgive myself.

| TOTALLY AGREE | AGREE VERY MUCH | AGREE SLIGHTLY | NEUTRAL | DISAGREE SLIGHTLY | DISAGREE VERY MUCH | TOTALLY DISAGREE |

21. Many of my past actions have been intended to prevent harm to others.

| TOTALLY AGREE | AGREE VERY MUCH | AGREE SLIGHTLY | NEUTRAL | DISAGREE SLIGHTLY | DISAGREE VERY MUCH | TOTALLY DISAGREE |

22. I have to make sure other people are protected from all of the consequences of things I do.

| TOTALLY AGREE | AGREE VERY MUCH | AGREE SLIGHTLY | NEUTRAL | DISAGREE SLIGHTLY | DISAGREE VERY MUCH | TOTALLY DISAGREE |

23. Other people should not rely on my judgement.

| TOTALLY AGREE | AGREE VERY MUCH | AGREE SLIGHTLY | NEUTRAL | DISAGREE SLIGHTLY | DISAGREE VERY MUCH | TOTALLY DISAGREE |

24. If I cannot be <u>certain</u> I am blameless, I feel that I am to blame.

| TOTALLY AGREE | AGREE VERY MUCH | AGREE SLIGHTLY | NEUTRAL | DISAGREE SLIGHTLY | DISAGREE VERY MUCH | TOTALLY DISAGREE |

25. If I take sufficient care then I can prevent any harmful accidents.

| TOTALLY AGREE | AGREE VERY MUCH | AGREE SLIGHTLY | NEUTRAL | DISAGREE SLIGHTLY | DISAGREE VERY MUCH | TOTALLY DISAGREE |

26. I often think that bad things will happen if I am not careful enough.

| TOTALLY AGREE | AGREE VERY MUCH | AGREE SLIGHTLY | NEUTRAL | DISAGREE SLIGHTLY | DISAGREE VERY MUCH | TOTALLY DISAGREE |

Responsibility Interpretations Questionnaire (RIQ)

We are interested in your reaction to intrusive thoughts that you have had in the **last 2 weeks**. Intrusive thoughts are thoughts that suddenly enter your mind, may interrupt what you are thinking or doing and tend to recur on separate occasions. They may occur in the form of words, mental image, or an impulse (a sudden urge to carry out some action). We are interested in those intrusive thoughts that are unacceptable. Research has shown that most people experience or have experienced such thoughts which they find unacceptable in some way, at some time in their lives to a greater or lesser degree, so there is nothing unusual about this.

Some examples of unpleasant intrusions are:

Repeated image of attacking someone
Suddenly thinking that your hands are dirty and you may cause contamination
Suddenly thinking you might not have turned off the gas, or that you left a door unlocked
Repeated senseless images of harm coming to someone you love
Repeated urge to attack or harm somebody (even though you would never do this)

These are just a few examples of intrusions to give you some idea of what we are looking at; people vary tremendously in the type of thoughts that they have.

IMPORTANT

Think of INTRUSIONS OF THE TYPE DESCRIBED ABOVE that you have had in the last 2 weeks, and answer the following questions with that intrusion in mind. The questions do NOT relate to all thoughts but specifically to your negative intrusions.

Please write down intrusions that you have had in the last 2 weeks:

This questionnaire has two parts:

Overleaf are some ideas that may go through your mind **when you are bothered by worrying intrusive thoughts which you know are probably senseless or unrealistic**. Think of times when you were bothered by intrusive thoughts, impulses and images **in the last 2 weeks**.

APPENDIX

A. Frequency

Indicate <u>how often</u> each of the ideas listed below occurred <u>when you were bothered by these intrusive thoughts, impulses or images</u>; circle the digit that most accurately describes the frequency of the occurrence of the ideas using the following scale:

Over the <u>LAST TWO WEEKS</u>:

0 = Idea never occurred
1 = Idea rarely occurred
2 = Idea occurred during about half of the times when I had worrying intrusive thoughts
3 = Idea usually occurred
4 = Idea always occurred when I had worrying intrusive thoughts

<u>F1</u>	never occurred	rarely occurred	half the time	usually occurred	always occurred
If I don't resist these thoughts it means I am being irresponsible	0	1	2	3	4
I could be responsible for serious harm	0	1	2	3	4
I cannot take the risk of this thought coming true	0	1	2	3	4
If I don't act now then something terrible will happen and it will be my fault	0	1	2	3	4
I need to be certain something awful won't happen	0	1	2	3	4
I shouldn't be thinking this type of thing	0	1	2	3	4
It would be irresponsible to ignore these thoughts	0	1	2	3	4
I'll feel awful unless I do something about this thought	0	1	2	3	4
Because I've thought of bad things happening then I must act to prevent them	0	1	2	3	4
Since I've thought of this I must want it to happen	0	1	2	3	4
Now I've thought of things which could go wrong I have a responsibility to make sure I don't let them happen	0	1	2	3	4
Thinking this could make it happen	0	1	2	3	4
I must regain control of my thoughts	0	1	2	3	4
This could be an omen	0	1	2	3	4
It's wrong to ignore these thoughts	0	1	2	3	4
Because these thoughts come from my own mind, I must want to have them	0	1	2	3	4

Now rate these items:

F2

	never occurred	rarely occurred	half the time	usually occurred	always occurred
Thoughts can NOT make things happen	0	1	2	3	4
This is just a thought so it doesn't matter	0	1	2	3	4
Thinking of something happening doesn't make me responsible for whether it happens	0	1	2	3	4
There's nothing wrong with letting such thoughts come and go naturally	0	1	2	3	4
Everybody has horrible thoughts sometimes, so I don't need to worry about this one	0	1	2	3	4
Having this thought doesn't mean I have to do anything about it	0	1	2	3	4

B. Belief

Over the last two weeks. When you were bothered by these worrying intrusive thoughts, how much did you **believe** each of these ideas to be true? Rate the belief you had of these ideas when you had the intrusions, using the following scale; mark the point on the line that most accurately applies to your belief at the time of the intrusion.

B1

	I did not believe this idea at all — I as completely convinced this idea was true
If I don't resist these thoughts it means I am being irresponsible	0 10 20 30 40 50 60 70 80 90 100
I could be responsible for serious harm	0 10 20 30 40 50 60 70 80 90 100
I can not take the risk of this thought coming true	0 10 20 30 40 50 60 70 80 90 100
If I don't act now then something terrible will happen and it will be my fault	0 10 20 30 40 50 60 70 80 90 100
I need to be certain something awful won't happen	0 10 20 30 40 50 60 70 80 90 100
I should not be thinking this kind of thing	0 10 20 30 40 50 60 70 80 90 100
It would be irresponsible to ignore these thoughts	0 10 20 30 40 50 60 70 80 90 100
I'll feel awful unless I do something about this thought	0 10 20 30 40 50 60 70 80 90 100
Because I've thought of bad things happening then I must act to prevent them	0 10 20 30 40 50 60 70 80 90 100
Since I've had this thought I must want it to happen	0 10 20 30 40 50 60 70 80 90 100

B1

	I did not believe this idea at all										I as completely convinced this idea was true

Now I've thought of bad things which could go wrong I have a responsibility to make sure I don't let them happen

0 10 20 30 40 50 60 70 80 90 100

Thinking this could make it happen

0 10 20 30 40 50 60 70 80 90 100

I must regain control of these thoughts

0 10 20 30 40 50 60 70 80 90 100

This could be an omen

0 10 20 30 40 50 60 70 80 90 100

It's wrong to ignore these thoughts

0 10 20 30 40 50 60 70 80 90 100

Because these thoughts come from my mind, I must want to have them

0 10 20 30 40 50 60 70 80 90 100

Now rate these items:

B2

	I did not believe this idea at all										I as completely convinced this idea was true

Thoughts can NOT make things happen

0 10 20 30 40 50 60 70 80 90 100

This is just a thought so it doesn't matter

0 10 20 30 40 50 60 70 80 90 100

Thinking of something happening doesn't make me responsible for whether it happens

0 10 20 30 40 50 60 70 80 90 100

There's nothing wrong with letting thoughts like this come and go naturally

0 10 20 30 40 50 60 70 80 90 100

Everybody has horrible thoughts sometimes, so I don't need to worry about this one

0 10 20 30 40 50 60 70 80 90 100

Having this thought doesn't mean I have to do anything about it

0 10 20 30 40 50 60 70 80 90 100

Thought-Action Fusion Scale (TAF Scale)

Do you disagree or agree with the following statements?	Disagree Strongly	Disagree	Neutral	Agree	Agree Strongly
1. Thinking of making an extremely critical remark to a friend is almost as unacceptable to me as actually saying it	0	1	2	3	4
2. If I think of a relative/friend losing their job, this increases the risk that they will lose their job	0	1	2	3	4
3. Having a blasphemous thought is almost as sinful to me as a blasphemous action	0	1	2	3	4
4. Thinking about swearing at someone else is almost as unacceptable to me as actually swearing	0	1	2	3	4
5. If I think of a relative/friend being in a car accident, this increases the risk that he/she will have a car accident	0	1	2	3	4
6. When I have a nasty thought about someone else, it is almost as bad as carrying out a nasty action	0	1	2	3	4
7. If I think of a friend/relative being injured in a fall, this increases the risk that he/she will have a fall and be injured	0	1	2	3	4
8. Having violent thoughts is almost as unacceptable to me as violent acts	0	1	2	3	4
9. If I think of a relative/friend falling ill this increases the risk that he/she will fall ill	0	1	2	3	4
10. When I think about making an obscene remark or gesture in church, it is almost as sinful as actually doing it	0	1	2	3	4
11. If I wish harm on someone, it is almost as bad as doing harm	0	1	2	3	4
12. If I think of myself being injured in a fall, this increases the risk that I will have a fall and be injured	0	1	2	3	4

Do you disagree or agree with the following statements?	Disagree Strongly	Disagree	Neutral	Agree	Agree Strongly
13. When I think unkindly about a friend, it is almost as disloyal as doing an unkind act	0	1	2	3	4
14. If I think of myself being in a car accident, this increases the risk that I will have a car accident	0	1	2	3	4
15. If I think about making an obscene gesture to someone else, it is almost as bad as doing it	0	1	2	3	4
16. If I think of myself falling ill, this increases the risk that I will fall ill	0	1	2	3	4
17. If I have a jealous thought, it is almost the same as making a jealous remark	0	1	2	3	4
18. Thinking of cheating in a personal relationship is almost as immoral to me as actually cheating	0	1	2	3	4
19. Having obscene thoughts in a church is unacceptable to me	0	1	2	3	4

Yale-Brown Obsessive Compulsive Scale (Y-BOCS)

Y-BOCS SYMPTOM CHECKLIST (Clinician Version; from Revised Y-BOCS; 11/13/00)

Instructions: Check all that apply, but clearly mark the principal current (last 30 days) symptoms with a "P". Rater must ascertain whether the reported behaviors are bona fide symptoms of OCD, and not symptoms of another disorder such as Specific Phobia or Trichotillomania. Items marked with an asterisk "*" may or may not be OCD phenomena. Do not read out loud the category headings (e.g., "Violent Obsessions") to the patient. These terms are for the convenience of the rater in organizing the themes of the material but may confuse or offend the patient. Abbreviations: OCD, obsessive-compulsive disorder; OCPD, obsessive-compulsive personality disorder; BDD, body dysmorphic disorder; TS, Tourette's Syndrome; GAD, generalized anxiety disorder.

OBSESSIONS

Last 30 days	Past	Contamination Obsessions
		001. **Concern with dirt or germs.**
		002. **Excessive concern with environmental contaminants.** Examples: asbestos, radiation, pesticides or toxic waste.
		003. **Excessive concern with household items.** Examples: cleansers, solvents.
		004. **Concerns or disgust with bodily waste or secretions.** Examples: urine, feces, or saliva.
		005. **Fear of blood.*** Specify whether fear is a) related to blood-borne illnesses like AIDS or hepatitis or b) cued by just the sight of blood, which may result in a vasovagal response as in a *Specific Phobia.
		006. **Bothered by sticky substances or residues.** Examples: adhesives, chalk dust, or grease.
		007. **Excessive concern with animals or insects*** Distinguish from *Specific Phobia.
		008. **Concerned will get ill because of contaminants.** Examples: AIDS or cancer.
		009. **Concerned will get others ill by spreading contaminants.**
		010. **No concern with consequences of contamination other than how it might feel.**
		011. **Excessive concern with becoming pregnant or of making someone pregnant.**
		012. **Concerned with having an illness or disease.*** Where to draw the line between somatic obsessions and the somatic preoccupations of *Hypochondriasis is not always evident. Factors that point to OCD are presence of multiple obsessions, compulsions not limited to seeking reassurance, and persistence of symptoms.

Last 30 days	Past	Contamination Obsessions (continued)
		013. **Fear of eating certain foods.*** Examples: excessive concern about risks of certain foods or food preparations. *Distinguish from anorexia nervosa in which concern is gaining weight.
		014. **Other**

Last 30 days	Past	Safety/Harm/Violent Obsessions
		015. **Fear might be harmed because not careful enough.** Exclude contamination obsessions.
		016. **Fear might harm self on impulse.*** This item involves unwanted impulses or inexplicable acts. Examples: fear of stabbing self with a knife, jumping in front of a car, leaping out an open window, or swallowing poison. *Distinguish from suicidal ideation secondary to depression.
		017. **Fear might harm others because not careful enough.** Examples: parked car rolling down hill, hit a pedestrian because not paying attention, customer gets injured because you gave him wrong materials or information.
		018. **Fear might harm others on impulse.*** Examples: physically harming loved ones, stabbing or poisoning dinner guests, pushing stranger in front of a train. *Distinguish from homicidal intent.
		019. **Fear of being responsible for terrible events.** Examples: fire, burglary, flooding house, company going bankrupt, pipes freezing.
		020. **Fear of blurting out obscenities or insults.** Examples: shouting blasphemies in church, yelling fire in the movie theatre, writing obscenities in a business letter.
		021. **Fear of doing something else embarrassing.*** Examples: taking off clothes in public, walking out with unpaid merchandise. *Distinguish from Social Phobia.
		022. **Violent or horrific images.** Examples: intrusive and disturbing images of car crashes or disfigured people.
		023. **Other.**

Last 30 days	Past	Religious, Scrupulous, Sexual, and Morbid Obsessions
		024. **Excessive concern with right/wrong.** For example, worries about always doing "the right thing", unfounded worries about lying or cheating.
		025. **Concern with sacrilege and blasphemy.** Examples: intrusive unacceptable thoughts or images about God or religion. Concerns about adherence to religious principles exceed those of religious peer group.
		026. **Excessive fears of Satan or demonic possession.** Examples: fears triggered by "Red Devil" paint, sports teams with word devil in them; apostrophe (signifies "possession"), "666", pentangles.
		027. **Forbidden or improper sexual thoughts, images, or impulses.*** Examples: unwanted sexual thoughts about family members; images of unacceptable acts. *Distinguish from Paraphilias by asking about fantasy life.
		028. **Fear might act on unacceptable sexual impulses.*** Examples: concerned that might "snap" and commit sexual assault *Distinguish from Paraphilias.
		029. **Unfounded concerns about gender identity.** Examples: man repeatedly wonders if he's gay even though there is every reason to believe he is heterosexual.
		030. **Excessive fear of death.** Examples: fears triggered by cemeteries, funerals/funeral parlors, hearses, the color black (signifies mourning).
		031. **Other.**

Last 30 days	Past	Symmetry, Order, Exactness, and "Just Right" Obsessions
		032. **Need for symmetry or exactness.*** Examples: certain things can't be touched or moved, clothes organized in closet alphabetically, bothered if pictures are not straight or canned goods not lined up *Distinguish from OCPD in which perfectionism is less dramatic.
		033. **Exactness in dressing.** Examples: excessive concern about appearance of clothing such as wrinkles, lint, loose threads; may not wear garments out of concern they will become worn.
		034. **Symmetry in dressing.** . Examples: bothered if stockings are not at the same height or shoe laces not tied at the same tension.

Last 30 days	Past	Symmetry, Order, Exactness, and "Just Right" Obsessions (continued)
		035. **Exactness or symmetry in grooming.** Examples: bothered if hair not parted exactly straight or hair not precisely same length on each side of the head.
		036. **Fear of saying the wrong thing or not saying it "just right".** Example: patient may appear to have thought-blocking because she is reviewing every interpretation of what she is about to say.
		037. **Need for exactness (items 32–36) related to feared consequences.** Example: something terrible may happen if things aren't in their proper place.
		038. **Need for exactness (items 32–36) <u>unrelated</u> to feared consequences.** Examples: can't explain what might happen if things aren't in their proper place; feels discomfort unless things are just right. N.B. If some obsessions with order and symmetry are associated with feared consequences and others aren't, endorse both items 37 and 38.
		039. **Excessively bothered by things not sounding "just right."** Examples: readjusting stereo system until it sounds "just right"; asks family members to say things in just the right way.
		040. **Finds certain sounds irritating.*** Examples: "sh" sound, lisps, static/noise, sniffing/coughing, ticking clocks, dripping water. *Distinguish from irritability not specific to OCD.
		041. **Need to know or remember.** Examples: needing to remember insignificant things like license plate numbers, bumper stickers, advertising slogans, names of actors.
		042. **Other.**

Last 30 days	Past	Hoarding/Saving Obsessions
		043. **Need to hoard or save things.*** Examples: afraid that something valuable might be discarded with recycled newspapers even though all valuables are locked up in the safe. *Distinguish from hobbies and concern with objects of monetary or sentimental value. Hoarding can be present in OCPD, but if pronounced it is usually better explained by OCD.
		044. **Fear of losing objects or information.**
		045. **Fear of losing people.** Example: otherwise rational man feared "losing" his 5-year old daughter when mailing envelopes.

Last 30 days	Past	Hoarding/Saving Obsessions (continued)
		046. **Fear of losing something symbolic.** Example: patient concerned that her "essence" would be left behind when getting up from a chair.

Last 30 days	Past	Other Obsessions
		047. **Pathological doubting.** Examples: after completing a routine activity patient wonders whether he performed it correctly or did it at all; may not trust his memory or his own senses (i.e., "his mind doesn't trust what his eyes see.").
		048. **Pathological indecisiveness.*** Examples: continual weighing of pros and cons about nonessentials like which clothes to put on in the morning or which brand of cereal to buy. Differentiate from worries about real-life decisions characteristic of *GAD.
		049. **Excessive concern with functioning of or injury to a body part.*** Examples: protecting face or eyes from damage; obsessed with mechanical functioning of feet. *In most cases of preoccupations with physical appearance, BDD is most appropriate diagnosis.
		050. **Colors with special significance.** Examples: black connected with death, red associated with blood and injury.
		051. **Superstitious fears.** Examples: black cats, breaking mirror, stepping on side walk cracks, spilling salt, omens.
		052. **Lucky or unlucky numbers.** Example: the numbers thirteen. N.B. The reliability item of the Revised Y-BOCS is not numbered.
		053. **Intrusive meaningless thoughts or images.**
		054. **Intrusive nonsense sounds, words, or music.** Examples: songs or music with no special significance play over like a broken record.

COMPULSIONS

Last 30 days	Past	Cleaning Compulsions
		055. **Excessive or ritualized handwashing.** Examples: washes hands like surgeon scrubbing for the operating room, uses harsh detergents or very hot water.
		056. **Excessive or ritualized showering, bathing, toothbrushing, grooming, or toilet routine.**

Last 30 days	Past	Cleaning Compulsions (continued)
		057. **Cleaning of household items or other inanimate objects.** Examples: floors kept so clean you can eat off them; prolonged vacuuming; daily thorough washing of car tires.
		058. **Cleaning of pets or things they contacted.** Examples: frequent shampooing of dog and ritualized scouring of kitty litterbox.
		059. **Other measures to prevent or remove contact with contaminants.** Examples: wears rubber gloves, doesn't shake hands, has one clean and one dirty hand, won't go near anyone who seems to have a cut, won't sit down in a chair that has a red spot (possibly blood). Some of the compulsions listed here may overlap with avoidance behavior. If in doubt, count as compulsions (symptoms items 56 and/or 57) and as avoidance behavior under Severity item 11.
		060. **Ritualized avoidance to prevent contamination.** Examples: avoids public restrooms, stays at least 1 mile from chemical factories, won't open letters postmarked from New Jersey.

Last 30 days	Past	Checking Compulsions
		061. **Checking locks, stove, appliances, emergency brake, faucets, etc.**
		062. **Checking that did not/will not harm others.**
		063. **Checking that did not/will not harm self.**
		064. **Checking that nothing terrible did/will happen.**
		065. **Checking that did not make mistake.**
		066. **Checking tied to somatic obsessions.*** Examples: repeatedly probing groin to see if hernia is present; scrutinizing skin for signs of cancer; excessive exploration of lymph nodes. *Distinguish from Hypochondriasis.
		067. **Checking personal appearance.*** Example: looking in mirror to see if hair is combed evenly or there are signs of disease or contamination. Distinguish from *BDD in which concern is with perceived defects in appearance.
		068. **Other.**

Last 30 days	Past	Arranging, Counting, & Repeating Rituals
		069. **Need to repeat routine activities.** Examples: taking clothes on/off; relighting cigarette, turning car on/off, in/out chair, up/down stairs; may have to repeat a certain number of times.
		070. **Need to repeat boundary crossings.** Examples: going through doorway, crossing state lines; may get stuck trying to enter a building.
		071. **Evening up behaviors.** Examples: movement on right side of body has to be balanced with same movement on left side; adjusts height of stockings, tension of shoe laces.
		072. **Re-reading* or re-writing.** Distinguish from *dyslexia.
		073. **Counting compulsions.** Examples: counting things like ceiling or floor tiles, books in a bookcase, words in a sentence.
		074. **Ritualized routines.** Example: may have to put clothes on in a certain order or can only go to bed after following an elaborate series of steps.
		075. **Excessive religious rituals.** Example: Repeating prayers or passages from the Bible an inordinate number of times.
		076. **Ordering or arranging compulsions.** Example: straightening piles of stationery on a desktop or adjusting books in a bookcase.
		077. **Repeating what someone else has said.*** Example: word, phrase, or sound. *Distinguish from echolalia of TS.
		078. **Having to say something over and over again in just the same way.**
		079. **Asking for reassurance.** Example: repeatedly asking spouse that they performed a routine correctly.
		080. **Ritualized eating behaviors.*** Examples: arrange or eat food in particular way or a specific order to avert a feared consequence other than gaining weight as in *anorexia nervosa.
		081. **Other.**

Last 30 days	Past	Hoarding/Collecting Compulsions
		082. **Saves or collects useless items.** Examples: piles up old newspapers, collects useless objects; house can become obstacle course with piles of trash. *Distinguish from hobbies and concern with objects of monetary or sentimental value.

Last 30 days	Past	Hoarding/Collecting Obsessions (continued)
		083. **Picks up things from the street.** Examples: shards of broken glass, nails, pieces of paper with writing on them.
		084. **Examines things that leave one's possession. Examples: sifts through garbage, ritual for washing off dinner plates to separate waste from accidentally lost items; won't throw out used disposable vacuum bags or the kitty litter; repeatedly checks wallet or pocketbook to make sure nothing was lost, reopens letters before they are mailed.**
		085. **Buys certain number of things.** Examples: always buys exactly three of any one item.
		086. **Buys extra items.*** Examples: at store sales may buy a few extra items in case they might be needed for future. *May not be symptom of OCD unless urge is strong and behavior has deleterious consequences for the individual (e.g., wastes a lot of money, or accumulates closets full of unnecessary items.

Last 30 days	Past	Other Compulsions
		087. **Need to tell, ask or confess things.** Examples: confessing to sins or wrongs that didn't commit; feels must describe every detail so that nothing is left out; repeats the same question in different ways to make sure it was understood.
		088. **Need to do something until it feels "just right."** Examples: tightens nuts until they break, combs hair until it feels just right, doesn't let go of handshake until feels a "click" that it's OK. Has no specific feared consequences in mind.
		089. **Need to touch, tap, or rub.*** Examples: urge to touch or run finger along surfaces or edges, lightly touches other people; taps a certain number of times; rubs against soft materials. May be difficult to distinguish from complex motor tics of *TS. If behaviors are preceded by an obsessive thought, endorse as compulsions here.
		090. **Staring or blinking rituals.*** May be difficult to distinguish from motor tics of *TS. If patient says has to blink a certain number or times or stare until a bad thought goes away, endorse as compulsions here.
		091. **Measures (excluding checking) to prevent harm to self.**
		092. **Measures (excluding checking) to prevent harm to others.**

Last 30 days	Past	Other Compulsions (continued)
		093. **Measures (excluding checking) to prevent terrible consequences.**
		094. **Measures (excluding checking) to relieve discomfort.** Example: turns light switch on/off until bad feeling dissipates—has no specific feared consequences in mind.
		095. **Superstitious behaviors.** Examples: steps over sidewalk cracks, spits after having a bad thought; makes sure sentences never contain 13 words; makes sign of the cross before dialing area code for New Jersey.
		096. **Mental rituals (other than checking or counting).** Examples: silently reciting prayers or nonsense words to neutralize bad thoughts.
		097. **Pervasive slowness.** Extensive difficulty in starting, executing, and finishing a wide range of routines tasks. In extreme cases, may be unable to complete tasks without assistance and may become "paralyzed". *Distinguish from psychomotor retardation secondary to depression or as a sign of Parkinson's Disease.
		098. **Hairpulling.*** Examples: Urge to pull hair from scalp or face for a certain reason, such as, making moustache or eyebrows even, or to neutralize a bad thought. May be difficult to distinguish from *Trichotillomania, which should not be rated as a form of OCD. In general, hairpulling in Trichotillomania is best described as a habit.
		099. **Compulsions by proxy.** Insists that family members carry out rituals on the patient's behalf. May overlap with avoidance behavior.
		100. **Ritualized avoidance.** Examples: stays at least 1 mile away from chemical factories, won't buy or touch anything that comes from New Jersey.
		101. **Ritualized body movements.** Examples: particular gestures or movements that must be done in just the right manner.
		102. **Other.**

Y-BOCS Symptom Checklist © 2000 Wayne Goodman. Reprinted with permission.

Y-BOCS TARGET SYMPTOM LIST

OBSESSIONS:

1. _____
_____

2. _____
_____

3. _____
_____

4. _____
_____

COMPULSIONS:

1. _____
_____

2. _____
_____

3. _____
_____

4. _____
_____

AVOIDANCE:

1. _____
_____

2. _____
_____

3. _____
_____

4. _____
_____

APPENDIX

Yale–Brown Obsessive Compulsive Scale (Y-BOCS)

"I am now going to ask several questions about your obsessive thoughts." [Make specific reference to the patient's target obsessions.]

1. TIME OCCUPIED BY OBSESSIVE THOUGHTS

   Q: How much of your time is occupied by obsessive thoughts? [When obsessions occur as brief, intermittent intrusions, it may be difficult to assess time occupied by them in terms of total hours. In such cases, estimate time by determining how frequently they occur. Consider both the number of times the intrusions occur and how many hours of the day are affected. Ask:] How frequently do the obsessive thoughts occur? [Be sure to exclude ruminations and preoccupations which, unlike obsessions, are ego-syntonic and rational (but exaggerated).]

   0 = None.

   1 = Mild, less than 1 hr/day or occasional intrusion.

   2 = Moderate, 1 to 3 hrs/day or frequent intrusion.

   3 = Severe, greater than 3 and up to 8 hrs/day or very frequent intrusion.

   4 = Extreme, greater than 8 hrs/day or near constant intrusion.

1b. OBSESSION-FREE INTERVAL (not included in total score)

   Q: On the average, what is the longest number of consecutive waking hours per day that you are completely free of obsessive thoughts? [If necessary, ask:] What is the longest block of time in which obsessive thoughts are absent?

   0 = No symptoms.

   1 = Long symptom-free interval, more than 8 consecutive hours/day symptom-free.

   2 = Moderately long symptom-free interval, more than 3 and up to 8 consecutive hours/day symptom-free.

   3 = Short symptom-free interval, from 1 to 3 consecutive hours/day symptom-free.

   4 = Extremely short symptom-free interval, less than 1 consecutive hour/day symptom-free.

2. INTERFERENCE DUE TO OBSESSIVE THOUGHTS

   Q: How much do your obsessive thoughts interfere with your social or work (or role) functioning? Is there anything that you don't do because of them? [If currently not working determine how much performance would be affected if patient were employed.]

   0 = None.

   1 = Mild, slight interference with social or occupational activities, but overall performance not impaired.

   2 = Moderate, definite interference with social or occupational performance, but still manageable.

   3 = Severe, causes substantial impairment in social or occupational performance.

   4 = Extreme, incapacitating.

3. DISTRESS ASSOCIATED WITH OBSESSIVE THOUGHTS

   Q: How much distress do your obsessive thoughts cause you?

   [In most cases, distress is equated with anxiety; however, patients may report that their obsessions are "disturbing" but deny "anxiety." Only rate anxiety that seems triggered by obsessions, not generalized anxiety or anxiety associated with other conditions.]

0 = None
1 = Mild, not too disturbing
2 = Moderate, disturbing, but still manageable
3 = Severe, very disturbing
4 = Extreme, near constant and disabling distress

4. RESISTANCE AGAINST OBSESSIONS

Q: How much of an effort do you make to resist the obsessive thoughts? How often do you try to disregard or turn your attention away from these thoughts as they enter your mind? [Only rate effort made to resist, not success or failure in actually controlling the obsessions. How much the patient resists the obsessions may or may not correlate with his/her ability to control them. Note that this item does not directly measure the severity of the intrusive thoughts; rather it rates a manifestation of health, i.e., the effort the patient makes to counteract the obsessions by means other than avoidance or the performance of compulsions. Thus, the more the patient tries to resist, the less impaired is this aspect of his/her functioning. There are "active" and "passive" forms of resistance. Patients in behavioral therapy may be encouraged to counteract their obsessive symptoms by not struggling against them (e.g., "just let the thoughts come"; passive opposition) or by intentionally bringing on the disturbing thoughts. For the purposes of this item, consider use of these behavioral techniques as forms of resistance. If the obsessions are minimal, the patient may not feel the need to resist them. In such cases, a rating of "0" should be given.]

0 = Makes an effort to always resist, or symptoms so minimal doesn't need to actively resist
1 = Tries to resist most of the time
2 = Makes some effort to resist
3 = Yields to all obsessions without attempting to control them, but does so with some reluctance
4 = Completely and willingly yields to all obsessions

5. DEGREE OF CONTROL OVER OBSESSIVE THOUGHTS

Q: How much control do you have over your obsessive thoughts? How successful are you in stopping or diverting your obsessive thinking? Can you dismiss them? [In contrast to the preceding item on resistance, the ability of the patient to control his obsessions is more closely related to the severity of the intrusive thoughts.]

0 = Complete control
1 = Much control, usually able to stop or divert obsessions with some effort and concentration.
2 = Moderate control, sometimes able to stop or divert obsessions.
3 = Little control, rarely successful in stopping or dismissing obsessions, can only divert attention with difficulty.
4 = No control, experienced as completely involuntary, rarely able to even momentarily alter obsessive thinking.

"The next several questions are about your compulsive behaviors." [Make specific reference to the patient's target compulsions.]

6. TIME SPENT PERFORMING COMPULSIVE BEHAVIORS

Q: How much time do you spend performing compulsive behaviors? [When rituals involving activities of daily living are chiefly present, ask:] How much longer than most people does it take to complete routine activities because of your rituals? [When compulsions occur as brief, intermittent behaviors, it may difficult to assess time spent performing them in terms of total hours. In such cases, estimate time by determining how frequently they are performed. Consider both the number of times compulsions are performed and how many hours of the day are affected. Count separate occurrences of compulsive behaviors, not number of repetitions; e.g., a patient who goes into the bathroom 20 different times a day to wash his hands 5 times very quickly, performs compulsions 20 times a day, not 5 or $5 \times 20 = 100$. Ask:] How frequently do you perform compulsions? [In most cases compulsions are observable behaviors (e.g., hand washing), but some compulsions are covert (e.g., silent checking).]

0 = None
1 = Mild (spends less than 1 hr/day performing compulsions), or occasional performance of compulsive behaviors.
2 = Moderate (spends from 1 to 3 hrs/day performing compulsions), or frequent performance of compulsive behaviors.
3 = Severe (spends more than 3 and up to 8 hrs/day performing compulsions), or very frequent performance of compulsive behaviors.
4 = Extreme (spends more than 8 hrs/day performing compulsions), or near constant performance of compulsive behaviors (too numerous to count).

6b. COMPULSION-FREE INTERVAL (not included in total score)
Q: On the average, what is the longest number of consecutive waking hours per day that you are completely free of compulsive behavior? [If necessary, ask:] What is the longest block of time in which compulsions are absent?

0 = No symptoms.
1 = Long symptom-free interval, more than 8 consecutive hours/day symptom-free.
2 = Moderately long symptom-free interval, more than 3 and up to 8 consecutive hours/day symptom-free.
3 = Short symptom-free interval, from 1 to 3 consecutive hours/day symptom-free.
4 = Extremely short symptom-free interval, less than 1 consecutive hour/day symptom-free.

7. INTERFERENCE DUE TO COMPULSIVE BEHAVIORS
Q: How much do your compulsive behaviors interfere with your social or work (or role) functioning? Is there anything that you don't do because of the compulsions? [If currently not working determine how much performance would be affected if patient were employed.]

0 = None
1 = Mild, slight interference with social or occupational activities, but overall performance not impaired
2 = Moderate, definite interference with social or occupational performance, but still manageable
3 = Severe, causes substantial impairment in social or occupational performance
4 = Extreme, incapacitating

8. DISTRESS ASSOCIATED WITH COMPULSIVE BEHAVIOR
Q: How would you feel if prevented from performing your compulsion(s)? [Pause] How anxious would you become? [Rate degree of distress patient would experience if performance of the compulsion were suddenly interrupted without reassurance offered. In most,

but not all cases, performing compulsions reduces anxiety. If, in the judgment of the interviewer, anxiety is actually reduced by preventing compulsions in the manner described above, then ask:] How anxious do you get while performing compulsions until you are satisfied they are completed?

0 = None
1 = Mild only slightly anxious if compulsions prevented, or only slight anxiety during performance of compulsions
2 = Moderate, reports that anxiety would mount but remain manageable if compulsions prevented, or that anxiety increases but remains manageable during performance of compulsions
3 = Severe, prominent and very disturbing increase in anxiety if compulsions interrupted, or prominent and very disturbing increase in anxiety during performance of compulsions
4 = Extreme, incapacitating anxiety from any intervention aimed at modifying activity, or incapacitating anxiety develops during performance of compulsions

9. RESISTANCE AGAINST COMPULSIONS
Q: How much of an effort do you make to resist the compulsions? [Only rate effort made to resist, not success or failure in actually controlling the compulsions. How much the patient resists the compulsions may or may not correlate with his ability to control them. Note that this item does not directly measure the severity of the compulsions; rather it rates a manifestation of health, i.e., the effort the patient makes to counteract the compulsions. Thus, the more the patient tries to resist, the less impaired is this aspect of his functioning. If the compulsions are minimal, the patient may not feel the need to resist them. In such cases, a rating of "0" should be given.]

0 = Makes an effort to always resist, or symptoms so minimal doesn't need to actively resist
1 = Tries to resist most of the time
2 = Makes some effort to resist
3 = Yields to almost all compulsions without attempting to control them, but does so with some reluctance
4 = Completely and willingly yields to all compulsions

10. DEGREE OF CONTROL OVER COMPULSIVE BEHAVIOR
Q: How strong is the drive to perform the compulsive behavior? [Pause] How much control do you have over the compulsions? [In contrast to the preceding item on resistance, the ability of the patient to control his compulsions is more closely related to the severity of the compulsions.]

0 = Complete control
1 = Much control, experiences pressure to perform the behavior but usually able to exercise voluntary control over it
2 = Moderate control, strong pressure to perform behavior, can control it only with difficulty
3 = Little control, very strong drive to perform behavior, must be carried to completion, can only delay with difficulty
4 = No control, drive to perform behavior experienced as completely involuntary and overpowering, rarely able to even momentarily delay activity

Measures for Posttraumatic Stress Disorder

Accident Fear Questionnaire (AFQ)

Date of the accident (day/month/year)   ____/____/____

The following questions are about your motor vehicle accident and your reactions to it. This questionnaire only applies to you if you remember the accident.

	(Please circle)
Were you in a car, truck or on a cycle or a pedestrian?	YES / NO
Were you a passenger or the driver?	YES / NO
During the accident, did you fear for your life?	YES / NO
During the accident, did you see anyone injured or killed?	YES / NO
During the accident, did you lose consciousness?	YES / NO

Since the accident,

Do you have nightmares about the accident?	YES / NO
Are you nervous before trips?	YES / NO
Do you easily get upset in the car?	YES / NO
Do you tell the driver what to do?	YES / NO
Do you drive less than you used to?	YES / NO
Do you expect another accident soon?	YES / NO
Would most people feel after an accident the way you do?	YES / NO

Instructions: How much do you avoid the situations listed below because of fear or distress? For each question, please pick a number from the scale below to show how much you avoid the situation. Then write the number on the line opposite the situation.

0	1	2	3	4	5	6	7	8
Would not avoid it		*would sometimes avoid it*				*would often avoid it*		*would always avoid it*

Since your accident, do you avoid:

Driving as a passenger . . . . ____

Driving yourself . . . . ____

Riding in a particular seat . . . . ____

Driving on certain roads . . . . ____

Riding with certain drivers . . . . ____

Driving in certain weather conditions . . . . ____

Hearing news of accidents . . . . ____

Seeing wounds and injuries . . . . ____

Crossing streets alone . . . . ____

Riding a bus or streetcar . . . . ____

To what extent does physical illness such as back pain or stomach problems interfere with your life? (Please circle the most appropriate number, from 0 for "not at all" to 8 for "severe").

0   1   2   3   4   5   6   7   8

From Kuch, K., Cox, B.J., & Direnfeld, D.M. (1995). A brief self-rating scale for PTSD after road vehicle accident. *Journal of Anxiety Disorders*, *9*, 503–514. Reprinted with permission from Elsevier Science and Klaus Kuch, M.D.

Dissociative Experiences Scale (DES)

DIRECTIONS: This questionnaire consists of twenty-eight questions about experiences that you may have in your daily life. We are interested in how often you have these experiences. It is important, however, that your answers show how often these experiences happen to you when you **are not** under the influence of alcohol or drugs. To answer the questions, please determine to what degree the experience described in the question applies to you and circle the number to show what percentage of the time you have the experience.

EXAMPLE:

0%	10	20	30	40	50	60	70	80	90	100%
(never)										(always)

1. Some people have the experience of driving or riding in a car or bus or subway and suddenly realizing that they don't remember what has happened during all or part of the trip. Circle a number to show what percentage of the time this happens to you.

0%	10	20	30	40	50	60	70	80	90	100%

2. Some people find that sometimes they are listening to someone talk and they suddenly realize that they did not hear part or all of what was said. Circle a number to show what percentage of the time this happens to you.

0%	10	20	30	40	50	60	70	80	90	100%

3. Some people have the experience of finding themselves in a place and having no idea how they got there. Circle a number to show what percentage of the time this happens to you.

0%	10	20	30	40	50	60	70	80	90	100%

4. Some people have the experience of finding themselves dressed in clothes that they don't remember putting on. Circle a number to show what percentage of the time this happens to you.

0%	10	20	30	40	50	60	70	80	90	100%

5. Some people have the experience of finding new things among their belongings that they do not remember buying. Circle a number to show what percentage of the time this happens to you.

0%	10	20	30	40	50	60	70	80	90	100%

6. Some people sometimes find that they are approached by people that they do not know who call them by another name or insist that they have met them before. Circle a number to show what percentage of the time this happens to you.

0%	10	20	30	40	50	60	70	80	90	100%

7. Some people sometimes have the experience of feeling as though they are standing next to themselves or watching themselves do something and they actually see themselves as if they were looking at another person. Circle a number to show what percentage of the time this happens to you.

0%	10	20	30	40	50	60	70	80	90	100%

8. Some people are told that they sometimes do not recognize friends or family members. Circle a number to show what percentage of the time this happens to you.

0%	10	20	30	40	50	60	70	80	90	100%

9. Some people find that they have no memory for some important events in their lives (for example, a wedding or graduation). Circle a number to show what percentage of the time this happens to you.

0%   10   20   30   40   50   60   70   80   90   100%

10. Some people have the experience of being accused of lying when they do not think that they have lied. Circle a number to show what percentage of the time this happens to you.

0%   10   20   30   40   50   60   70   80   90   100%

11. Some people have the experience of looking in a mirror and not recognizing themselves. Circle a number to show what percentage of the time this happens to you.

0%   10   20   30   40   50   60   70   80   90   100%

12. Some people have the experience of feeling that other people, objects, and the world around them are not real. Circle a number to show what percentage of the time this happens to you.

0%   10   20   30   40   50   60   70   80   90   100%

13. Some people have the experience of feeling that their body does not seem to belong to them. Circle a number to show what percentage of the time this happens to you.

0%   10   20   30   40   50   60   70   80   90   100%

14. Some people have the experience of sometimes remembering a past event so vividly that they feel as if they were reliving that event. Circle a number to show what percentage of the time this happens to you.

0%   10   20   30   40   50   60   70   80   90   100%

15. Some people have the experience of not being sure whether things that they remember happening really did happen or whether they just dreamed them. Circle a number to show what percentage of the time this happens to you.

0%   10   20   30   40   50   60   70   80   90   100%

16. Some people have the experience of being in a familiar place but finding it strange and unfamiliar. Circle a number to show what percentage of the time this happens to you.

0%   10   20   30   40   50   60   70   80   90   100%

17. Some people find that when they are watching television or a movie they become so absorbed in the story that they are unaware of other events happening around them. Circle a number to show what percentage of the time this happens to you.

0%   10   20   30   40   50   60   70   80   90   100%

18. Some people find that they become so involved in a fantasy or daydream that it feels as though it were really happening to them. Circle a number to show what percentage of the time this happens to you.

0%   10   20   30   40   50   60   70   80   90   100%

19. Some people find that they sometimes are able to ignore pain. Circle a number to show what percentage of the time this happens to you.

0%   10   20   30   40   50   60   70   80   90   100%

20. Some people find that that they sometimes sit staring off into space, thinking of nothing, and are not aware of the passage of time. Circle a number to show what percentage of the time this happens to you.

0%　　10　　20　　30　　40　　50　　60　　70　　80　　90　　100%

21. Some people sometimes find that when they are alone they talk out loud to themselves. Circle a number to show what percentage of the time this happens to you.

0%　　10　　20　　30　　40　　50　　60　　70　　80　　90　　100%

22. Some people find that in one situation they may act so differently compared with another situation that they feel almost as if they were two different people. Circle a number to show what percentage of the time this happens to you.

0%　　10　　20　　30　　40　　50　　60　　70　　80　　90　　100%

23. Some people sometimes find that in certain situations they are able to do things with amazing ease and spontaneity that would usually be difficult for them (for example, sports, work, social situations, etc.). Circle a number to show what percentage of the time this happens to you.

0%　　10　　20　　30　　40　　50　　60　　70　　80　　90　　100%

24. Some people sometimes find that they cannot remember whether they have done something or have just thought about doing that thing (for example, not knowing whether they have just mailed a letter or have just thought about mailing it). Circle a number to show what percentage of the time this happens to you.

0%　　10　　20　　30　　40　　50　　60　　70　　80　　90　　100%

25. Some people find evidence that they have done things that they do not remember doing. Circle a number to show what percentage of the time this happens to you.

0%　　10　　20　　30　　40　　50　　60　　70　　80　　90　　100%

26. Some people sometimes find writings, drawings, or notes among their belongings that they must have done but cannot remember doing. Circle a number to show what percentage of the time this happens to you.

0%　　10　　20　　30　　40　　50　　60　　70　　80　　90　　100%

27. Some people sometimes find that they hear voices inside their head that tell them to do things or comment on things that they are doing. Circle a number to show what percentage of the time this happens to you.

0%　　10　　20　　30　　40　　50　　60　　70　　80　　90　　100%

28. Some people sometimes feel as if they are looking at the world through a fog so that people and objects appear far away or unclear. Circle a number to show what percentage of the time this happens to you.

0%　　10　　20　　30　　40　　50　　60　　70　　80　　90　　100%

From Bernstein, E.M., & Putnam, F.W. (1986). Development, reliability and validity of a dissociation scale. *Journal of Nervous and Mental Disease, 174*, 727–735, and Carlson, E.B., & Putnam, F.W. (1993). An update on the Dissociative Experiences Scale. *Dissociation, 6*, 16–27. Reprinted with permission from Lippincott, Williams & Wilkins, Ridgeview Institute, and Eve Bernstein Carlson, Ph.D.

Impact of Event Scale (IES)

On _____ you experienced _____
    (date)   (life event)

Below is a list of comments made by people after stressful life events. Please check each item, indicating how frequently these comments were true for you *DURING THE PAST SEVEN DAYS*. If they did not occur during that time, please mark the "not at all" column.

FREQUENCY

	Not at All	Rarely	Sometimes	Often
1. I thought about it when I didn't mean to.				
2. I avoided letting myself get upset when I thought about it or was reminded of it.				
3. I tried to remove it from memory.				
4. I had trouble falling asleep or staying asleep, because of pictures or thoughts about it that came into my mind.				
5. I had waves of strong feelings about it.				
6. I had dreams about it.				
7. I stayed away from reminders of it.				
8. I felt as if it hadn't happened or it wasn't real.				
9. I tried not to talk about it.				
10. Pictures about it popped into my mind.				
11. Other things kept making me think about it.				
12. I was aware that I still had a lot of feelings about it, but I didn't deal with them.				
13. I tried not to think about it.				
14. Any reminder brought back feelings about it.				
15. My feelings about it were kind of numb.				

From Horowitz, M., Wilner, N., & Alvarez, W. (1979). Impact of Event Scale: A measure of subjective stress. *Psychosomatic Medicine, 41*, 209–218. Reprinted with permission from Lippincott, Williams & Wilkins, and Mardi Horowitz, M.D.

Los Angeles Symptom Checklist (LASC)

Below is a list of problems. Rate each one on a scale of 0 to 4 according to how much of a problem that item is for you. A rating of zero would mean that the item is not a problem for you; one, a slight problem; two, a moderate problem; three, a serious problem; and four, an extreme problem.

0	1	2	3	4
Not a problem	Slight problem	Moderate problem	Serious problem	Extreme problem

_____ 1. difficulty falling asleep

_____ 2. abusive drinking

_____ 3. severe headaches

_____ 4. restlessness

_____ 5. nightmares

_____ 6. difficulty finding a job

_____ 7. difficulty holding a job

_____ 8. irritability

_____ 9. pervasive disgust

_____ 10. momentary blackouts

_____ 11. abdominal discomfort

_____ 12. management of money

_____ 13. trapped in an unsatisfying job

_____ 14. physical disabilities or medical problems. Explain: _____
_____

_____ 15. hostility/violence

_____ 16. marital problems

_____ 17. easily fatigued

_____ 18. drug abuse

_____ 19. inability to express feelings

_____ 20. tension and anxiety

_____ 21. no leisure activities

_____ 22. suicidal thoughts

_____ 23. vivid memories of unpleasant prior experiences

_____ 24. excessive eating

_____ 25. difficulty concentrating

_____ 26. dizziness/fainting

_____ 27. sexual problems

_____ 28. waking during the night

_____ 29. difficulty with memory

_____ 30. marked self-consciousness

_____ 31. depression

_____ 32. inability to make and keep same sex friends

_____ 33. inability to make and keep opposite sex friends

_____ 34. excessive jumpiness

_____ 35. waking early in the morning

_____ 36. loss of weight/appetite

_____ 37. heart palpitations

_____ 38. panic attacks

_____ 39. problems with authority

_____ 40. avoidance of activities that remind you of prior unpleasant experiences

_____ 41. trouble trusting others

_____ 42. loss of interest in usual activities

_____ 43. feeling emotionally numb

How long have you been bothered by these symptoms? _____

Civilian Mississippi Scale

Please circle the number that best describes how you feel about each statement.

1. In the past, I had more close friends than I have now.

1	2	3	4	5
Not at all True	Slightly True	Somewhat True	Very True	Extremely True

2. I feel guilt over things that I did in the past.

1	2	3	4	5
Never True	Rarely True	Sometimes True	Usually True	Always True

3. If someone pushes me too far, I become verbally or physically aggressive.

1	2	3	4	5
Very Unlikely	Unlikely	Somewhat Un-likely	Very Likely	Extremely Likely

4. If something happens that reminds me of the past, I become very distressed and upset.

1	2	3	4	5
Never	Rarely	Sometimes	Frequently	Very Frequently

5. The people who know me best are afraid of me.

1	2	3	4	5
Never True	Rarely True	Sometimes True	Frequently True	Very Frequently True

6. I am able to get emotionally close to others.

1	2	3	4	5
Never	Rarely	Sometimes	Frequently	Very Frequently

7. I have nightmares of experiences in my past that really happened.

1	2	3	4	5
Never	Rarely	Sometimes	Frequently	Very Frequently

8. When I think of some of the things that I did in the past, I wish I were dead.

1	2	3	4	5
Never True	Rarely True	Sometimes True	Frequently True	Very Frequently True

9. It seems as if I have no feelings.

1	2	3	4	5
Not at all True	Rarely True	Sometimes True	Frequently True	Very Frequently True

10. Lately, I have felt like killing myself.

1	2	3	4	5
Not at all True	Slightly True	Somewhat True	Very True	Extremely True

11. I fall asleep, stay asleep, and feel rested when I awaken.

1	2	3	4	5
Never	Rarely	Sometimes	Frequently	Very Frequently

12. I wonder why I am still alive when others have died.

1	2	3	4	5
Never	Rarely	Sometimes	Frequently	Very Frequently

13. Being in certain situations makes me feel as though I am back in the past.

1	2	3	4	5
Never	Rarely	Sometimes	Frequently	Very Frequently

14. My dreams at night are so real that I waken in a cold sweat and force myself to stay awake.

1	2	3	4	5
Never	Rarely	Sometimes	Frequently	Very Frequently

15. I feel like I cannot go on.

1	2	3	4	5
Not at all True	Rarely True	Sometimes True	Very True	Almost Always True

16. I do not laugh or cry at the same things other people do.

1	2	3	4	5
Not at all True	Rarely True	Somewhat True	Very True	Extremely True

17. I still enjoy doing many things that I used to enjoy.

1	2	3	4	5
Never True	Rarely True	Sometimes True	Very True	Always True

18. Daydreams are very real and frightening.

1	2	3	4	5
Never True	Rarely True	Sometimes True	Frequently True	Very Frequently True

19. I have found it easy to keep a job.

1	2	3	4	5
Not at all True	Slightly True	Somewhat True	Very True	Extremely True

20. I have trouble concentrating on tasks.

1	2	3	4	5
Never True	Rarely True	Sometimes True	Frequently True	Very Frequently True

21. I have cried for no good reason.

1	2	3	4	5
Never	Rarely	Sometimes	Frequently	Very Frequently

22. I enjoy the company of others.

1	2	3	4	5
Never	Rarely	Sometimes	Frequently	Very Frequently

23. I am frightened by my urges.

1	2	3	4	5
Never	Rarely	Sometimes	Frequently	Very Frequently

24. I fall asleep easily at night.

1	2	3	4	5
Never	Rarely	Sometimes	Frequently	Very Frequently

25. Unexpected noises make me jump.

1	2	3	4	5
Never	Rarely	Sometimes	Frequently	Very Frequently

26. No one understands how I feel, not even my family.

1	2	3	4	5
Not at all True	Rarely True	Sometimes True	Very True	Extremely True

27. I am an easy-going, even-tempered person.

1	2	3	4	5
Never	Rarely	Sometimes	Usually	Very Much so

28. I feel there are certain things that I have done that I can never tell anyone, because no ever one would understand.

1	2	3	4	5
Not at all True	Slightly True	Somewhat True	Very True	Extremely True

29. There have been times when I used alcohol (or other drugs) to help me sleep or to make me forget about things that happened in the past.

1	2	3	4	5
Never	Infrequently	Sometimes	Frequently	Very Frequently

30. I feel comfortable when I am in a crowd.

1	2	3	4	5
Never	Rarely	Sometimes	Usually	Always

31. I lose my cool and explode over minor everyday things.

1	2	3	4	5
Never	Rarely	Sometimes	Frequently	Very Frequently

32. I am afraid to go to sleep at night.

1	2	3	4	5
Never	Rarely	Sometimes	Frequently	Almost Always

33. I try to stay away from anything that will remind me of things which happened in the past.

1	2	3	4	5
Never	Rarely	Sometimes	Frequently	Almost Always

34. My memory is as good as it ever was.

1	2	3	4	5
Not at all True	Rarely True	Somewhat True	Usually True	Almost Always True

35. I have a hard time expressing my feelings, even to the people I care about.

1	2	3	4	5
Not at all True	Rarely True	Sometimes True	Frequently True	Almost Always True

Reprinted with permission from Terence Keane, Ph.D.

Posttraumatic Cognitions Inventory (PTCI)

We are interested in the kind of thoughts which you may have had after a traumatic experience. Below are a number of statements that may or may not be representative of your thinking. Please read each statement carefully and tell us how much you AGREE or DISAGREE with each statement.
People react to traumatic events in many different ways. There are no right or wrong answers to these statements.

1 *Totally disagree*   5 *Agree slightly*
2 *Disagree very much*   6 *Agree very much*
3 *Disagree slightly*   7 *Totally agree*
4 *Neutral*

_____ 1. The event happened because of the way I acted.

_____ 2. I can't trust that I will do the right thing.

_____ 3. I am a weak person.

_____ 4. I will not be able to control my anger and will do something terrible.

_____ 5. I can't deal with even the slightest upset.

_____ 6. I used to be a happy person but now I am always miserable.

_____ 7. People can't be trusted.

_____ 8. I have to be on guard all the time.

_____ 9. I feel dead inside.

_____ 10. You can never know who will harm you.

_____ 11. I have to be especially careful because you never know what can happen next.

_____ 12. I am inadequate.

_____ 13. I will not be able to control my emotions, and something terrible will happen.

_____ 14. If I think about the event, I will not be able to handle it.

_____ 15. The event happened to me because of the sort of person I am.

_____ 16. My reactions since the event mean that I am going crazy.

_____ 17. I will never be able to feel normal emotions again.

_____ 18. The world is a dangerous place.

_____ 19. Somebody else would have stopped the event from happening.

_____ 20. I have permanently changed for the worse.

_____ 21. I feel like an object, not like a person.

_____ 22. Somebody else would not have gotten into this situation.

_____ 23. I can't rely on other people.

_____ 24. I feel isolated and set apart from others.

_____ 25. I have no future.

_____ 26. I can't stop bad things from happening to me.

_____ 27. People are not what they seem.

_____ 28. My life has been destroyed by the trauma.

_____ 29. There is something wrong with me as a person.

1 *Totally disagree*   5 *Agree slightly*
2 *Disagree very much*   6 *Agree very much*
3 *Disagree slightly*   7 *Totally agree*
4 *Neutral*

_____ 30. My reactions since the event show that I am a lousy coper.

_____ 31. There is something about me that made the event happen.

_____ 32. I will not be able to tolerate my thoughts about the event, and I will fall apart.

_____ 33. I feel like I don't know myself anymore.

_____ 34. You never know when something terrible will happen.

_____ 35. I can't rely on myself.

_____ 36. Nothing good can happen to me anymore.

PTSD Checklist-Civilian (PCL-C)

Instructions: Below is a list of problems and complaints that people sometimes have in response to stressful life experiences. Please read each one carefully, then circle one of the numbers to the right to indicate how much you have been bothered by that problem <u>in the past</u> <u>month</u>.

	Not at all	A little bit	Moderately	Quite a bit	Extremely
1. Repeated, disturbing memories, thoughts, or images of a stressful experience from the past?	1	2	3	4	5
2. Repeated, disturbing dreams of a stressful experience from the past?	1	2	3	4	5
3. Suddenly acting or feeling as if a stressful experience from the past were happening again (as if you were reliving it)?	1	2	3	4	5
4. Feeling very upset when something reminded you of a stressful experience from the past?	1	2	3	4	5
5. Having physical reactions (e.g. heart pounding, trouble breathing, sweating) when something reminded you of a stressful experience from the past?	1	2	3	4	5
6. Avoiding thinking or talking about a stressful experience from the past or avoiding having feelings related to it?	1	2	3	4	5
7. Avoiding activities or situations because they remind you of a stressful experience from the past?	1	2	3	4	5
8. Trouble remembering important parts of a stressful experience from the past?	1	2	3	4	5
9. Loss of interest in activities that you used to enjoy?	1	2	3	4	5
10. Feeling distant or cut off from other people?	1	2	3	4	5

APPENDIX

	Not at all	A little bit	Moderately	Quite a bit	Extremely
11. Feeling emotionally numb or being unable to have loving feelings for those close to you?	1	2	3	4	5
12. Feeling as if your future somehow will be cut short?	1	2	3	4	5
13. Trouble falling or staying asleep?	1	2	3	4	5
14. Feeling irritable or having angry outbursts?	1	2	3	4	5
15. Having difficulty concentrating?	1	2	3	4	5
16. Being "superalert" or watchful or on guard?	1	2	3	4	5
17. Feeling jumpy or easily startled?	1	2	3	4	5

APPENDIX

Reprinted with permission from Frank Weathers, Ph.D.

Purdue PTSD Scale-Revised (PPTSD-R)

These questions ask about your reactions to the event listed at the bottom of the previous page. Please answer each question for how often each reaction occurred <u>during</u> <u>the</u> <u>previous</u> <u>month</u>. Circle the appropriate letter for each question.

In <u>the last month</u>, how often ...

	not at all	sometimes			often
1. were you bothered by memories or thoughts of the event when you didn't want to think about it?	A	B	C	D	E
2. have you had upsetting dreams about the event?	A	B	C	D	E
3. have you suddenly felt as if you were experiencing the event again?	A	B	C	D	E
4. did you feel very upset when something happened to remind you of the event?	A	B	C	D	E
5. did you avoid activities or situations that might remind you of the event?	A	B	C	D	E
6. did you avoid thoughts or feelings about the event?	A	B	C	D	E
7. did you have difficulty remembering important aspects of the event?	A	B	C	D	E
8. did you react physically (heart racing, breaking out in a sweat) to things that reminded you of the event?	A	B	C	D	E

Since <u>the event</u> ...

	not at all	sometimes			often
9. have you lost interest in one or more of your usual activities (e.g., work, hobbies, entertainment)?	A	B	C	D	E
10. have you felt unusually distant or cut off from people?	A	B	C	D	E
11. have you felt emotionally "numb" or unable to respond to things emotionally the way you used to?	A	B	C	D	E
12. have you been less optimistic about your future?	A	B	C	D	E
13. have you had more trouble sleeping?	A	B	C	D	E
14. have you been more irritable or angry?	A	B	C	D	E
15. have you had more trouble concentrating?	A	B	C	D	E
16. have you found yourself watchful or on guard, even when there was no reason to be?	A	B	C	D	E
17. are you more jumpy or easily startled by noises?	A	B	C	D	E

Reprinted with permission from Dean Lauterbach, Ph.D.

Short Screening Scale for DSM-IV PTSD

1. Did you avoid being reminded of this experience by staying away from certain places, people or activities? (REMIND RESPONDENT OF LIFE EVENT IF NECESSARY.)

   1. YES

   2. NO

2. Did you lose interest in activities that were once important or enjoyable? (REMIND RESPONDENT OF LIFE EVENT IF NECESSARY.)

   1. YES

   2. NO

3. Did you begin to feel more isolated or distant from other people? (REMIND RESPONDENT OF LIFE EVENT IF NECESSARY.)

   1. YES

   2. NO

4. Did you find it hard to have love or affection for other people? (REMIND RESPONDENT OF LIFE EVENT IF NECESSARY.)

   1. YES

   2. NO

5. Did you begin to feel that there was no point in planning for the future? (REMIND RESPONDENT OF LIFE EVENT IF NECESSARY.)

   1. YES

   2. NO

6. After this experience were you having more trouble than usual falling asleep or staying asleep? (REMIND RESPONDENT OF LIFE EVENT IF NECESSARY.)

   1. YES

   2. NO

7. Did you become jumpy or get easily startled by ordinary noises or movements? (REMIND RESPONDENT OF LIFE EVENT IF NECESSARY.)

   1. YES

   2. NO

Reprinted with permission from the authors of the Diagnostic Interview Schedule for DSM-IV (DIS-IV): Lee Robins, Linda Cottler, Kathleen Bucholz, and Wilson Compton, and with permission from Naomi Breslau.

Stanford Acute Stress Reaction Questionnaire (SASRQ)

DIRECTIONS: Recall the stressful events that occurred during _____
Briefly describe the one event that was most disturbing below:

_____

_____

_____

_____

How disturbing was this event to you? (Please mark one):

Not at all disturbing   _____
Somewhat disturbing   _____
Moderately disturbing   _____
Very disturbing   _____
Extremely disturbing   _____

DIRECTIONS: Below is a list of experiences people sometimes have during and after a stressful event. Please read each item carefully and decide how well it describes your experience during _____ described above. Refer to this event in answering the items that mention "the stressful event." Use the 0–5 point scale shown below and circle the number that best describes your experience.

0	1	2	3	4	5
not experienced	very rarely experienced	rarely experienced	sometimes experienced	often experienced	very often experienced

1. I had difficulty falling or staying asleep. 0 1 2 3 4 5

2. I felt restless. 0 1 2 3 4 5

3. I felt a sense of timelessness. 0 1 2 3 4 5

4. I was slow to respond. 0 1 2 3 4 5

5. I tried to avoid feelings about the event. 0 1 2 3 4 5

6. I had repeated distressing dreams of the stressful event. 0 1 2 3 4 5

7. I felt extremely upset if exposed to events that reminded me of an aspect of the stressful event. 0 1 2 3 4 5

8. I would jump in surprise at the least thing. 0 1 2 3 4 5

9. The stressful event made it difficult for me to perform work or other things I needed to do. 0 1 2 3 4 5

10. I did not have the usual sense of who I am. 0 1 2 3 4 5

11. I tried to avoid activities that reminded me of the stressful event. 0 1 2 3 4 5

12. I felt hypervigilant or "on edge." 0 1 2 3 4 5

13. I experienced myself as though I were a stranger. 0 1 2 3 4 5

14. I tried to avoid conversations about the event. 0 1 2 3 4 5

15. I had a bodily reaction when exposed to reminders of the stressful event. 0 1 2 3 4 5

0	1	2	3	4	5
not experienced	very rarely experienced	rarely experienced	sometimes experienced	often experienced	very often experienced

16. I had problems remembering important details about the stressful event.　　0 1 2 3 4 5

17. I tried to avoid thoughts about the stressful event.　　0 1 2 3 4 5

18. Things I saw looked different to me from how I know they really looked.　　0 1 2 3 4 5

19. I had repeated and unwanted memories of the event.　　0 1 2 3 4 5

20. I felt distant from my own emotions.　　0 1 2 3 4 5

21. I felt irritable or had outbursts of anger.　　0 1 2 3 4 5

22. I avoided contact with people who reminded me of the stressful event.　　0 1 2 3 4 5

23. I would suddenly act or feel as if the stressful event were happening again.　　0 1 2 3 4 5

24. My mind went blank.　　0 1 2 3 4 5

25. I had amnesia for large periods of the event.　　0 1 2 3 4 5

26. The stressful event caused problems in my relationships with other people.　　0 1 2 3 4 5

27. I had difficulty concentrating.　　0 1 2 3 4 5

28. I felt estranged or detached from other people.　　0 1 2 3 4 5

29. I had a vivid sense that the event was happening all over again　　0 1 2 3 4 5

30. I tried to stay away from places that remind me of the event.　　0 1 2 3 4 5

How many days did you experience the worst symptoms of distress? (Please mark one):

none _____
one _____
two _____
three _____
four _____
five or more _____

Reprinted with permission from Etzel Cardeña, Ph.D.

Traumatic Events Questionnaire (TEQ)

DIRECTIONS: This questionnaire is comprised of a variety of traumatic events which you may have experienced. For each of the following "numbered" questions, indicate whether or not you experienced the event. If you have experienced one of the events, circle "Yes" and complete the "lettered" items immediately following it that ask for more details. If you have not experienced the event, circle "No" and go to the next "numbered" item.

No Yes 1. **Have you been in or witnessed a serious industrial, farm, or car accident, or a large fire or explosion?**

    a. How many times? Once ☐ twice ☐ three + ☐

    b. How old were you at that time(s)? 1st _____ 2nd _____ 3rd _____

    c. Were you injured?

    Not at all   Severely

      1 2 3 4 5 6 7

    d. Did you feel your life was threatened?

    Not at all   Extremely

      1 2 3 4 5 6 7

    e. How traumatic **was** this for you at that time?

    Not at all   Extremely

      1 2 3 4 5 6 7

    f. How traumatic **is** this for you now?

    Not at all   Extremely

      1 2 3 4 5 6 7

    g. What was the event? _____

No Yes 2. **Have you been in a natural disaster such as a tornado, hurricane, flood or major earthquake?**

    a. How many times? Once ☐ twice ☐ three + ☐

    b. How old were you at that time(s)? 1st _____ 2nd _____ 3rd _____

    c. Were you injured?

    Not at all   Severely

      1 2 3 4 5 6 7

    d. Did you feel your life was threatened?

    Not at all   Extremely

      1 2 3 4 5 6 7

    e. How traumatic **was** this for you at that time?

    Not at all   Extremely

      1 2 3 4 5 6 7

    f. How traumatic **is** this for you now?

    Not at all   Extremely

      1 2 3 4 5 6 7

    g. What was the event? _____

No Yes **3. Have you been a victim of a violent crime such as rape, robbery, or assault?**

a. How many times? Once ☐ twice ☐ three + ☐

b. How old were you at that time(s)? 1st _____ 2nd _____ 3rd _____

c. Were you injured?

Not at all   Severely
1 2 3 4 5 6 7

d. Did you feel your life was threatened?

Not at all   Extremely
1 2 3 4 5 6 7

e. How traumatic **was** this for you at that time?

Not at all   Extremely
1 2 3 4 5 6 7

f. How traumatic **is** this for you now?

Not at all   Extremely
1 2 3 4 5 6 7

g. What was the crime? _____

No Yes **4. As a child, were you the victim of either physical or sexual abuse?**

a. How old were you when it began? _____

b. How old were you when it ended? _____

c. Were you injured?

Not at all   Severely
1 2 3 4 5 6 7

d. Did you feel your life was threatened?

Not at all   Extremely
1 2 3 4 5 6 7

e. How traumatic **was** this for you at that time?

Not at all   Extremely
1 2 3 4 5 6 7

f. How traumatic **is** this for you now?

Not at all   Extremely
1 2 3 4 5 6 7

g. Was the assailant male or female? Male ☐ Female ☐

h. Check (✓) all categories that describe the experience ...
☐ physical abuse
☐ there was sexual penetration of the mouth, anus or vagina
☐ there was no sexual penetration, but the assailant attempted to force you to complete such an act
☐ there was some other form of sexual contact e.g., touched your sexual organs, or forced to touch assailant's sexual organs
☐ no sexual contact occurred, however, the assailant attempted to touch your sexual organs, or make you touch his/her sexual organs

No Yes 5. **As an adult, have you had any unwanted sexual experiences that involved the threat or use of force?**

a. How many times? Once ☐   twice ☐   three + ☐

b. How old were you at that time(s)? 1st _____ 2nd _____ 3rd _____

c. Were you injured?

Not at all   Severely
 1   2   3   4   5   6   7

d. Did you feel your life was threatened?

Not at all   Extremely
 1   2   3   4   5   6   7

e. How traumatic **was** this for you at that time?

Not at all   Extremely
 1   2   3   4   5   6   7

f. How traumatic **is** this for you now?

Not at all   Extremely
 1   2   3   4   5   6   7

g. Was the assailant male or female? Male ☐ Female ☐

h. Check (✓) all categories that describe the experience ...

☐ there was sexual penetration of the mouth, anus or vagina

☐ there was no sexual penetration, but the assailant attempted to force you to complete such an act

☐ there was some other form of sexual contact e.g., touched your sexual organs, or forced to touch assailant's sexual organs

☐ no sexual contact occurred, however, the assailant attempted to touch your sexual organs, or make you touch his/her sexual organs

No Yes 6. **As an adult, have you ever been in a relationship in which you were abused either physically or otherwise?**

a. How old were you when it began? _____

b. How old were you when it ended? _____

c. Were you injured?

Not at all   Severely
 1   2   3   4   5   6   7

d. Did you feel your life was threatened?

Not at all   Extremely
 1   2   3   4   5   6   7

e. How traumatic **was** this for you at that time?

Not at all   Extremely
 1   2   3   4   5   6   7

f. How traumatic **is** this for you now?

Not at all   Extremely
 1   2   3   4   5   6   7

No Yes   **7. Have you witnessed someone who was mutilated, seriously injured, or violently killed?**

→ a. How many times? Once ☐ twice ☐ three + ☐

b. How old were you at that time(s)? 1st _____ 2nd _____ 3rd _____

c. Were you injured?

Not at all   Severely
1   2   3   4   5   6   7

d. Did you feel your life was threatened?

Not at all   Extremely
1   2   3   4   5   6   7

e. How traumatic **was** this for you at that time?

Not at all   Extremely
1   2   3   4   5   6   7

f. How traumatic **is** this for you now?

Not at all   Extremely
1   2   3   4   5   6   7

No Yes   **8. Have you been in serious danger of losing your life or of being seriously injured?**

→ a. How many times? Once ☐ twice ☐ three + ☐

b. How old were you at that time(s)? 1st _____ 2nd _____ 3rd _____

c. Were you injured?

Not at all   Severely
1   2   3   4   5   6   7

d. Did you feel your life was threatened?

Not at all   Extremely
1   2   3   4   5   6   7

e. How traumatic **was** this for you at that time?

Not at all   Extremely
1   2   3   4   5   6   7

f. How traumatic **is** this for you now?

Not at all   Extremely
1   2   3   4   5   6   7

g. What was the event? _____

No Yes 9. Have you received news of the mutilation, serious injury, or violent or unexpected death of someone close to you?

    a. How many times? Once ☐   twice ☐   three + ☐

    b. How old were you at that time(s)? 1st _____ 2nd _____ 3rd _____

    c. What relation was this person to you? _____

    Not at all   Severely
       1   2   3   4   5   6   7

    d. Did you feel your life was threatened?

    Not at all   Extremely
       1   2   3   4   5   6   7

    e. How traumatic **was** this for you at that time?

    Not at all   Extremely
       1   2   3   4   5   6   7

    f. How traumatic **is** this for you now?

    Not at all   Extremely
       1   2   3   4   5   6   7

No Yes 10. Have you ever had any other very traumatic event like these?

    a. How many times? Once ☐   twice ☐   three + ☐

    b. How old were you at that time(s)? 1st _____ 2nd _____ 3rd _____

    c. Were you injured?

    Not at all   Severely
       1   2   3   4   5   6   7

    d. Did you feel your life was threatened?

    Not at all   Extremely
       1   2   3   4   5   6   7

    e. How traumatic **was** this for you at that time?

    Not at all   Extremely
       1   2   3   4   5   6   7

    f. How traumatic **is** this for you now?

    Not at all   Extremely
       1   2   3   4   5   6   7

    g. What was the event? _____

APPENDIX

No Yes 11. Have you had any experiences like these that you feel you can't tell about (note: you don't have to describe the event)?

           ⟶ a. How many times? Once ☐ twice ☐ three + ☐

               b. How old were you at that time(s)? 1st _____ 2nd _____ 3rd _____

               c. Were you injured?

                   Not at all   Severely

                     1 2 3 4 5 6 7

               d. Did you feel your life was threatened?

                   Not at all   Extremely

                     1 2 3 4 5 6 7

               e. How traumatic **was** this for you at that time?

                   Not at all   Extremely

                     1 2 3 4 5 6 7

               f. How traumatic **is** this for you now?

                   Not at all   Extremely

                     1 2 3 4 5 6 7

If you answered "Yes" to one or more of the questions above, which was the **MOST** traumatic thing to have happened to you? Fill in the number of the question (e.g., #2 for natural disaster). _____

Did you answer **Yes** to more than one question above while thinking about the same event? Yes ☐ No ☐
If yes, which items refer to the same event? _____

Go on to the next page and answer the PTSD Checklist based on your responses to the **most traumatic event** you reported (you won't need to give any more details about the event).

If you answered "No" to all questions, describe briefly the most traumatic thing to happen to you

_____

_____

_____

_____

a. How many times? Once ☐   twice ☐   three + ☐

b. How old were you at that time(s)? 1st _____ 2nd _____ 3rd _____

c. Were you injured?

Not at all   Severely
    ⋅ 1   2   3   4   5   6   7

d. Did you feel your life was threatened?

Not at all   Extremely
       1   2   3   4   5   6   7

e. How traumatic **was** this for you at that time?

Not at all   Extremely
       1   2   3   4   5   6   7

f. How traumatic **is** this for you now?

Not at all   Extremely
       1   2   3   4   5   6   7

Go on to the next page and answer the PTSD Checklist based on this event.

Reprinted with permission from Dean Lauterbach, Ph.D.

Appendix C
Glossary

Sharon L. Foster and Arthur M. Nezu

Concurrent validity
> The extent to which scores on a target measure can be used to predict an individual's score on a measure of performance collected at the same time as the target measure.

Construct validity
> The extent to which scores on a measure enter into relationships in ways predicted by theory or by previous investigations. Examinations of construct validity address the meaning of scores on a measure, and are relevant to the issue of whether the instrument assesses what it purports to assess. Construct validity has several specific subtypes; other investigations that speak to construct validity, but do not fall into any of the specific subtypes, are generally called "investigations of construct validity."

Content validity
> Whether the measure appropriately samples or represents the domain being assessed. Substantiation of content validity requires systematic, replicable development of the assessment device, often with formal review by clients or experts to ensure appropriate material is included and excluded.

Convergent validity
> The extent to which scores on the target measure correlate with scores on measures of the same construct.

Criterion-related validity
> The extent to which test scores can be used to predict an individual's performance on some important task or behavior. Examinations of criterion-related validity speak to the utility of scores on a measure rather than to their meaning. Often one ideally would like a perfect match between scores on that target measure and those on the criterion measure. There are two subtypes of criterion-related validity—concurrent validity and predictive validity.

Discriminant validity
> The extent to which scores on a measure are unrelated to scores on measures assessing other, theoretically unrelated constructs.

Discriminative validity
> The extent to which scores on a measure distinguish between groups known or suspected to differ on the construct assessed by the target measure.

Internal consistency

A form of reliability indicating the extent to which different item groupings produce consistent scores on a measure, usually measured by (Cronbach's) coefficient alpha or KR-20.

Interrater reliability

The extent to which two individuals who rate (score, or observe) the same person (or stimulus material) score the person (person's behavior, or stimulus material) consistently; usually established by having two independent observers or raters evaluate the same stimulus material at approximately the same time.

Predictive validity

The extent to which scores on a target measure can be used to predict an individual's score on a measure of performance collected some time after the target measure (i.e., in the future).

Sensitivity

The level at which a measure accurately identifies individuals who have a given characteristic in question using a given criterion or cutoff score (e.g., the proportion of people with major depression who are correctly identified as depressed by their score on a given measure of depression).

Specificity

The degree to which a measure accurately identifies people who do not have a characteristic that is being measured (e.g., the proportion of people who do not have a diagnosis of major depression and who are correctly identified as not depressed by their score on a given measure of depression).

Test–retest reliability

The extent to which scores on a measure are consistent over a specified period of time, established by administering the same instrument on two separate occasions.

Treatment sensitivity

Whether the measure is sensitive to changes produced by treatment that have been documented or corroborated by other measures. Note that a measure can have good content and construct validity, but still not be sensitive to treatment effects.

Reprinted from: Nezu, A. M., Ronan, G. F., Meadows, E. A., & McClure, K. S. (2000). *Practitioner's guide to empirically based measures of depression.* New York: Kluwer Academic / Plenum Publishers.

Author Index

Printed in the United States
77262LV00003B/1-20

9 780306 465826